Surface chang

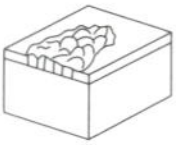

ssue

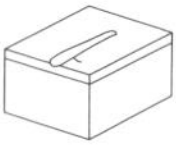

Scratch mark (a sign of itching = pruritus)

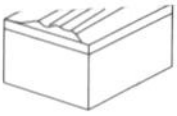

Lichenification

Thickening of the epidermis with exaggerated skin markings (bark-like) usually due to repeated scratching or rubbing

Vascular changes

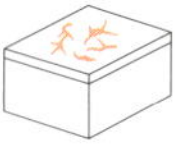

Telangiectasia

Easily visible superficial blood vessels (blanches)

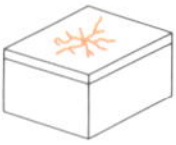

Spider naevus

A single telangiectatic arteriole in the skin

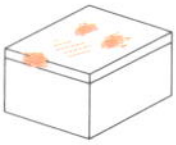

Purpura

(non-blanching): extravasation of blood into skin (usually around 2mm in diameter)

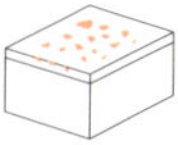

Petechiae

Pin-head sized areas of purpura

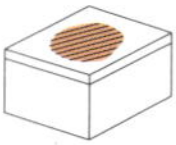

Ecchymosis

A 'bruise'. Purpura >2mm diameter

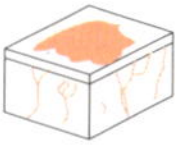

Erythema

Blanching reddening of the skin due to local vasodilatation

Further terminology

- Eruption: rash.
- Cyst: an epithelial-lined cavity filled with fluid or semisolid material.
- Milium (milia): the tiny firm white papule is an intradermal cyst.
- Open comedone: dark plugged dilated pilosebaceous orifice (blackhead).
- Closed comedone: pale pinhead-sized papule in pilosebaceous orifice (whitehead).
- Hyperkeratotic: thickened horny layer, difficult to detach scale.
- Scar: dermal fibrous tissue replaces normal architecture.
- Haematoma: localized deep swelling from bleeding.
- Hyperpigmented (dark): usually increased melanin or iron in skin.
- Depigmented: lost all pigment, e.g. vitiligo.
- Hypopigmented (pale): less melanin or colour obscured, e.g. by oedema.
- Morbilliform rash: erythematous macules and papules of 2–10mm in diameter with tendency to confluence (as in measles).
- Cribriform: spaces, perforations, or holes like a sieve. Often applied to the pattern of scarring seen in pyoderma gangrenosum.

OXFORD MEDICAL PUBLICATIONS

Oxford Handbook of
Medical Dermatology

Published and forthcoming Oxford Handbooks

Oxford Handbook for the Foundation Programme 2e
Oxford Handbook of Acute Medicine 3e
Oxford Handbook of Anaesthesia 2e
Oxford Handbook of Applied Dental Sciences
Oxford Handbook of Cardiology
Oxford Handbook of Clinical and Laboratory Investigation 2e
Oxford Handbook of Clinical Dentistry 4e
Oxford Handbook of Clinical Diagnosis 2e
Oxford Handbook of Clinical Examination and Practical Skills
Oxford Handbook of Clinical Haematology 3e
Oxford Handbook of Clinical Immunology and Allergy 2e
Oxford Handbook of Clinical Medicine—Mini Edition 7e
Oxford Handbook of Clinical Medicine 7e
Oxford Handbook of Clinical Pharmacy
Oxford Handbook of Clinical Rehabilitation 2e
Oxford Handbook of Clinical Specialties 8e
Oxford Handbook of Clinical Surgery 3e
Oxford Handbook of Complementary Medicine
Oxford Handbook of Critical Care 3e
Oxford Handbook of Dental Patient Care 2e
Oxford Handbook of Dialysis 3e
Oxford Handbook of Emergency Medicine 3e
Oxford Handbook of Endocrinology and Diabetes 2e
Oxford Handbook of ENT and Head and Neck Surgery
Oxford Handbook of Expedition and Wilderness Medicine
Oxford Handbook of Gastroenterology and Hepatology
Oxford Handbook of General Practice 3e
Oxford Handbook of Genetics
Oxford Handbook of Genitourinary Medicine, HIV and AIDS
Oxford Handbook of Geriatric Medicine
Oxford Handbook of Infectious Diseases and Microbiology
Oxford Handbook of Key Clinical Evidence
Oxford Handbook of Medical Sciences
Oxford Handbook of Nephrology and Hypertension
Oxford Handbook of Neurology
Oxford Handbook of Nutrition and Dietetics
Oxford Handbook of Obstetrics and Gynaecology 2e
Oxford Handbook of Occupational Health
Oxford Handbook of Oncology 2e
Oxford Handbook of Ophthalmology
Oxford Handbook of Paediatrics
Oxford Handbook of Palliative Care 2e
Oxford Handbook of Practical Drug Therapy
Oxford Handbook of Pre-Hospital Care
Oxford Handbook of Psychiatry 2e
Oxford Handbook of Public Health Practice 2e
Oxford Handbook of Reproductive Medicine and Family Planning
Oxford Handbook of Respiratory Medicine 2e
Oxford Handbook of Rheumatology 2e
Oxford Handbook of Sport and Exercise Medicine
Oxford Handbook of Tropical Medicine 3e
Oxford Handbook of Urology 2e

Oxford Handbook of Medical Dermatology

Susan Burge

Consultant Dermatologist
Oxford Radcliffe Hospitals NHS Trust
and Associate Director of Clinical Studies
University of Oxford, Oxford, UK

with

Dinny Wallis

Specialty Registrar, Rheumatology
Royal National Hospital for Rheumatic Diseases
Bath, UK

OXFORD
UNIVERSITY PRESS

OXFORD
UNIVERSITY PRESS

Great Clarendon Street, Oxford OX2 6DP

Oxford University Press is a department of the University of Oxford.
It furthers the University's objective of excellence in research, scholarship,
and education by publishing worldwide in

Oxford New York

Auckland Cape Town Dar es Salaam Hong Kong Karachi
Kuala Lumpur Madrid Melbourne Mexico City Nairobi
New Delhi Shanghai Taipei Toronto

With offices in

Argentina Austria Brazil Chile Czech Republic France Greece
Guatemala Hungary Italy Japan Poland Portugal Singapore
South Korea Switzerland Thailand Turkey Ukraine Vietnam

Oxford is a registered trade mark of Oxford University Press
in the UK and in certain other countries

Published in the United States
by Oxford University Press Inc., New York

First edition published 2011

British Library Cataloguing in Publication Data
Data available

Library of Congress Cataloging in Publication Data
Data available

Typeset by Glyph International, Bangalore, India
Printed in China
on acid-free paper through
Asia Pacific Offset

ISBN 978–0–19–955832–2

10 9 8 7 6 5 4 3 2 1

Foreword

Dr Susan Burge and I first (really) met as senior registrars to the Department of Dermatology in Oxford in 1981. It soon became apparent to me that Susan's most commonly asked question was 'why?', always spoken in a most expressive Northern Irish accent. Usually there was no easy answer which of course indicated why she had asked the question in the first place. If an answer was preferred it had to make sense, be logical and simple. Any flannel would meet with short shrift! This story reflects the (senior) author's enquiring mind and need for knowledge to be imparted in a sound, simple and logical way. It therefore comes as no surprise that the format of the new textbook is prompted by questions: What should I look for? What should I do?

Dermatology is arguably the most clinical of all medical specialties because it relies less on investigation and more on good old fashioned observation and interpretation of symptoms and signs for diagnosis. Dermatology practice is sometimes criticized for being simply a 'spot diagnosis' and for using outdated Latin terminology. The diagnosis and management of skin disease, however, demands a logical ordering and structuring of clinical information in such a way that makes it a most stimulating intellectual exercise which has few equals among other medical specialties.

In this new book Susan and Dinny, who is currently in specialist training in rheumatology, bring a refreshingly new approach to learning dermatology. The combination of old and young authors (forgive me Susan!) brings a nice balance of wisdom and practicality—exactly what the junior doctor requires.

Professor Peter Mortimer
Professor of Dermatological Medicine to the University of London,
Consultant Skin Physician to St George's Hospital, London,
and the Royal Marsden Hospital,
London

Preface

The approach to skin problems should be as logical as the approach to any other medical condition. This handbook will help you to take a step-by-step approach at the bedside and make sense of problems such as rashes, skin tumours, or leg ulcers. It is written primarily for doctors working in hospitals, but it includes much that will be of value to those working in the community and to medical students who want to know more about the skin. The focus is unashamedly on medical rather than surgical dermatology. A handbook cannot 'cover' dermatology (> 2500 diagnoses), but we discuss common conditions with a medical flavour, and include some rarities that we hope will fascinate you or perhaps inspire you to read more. The chapters on skin problems in the medical specialities should be of particular interest to physicians working in those disciplines. The insights into the structure and function of the skin may also help you to care for your own skin!

We provide a framework for analysing clinical signs so that you can develop your diagnostic expertise. Lists of causes of problems such as itch, red faces, red legs, scaly rashes, leg ulcers, funny nails, and too much or too little hair will help you to reach a diagnosis and references will guide you to the appropriate section of the book for more information. Illustrations complement the text, but the emphasis is on enabling you to make sense of the findings using clinical skills rather than matching findings to pictures.

Common skin conditions (including those in childhood, pregnancy, and old age) are discussed. Each topic includes answers to the questions 'What should I ask?' 'What should I look for?' 'What should I do?' We suggest tools that will help you to evaluate the impact of skin conditions. Bedside procedures, such as measuring the ABPI, applying dressings, and skin biopsy, are described clearly. The section on emergency dermatology will help you to recognize and manage life-threatening problems such as necrotizing fasciitis, toxic epidermal necrolysis, and purpura fulminans. We introduce skin conditions that you may encounter when working in specialities such as rheumatology, haematology, nephrology, endocrinology, and gastroenterology. Finally the section on medical management includes descriptions of topical treatments, occlusion, and wet dressings as well as some systemic drugs.

We hope that you will find this little book useful when you are asked to see someone with a puzzling skin problem and that there will be a place for it on your desk, in the outpatient clinic, or on the ward—and a niche for it in your backpack.

Acknowledgements

First and foremost SB would like to thank all the Oxford dermatology trainees who inspired the book, advised on the content when it was no more than a pipe-dream, and patiently went through the early drafts. The chapters became required reading for the regular Tuesday morning DONUT rounds. We would also like to thank Adam Wallis for advice on radiological matters and James Burge for teaching SB how to draw in PowerPoint.

We are very grateful to the colleagues who reviewed individual chapters especially:
Elise Olsen (Hair problems)
Sheru George (Photodermatology)
Tim Littlewood (Haematology)
Chris Winearls (Renal disease)
Chris Alcock (Radiotherapy)
James Burge (Neurology)
Jonathan Price and Chris Bass (Psychiatry)
Vanessa Venning (Blisters)
Richard Turner (Tumours)
Graham Ogg (Immune system)

It has been a pleasure to work with the staff of OUP, especially Anna Winstanley and Kate Wanwimolruk, who were always helpful and eminently practical.

Finally special thanks go to Peter Burge for encouragement, endless cups of tea, advice on use of English, and enthusiastic wielding of the 'red pen' when proofreading.

Contents

Symbols and abbreviations

►►	don't dawdle—act now
💣	incendiary (controversial) topic
△	rare but fascinating
⚠	caution/warning
📖	cross reference
>	greater than
<	less than
🖱	website
6-MP	6-mercaptopurine
AAT	alpha-1-antitrypsin
ABPI	ankle–brachial pressure index
ACE	angiotensin-converting enzyme
ACTH	adrenocorticotropic hormone
AGEP	acute generalized exanthematous pustulosis
AMP	antimicrobial peptide
ANA	antinuclear antibody
ANCA	antineutrophil cytoplasmic antibodies
APECED	autoimmune polyendocrinopathy–candidiasis–ectodermal dystrophy
AST	aspartate transferase
BCC	basal cell cancer
BCG	Bacille Calmette-Guérin
BMZ	basement membrane zone
BP	bullous pemphigoid
bpm	beats per minute
BSA	body surface area
CCLE	chronic cutaneous lupus erythematosus
CINCA	chronic infantile neurological cutaneous and articular syndrome
CLASI	Cutaneous Lupus Disease Activity and Severity Index
CNS	central nervous system
CRP	C-reactive protein
CT	computed tomography
CVA	cerebrovascular accident
CVP	central venous pressure
CXR	chest radiograph

Dg	desmoglein
DH	dermatitis herpetiformis
DIC	disseminated intravascular coagulation
DIP	distal interphalangeal
DLE	discoid lupus erythematosus
DLQI	Dermatology Life Quality Index
DMSO	dimethyl sulphoxide
DRESS	drug rash, eosinophilia, and systemic symptoms
DSSI	Dermatomyositis Skin Severity Index
DVT	deep vein thrombosis
EAC	erythema annulare centrifugum
EB	epidermolysis bullosa
EBA	epidermolysis bullosa acquisita
EC	engraftment syndrome
ECG	electrocardiogram
ECP	extracorporeal photophoresis
ELR	eruption of lymphocyte recovery
EM	erythema multiforme
EN	erythema nodosum
ENA	extractable nuclear antigen
ENT	ear, nose, and throat
EPP	erythropoietic protoporphyria
EPS	elastosis perforans serpiginosa
ESR	erythrocyte sedimentation rate
ET	epidermolytic toxin
FBC	full blood count
FGFR	fibroblast growth factor receptor
FMF	familial Mediterranean fever
FTU	finger-tip unit
G6PD	glucose-6-phosphate dehydrogenase
G-CSF	granulocyte colony-stimulating factor
GFR	glomerular filtration rate
GP	general practitioner
GT	glutamyl transpeptidase
GTN	glyceryl trinitrate
GVHD	graft versus host disease
HAART	highly active antiretroviral therapy
HCV	hepatitis C virus
HDL	high-density lipoprotein
HDU	high dependency unit

HFE	hereditary haemochromatosis
HIDS	hyperimmunoglobulin D syndrome
HIV	human immunodeficiency virus
HPV	human papillomas virus
HSCT	haemopoietic stem cell transplant
IBD	inflammatory bowel disease
ICU	intensive care unit
IgE	immunoglobulin E
IL	interleukin
ILVEN	inflammatory linear verrucous epidermal naevus
IM	intramuscular
IMF	immunofluorescence
IP	incontinentia pigmenti
IRIS	immune reconstitution inflammatory syndrome
IV	intravenous
KOH	potassium hydroxide
KP	Kaposi's sarcoma
LDL	low-density lipoprotein
LE	lupus erythematosus
LEOPARD	lentigines, electrocardiographic cardiac conduction defects, ocular telorism, pulmonary stenosis, abnormalities of genitalia, retardation of growth, deafness
LFT	liver function test
LP	lichen planus
LPC	liquor picis carbonis
LPP	lichen planopilaris
mcg	microgram(s)
MCP	metacarpophalangeal
MED	minimal erythema dose
MF	mycosis fungoides
mg	milligram(s)
MHC	major histocompatibility complex
min	minute(s)
mL	millilitre(s)
mm	millimetre(s)
MRI	magnetic resonance imaging
MRSA	meticillin-resistant *Staphylococcus aureus*
NF	neurofibromatosis
NG	nasogastric
NHS	National Health Service

NOMID	neonatal-onset multisystem inflammatory disease
NSAID	non-steroidal anti-inflammatory drug
PAN	polyarteritis nodosa
PAPA	pyogenic arthritis, pyoderma gangrenosum, and acne
PASI	Psoriasis Area and Severity Index
PCOS	polycystic ovary syndrome
PCP	*Pneumocystis jiroveci (carinii)* pneumonia
PCR	polymerase chain reaction
PCT	porphyria cutanea tarda
PDT	photodynamic therapy
PEX	pseudoxanthoma elasticum
PHACE(S)	posterior fossa malformations, facial haemangioma, arterial abnormalities, coarctation of the aorta, and eye abnormalities (sternal clefting and/or supraumbilical raphe)
PIIINP	type 3 procollagen aminoterminal propeptide
PIP	proximal interphalangeal
PLE (PMLE)	polymorphic light eruption
PMH	past medical history
POEMS	polyneuropathy, organomegaly, endocrinopathy, monoclonal gammopathy, skin changes
prn	as needed
PTH	parathyroid hormone
PVL	Panton–Valentine leucocidin
PWS	port-wine stain
RA	rheumatoid arthritis
RAST	radioallergosorbent test
s	second(s)
SAPHO	synovitis, acne, pustulosis, hyperostosis, osteitis
SC	subcutaneous
SCC	squamous cell cancer
SCLE	subacute cutaneous lupus erythematosus
SCTE	stem cell transplantation erythema
SDRIFE	symmetrical drug-related intertriginous and flexural erythema
SHBG	sex hormone-binding globulin
SJS	Stevens–Johnson syndrome
SLE	systemic lupus erythematosus
SPF	sun protection factor
SSSS	staphylococcal scalded skin syndrome
TB	tuberculosis

TEN	toxic epidermal necrolysis
TNFα	tumour necrosis factor alpha
TORCH	toxoplasmosis, other, rubella, cytomegalovirus, herpes simplex
TPMP	thiopurine methyltransferase
TPN	total parenteral nutrition
TRAPS	TNF receptor-associated periodic fever syndrome
TSS	toxic shock syndrome
UDCA	ursodeoxycholic acid
UK	United Kingdom
USA	United States of America
UV	ultraviolet
UVR	ultraviolet radiation
VLDL	very low-density lipoprotein
WBC	white blood cell
WHO	World Health Organization
WSP	white soft paraffin
XP	xeroderma pigmentosum

Definitions

Isomorphic response (Köbner phenomenon): appearance of new lesions of a pre-existing disorder at a site of injury.

Isotopic response: occurence of a new skin disorder exactly at the site of another unrelated and already healed skin disorder.

Pathergy test: hyper reactivity of the skin to needle prick.

Chapter 1

Structure and function of the skin

Contents

Relevant pages in other chapters

📖 Chapter 13, Adhesion in the epidermis, p.242 for a discussion of adhesion within the epidermis and at the basement membrane zone.

📖 Chapter 16, p.300 and p.316 for pigmentation, melanocytes, and sun protection.

Introduction

The skin is the largest organ in the body and the heaviest—an adult's skin weighs 4–5kg. Skin is by no means an inert barrier, but plays an active part in defending each of us against the insults (microbial, physical, and chemical) hurled at us by the outside environment.

In this chapter we aim to give you some insight into what your skin is doing for you, in the hope that this will encourage you to care for the skin of your patients (and your own skin) with the respect it deserves. An understanding of cutaneous physiology will also help you to analyse what has gone wrong or what might happen in patients with skin problems, including skin failure.

We discuss the structure of the skin and consider how this finely tuned organ functions as a barrier ('keeping the inside in and the outside out') and reduces water loss, is part of the immune system, is a metabolic organ synthesizing vitamin D and cytokines, regulates body temperature, and senses noxious stimuli (skin on the tips of your fingers is particularly sensitive—Box 1.1).

Most of us will, at some stage, worry about the appearance of our skin, hair, and/or nails. 'Looking good' gives us confidence and we may try to enhance the appearance (or smell) of our skin if we want to display ourselves to make a positive impression or attract a sexual partner. It is no surprise that fortunes are spent on lotions, potions, and procedures designed to conceal blemishes (actual or imagined) and to restore the appearance of youth. The psychological aspects of skin problems are discussed in more detail in 📖 Chapter 28, p.528.

Box 1.1 Dermatoglyphics (fingerprints)

- Fingertips, palms, soles, and toes are covered with a pattern of epidermal ridges called dermatoglyphics.
- The three basic patterns (loops, arches, and whorls) are unique to each individual.
- Characteristic dermatoglyphic patterns accompany many chromosomal abnormalities.
- The ridges amplify vibrations when your finger brushes across a rough surface.
- The ridges enhance grip.

Summary of functions of the skin

Prevention of water loss

- Stratum corneum—overlapping cells and intercellular lipid.

Immune defence

- Structural integrity of stratum corneum.
- Keratinocytes produce antimicrobial peptides (defensins and cathelicidins).
- Langerhans cells trap antigens and migrate to lymph nodes where antigens are presented to T-cells—see 📖 p.14.
- Cytokines secreted by lymphocytes, macrophages, and keratinocytes regulate inflammatory and immune responses.
- Acid pH of sweat.
- Fungistatic activity of sebaceous secretions.

Protection against UV damage

- Melanin synthesized by melanocytes helps to protect keratinocyte nuclei from the harmful effects of UV radiation by absorbing and scattering the rays, and by scavenging free radicals—see 📖 Chapter 16, p.300.
- UV-damaged DNA is repaired by enzymes—see 📖 Chapter 16, p.300.

Temperature regulation

- Vasoconstriction and vasodilation control the flow of blood and transfer of heat to the body surface.
- Evaporation of sweat cools the body.

Synthesis of vitamin D

- Skin is the primary source of vitamin D. 7-Dehydrocholesterol is photoactivated to cholecalciferol (vitamin D_3), which is metabolized in the liver to 25-(OH)D_3 and in the kidney to the active form of vitamin D, (1,25-$(OH)_2D_3$) calcitriol. Only small amounts of vitamin D are obtained from the diet. Vitamin D is required for calcium absorption and has essential roles in bone metabolism, neuromuscular function, and immune function. Deficiency can lead to rickets (in children), osteomalacia, and osteoporosis.

Sensation

- Free nerve endings detect potentially harmful stimuli (heat, pain).
- Specialized end organs detect pressure, vibration, and touch (Box 1.1).
- Autonomic nerves supply blood vessels, sweat glands, and arrector pili muscles.

Aesthetic

- The skin has an important role in social interaction.

Epidermis

The epidermis originates from embryonic neuroectodermal cells. The epidermis is a stratified squamous epithelium composed of layers of keratinocytes that differentiate as they move towards the skin surface (see 📖 Box 1.2, p.6). The epidermis is attached to an underlying collagenous dermis, which contains the blood vessels that nourish the epidermis. Downward projections of epidermal rete pegs interlock with upward projecting dermal papillae, stabilizing the structure and making it difficult to shear the epidermis from the dermis (Fig. 1.1).

Structure of the epidermis (Fig. 1.2)

- A single layer of columnar keratinocytes in the deepest layer of the epidermis (basal layer) is attached to a basement membrane that is an interface between the epidermis and the underlying dermis. The basal cells are anchored to the basement membrane by adhesion junctions called hemidesmosomes—see 📖 p.242.
- Regeneration of epidermis (and hair follicles—see 📖 p.10) depends on populations of epidermal stem cells.
- The middle layers of the epidermis (spinous or prickle cell layers) have a spiky appearance under a light microscope because of the intercellular junctions (desmosomes) that are the main adhesive force between adjacent keratinocytes—see 📖 p.242.
- The outermost horny layer or stratum corneum is composed of layers of flattened keratinocytes (corneocytes) locked together by modified desmosomes (corneodesmosomes) in a lipid matrix.
- All keratinocytes contain keratin intermediate filaments, but the structure of the keratins changes as the cells differentiate—see 📖 Box 1.2, p.6.
- Melanocytes are dendritic cells that are interspersed amongst the basal keratinocytes—see 📖 p.12.
- Epidermal Langerhans cells (dendritic antigen-presenting cells) are found throughout the epidermis—see 📖 p.14.
- Migratory leucocytes are present in small numbers in the epidermis.

Proliferation and shedding

- The thickness of normal epidermis (0.05–0.1mm) is regulated by the balance between proliferation of basal keratinocytes and shedding of cells at the surface (desquamation).
- It takes about 40 days for a keratinocyte to move upwards from the basal layer to the horny layer where, after proteolytic breakdown of adhesion junctions, the cells flake off (desquamate)—see 📖 Box 1.2, p.6.
- Cornification and desquamation are regulated by the activity of epidermal proteases and their inhibitors.

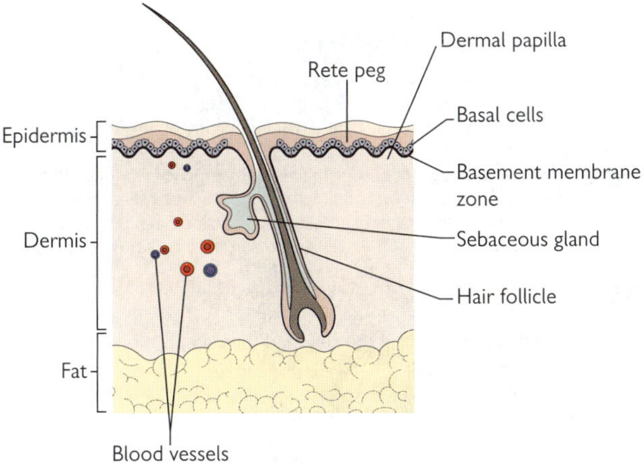

Fig. 1.1 Diagram of skin: epidermis, dermis, and fat.

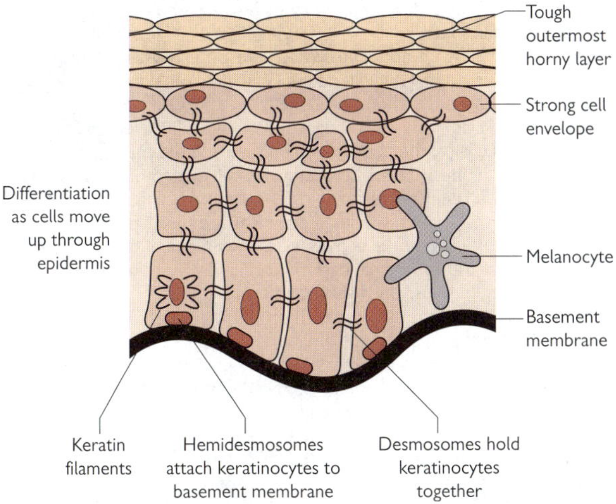

Fig. 1.2 Structure of epidermis.

Differentiation and the skin barrier

Box 1.2 Keeping the outside out

- Each keratinocyte has a cytoskeleton of microfilaments containing actin, microtubules containing tubulin, and intermediate keratin filaments composed of type I and type II keratins (from the Greek 'keras' meaning horn).
- Keratinocytes are held together mainly by desmosomes (see 🕮 Fig. 1.2, p.5). A glycoprotein intercellular substance aids cell cohesion. In acute eczema, hyaluronan secreted by keratinocytes into the intercellular space takes up water and may dilute noxious chemicals (see 🕮 p.200).
- Keratinocytes change (differentiate) as they move from the basal layer towards the skin surface:
  - The types of keratins in the cells and the composition of the desmosomes change.
  - A protein called filaggrin aggregates and cross-links the keratin filaments, giving the keratinocytes internal strength.
  - The cell envelope is strengthened by calcium-dependent cross-linking of proteins such as involucrin and loricrin that is catalysed by transglutaminase-1 (TGM1). Mutations in *TGM1* cause ichthyosis (abnormalities in both cell envelope and desquamation).
  - Lipid is synthesized by keratinocytes and accumulates in the intercellular space.
  - By the time the keratinocytes reach the outermost horny layer, they have lost their nuclei and subcellular organelles and are densely packed with keratin filaments.
- The outermost horny layer is composed of about 20 layers of flattened horny cells (corneocytes) with tough insoluble cell membranes (cornified envelopes) that are locked together by corneodesmosomes and a thick intercellular layer of lipids (like mortar). This impermeable layer enables the skin to withstand chemical and mechanical injury and restricts loss of water and electrolytes. Darkly pigmented skin seems to provide a better epidermal barrier than lightly pigmented skin—the stratum corneum is less permeable and more cohesive.
- The permeability of the skin depends primarily on the balance between intercellular cohesion and desquamation in the stratum corneum. Serine proteases such as kallikreins degrade corneodesmosomes so the cells can desquamate. Protease activity is controlled by inhibitors such as lymphoepithelial Kazal-type 5 serine protease inhibitor (LEKTI). In Netherton's syndrome, mutations in the *SPINK5* gene encoding LEKTI lead to defective LEKTI expression, unregulated proteolytic activity, increased desquamation, and highly permeable skin (see 🕮 Box 31.10, p.555).

Further reading

Cork MJ *et al. J Invest Dermatol* 2009; **129:**1892–908.

Dermis and glands

The dermis is a layer of connective tissue beneath the epidermis. A layer of subcutaneous fat separates the dermis from underlying fascia and muscle. The dermis has a rich supply of blood vessels, lymphatics, nerves, and sensory receptors. The thickness of the dermis varies with body site and may measure as much as 5mm on the back.

Structural components

- Collagen, mainly type I but some type III, gives the dermis tensile strength. Ageing skin is characterized by reduced collagen synthesis and increased collagen breakdown by matrix metalloproteinases.
- Elastic fibres, containing a core of elastin, supply elasticity and resilience, but elastin functions poorly in aged skin.
- Ground substance of proteoglycans and glycoproteins that binds water and hydrates the dermis.
- Skin appendages: hair follicles, sebaceous glands, eccrine sweat glands, and apocrine sweat glands—see 🕮 p.9 and p.10.
- Blood vessels: superficial and deep vascular plexus. Vasodilatation and vasoconstriction help to regulate heat loss.
- Lymphatics: afferent capillaries in dermal papillae pass via a superficial plexus to deeper horizontal plexuses and collecting lymphatics—see 🕮 immune system p.14.
- Nerve fibres: most sensory nerves end in the dermis, but a few penetrate the epidermis. Free nerve endings detect heat and pain; Pacinian corpuscles detect pressure and vibration, and Meissner corpuscles detect pressure and touch. Autonomic innervation is cholinergic to the eccrine sweat glands; adrenergic to eccrine and apocrine glands, arterioles, and arrector pili muscle.

Cellular components

- Fibroblasts synthesize proteins such as collagen and elastin as well as the glycosaminoglycans in dermal ground substance.
- Dendritic cells (dermal dendritic cells) are involved in antigen presentation—see 🕮 p.14.
- Macrophages scavenge cell debris and foreign material.
- Mast cells: a few near blood vessels. Granules contain inflammatory mediators such as histamine, prostaglandins, leukotrienes, and other chemokines that may be involved in inflammatory responses.

Langer's lines

Langer's lines (cleavage lines) correspond to the alignment of collagen fibres within the dermis. They define the direction along which the skin has the least flexibility. Surgical incisions carried out parallel to Langer's lines heal with less scarring than those made across the lines.

Eccrine glands

- Eccrine glands cover most of the body surface, but are most numerous on palms and soles.
- A secretory coil deep in the dermis is attached to a duct that conveys sweat to the surface of the skin.
- Glands are innervated by the sympathetic nervous system.
- Eccrine glands secrete water, electrolytes, lactate, urea, and ammonia.
- Sweating helps to regulate body temperature.
- Sweat may have antimicrobial properties.

Apocrine glands

- Apocrine glands are found mainly in the axillae, anogenital region, female breast, eyelids, and external auditory canal.
- A secretory coil in the deep dermis leads to a duct which opens into the upper portion of a hair follicle.
- The glands produce an oily secretion of protein, carbohydrate, ammonia, and lipid.
- Apocrine glands become active at puberty.
- Secretion is controlled by sympathetic nerve fibres.
- The action of bacteria on secretions produces body odour.

Sebaceous glands

- Sebaceous glands are associated with the upper portion of each hair follicle. The hair follicle and associated gland is known as a pilosebaceous unit. See 📖 Fig.1.3, p.11.
- Size of glands varies at different body sites. The largest glands are on face and upper trunk (sites prone to acne).
- Sebocytes secrete lipid-rich sebum with emollient as well as antimicrobial properties.
- Sebum in the sebaceous duct enters the upper portion of the hair follicle and protects the surface of the skin.

Hair and nails

Hair

- Hair is found all over the body, except for palms and soles, but the density and size of hair follicles vary at different sites.
- The hair follicle opens onto the surface of the epidermis and is a potential portal of entry for pathogenic microbes.
- The size of the follicle determines the size of the hair shaft (the product of the follicle). Short, fine, soft, unpigmented vellus hair covers most of the body (you can just feel the vellus hair on your forehead) and coarse, pigmented terminal hair grows at sites such as scalp, eyebrows, eyelashes, limbs, genitalia, and axillae. Androgens influence hair type—some vellus hair changes to terminal hair in hirsutes—see 🕮 p.440.
- The cylindrical follicular root sheath moulds the shape of the hair shaft.
- A bulge region in the mid-portion of the root sheath contains epithelial hair follicle stem cells from which the follicle arises; see Fig. 1.3. These stem cells regulate the hair cycle; see Box 1.3. Damage to stem cells may contribute to irreversible hair loss (scarring alopecia) in inflammatory conditions such as cutaneous lupus erythematosus (LE).
- The hair shaft arises from dividing cells in the bulb at the bottom of the follicle. The shaft gradually keratinizes, producing a highly cohesive structure, as it moves up through the follicle root sheath. Blood vessels and sensory nerves in the associated dermal papilla supply the cells of the hair bulb; see Fig. 1.3.
- Melanocyte stem cells are found in the bulge region from where they migrate to the bulb.
- The arrector pili muscles attach to the mid-portion of follicles. These smooth muscles, supplied by adrenergic nerves, make hair 'stand on end' in the cold or during emotional stress (goose pimples).
- The sebaceous and apocrine ducts penetrate the follicular root sheath at the start of the upper third of the follicle.

Nails

- A nail is a plate of keratinized cells (onychocytes) with a free edge.
- The nail plate is formed by specialized keratinocytes in the nail matrix, which lies under the proximal nail fold and extends distally to the lunula but proximally to the insertion of the extensor tendon.
- The nail plate grows forward over a nail bed which is tightly connected to the nail plate.
- Lateral and proximal nail folds cover the sides and base of the nail plate. The cuticle forms a seal between the nail plate and the proximal nail fold.
- Fingernails grow by about 1mm per week (toenails more slowly). If growth in the matrix is slowed by serious illness or by drugs, horizontal lines or dents appear at the same place in all the nail plates (Beau's lines). The lines will only become apparent some 8–12 weeks after the insult when the nail plate emerges from under the cuticle.

See 🕮 Fig. 3.3, p.47 for a diagram of a normal nail.

Box 1.3 The hair follicle cycle

- Hair grows 0.3–0.4mm/day. About 90% of the 100,000 scalp hairs are growing. Each hair follicle cycles through phases of:
  - Growth (anagen): active phase of hair production (2–6 years on the scalp). The length of hair is determined by the duration of anagen. The duration of anagen is determined by your genes. 85% of scalp hairs are in anagen.
  - Involution (catagen): conversion from active growth to resting phase (2–4 weeks).
  - Rest (telogen): 15% of scalp hairs are in telogen (2–4 months).
- At the end of telogen, hair is shed and a new cycle starts. It is normal to lose 100–150 scalp hairs a day.
- Each hair follicle cycle is independent of neighbouring follicles so humans do not moult, unlike many other mammals.

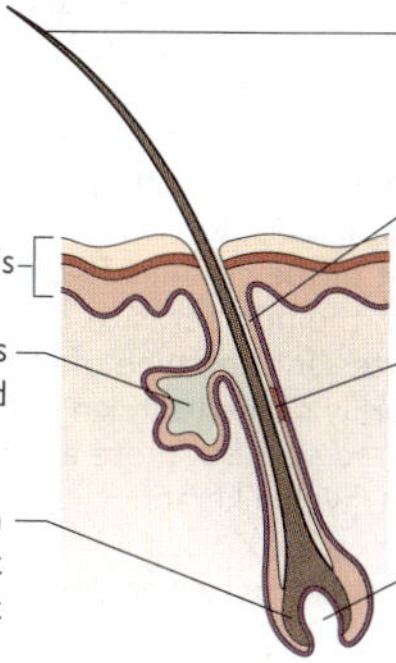

Fig. 1.3 Structure of a hair follicle.

Further reading

Harries MJ *et al. Autoimmun Rev* 2009; **8:**478–83.

Melanocytes and colour

Melanin, synthesized by melanocytes, provides some defence against ultraviolet radiation (UVR) as well as giving colour to skin and hair. Skin colour and ease of tanning are important determinants of the risk of skin cancer—see p.300 and p.324, Chapters 16 and 17.

- Melanocytes are dendritic cells that migrate from the neural crest to the epidermis and hair follicles in the third month of fetal development.
- Melanocytes are interspersed amongst the basal keratinocytes in the epidermis. Melanocyte stem cells are found in the bulge region of hair follicles from where they migrate to the hair bulb. See Fig. 1.3, p.11
- Melanocytes synthesize both brown/black eumelanin and red/yellow phaeomelanin from tyrosine.
- Melanin is passed in packages (melanosomes) along dendritic processes into keratinocytes (see Fig. 1.2, p.5), where the melanosomes sit in a cap or 'parasol' over the upper sun-exposed side of the keratinocyte nucleus. Each melanocyte links to a number of keratinocytes forming an epidermal melanin unit. Melanin provides some UV protection by absorbing visible light as well as UV radiation—see p.300.
- UVR induces tanning by stimulating oxidation of pre-existing melanin, by triggering the synthesis of new melanin, and by changing the distribution of melanosomes—see p.300.
- Melanin is the main determinant of the colour of skin and hair; see Box 1.4. The colour depends on the number, size, and distribution of melanosomes within keratinocytes and the type of melanin, rather than the number of melanocytes. Darkly pigmented skin has similar numbers of melanocytes to lightly pigmented skin, but more and slightly differently packaged melanin (melanosomes) within keratinocytes.
- Skin colour is not uniform—see Box 1.5, p.13.
- Darkly pigmented skin seems to have better epidermal barrier function than lightly pigmented skin—see Box 1.2, p.6.
- Genetic variation in the amino acid sequence of the melanocortin 1 receptor (MC1R) is a major determinant of skin and hair colour. Some variants, e.g. red-heads, do not tan in response to sun.
- The first step in the synthesis of melanin is hydroxylation of tyrosine to dopaquinone. Oculocutaneous albinism is caused by abnormalities in the function of tyrosinase or other enzymes in the synthetic pathway of melanin.
- Defective migration of melanocytes from the neural crest or abnormalities in the maturation or trafficking of melanosomes may present as a pigmentary disorder.
- Depletion of melanocyte stem cells in hair follicles may contribute to age-related greying of hair.

Box 1.4 Skin colour

- The colour of normal skin comes from a mixture of pigments, but melanin is the main contributor to skin colour.
- Oxyhaemoglobin in the blood gives untanned Caucasian skin a pink colour.
- Carotene in subcutaneous fat and the horny layer of the epidermis adds a yellow hue to normal skin.
- Abnormalities in skin colour may result from imbalance of pigments (e.g. in cyanosis, chloasma, and carotenaemia) or the presence of abnormal pigments (e.g. haemosiderin).
- Genetic abnormalities in the synthetic pathway of melanin present with abnormal skin colour.
- Postinflammatory hypo-or hyperpigmentation is common, particularly in dark-coloured skins.
- Damage to the basal layer of the epidermis (interface or lichenoid reaction) is associated with the release of melanin into the dermis and hyperpigmentation.

Box 1.5 Pigmentary demarcation lines (Voigt–Futcher lines)

Dorsal skin surfaces are more pigmented than ventral surfaces. Lines of demarcation between darker dorsal and paler ventral surfaces are apparent in about 20% of people with dark skins. The lines, which are symmetrical and bilateral, are present from infancy and have no clinical significance.

- Type A: vertical line on the lateral aspect of the upper arm that may extend into the pectoral region (most common).
- Type B: curved line on the back of the thigh (posteromedial) that extends from the perineum to the popliteal fossa and occasionally the ankle.
- Type C: vertical or curved hypopigmented band on the mid-chest (contains two parallel lines).
- Type D: vertical line on posteromedial area of spine.
- Type E: bilateral hypopigmented streaks, bands, or patches on the upper chest in the zone between the mid-third of the clavicle and the periareolar skin.

Facial patterns, which appear around puberty, have been described in the Indian sub-population:

- Type F: 'V' shaped hyperpigmented lines between the malar prominence and the temple.
- Type G: 'W' shaped hyperpigmented lines between the malar prominence and the temple.
- Type H: linear bands of hyperpigmentation from the angle of the mouth to the lateral aspects of the chin.

Somani VK *et al. Indian J Dermatol Venereol Leprol* 2004; **70:**336–41.

Further reading

Lin JY and Fisher DE. *Nature* 2007; **445:**843–50.

Skin immune system

The skin immune system (both innate and adaptive) provides a vital defence against external cutaneous pathogens or physical injury.

Keratinocytes

Keratinocytes respond to cutaneous injury or infection by releasing antimicrobial peptides (AMPs) such as β-defensins and cathelicidins that have broad-spectrum antimicrobial activity against bacteria, fungi, and viruses. AMPs may also reduce the likelihood of microbes entering the skin through follicular openings. AMPs are part of the innate immune system; see Box 1.6. Keratinocytes can also produce a wide range of cytokines: pro- or anti-inflammatory, immunomodulatory, and immunosuppressive. Cathelicidins induce the production of proinflammatory cytokines that enhance cell migration and promote wound healing. Vitamin D_3 seems to be involved in the regulation of cathelicidin expression in the epidermis. Keratinocytes are also able to present antigens to T-cells.

Dendritic cells

Dendritic antigen-presenting cells, such as epidermal Langerhans cells and dermal dendritic cells, express major histocompatibility complex (MHC) class II antigens on their surface and 'police' the skin. They are part of the first line of defence if the skin is breached. The cells trap, ingest, process, and present antigens, in association with MHC class II, to the receptors of T-cells.

Lymphatics

Epidermal Langerhans cells and dermal dendritic cells that have trapped antigens migrate via afferent lymphatics to draining lymph nodes, where the processed antigen is presented to naïve T-cells that have the receptor that will bind that antigen. This triggers the generation of activated and memory T-cells imprinted with specific combinations of adhesion molecules and chemokine receptors that target their migration to the skin.

T-cells

Memory T-cells patrol the body for foreign antigens, recirculating through lymph nodes, lymphatics, blood vessels, and specific tissue. Memory T-cells for cutaneous antigens recirculate through the skin. Trafficking is aided by endothelial adhesion molecules that tether flowing T-cells so they can migrate through endothelial junctions as well as chemokine gradients that direct migration in the skin.

The receptor of each memory T-lymphocyte will bind to a specific antigen presented on the surface of target cells in association with MHC class I (for CD8+ T-cells) or class II (for CD4+ T-cells). The antigen–MHC complex interacts with the T-cell receptor which, along with co-stimulatory molecules, triggers release of cytokines that attract more lymphocytes into the skin to augment the inflammatory response.

Box 1.6 What is the innate immune system?

The innate immune system is a first line of defence against environmental insults. The response is rapid and efficient, but is less specific than adaptive immunity and does not improve with repeated exposure.

Receptors (transmembrane and intracellular), such as Toll-like receptors, recognize highly conserved molecular patterns that are common to many classes of pathogen, e.g. components of the wall of microbes.

Activated receptors stimulate the production of cytokines, chemokines, and antimicrobial peptides. Immune cells, such as natural killer cells, and neutrophils are activated and recruited to the site of injury or infection. This innate response kills pathogens, promotes angiogenesis, and initiates repair after injury.

The major components of the skin innate immune system are:

- Intact physical barrier: stratum corneum and intercellular junctions.
- Antigen-presenting cells, keratinocytes, mast cells, and neutrophils.
- Antimicrobial peptides, cytokines, and chemokines.

Further reading

Sigmundsdottir H and Butcher EC. *Nature Immunology* 2008; **9**:981–7.

The history in dermatology

Contents

Relevant pages in other chapters

The history in psoriasis 📖 p.180
The history in leg ulcers 📖 p.274
Pain 📖 p.284
Clinical approach in drug reactions 📖 p.346
History in blisters 📖 p.246

The dermatological history: 1

Setting the scene

Introduce yourself, make the patient comfortable, ensure privacy (difficult on a ward), and allow sufficient time to establish rapport and for the patient to explain what has happened. Remember that skin problems can be embarrassing. Your history will be guided by the nature of the problem—a rash, a leg ulcer, or a skin tumour—but 'Please tell me about your skin problem' is a good opening question.

Finding out what the patient means

Clarify what the patient means by words such as blemish, wheal, hive, scar, or blister. Patients, as well as many doctors, find it difficult to describe rashes. You may think that you know what is meant, but make sure you use these words to describe the same thing as the patient. For example, some people call any raised lesion a 'blister', but do not mean a bump filled with clear fluid; and people may use the word 'scar' to describe postinflammatory pigmentation without any dermal damage. Even 'sunburn' means different things to different people. Some people use this term to describe getting a suntan.

Sometimes the rash will have changed or even disappeared and you will have nothing but the patient's description to help you make a diagnosis, so the description should be as accurate as possible; see Box 2.1.

Getting on the same wavelength

Clarify the patient's preconceptions about the cause of the problem as well as their expectations of the consultation and your role.

It is helpful to know more about the patient's perception of the current severity of the condition, particularly in those with fluctuating inflammatory rashes. This may differ markedly from your own assessment (see Box 2.2).

Symptoms, causation, and impact

'How does your rash/skin condition bother you?' is another good open question to start off the discussion—see Box 2.3.

Document the relationship of the condition to work, hobbies, and drugs including herbal medicines and health foods.

Skin conditions can be both disfiguring and embarrassing, and treatments can be messy, unpleasant, and time consuming, so find out how the skin condition is affecting the life of the patient as well as that of the family or carers.

More information about questions to ask in specific circumstances is given later in this chapter.

Box 2.1 Questions to ask when exploring the appearance of a rash

- Where the rash started, what the rash looked like at the onset, and how it evolved.
- If the surface of the rash is smooth or scaly, or the rash is flat or raised.
- The colour of the rash: if red, did the patient notice what happened if he/she applied light pressure, i.e. did it blanch, suggesting an erythema as opposed to purpura?
- If the rash is persistent or if lesions come and go.
- If transient—how long do individual lesions last and when they fade, what does the skin look like? Are there any changes in skin colour or any marking (scarring)?
- Are hair, nails, or mucosal surfaces affected?

Box 2.2 Grading the skin condition: the patient's perception

It helps to have some insight into the patient's perception of the severity of his/her skin condition as it is *now*. Ask the patient to grade the condition:

'You have explained that your rash/skin condition can vary a bit. I would like to get a feel how bad it is for you today by asking you to grade your skin condition. Let us say that a grade of 10 means it is the worst it has ever been for you and zero means that you have no skin problem. What grade would you give your skin today?'

Box 2.3 Questions to ask when exploring the symptoms and impact of a skin condition

- What does the rash feel like? Is the skin tender, itchy, or painful?
- What brings on the itch/pain? What does the patient do about it?
- Itch—try to quantify the impact. Does it affect sleep or concentration?
- Is anyone else itchy? Ask about family and all close contacts, e.g. sexual partner (could it be scabies?).
- Pain: what is the character of the pain? Sharp, dull, throbbing, paraesthesiae, continuous, or intermittent?
- Does the skin ooze clear fluid, pus, or blood?
- Is the skin fragile, does the skin bruise easily, or does the skin blister?
- Has the patient noticed any smell from the skin (ulcer)? Patients usually welcome a chance to discuss this awkward and embarrassing symptom provided you introduce the subject in a sensitive manner.
- What makes the rash better or worse? Is there any relationship to recent travel, work, or hobbies? Does the problem improve or worsen at the weekends or in holidays? Does sunlight make a difference? Any relationship to cosmetics being used or to drugs/health foods?
- How does the skin condition affect activities of everyday living—school, work, or social?
- How long does it take to apply treatments and what is treatment costing?
- Is the skin condition affecting mood?
- Are carers coping, for example, the parents of a child with eczema?

The dermatological history: 2

Drug history

- What has been prescribed, purchased, begged, or borrowed? Patients may be using a variety of topical preparations, some of which they will not regard as medicaments at all—and they will probably not remember all the names.
- Is the product an ointment (greasy, petroleum jelly-like, sits on the surface of the skin), a cream (white, 'disappears into the skin'), a gel, a foam, or a lotion (liquid)?
- What does the patient do with the treatment? How much is used—how long does the tube or tub last? Where, and how often, is it applied? If the patient has more than one topical preparation, how and where are they used: at the same time or at different times?
- Is any moisturizer being used and how often is it applied?
- What soaps, cosmetics, or other toiletries are used?
- Is anything added to the bath, e.g. bath salts?
- Is the patient taking other drugs, including recreational drugs, and how does the use of these relate to the onset of the rash?

Past medical history

- Enquire about previous skin problems, in particular has the patient had a similar skin condition before and, if so, how long did it last and what was done?
- Is there a history of atopy such as infantile eczema or 'dry skin', asthma, or hay fever?
- Document other medical conditions.

Allergies

- Has the patient noticed 'reactions' when anything is in contact with the skin, e.g. topical medicaments, jewellery (usually nickel allergy), cosmetics, or perfumes? What sort of reaction and how long did it last? Has allergy been investigated by patch or prick testing?
- Have there been 'reactions' to oral medications? What happened and what was done?
- Ensure you know what the patient means if he/she uses the term 'allergy'.

Social and personal history

Explore lifestyle exposure to nicotine and alcohol, sexual history, travel, hobbies, and occupation.

Family history

- Does anyone at home have a similar skin problem? Scabies and skin infections are contagious. Other skin conditions, such as atopic eczema or psoriasis, may have a strong genetic predisposition.
- Draw a family tree if you think that you are dealing with an inherited condition.

Functional enquiry

Complete the history with a review of all systems (functional enquiry). Itching, ulcers, or purpuric rashes can be manifestations of a systemic disease. A careful history may provide clues to a diagnosis, such as underlying malignancy or connective tissue disease, and guide the examination as well as investigation.

Patients do not always volunteer such additional information without prompting, because they do not relate the skin problem to their other symptoms.

The history in patients with allergy

Type I hypersensitivity

Urticaria (hives, wheals, welts) is an immediate type I hypersensitivity reaction that may occur on its own or in association with angio-oedema and/or anaphylaxis. Urticaria is more common in atopics.

Acute urticaria may be triggered by drugs, e.g. penicillin, or foods, e.g. peanuts, fish. The patient can often identify the allergen. In contrast, it is difficult to pinpoint the trigger in most patients with chronic urticaria. Physical urticarias can be triggered by firm pressure (dermographism), heat, cold, sun, or exercise.

The wheals of urticaria are secondary to dermal oedema. They are raised, smooth, erythematous and, usually, itchy. Angio-oedema implies oedema of deep dermis and subcutaneous tissues as well as mucosal and submucosal oedema. Patients describe the sudden onset of large tender swellings involving skin, mucosa, and submucosal tissues. See 🕮 p.98.

The history should be directed at finding out exactly what happened to confirm the diagnosis of urticaria and/or angio-oedema, as the rash may not be present when you see the patient (see Boxes 2.4 and 2.5). Does the patient have one or both problems? ⚠ Rarely, angio-oedema can be caused by a deficiency of C1 esterase inhibitor (inherited or acquired) but these patients do *not* have urticaria. See 🕮 p.98.

Prick testing may be helpful to investigate the cause in some cases of acute urticaria, particularly if there is a history suggesting food allergy, but such testing is most unlikely to be helpful in chronic urticaria.

Irritant contact dermatitis or type IV hypersensitivity

Dermatitis (eczema) caused by an external agent is known as contact dermatitis. Contact dermatitis may be irritant or, less often, allergic.

Irritant contact dermatitis is caused by chronic exposure to irritants (wet work, detergents, chemicals) and is most common in individuals with atopic eczema, who already have a poorly functioning skin barrier.

Allergic contact dermatitis is a type IV hypersensitivity. The patient has to be sensitized by prior exposure to the allergen, sometimes for months or years, before the onset of allergy. The eczematous response is maximal 5–7 days after exposure to the allergen. Allergic contact dermatitis is less common in children than in adults. An irritant contact dermatitis is more common than allergy.

If you suspect an allergic contact dermatitis, direct your history towards elucidating the cause (see Box 2.6) by exploring the relationship of the rash to activities (work, hobbies). Patch testing is the investigation of choice.

A secondary allergic contact dermatitis may complicate the picture in an individual with longstanding dermatitis of another type, particularly when many different medicaments or over-the-counter preparations have been used over a prolonged period. Consider this possibility in individuals with chronic problems such as leg ulcers, pruritus ani, hand dermatitis, facial dermatitis, or otitis externa.

Box 2.4 The history in suspected urticaria

- Triggers?
- Confirm the diagnosis by asking about the appearance and behaviour of the rash:
  - Urticarial wheals are raised pink papules or plaques.
  - The wheals may be itchy.
  - The surface of the skin is smooth.
  - The wheals are erythematous, i.e. blanch with light pressure.
  - Individual wheals generally last no more than 24 h (48 h at the very most).
  - Wheals come and go in different places.
  - Wheals fade to leave normal skin.
- What happens if skin is rubbed—does it wheal up? = dermographism

See 📖 Chapter 11, p.212 and p.214.

Box 2.5 The history in suspected angio-oedema

- Triggers? Dental procedures or vaginal pressure during sexual intercourse may precipitate attacks of angio-oedema in people with C1 esterase inhibitor deficiency. These patients do not develop urticaria, only angio-oedema.
- The patient may describe one or more of these problems:
  - Sudden onset of deep tender swellings of hands, feet, and genitals.
  - Swelling of lips, tongue, and/or larynx.
  - Puffiness around eyes and lips.
  - Difficulty swallowing or difficulty breathing.
  - Stridor or wheeze.
- Gastrointestinal symptoms such as vomiting or abdominal pain occur in patients with C1 esterase inhibitor deficiency.

See 📖 Chapter 5, p.98 and Chapter 11, p.212.

Box 2.6 The history in suspected contact dermatitis

- Remember that the allergen may be a product that the patient has used for some time.
- Document the symptoms (itch?) and appearance (red, scaly blisters?).
- Explore the patient's occupation and hobbies in detail. Find out exactly what they do and what they are in contact with. Do they protect the skin, e.g. with gloves?
- Does the rash improve at weekends or during holidays?
- Is the skin exposed to any prescribed topical medicaments or over-the-counter remedies and how long have they been used?
- How does the patient care for his/her skin—what is used to wash the skin or to moisturize? What cosmetics are being applied?
- Is the patient atopic? Atopy is linked to a predisposition to an irritant contact dermatitis (dry skin with poor barrier function is easily irritated).

See 📖 Chapter 10, p.200.

The history in patients with hair loss

Hair loss is a cause of great distress and may be difficult or impossible to reverse. Androgenetic alopecia is patterned in men (male-pattern baldness) with loss being most marked on the vertex of the scalp and/or the temples. Women with androgenetic alopecia describe diffuse thinning.

The commonest cause of sudden diffuse shedding is telogen effluvium (see Box 2.7)—a great diagnosis to make because you can reassure your patient that he/she will not lose all their hair and that the hair will grow back. Drugs are another cause of reversible hair loss—see Box 2.8.

What should I ask the patient?

- When did problem start? Has this happened before?
- Establish if hair was shed suddenly or gradually.
- Is the loss diffuse or in patches?
- Is loss complete, leaving bald patches, or partial?
- Is hair being lost at other sites, e.g. eyebrows, eyelashes, axillae? Alopecia areata can be widespread—alopecia totalis (all scalp hair) or universalis (all body hair).
- Are teeth or nails abnormal (indication of an ectodermal problem)?
- Is the patient still shedding excess hair? Remember it is normal to shed 100–150 hairs a day and this may appear to be a lot to an anxious patient, particularly if the hair is long.
- Is the loss associated with other symptoms such as itching or scaling? Eczema and psoriasis are not usually associated with hair loss, but fungal infections certainly are. Some fungal infections cause no inflammation and minimal scale.
- How does the patient care for the hair—hot combs, perms, hair straighteners, colouring?
- Is the hair ever tied back tightly and for how long each day?
- Does the patient pull or pluck the hair?
- Did the patient start any new medications prior to the hair loss? See Box 2.8.
- Any exposure to radiation?
- Is there a family history of hair loss?
- Do close contacts have similar problems?
- Was there was an event 8–12 weeks prior to the onset of loss, e.g. serious illness that might have triggered a telogen effluvium? See Box 2.7.
- Has the patient just had a baby? The growing phase (anagen) is prolonged in pregnancy, but hair is shed postpartum.
- Has the patient any other medical problems? Iron deficiency and thyroid disease (hypo- and hyperthyroidism) may be associated with diffuse hair loss.

Box 2.7 The hair cycle and telogen effluvium

Hair grows 0.3–0.4mm a day but growth is asynchronous. About 90% of the 100,000 scalp hairs are growing. Each hair follicle cycles through phases of growth (anagen), involution (catagen), and rest (telogen)—see 📖 p.10. At the end of the telogen phase, hair is shed and a new cycle is initiated. It is normal to shed 100–150 hairs per day.

Telogen effluvium, 2–3 months after an insult such as severe illness or major surgery, is a common cause of acute diffuse hair loss. The hair follicle switches from a growing phase into a resting phase and then the hair is shed, when the new hair starts to form.

Box 2.8 Drugs causing reversible hair loss

- Anticoagulants
- Antineoplastic agents
- Antiretroviral drugs
- Oral contraceptives
- Progestin-releasing implants
- Gonadotropin-releasing hormone agonist
- Antioestrogens and aromatase inhibitors
- Esterified oestrogens–methyltestosterone replacement therapy
- Extracorporeal membrane oxygenation
- Immunosuppressive drugs
- Interferons
- Minoxidil
- Psychotropic drugs:
    - Antidepressants
    - Anxiolytics
    - Dopaminergic therapy
    - Mood stabilizers
- Retinol (vitamin A)/retinoids.

The history in patients with skin tumours

Skin cancers are the commonest type of cancer. The non-melanocytic skin cancers, basal cell cancer (BCC; the commonest skin cancer) and squamous cell cancer (SCC), are more common than the melanocytic cancer, malignant melanoma, but all are rising in incidence.

Most elderly patients have sun-damaged skin and are at risk of skin cancer. In any patient with a cutaneous tumour or an isolated scaly lesion, the history should include specific questions that will help you to decide if this patient is likely to have a skin cancer.

Sun damage and skin cancers are discussed in more detail in 📖 Chapter 16, p.300 and p.314 and Chapter 17, p.319.

The history

Find out

- How long the patient has had the lesion(s).
- If it is changing (many skin cancers grow slowly and the patient may not have noticed any recent change).
- If the patient is aware of any reason for the 'bump' to have changed, e.g. a history of trauma.
- If it is symptomatic—most skin cancers do not itch or cause pain but some SCCs can be tender.
- If there was any pre-existing mark such as a brown 'spot' or 'mole', but most malignant melanomas arise de novo, not in a pre-existing melanocytic lesion.

Risk factors

Document

- The skin phototype—what happens to the patient's skin in the sun? See Table 2.1.
- History of sunburn, particularly in childhood.
- Chronic sun exposure—explore occupation, hobbies, holiday destinations, time spent in hot climates, e.g. military service or living abroad in childhood.
- Previous skin cancers.
- Family history of skin cancers.
- Immunosuppression such as HIV or exposure to immunosuppressive drugs. Chronic immunosuppression increases the risk of skin cancer.
- Exposure to carcinogens such as industrial tars or oils, pipe smoking, especially the clay pipes still smoked in India (SCC of lower lip), X-irradiation, or arsenic (a constituent of some old-fashioned 'tonics' such as Fowler's solution; a contaminant in drinking water drawn from wells in Bangladesh and parts of India and elsewhere, e.g. Taiwan).

Skin phototype

Skin phototype affects the likelihood of burning in the sun as well as the risk of skin cancer.

Table 2.1 Fitzpatrick classification

Skin type	Response of skin to sun	Appearance
I	Always burns, never tans	White or pale skin, many freckles, blond or red hair, blue or green eyes
II	Burns easily, tans poorly	Pale skin, possibly some freckles, blond hair, blue or green eyes
III	Sometimes burns, tans lightly	Darker white skin, dark hair, brown eyes
IV	Burns minimally, tans easily	Olive skin, brown or black hair, brown eyes. Mediterranean
V	Rarely burns, always tans	Naturally black-brown skin. Often has dark brown eyes and hair. Asian, Latin American, Middle Eastern
VI	Never burns, tans darkly	Naturally black-brown skin. Usually has black-brown eyes and hair. Black African

The history in photosensitivity

Photosensitivity is defined as an abnormal cutaneous response involving the interaction between photosensitizing substances and sunlight or filtered or artificial light. People who are photosensitive are easily sunburned. The skin is uncomfortable or develops a rash when exposed to sunlight or filtered or artificial light. You may suspect photosensitivity from the history or if you find a rash predominantly on sun-exposed surfaces (see examination). Photosensitivity is most often an acquired problem—see Boxes 2.9 and 2.10. Sometimes conditions such as atopic eczema or psoriasis are made worse by sunlight (photoaggravated).

What should I ask?

Specific questions will help you to pinpoint the type and cause of the photosensitivity.

- At what age did the problem start?
- Were any drugs or topical agents started prior to the onset of the problem? Most cases will present within 6 weeks of starting the drug, but drugs started in late autumn may not cause a rash until the following spring or summer.
- What are the symptoms—itch, pain, burning?
- Is there a rash, what is the distribution, and what does it look like—redness, swelling, blisters, pigmentation?
- How quickly does the problem occur after exposure to sunlight?
- How long does the problem persist—minutes, hours, or days?
- Does the rash leave any pigmentation when it fades?
- What time of year does the problem present—is there any seasonal variation? Symptoms usually commence in the spring.
- What sort of exposure is required to trigger the problem?
    - How much exposure is required to cause the rash?
    - Does sunlight in the UK produce the eruption or does it only happen when the patient is abroad?
    - Does it happen if the light comes through glass, e.g. when sitting next to a window or when driving? UVB, unlike UVA or visible light, cannot penetrate glass. See 📖 p.300.
    - Does lying on a sunbed (UVA) trigger the problem?
- Is there any evidence of 'hardening', i.e. does the skin become tolerant after repeated exposures to sunlight or a sunbed? Paradoxically some problems improve as summer progresses and the rash may spare chronically exposed skin on the face.
- Are antihistamines, sunscreen creams, or clothing protective?
- What impact does the problem have on quality of life?
- Is there a history of skin cancer and did skin cancers occur at an earlier age than one would expect, given the skin type and history of sun exposure? Some photosensitive patients are more prone to skin cancers.
- What hobbies or occupation does the patient have?
- Is there a family history of photosensitivity?

Box 2.9 Types of photosensitivity

Primary photosensitivity (uncommon or rare)
- Idiopathic photodermatoses.
- Cutaneous porphyrias.
- Genophotodermatoses: very rare.

Acquired photosensitivity: phototoxicity or photoallergy
- Drug induced (commonest cause of photosensitivity).
- Contact photosensitivity:
  - Soaps, tars, perfumes.
  - Phytophotodermatitis (plants containing psoralen).

Box 2.10 Drugs that cause photosensitivity

Phototoxicity: common, erythematous like an exaggerated sunburn.
- Phenothiazines, amiodarone, thiazides, NSAIDs, quinine, tetracyclines, sulphonamides, retinoids, psoralens.

Photoallergy: eczematous scaly rash, may not occur on first exposure.
- Sulphonamides, phenothiazines, thiazides.

Lupus erythematosus
- Hydralazine, procainamide, thiazides.

Pseudoporphyria
- Furosemide, nalidixic acid, amiodarone, ciprofloxacin, bumetanide, NSAIDs.

Lichen planus (may be photoaggravated)
- Thiazides, quinine.

Pellagra
- Isoniazid.

See 🕮 Box 4.6, p.71, and Chapter 16 for more information.

Why the skin condition has not responded to treatment

Patients often say that the treatment 'has not worked'. It is important to explore exactly what is meant by this statement. It is not much fun using messy ointments and some people, particularly the elderly and those living alone, may find it difficult to apply the treatment. It is hardly surprising if patients do not adhere to treatment plans.

What should I ask the patient?

- What the patient means by the phrase 'has not worked'—are the patient's expectations realistic? Most skin conditions can be controlled, but cure is the exception rather than the rule.
- Has the patient given the treatment enough time to 'work'? It may take 3 or 4 months before some treatments have a maximal effect.
- If the patient has stopped the treatment, what was the reason? Were there any problems applying the treatment or reactions to the treatment? Was the patient under the impression that it was a 'course' of treatment that would be stopped rather than ongoing treatment?
- Did the patient collect the prescribed medicaments or more medicaments from the GP after the initial prescription?
- What was prescribed? It is not sufficient to know the name. You need more information before agreeing with the patient that 'it does not work'. See Box 2.11. It will help if the patient can show you the preparations being used—they may not be what you think were prescribed!
- When, where, and how the preparation is applied? Ask open questions to find out exactly what the patient is doing: 'Tell me more about how you use your treatment'.
- How much is being applied and how often? Under-use is common.
    - Steroid phobia is a common cause of treatment failure. How long does the 30g or 100g tube of steroid ointment last?
    - Emollients should be used liberally and frequently. Was the patient given a 500g tub?
- It can be particularly confusing for the patient if several topical preparations were prescribed. Are they to be used at the same time or sequentially; all over the skin or just on localized areas?
- Has anyone shown the patient how to use the treatment? There is a knack to applying topical medicaments. Ideally all patients with chronic skin problems would see a dermatology nurse. The nurse can answer questions, explain (again) what the treatment is likely to do, and show the patient (or carer) how to use the treatments. If you do not have access to a dermatology nurse, you should be prepared to demonstrate the treatments yourself.

Box 2.11 Questions to ask when exploring what was prescribed

- Is the product a cream, an ointment, or a lotion?
- Ointments have fewer preservatives and are less likely to irritate the skin than creams. They are also more effective than creams in dry scaly conditions. But some people stop treatment because they dislike the feel of the greasy film left on the surface of the skin or the mess left on clothes. They may also have the erroneous perception that the ointment does not 'get into the skin'. The answer may be to use an ointment in the evenings and a cream in the daytime. Some people find the skin is itchier under an occlusive ointment than under a cream.
- Preservatives in creams can sting inflamed skin or cause transient erythema. People who misinterpret these problems as a sign of 'allergy' will stop the treatment.
- Was the patient prescribed enough of the preparation? Hopefully a 500g tub of moisturizer (emollient) rather than a small tube? Most medicaments come in 30g or 100g tubes.

Assessing the impact of skin conditions

Impact of skin diseases

Our appearance affects the way we feel about ourselves and how well we function. The skin is always on show, particularly on the face and hands. If we think that we 'look good', we are more likely to 'feel good' and have confidence.

The psychosocial and physical impact of highly visible, inflammatory skin diseases such as psoriasis, acne, or atopic eczema may be profound. Skin diseases disrupt school, work, and social life. Low self-esteem, common in teenagers with acne, may affect relationships with the opposite sex as well as prospects of employment. Inherited skin diseases, such as epidermolysis bullosa or ichthyosis, may be even more devastating. Patients, their families, and friends may find it difficult to cope.

Patients with chronic scaly skin conditions may also have a deep-seated, and probably quite irrational, fear of being contagious. 'I feel like a leper'. This may be reinforced by the reaction of family and/or friends, who have an equally deep-seated fear of 'catching something'. The patient withdraws from physical and social contact.

Skin conditions in patients with other medical problems may be the 'last straw'. For example, the intractable itching in chronic liver or renal failure can be more difficult to control than pain; photosensitivity in diseases such as systemic lupus erythematosus (SLE) or porphyria may have a major impact on normal daily activities; and hair loss or pigmentary changes may be disabling and highly visible adverse effects of drugs such as chemotherapeutic agents (see 🕮 p.358) or the result of conditions such as chronic graft-versus-host disease (GVHD) (see 🕮 p.496).

Quality of life

Consider measuring quality of life objectively using a validated questionnaire such the Dermatology Life Quality Index (DLQI) (🔗 www.dermatology.org.uk)—see 🕮 Fig. 2.1, p.34 and Box 2.12, p.35. This tool will give you insight into patients' perceptions of the impact of their skin conditions on their lives and also help you to assess the effectiveness of interventions such as education, counselling, and, of course, treatment. The reaction of patients is not predictable and sometimes may seem out of proportion to the severity of the skin disease. The DLQI provides insight into that reaction.

The DLQI is self-explanatory and can be handed to the patient before the consultation. It takes only 1 or 2min to complete. It is designed for patients over the age of 16 years. A similar questionnaire has been validated for use in children. Skindex is another well-studied dermatology-specific health-related quality of life instrument that can be self-administered.

Itch severity scale

Itch is the most common symptom in dermatology and severe itch may be extremely debilitating. A questionnaire (completed by the patient) quantifies how much of the day itch is a problem, the quality of itch, the intensity of itch, and the impact of itch (including impact on sleep).

Further reading

Chren MM *et al. J Invest Dermatol* 1996; **107:**707–13.
Finlay AY and Khan GT *Clin Exp Dermatol* 1994; **19:**210–16.
Hongbo Y *et al. J Invest Dermatol* 2005; **125:**659–64.
Majeski CJ *et al. Br J Dermatol* 2007; **156:**667–73 (itch severity scale).

DERMATOLOGY LIFE QUALITY INDEX

DLQI

Hospital No: Date:
Name: Score:
Address: Diagnosis:

The aim of this questionnaire is to measure how much your skin problem has affected your life OVER THE LAST WEEK. Please tick one box for each question.

1. Over the last week, how **itchy**, **sore**, **painful** or **stinging** has your skin been?
Very much ❒
A lot ❒
A little ❒
Not at all ❒

2. Over the last week, how **embarrassed** or **self conscious** have you been because of your skin?
Very much ❒
A lot ❒
A little ❒
Not at all ❒

3. Over the last week, how much has your skin interfered with you going **shopping** or looking after your **home** or **garden**?
Very much ❒
A lot ❒
A little ❒
Not at all ❒ Not relevant ❒

4. Over the last week, how much has your skin influenced the **clothes** you wear?
Very much ❒
A lot ❒
A little ❒
Not at all ❒ Not relevant ❒

5. Over the last week, how much has your skin affected any **social** or **leisure** activities?
Very much ❒
A lot ❒
A little ❒
Not at all ❒ Not relevant ❒

6. Over the last week, how much has your skin made it difficult for you to do any **sport**?
Very much ❒
A lot ❒
A little ❒
Not at all ❒ Not relevant ❒

7. Over the last week, has your skin prevented you from **working** or **studying**?
Yes ❒
No ❒ Not relevant ❒

If "No", over the last week how much has your skin been a problem at **work** or **studying**?
A lot ❒
A little ❒
Not at all ❒

8. Over the last week, how much has your skin created problems with your **partner** or any of your **close friends** or **relatives**?
Very much ❒
A lot ❒
A little ❒
Not at all ❒ Not relevant ❒

9. Over the last week, how much has your skin caused any **sexual difficulties**?
Very much ❒
A lot ❒
A little ❒
Not at all ❒ Not relevant ❒

10. Over the last week, how much of a problem has the **treatment** for your skin been, for example by making your home messy, or by taking up time?
Very much ❒
A lot ❒
A little ❒
Not at all ❒ Not relevant ❒

Please check you have answered EVERY question. Thank you.

Fig. 2.1 Dermatology Life Quality Index© (DLQI). AY Finlay and GK Khan, April 1992. Reproduced from Finlay AY, Khan GK, *Exp Dermatol* 1994, **19:**210–6, with kind permission of Wiley-Blackwell.

Box 2.12 Calculating and interpreting the DLQI score

Very much scored 3;
A lot scored 2;
A little scored 1;
Not at all scored 0;
Not relevant scored 0.
Sum the score of the answers.
0–1 = no effect on patient's life;
2–5 = small effect on patient's life;
6–10 = moderate effect on patient's life;
11–20 = very large effect on patient's life;
21–30 = extremely large effect on patient's life.

Skin and the psyche

Impact of skin disease on mood

People with skin disease may feel shame or embarrassment and have poor self-image or low self-esteem. 10% of people with psoriasis have had suicidal thoughts. Some patients become increasingly introspective, isolated, and depressed. Treatments prescribed for the skin condition, such as systemic corticosteroids, can also affect mood.

But anxiety or depression may be quite unrelated to skin disease and the potential link between the mood change and the skin problem should be explored in the history.

Dysmorphophobia and dermatological non-disease

Each of us has a clear idea of how we look, but some individuals have a distorted body image.

Dysmorphophobia (body dysmorphic disorder) is a psychiatric condition in which patients have an unshakeable belief that they have a major flaw in their appearance. If present, the lesion is trivial but some patients have no visible pathology (dermatological non-disease). Most patients lack insight into their behaviour, but want a dermatological answer to the intractable problem.

Before diagnosing dysmorphophobia or dermatological non-disease, it is important to be clear what the patient is describing and what they are doing to their skin—e.g. picking may scar skin, hair plucking induces folliculitis. Many inflammatory skin conditions do fluctuate in severity and some, such as urticaria, may disappear completely.

Ask the patient to grade the skin problem as it is today with 10 being the worst possible and zero being normal skin. If the patient says it is dreadful and gives the problem a grade of 10, yet you can see no gross pathology, it is likely that your patient is delusional—see 📖 p.528.

Delusions of parasitosis

The patient believes that he/she is infested and quite often will have convinced other members of the family that this is the case. He/she may describe a crawling or biting sensation, lumps on the skin, and digging out the 'parasites' to provide relief. You may be given a bag or box containing specimens of these 'parasites' (fragments of skin scale, crust, or hair). See 📖 Delusions, p.528 for more information.

Chapter 3

The dermatological examination

Contents

Relevant pages in other chapters

Signs of photosensitivity 🕮 Box 4.6, p.71
Blister 🕮 p.246
Examination of leg ulcer 🕮 p.276

Preparation

Get the basics right and examination of the skin will be much easier. You should inspect all the skin and aim to describe the signs just as accurately as you would signs in the respiratory or cardiovascular systems. You should be able to interpret what you see and although you may not reach a diagnosis, try to pull together a reasonable differential.

Explain what you would like to do and obtain the patient's consent to examine all the skin, not just the areas that that seem to be affected. Ensure the patient is warm and comfortable. You will need to expose the skin, but you can do this in stages, so have a sheet or blanket to hand so that you can cover the patient. Ask if the skin is tender before you begin.

Remember to examine the nails, the scalp, the hair, and the mucous membranes as well as the skin. Look under dressings and invite patients to remove make-up, dentures, or wigs. You may need a chaperone, particularly if you are going to examine sensitive areas such as the genitalia. You may also need a nurse to help you with dressings.

Can you see?

Lighting in most clinical areas is inadequate for examining the skin. Ideally you should be working in bright ambient lighting that is equivalent to daylight, and you should have access to mobile supplementary illumination for some tasks, e.g. inspecting inside the mouth or illuminating awkward skin folds.

Magnification

Some dermatologists use a hand lens or magnifying loupes for close inspection of skin lesions. You will need some form of magnification if you wish to assess the small blood vessels in the nail folds. You can use an ophthalmoscope with a drop of immersion oil, but a dermatoscope is even better. A dermatoscope can also confirm the diagnosis of scabies by revealing mites in burrows. A dermatoscope is used for assessing pigmented lesions, but it takes expertise to interpret the signs—see 🕮 p.568.

Wood's light (black light)

A Wood's light emitting UVR in the long-wave UVA region may be used in the assessment of hypo-or hyperpigmentation or some cutaneous infections—see 🕮 p.568.

Recording the rash

Draw pictures or use a body map to show the distribution of any rash or tumours (Fig. 3.1). It may be helpful to record the appearance of a rash or tumour photographically, but do obtain consent before you take clinical photographs.

Use simple diagrams to show your findings

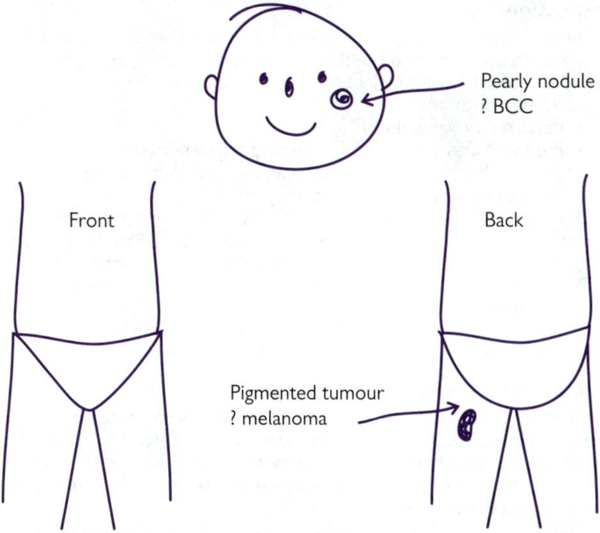

Fig. 3.1 Recording signs.

Rashes

Inspection

- Start by inspecting the patient from the end of the examination couch or bed to assess general health. Is this a life-threatening problem, is the patient unwell (septic, malnourished) or looking healthy?
- Decide if the rash is:
  - Localized or generalized.
  - Predominantly symmetrical suggesting a systemic (endogenous) cause or asymmetrical suggesting an external cause such as infection, trauma, or a contact dermatitis.
- Does the rash have a predilection for certain areas, e.g. extensor surfaces, flexural surfaces, light-exposed skin (see 📖 Box 4.6, p.71), or the extremities—fingers, toes, ears, and nose (an acral distribution).
- Does the rash demonstrate the Köbner phenomenon (show a predilection for scars or areas of trauma)?
- Are lesions grouped, scattered, generalized, linear, annular (in a ring), reticulate (net-like), or serpiginous (snake-like)? See Fig. 3.2.

Palpation and interpreting the signs

Now look more closely at the individual lesions and be prepared to feel the skin, but do ask the patient if the rash is tender before you begin. Try to describe a primary lesion as precisely as possible and decide whether the problem is predominantly epidermal or dermal. Ask yourself the following questions:

- How does the rash start and what shape are the primary lesions?
- Is the border well-demarcated or indistinct?
- Is the surface scaly indicating epidermal pathology or smooth suggesting predominantly dermal pathology? Don't be afraid to gently scratch the surface of the skin with your fingernail.
- Are the lesions raised or flat? Palpate to answer this question.
- What colour is the rash? Does redness blanch with gentle pressure indicating erythema (increased blood in small vessels) or persist indicating purpura (leakage of blood from the vessels into the dermis)?
- Is the involved skin hotter or cooler than normal?
- If there are blisters, what size are they? Do they rupture easily suggesting an intraepidermal blister or are they tense with a thick roof suggesting a subepidermal blister with the whole of the epidermis forming the roof?—see 📖 Fig. 13.1, p.241. Any milia? These tiny (<3mm), white, intradermal keratinous cysts are sometimes found in subepidermal blistering diseases.
- Are there excoriations or erosions secondary to scratching?
- Is the skin thickened (lichenified) suggesting chronic rubbing?
- What happens as lesions evolve? Ask the patient to show you lesions at different stages. Do lesions leave any colour change or scars?
- Is the problem malodorous, suggesting anaerobic infection?

See 📖 inside front cover for terminology.

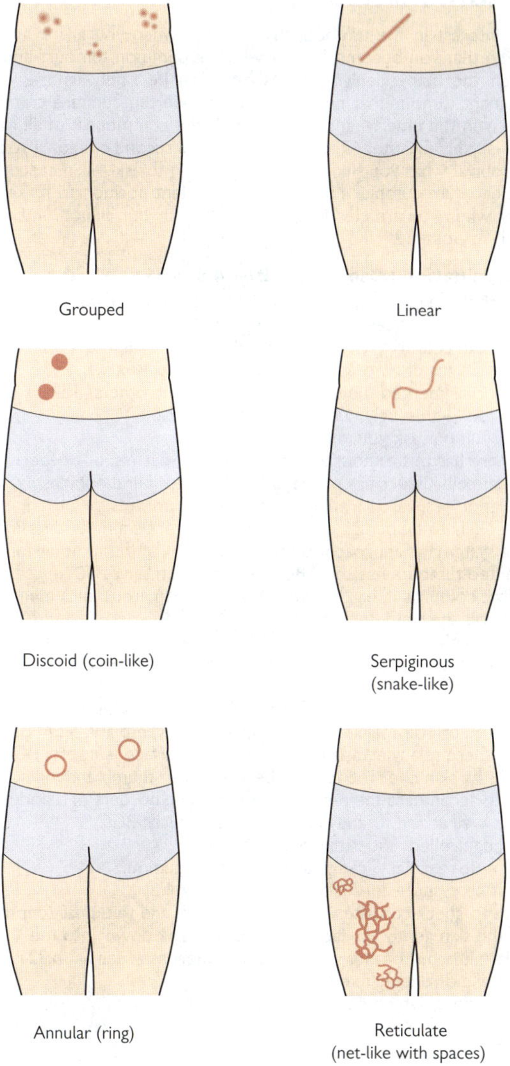

Fig. 3.2 Diagram of signs in the skin and patterns.

Skin tumours

Take an interest in the tumours that you see when you are examining patients so that you become familiar with the common tumours and can distinguish the many benign 'bumps' that can be safely ignored from the malignant tumour that needs treatment. Skin tumours are common, particularly in the elderly, and skin cancer is the commonest of all malignancies—see 🕮 Chapter 17, pp.324–330. Seek a second opinion if you are not sure about what you find. Don't be ashamed to ask—skin cancers diagnosed early are curable. You are in an excellent position to make that diagnosis, when you are clerking patients. Record your clinical findings as accurately as possible.

The examination (also see 🕮 Box 4.8, p.81)

- Check all the skin, taking a particular interest in your patient's back—he/she can't see it.
- Record skin colouring (skin phototype)—see 🕮 Table 2.1, p.27.
- Are there signs of chronic sun damage?—see 🕮 Box 3.1, p.43.
- Does one pigmented tumour stand out from the others? Take a careful look—this 'ugly duckling' may be malignant.
- For any tumour ask yourself:
    - Where has this tumour arisen—epidermis, dermis, or deeper?
    - What cells/tissues are probably involved, e.g. keratinocytes, melanocytes, vascular, fibroblasts, neural, lipocytes, or other?
    - Is it likely to be benign or malignant (might it be a metastasis)?
- Take a systematic approach to the examination of the tumour: for pigmented tumours use the ABCDEF criteria on 🕮 p.330.
    - What colour is it, e.g. brown, purple, erythematous, or a mix?
    - What is the diameter?
    - Is the outline regular or irregular?
    - Is the surface smooth, shiny (pearly), crusted, keratotic, or ulcerated?
    - Has it a punctum? Seen in epidermoid cysts and other tumours centred on hair follicles, such as sebaceous hyperplasia—see Box 3.1.
    - Are there telangiectasia running over the surface (suggests BCC)?
- Stretch the skin over the tumour between your thumb and index finger to accentuate the pearly appearance and borders of a nodular BCC as well as the thready margin of a superficial BCC.
- Is the edge rolled, undermined, or indurated?
- Could it be vascular—can you compress the tumour?
- Might it be cystic—does it transilluminate?
- Palpate to check consistency (soft, firm, hard) and thickness (depth).
- Pinch the skin gently on each side—does it 'sink down' into the dermis?—the button-hole sign in dermatofibromas; see 🕮 p.321.
- Is it mobile or deeply fixed?
- Check regional lymph nodes if you suspect malignancy.

Chronic sun damage (photoageing)

Patients with fair skin, blue eyes, and blond or red hair are most at risk of sun damage and skin cancer. UVR is responsible for many of the signs we associate with old age, including coarse wrinkles and blotchy abnormal pigmentation.

Sun damaged skin looks old—perhaps the most effective message to give to those addicted to 'cooking' themselves on beaches!

Box 3.1 Signs of chronic sun damage

- Solar lentigines: persistent flat brown spots (liver spots) on exposed skin, e.g. backs of hands, forearms, face.
- Easy bruising (senile purpura) which resolves leaving white stellate pseudoscars—most obvious on forearms and backs of hands. Elastic tissue damaged by chronic sun exposure provides the small cutaneous blood vessels with inadequate support.
- Waxy coarse yellowish skin (solar elastosis) on forehead, temples, cheeks, and back of neck, associated with deep furrows.
- Sebaceous hyperplasia: scattered small yellowish papules on the face. Often misdiagnosed as BCC. Look for the central punctum.
- Favre–Racouchot syndrome: thick yellowish plaques (solar elastosis) studded with comedones (dilated follicles, blackheads) on the back of the neck and face, particularly the skin around the eyes.
- Telangiectasia on the side of the neck and cheeks.
- Hypopigmented macules alternating with areas of increased pigment—most obvious on forearms, bald scalp.
- Dry skin.
- Solar keratoses: erythematous or pigmented scaly areas on chronically sun exposed skin such as bald scalp, face, dorsum of hands.
- Skin cancers (BCC, SCC, malignant melanoma).

Scalp and hair

Examining the scalp is part of the general dermatological examination, but assumes particular importance in any patient who is complaining of hair thinning, excessive shedding, or balding (complete loss).

Hair loss (alopecia) may be caused by a variety of insults including fungal infections, drugs, or systemic disease. The loss may be diffuse or localized. Loss manifest by increased shedding may be apparent to the patient but not the physician. Normal hair density may be reduced by as much as 50% before thinning becomes obvious. The loss may affect hair elsewhere, e.g. eyelashes, eyebrows, beard hair, or body hair—see 🕮 p.88.

Your findings should help you to decide if the pathology is likely to be a non-scarring alopecia (you will still be able to see the hair follicles in the affected area) or scarring (the hair follicles cannot be seen easily).

What to look for: the scalp

- Is hair loss complete and/or is the hair density reduced? Is loss diffuse or patchy? Is there any sign of regrowth?
- Does the hair loss affect particular parts of the scalp, i.e. is it patterned? Androgenetic alopecia in men predominantly affects the vertex of the scalp and/or the temporal areas. Check the frontal hair line. See 🕮 p.446.
- Does the loss affect white hairs as well as pigmented hairs? White hairs are spared in alopecia areata—see 🕮 p.454.
- Does the scalp appear normal or is it erythematous or scaly? Are there pustules? Is there perifollicular erythema? Is there follicular plugging?
- Are there broken hairs? Is the texture of the hair shaft smooth or rough?
- Can you see exclamation mark hairs (short and tapering to a point) at the edge of patches of complete loss—pathognomonic of alopecia areata, but not found very often.
- Do you think there is scarring? See Box 3.2.

Hair pull and hair pluck

Telogen effluvium is a common cause of acute diffuse hair loss; 🕮 Box 2.7, p.25. The hair becomes less dense, but patients do not lose all their hair and the scalp looks entirely normal. In contrast, radiotherapy or drugs such as chemotherapeutic agents cause growing anagen hairs to fall out. Consider performing a hair pull or hair pluck—see Boxes 3.3 and 3.4.

What to look for: the hair shaft

You have examined the scalp, but you may also need to look at the morphology of individual hairs.

The hairs in some inherited ectodermal conditions are abnormal. Cut off a sample of a few hairs and examine the hair shafts under a light microscope (or send them to an expert). If the hair shafts are abnormal, does the patient have problems with other ectodermal tissues, e.g. nails, teeth, or sweat glands?

Box 3.2 Diagnosis of scarring alopecia

The diagnostic sign is loss of follicular ostia. Use a hand lens or dermatoscope to examine the involved areas of the scalp.

Other signs will depend on the cause but might include:

- Epidermal atrophy—shiny thin skin that wrinkles excessively if pinched gently.
- Perifollicular hyperkeratosis and perifollicular erythema.
- Boggy swelling and inflammation.
- Follicular plugging or prominent follicular openings without hair.
- Follicular pustules.
- Keloidal scarring.

To confirm of the diagnosis take 2 deep 4mm punch biopsies, orientated parallel to the hair shafts, from hair-bearing skin where disease is active clinically. Ask your pathologist to section one specimen vertically and the other horizontally.

Box 3.3 Hair pull

This test involves gently pulling a group of 25–50 hairs while running your fingers from the base to the terminal ends. Normally only 1 or 2 hair shafts are dislodged.

In active telogen effluvium, a gentle hair pull will yield at least 10 hairs with each pull. Light microscopy will demonstrate that these are in a telogen phase (see Box 3.4).

A gentle hair pull at the edge of a patch of alopecia areata will also remove hairs if the disease is active.

Box 3.4 Hair pluck or trichogram

A hair pluck involves removing a tuft of 10–20 hairs forcefully (use artery forceps).

The hairs are placed on a glass slide, covered with a glass coverslip, and the coverslip held in place by adhesive tape. Long hairs may be folded in a figure of eight to fit them under the coverslip. The hair shafts can be examined under the light microscope. Telogen hairs have club-shaped root 'bulbs' without much pigment. The growing anagen hairs have much smaller root bulbs. These bulbs tend to be soft and easily distorted and they may have tissue adhering to them (root sheaths).

The normal anagen/telogen ratio is 4:1. In telogen effluvium the ration is decreased or reversed. More than 25% of the hairs may be in telogen.

Nails

Inspection of finger- and toenails is an important part of the physical examination. Inspect the nail fold, the nail plate, and the nail bed (see Fig. 3.3).

Acquired changes may be a manifestation of drugs or systemic disease. Congenital problems may indicate a more widespread ectodermal problem that might also affect hair, teeth, and sweating. Nails may be partially absent, misshapen, or totally lost.

Equipment

Side-lighting makes it easier to pick up changes in surface of the nail plate. Consider magnification with an ophthalmoscope or a dermatoscope to look at the blood vessels in the nail fold.

What to look for

Inspect:

- Nail folds, both lateral and proximal. Is there erythema or swelling?
- Blood vessels in the proximal nail fold. You will need magnification to assess blood vessels—see 📖 p.38.
- Cuticle: is this present, intact, and firmly attached to the nail plate?
- Shape of the nail plates.
- Colour of the nail plates: punctate white areas are common in normal individuals; linear splinter haemorrhages near the distal free edge of the nail plate in 1 or 2 nails may be a sign of trauma. Is any colour change uniform or does it involve part of the nail?
- Surface of the nail plates: longitudinal grooves are common in the elderly, when they are of no significance.
- Thickness of the nail plates.
- Attachment of the nail plate to the underlying nail bed. Separation (onycholysis) may be caused by problems such as psoriasis.
- Nail beds (look beneath the nail plate). Is there hyperkeratosis or a tumour such as a subungual wart?

Interpretation

Which nails are involved?

The distribution of the nail problem, just as in the skin, will provide some guide to the likely cause. If the abnormality is widespread and symmetrical it is more likely to have an endogenous than an exogenous explanation.

If just a few nails appear abnormal, particularly if these are toenails, consider whether the changes might be due to trauma or a fungal infection. What does the patient do to his/her nails—biting, manicuring, trauma at work? If infection is a possibility you may wish to take nail clippings for mycological examination and culture—see 📖 p.574.

For more information about the causes of a nail dystrophy see 📖 p.90.

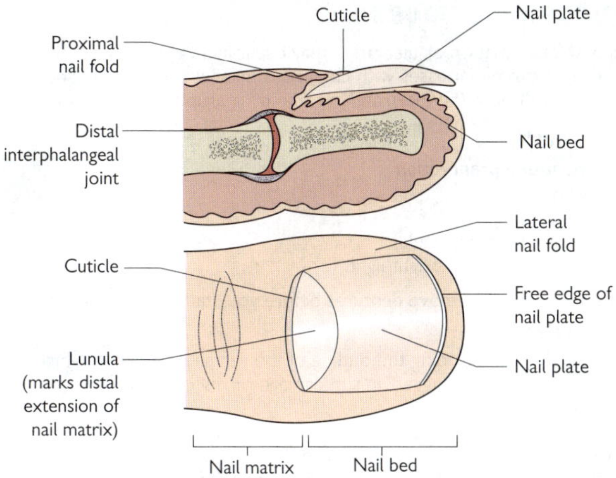

Fig. 3.3 Normal nail. Adapted with permission from De Berker D, Hair and nails. In Warrell, Firth, and Cox, *Oxford Textbook of Medicine* 5th edn, 2010. Oxford: Oxford University Press.

Mucosal surfaces

Mucosal inflammation or ulceration may occur in a variety of skin diseases as well as systemic diseases with cutaneous manifestations, including graft versus host disease (GVHD), and in some drug eruptions.

The mouth

Equipment and preparation

You will need:

- Gloves.
- 2 wooden tongue spatulas.
- A gauze swab and a bright light.

Ask the patient to remove dentures before you start the examination.

What to look for

- Assess the lips including the outline of the vermillion border, which may appear rather 'ragged' in sun damage or discoid lupus erythematosus.
- Palpate tumours or ulcers to assess infiltration.
- Are the lips swollen, scaly, or cracked?
- Lichen planus gives the lips a lacy white appearance.
- Look at the hard and soft palate.
- Check the attached gingiva for bright erythema (desquamative gingivitis), bleeding, or ulceration—seen in lichen planus or pemphigus.
- To examine the buccal mucosa, ask the patient to move his/her tongue across to one side of the mouth so that you can see the opposite side and repeat this for the other side. Use spatulas to help you to visualize the buccal mucosa. Are asymmetrical areas of erythema or ulcers adjacent to broken teeth? Are pigmented areas near teeth that are filled with amalgam?
- Grasp the tongue gently with a gauze swab and examine dorsal and ventral surfaces. Move the tongue to the right and left to examine the retromolar region ('the coffin trap' and a common site of oral cancer).
- Check the dentures if the signs suggest trauma.

Genitalia

In patients with oral mucosal lesions, you should examine the genitalia, where you may find similar mucosal signs. Sometimes these are not symptomatic or the patient may be too embarrassed to complain.

Assess the labia, the folds between them, and the clitoris. Inspect the scrotum and shaft of the penis. In uncircumcised patients, pull back the foreskin gently to check for tightening and to inspect the glans.

Inspect perianal skin and rectal mucosa.

What to look for

- Erythema, swelling, rashes, erosions, ulcers, or pigment change.
- Distortion of the normal anatomy or scarring. Does the foreskin retract normally? Are labia majora and minora visible or obliterated by scar tissue?
- Palpate to assess tenderness and infiltration.
- Discharge from vagina or penis?

The eye

The eye may be involved in a number of systemic diseases with cutaneous manifestations, including GVHD and connective tissue diseases, but pay particular attention to the eyes in any patient with a history of a red gritty eye, blisters, or mucosal ulcers.

What to look for

- Assess lids, e.g. the violaceous discoloration of dermatomyositis.
- Are eyelashes normal? These may be lost in alopecia areata.
- Is there blepharitis or are there chalazions, e.g. in rosacea?
- Is there ectropion—seen in chronic erythroderma?
- If a patient with ectropion closes the eye, is the cornea covered? If not, refer to an ophthalmologist.
- Is the eye red? See 📖 p.82 for causes of a red eye.
- Is the eye sticky?
- Is the patient photophobic?
- Is there subconjunctival blistering or scarring? Gently pull down the lower lid to see if the bulbar and lid conjunctival surfaces are adhering together because of scars (synechiae). This may be more obvious if you ask the patient to look laterally and then medially.

Assessing the severity of a rash

Clinicians should consider using an objective tool to assess and monitor the extent and severity of skin involvement in inflammatory conditions such as psoriasis, lupus erythematosus, or dermatomyositis, particularly when new therapies are being introduced. Objective scoring is equally important in patients with life-threatening problems such as toxic epidermal necrolysis (TEN).

The percentage of body surface area (BSA) affected can be calculated using the 'rule of nines' (Box 3.5), but this provides no other insight into severity. A number of instruments have been shown to be reliable in specific skin conditions. These clinical scoring systems supplement information provided by a tool like the DLQI that assesses the patient's perception of the impact of the condition on quality of life (see 📖 p.32). A few systems are mentioned here.

The Psoriasis Area Severity Index (PASI)

The PASI is probably one of the best known disease-specific tools for assessing an inflammatory skin disease. The clinician grades the inflammation, erythema, scale and thickness of plaques as well as the area of involvement. See 📖 p.186.

The Cutaneous Lupus Disease Activity and Severity Index (CLASI) and the Dermatomyositis Skin Severity Index (DSSI)

These indices have been validated by both dermatologists and rheumatologists. Changes in scores correlate well with changes in global assessments as well as with symptoms such as pain or itch. See 📖 Chapter 19, p.365.

SCORTEN

This severity-of-illness score was developed to predict mortality in toxic epidermolysis/Stevens–Johnson syndrome (SJS). 1 point is scored for each of the following criteria, if present at the time of admission:

- Age >40 years.
- Heart rate >120bpm.
- The presence of cancer or haematological malignancy.
- Involved BSA >10%.
- Serum urea >10mmol/L.
- Serum bicarbonate <20mmol/L.
- Serum glucose >14mmol/L.

The mortality rates for the total score are predicted as follows:

- Score 0–1: 3.2%
- Score of 2: 12.1%
- Score of 3: 35.3%
- Score of 4: 58.3%
- Score of ≥5: 90%.

Box 3.5 Rule of nines to calculate body surface area

The rule of nines was devised for determining the percentage of BSA involved in adults with thermal burns and is calculated as follows:

- Head and neck = 9%
- Anterior chest = 9%
- Posterior chest = 9%
- Anterior abdomen = 9%
- Posterior back and buttocks = 9%
- Upper limbs = 9% each
- Lower limbs = 18% each
- Perineum = 1%.

You can use the patient's palm to measure the BSA, as each palm (including the palmar surface of fingers and thumb) = 1% of total BSA. See Fig. 3.4.

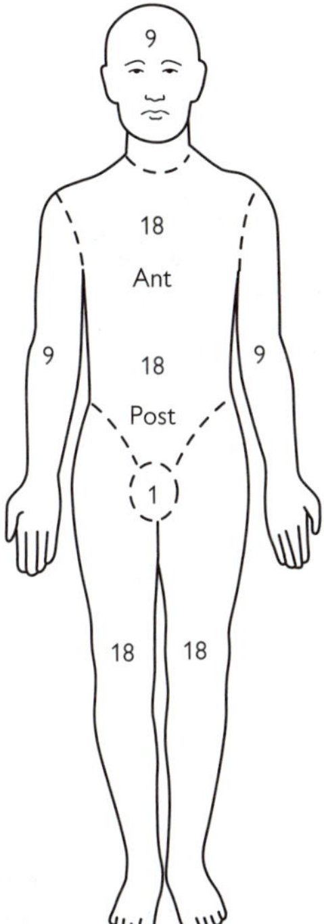

Rule of nines

Fig. 3.4 Wallace rule of nines. Reproduced with permission from Giele H and Cassell O. *Plastic and Reconstructive Surgery*, 2008. Oxford: Oxford University Press.

Chapter 4

What is the diagnosis?

Contents

Relevant pages in other chapters

Leg ulcers—see 📖 Boxes 15.1 and 15.2, p.275
Skin tumours—see Chapter 17, 📖 pp.319–40

Epidemiology of skin disease

The prevalence of the skin problems that you see will be influenced by the setting in which you are working—hospital or community, rural or urban, tropical or temperate, speciality or general—but always remember that common diseases are commonest! Atypical presentations of common skin diseases are much more frequent than typical presentations of rare skin diseases.

In the community you are more likely to come across skin infections, viral exanthems, skin tumours, and inflammatory dermatoses such as acne, eczema, psoriasis, or urticaria than manifestations of systemic disease. Chronic leg ulcers are common in primary and secondary care, as are drug eruptions. In secondary care, you may see manifestations of systemic disease and acute problems including conditions that cause skin failure.

But even in the hospital setting, please bear in mind what is common. Don't forget scabies as a cause of itching when you are caring for patients with chronic renal failure, many of whom are going to be itchy; remember fungal infections when you're looking at asymmetrical scaly rashes; exclude infection or trauma when you see blisters; and think of other causes of photosensitivity, for example, a photosensitizing drug, before diagnosing lupus erythematosus (LE).

What is common?

- Skin infections:
  - Bacterial cellulitis, impetigo
  - Viral: herpes simplex, varicella-zoster, warts, molluscum
  - Fungal: dermatophyte, yeast
- Skin infestations:
  - Scabies, fleas, lice
- Inflammatory diseases:
  - Acne
  - Eczema (dermatitis) of any type
  - Psoriasis
  - Urticaria
- Skin tumours:
  - Benign
  - Premalignant (solar keratoses, Bowen's disease)
  - Malignant (BCC, SCC malignant melanoma)
- Hair loss (alopecia) or gain (hirsutes, hypertrichosis)
- Chronic leg ulcers
- Pigment change (gain or loss).

Prevalence of skin disease

In 1975, the Lambeth Study of 2180 adults in the UK found that 55.5% of them had a skin condition. The prevalence of individual skin conditions in this community is shown on a bar chart in Fig. 4.1.

In developing countries skin diseases are a major burden, particularly in children. These are predominantly bacterial infections, fungal infections, and infestations.

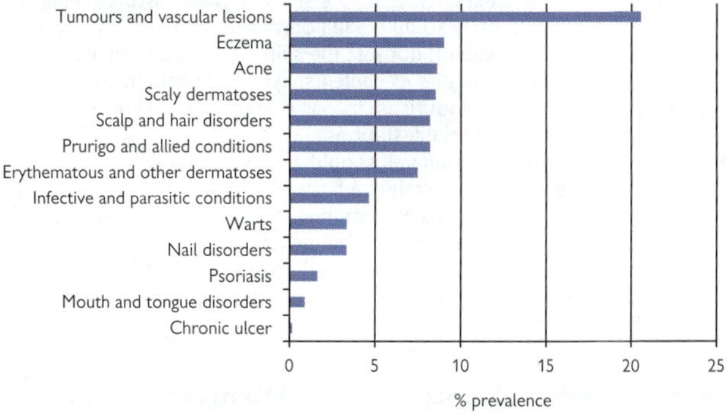

Fig. 4.1 Community prevalence of skin conditions. Data from Lambeth Study (Rea JN *et al. Br J Prev Soc Med* 1976; **30:**107–14).

Further reading

Williams HC. Epidemiology of skin disease. In: Burns T *et al.* (eds) *Rook's Textbook of Dermatology* 8th edn, 2010. Oxford: Blackwell Scientific Publications.

Reaching the diagnosis

The principles

- Read the introductory chapters on history and examination (📖 Chapters 2 and 3, p.17 and p.37), and approach assessment with structure and logic.
- The history is just as important as the physical examination, but experts often take short cuts, using the signs to guide history taking. If you are a novice, you should take a full dermatological history.
- Consider the whole patient, not just the skin—after all, dermatologists are physicians of the skin *and its contents*. Systemic problems such as immunosuppression, malnourishment, or rheumatological disease may have specific cutaneous manifestations.
- A rash in a patient who is unwell should alert you to a different differential diagnosis than a rash in a patient who is well—see 📖 p.58.
- Remember to check mucous membranes, hair, and nails as well as skin.
- Remove dressings so you can see what is beneath them.
- Integrate the information you gather and formulate a differential diagnosis, using analytical rules as well as pattern recognition—see Box 4.1.

Box 4.1 Analytical processing and pattern recognition

- Reaching a diagnosis depends partly on ordering and structuring information (analytical processing) and partly on pattern recognition.
- Experts use their knowledge and previous experience to integrate and make sense of clinical information.
- Pattern recognition ('spot diagnosis') is said to be an almost unconscious process that involves recognizing similarities between cases, based on the overall form of the cases. Expertise is equated with rapid, efficient, and accurate pattern recognition.
- Your skills in pattern recognition will improve when you have been exposed to many clinical examples of a condition and thought about their similarities. Concentrate on the variations in the presentation of common skin problems in the first instance. Why is this likely to be seborrhoeic dermatitis and not asteatotic eczema? What makes this venous stasis rather than a fungal infection? Read around the conditions that you see and discuss the variations you observe. Use your peers to help you to reflect on your findings.
- To develop your analytical skills, adopt an organized approach to each case so that you gather relevant information (experts know what questions to ask), detect important clinical signs (experts know what to look for), integrate the information, and formulate a differential diagnosis. The introductory chapters on history and examination will help you.
- Pattern recognition may have a powerful influence on the eventual diagnosis, but even experts use analytical rules as a safeguard against error.

A framework for analysing cutaneous signs

- Distribution: symmetrical (suggests an endogenous process) or asymmetrical (consider an external cause).
- Is there a predilection for certain sites, e.g. sun-exposed, acral (cold), flexures, extensors?
- What is the pattern, e.g. unilateral, generalized, grouped, linear (see 🕮 p.62), annular (ring-like), reticulate (may be vascular), serpiginous? (see 🕮 Fig. 3.2, p.41)
- Surface: scaly (epidermal problem—can scratch off scale), smooth (predominantly dermal), hyperkeratotic (thick horny layer, does not scratch off easily), or crusted (dried exudate—look underneath).
- Colour: erythema (blanches) or purpura (non-blanching).
- Hypo- or hyperpigmentation: this may be postinflammatory.
- Identify a primary lesion, e.g.:
  - Erythematous macules and papules: 2–10 mm in diameter, with tendency to confluence—morbilliform rash.
  - Erythematous scaly papules (papulosquamous rash) or scaly plaques.
  - Smooth papules or nodules (dermal involvement, e.g. granulomas).
  - Lichenoid papules: these have a purplish colour and relatively smooth surface.
  - Urticarial wheal: smooth raised erythematous papules or plaques that last no more than 48h and fade to leave normal skin.
  - Urticated erythema: smooth raised erythematous papules or plaques that persist for more than 48h.
  - Purpuric macules or papules.
  - Blister: is it thick-walled (subepidermal) or thin-walled and easy to rupture (intraepidermal)?
  - Pustule.
  - Thick plaque that feels as if the process extends below the dermis into subcutaneous tissue.
- What does the involved skin feel like—soft, firm, hard (like bone)?
- Identify secondary lesions:
  - Excoriations: sign of scratching.
  - Lichenification: sign of chronic rubbing.
  - Prurigo: nodular reaction to chronic rubbing, typically spares the middle of the back which cannot be reached easily.
  - Erosion, ulcer, or scar.

Generalized rash in a sick patient

Has the patient been travelling? Is the patient immunosuppressed or taking any medication? Has the patient a fever?

Generalized erythematous rash in a sick patient

- Drug rash, eosinophilia, and systemic symptoms (DRESS)—see 🕮 p.114.
- Infection—see Boxes 4.2 and 4.3.
- Erythroderma (red and scaly) secondary to drugs, eczema, psoriasis, or T-cell lymphoma but may be idiopathic—see 🕮 p.102.
- Acute GVHD—see 🕮 p.494.
- Early toxic epidermal necrolysis (TEN)—see 🕮 p.110.
- Toxic shock syndrome (TSS): may be rapidly fatal—see 🕮 p.95.

Anaphylactic reaction with urticaria

- Reaction to drugs, venoms, or foods—see 🕮 p.98.

Purpura in a sick patient

- Extensive irregularly outlined ecchymoses, bullae, and gangrene: disseminated intravascular coagulation (purpura fulminans): does the patient have meningococcal septicaemia? See 🕮 p.96.
- Other infection—see Box 4.4.
- Small-vessel cutaneous vasculitis secondary to infection, drugs, or a systemic vasculitis—see 🕮 p.406.
- Drug reaction: e.g. DRESS—see 🕮 p.114.

Widespread blisters and/or erosions in a sick patient

- Examine mucosal surfaces (ocular, oral, genital) for blisters or erosions.
- Blisters that rupture easily leaving erosions: consider staphylococcal scalded skin syndrome, SJS, TEN, DRESS, acute GVHD and pemphigus (may be secondary to drugs including angiotensin-converting enzyme (ACE) inhibitors). See 🕮 p.106, p.108.
- Generalized herpes simplex infection (eczema herpeticum) or herpes zoster. Vesicles evolve into pustules and become crusted—see 🕮 Box 5.11, p.107.
- Tense blisters: bullous pemphigoid but patients are usually systemically well, unless there is secondary infection—see 🕮 p.250.

Generalized pustules in a sick patient

- Herpes simplex infection in atopic patient (eczema herpeticum): vesicles evolve into vesicopustules—see 🕮 p.106.
- Varicella-zoster infection (chickenpox): vesicles evolve into vesicopustules—see 🕮 p.148.
- Bacterial infection.
- Sterile pustules: pustular psoriasis, acute generalized exanthematous pustulosis (AGEP) usually secondary to drugs—see 🕮 p.116.

See 🕮 Chapter 5, p.93 for dermatological emergencies.

Box 4.2 Some infections that may present with a morbilliform (measles-like) rash and fever: 📖 **Chapters 6 and 7, p.121 and p.141**

- Measles (rubeola): also cough, coryza, and Koplik's spots on buccal mucosa.
- Rubella (German measles).
- Erythema infectiosum (parvovirus B19). 'Slapped cheek' appearance on face of children.
- Roseola infantum (human herpesvirus 6, HHV-6) = exanthem subitum. Affects children.
- Enterovirus: may have pharyngitis.
- Infectious mononucleosis (Epstein–Barr virus, EBV): malaise, pharyngitis. A rash develops in 90% of patients with EBV who are treated with antibiotics such as amoxicillin.
- Leptospirosis.
- Acute retroviral syndrome (HIV).
- Secondary syphilis: weeks to months after initial chancre.
- Typhoid fever: vomiting, diarrhoea, pink papules on trunk = rose spots (culture of rose spots may yield *Salmonella typhi*).
- Streptococcal scarlet fever, staphylococcal toxic shock syndrome.

Box 4.3 Infections that may cause a morbilliform (measles-like) rash and fever in travellers

- Chikungunya fever: Asia, Africa, Indian Ocean.
- Dengue fever: South East Asia, Central America, South America, Caribbean, South East United States.
- West Nile virus: Asia, Africa Europe, south-eastern USA.
- O'nyong-nyong fever: sub-Saharan Africa.
- Mayaro virus: South America.
- Sindbis virus: Europe, Africa, Asia, Australia.
- Ross River disease: Australia, Papua New Guinea, Fiji, Samoa.

Box 4.4 Infections that may cause a purpuric rash and fever

- Meningococcal septicaemia.
- Rocky Mountain spotted fever: North America, Central America, and South America.
- Dengue fever: South East Asia, Central America, South America, Caribbean, south-eastern USA.
- Viral haemorrhagic fever: arbovirus infection; arenavirus infection.
- Yellow fever: sub-Saharan Africa, Amazon basin of South America.
- Epidemic louse-born typhus.
- Leptospirosis.
- Atypical measles.

Itch

Generalized itch

The history is crucial. You need to decide, for example, if the itch (pruritus not pruritis!) is a manifestation of a skin problem or an infestation, reflects an underlying systemic disease, or might be neuropathic or psychogenic in origin—see 🕮 Box 10.4, p.207 and Box 28.1, p.525. What is the character of the itch? Ask about symptoms such as burning, tingling, hypoaesthesia, or hyperalgesia that might suggest an underlying sensory neuropathy. How much impact is itch having on the patient? Is it disturbing sleep? Is anyone else itchy? Ask about drugs including substance abuse.

When you are examining the patient, decide what signs are secondary to scratching or rubbing (excoriations, lichenification, nodules, ulcers, scars) or if you can find evidence of a primary dermatosis. Patients cannot easily reach the middle of the upper back and usually this is spared if signs are just secondary to scratching. Look carefully for evidence of scabies (and look a second time if the patient returns still itching).

Primary skin condition—the differential includes

- Scabies (are any close contacts itchy?)—see 🕮 p.164.
- Eczema—see 🕮 p.197.
- Psoriasis—see 🕮 p.177.
- Urticaria (the rash may have gone by the time you see the patient). Ask about the rash and how it behaved. Scratch the skin to test for dermographism (a physical urticaria)—see 🕮 p.211, Fig. 11.2, p.215.
- Insect bites.
- Lichen planus.
- Prurigo nodularis—see 🕮 Fig. 10.6, p.207.
- The prodrome of bullous pemphigoid: look for urticated erythema and blisters—see 🕮 p.250.

Itch may be secondary to a systemic disease or drugs

Sensory neuropathy may cause itch or contribute to itch in some of these conditions—see 🕮 p.504. The differential includes:

- Pregnancy-related—see 🕮 p.540
- Iron deficiency anaemia.
- Hypo- or hyperthyroidism.
- Chronic renal failure.
- Biliary obstruction including primary biliary cirrhosis.
- Polycythaemia.
- Internal malignancy including Hodgkin's disease.
- Neuropathic. Centrally-driven neuropathic itch in association with brain tumours, strokes, spinal tumours, and multiple sclerosis. HIV and diabetes may be associated with neuropathic itch—see 🕮 p.504.
- Drugs may cause pruritus (see 🕮 Box 18.7, p.351) including:
  - Statins.
  - ACE inhibitors.
  - Opiates, barbiturates, and recreational drugs.
  - Antidepressants.
  - Oral retinoids.
- Hydroxyethyl starch used in many colloid expanders.

Localized itch

Skin that is persistently rubbed becomes thickened with increased markings (lichenified) or may become hyperpigmented, nodular, or even ulcerated. Consider:

- Contact dermatitis—see 🕮 p.200.
- Lichen simplex—see 🕮 p.206.
- Picker's nodule (localized prurigo nodularis)—see 🕮 p.206.
- Neuropathic itch such notalgia paraesthetica affecting lower border of the scapula or brachioradial pruritus affecting dorsolateral aspect of the arms—see 🕮 p.504 and Box 27.1, p.505.
- Trigeminal trophic syndrome—see Box 27.2, 🕮 p.505.

Linear patterns and sharp demarcations

If a rash is linear or displays a sharp cut-off, consider an external cause such as an excoriation, pressure of a waistband, or brushing against a plant (see 📖 Box 16.6, p.305). External agents usually produce strikingly asymmetrical rashes. Some inflammatory dermatoses such as lichen planus, psoriasis, or vitiligo demonstrate the Köbner phenomenon and the rash develops at sites of trauma, e.g. where skin has been scratched and some cutaneous infections may be auto-inoculated into a scratch, e.g. viral warts or molluscum contagiosum. Ask about trauma such as scratching.

Once you have excluded an outside cause, seek an internal explanation, remembering the comment of that distinguished skin pathologist, Ian Whimster: *'Some invisible intersegmental boundaries, whose existence we have been taught to expect by comparative anatomy and embryology, are only revealed by disease'.*

Venous or lymphatic drainage

Does the problem follow a vein or lymphatic? Stand the patient up to look for varicose veins. Conditions such as stasis dermatitis or vitiligo may follow varicose veins. Thrombophlebitis presents with tender nodules along a vein. The extending red line of lymphangitis is a typical finding in cellulitis, but other infections, including sporotrichosis, may spread along lymphatics as may a malignant infiltrate.

Dermatome

A dermatome is the cutaneous area supplied by 1 spinal dorsal nerve root. Almost all areas of skin are innervated by 2 or more spinal roots so that adjacent dermatomes overlap to a large and variable extent excluding those separated by the ventral axial line—see next section. Herpes zoster involves skin in a dermatomal pattern—see 📖 p.148. See 📖 Fig. 4.2, p.64.

Embryonic ventral axial line

The embryonic ventral axial line marks the border between the C5/C6 and C8/T1/T2 dermatomes. There is no crossover of sensory nerves or sensory function along this line that separates the cranial and caudal dermatomes. Contiguous dermatomes on either side of the ventral axial line are supplied from discontinuous spinal cord segments: C5 and C6 dorsal; and C8, T1, and T2 ventral (see 📖 Fig. 4.2, p.64).

Some morbilliform drug eruptions show a sharp 'drug line' that corresponds to this axial line with well-demarcated involvement of the T1, T2, T3 spinal nerve dermatomes, but sparing of the adjacent C5 nerve dermatome.

Pigmentary demarcation lines (Voigt–Futcher lines)—📖 Box 1.5, p.13

The demarcation between darker dorsal and paler ventral surfaces is apparent in about 20% of people with dark skins. Pigmentary demarcation lines in the upper limb that correspond to the ventral axial line (see previous section), were first described by Voigt and by Futcher. The lines are normal variants in skin colour that may appear pathological.

Blaschko's lines

These lines seem to correspond to the pathways followed by keratinocytes migrating from the neural crest during embryogenesis. Dermatoses following Blaschko's lines suggest keratinocyte mosaicism—see 📖 p.514 and Fig. 27.2, p.515, and inside front cover. The lines follow a V-shape over the spine, an S-shape on the front and sides of the trunk that is unlike dermatomes, and a linear pattern on the limbs.

A number of inflammatory conditions can follow Blaschko's lines including lichen striatus (self-limiting inflammatory rash of childhood), linear lichen planus, inflammatory linear verrucous epidermal naevus (ILVEN), and blashkitis (Blaschko dermatitis)—a rare, self-limiting linear or whorled itching erythematous papulovesicular eruption on trunk and limbs that may be the adult equivalent of lichen striatus. Rare inherited conditions with cutaneous features following Blaschko's lines include incontinentia pigmenti and Goltz syndrome—see 📖 p.518.

Embryonic cleft

Congenital anomalies in the midline may be associated with the lines of fusion between embryonic tissues.

Wallace's line

This demarcation line marks the anatomical boundary on the lateral aspect of palms and soles, where the glabrous (i.e. skin devoid of hair) plantar or palmar skin meets hair-bearing dorsal skin. Some inflammatory problems involving palms or soles such as lichen planus, pompholyx (vesicular eczema), or the erythematous rash of Kawasaki disease display a sharp cut-off at Wallace's line.

Langer's lines of cleavage

See 📖 p.8.

Further reading

Lee MW *et al. Clin Anat* 2008; **21:**363–73.

Shelley ED *et al. J Am Acad Dermatol* 1999; **40:**736–40.

Whimster IW. *Transact St Johns Hosp Dermatol Soc* 1968; **54:**11–41.

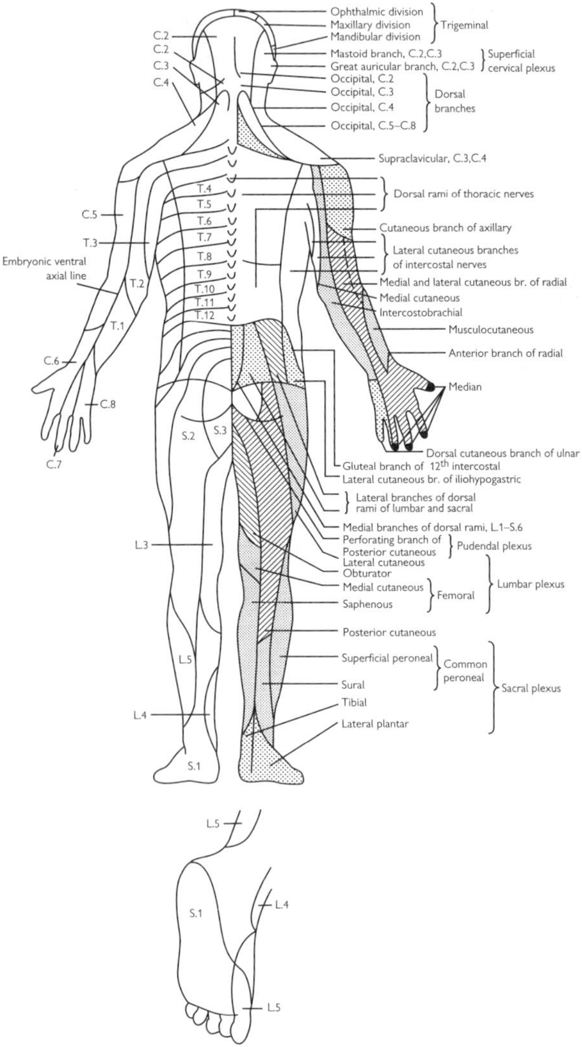

Fig. 4.2 Dermatomes, Reproduced with permission from Longmore, Wilkinson, and Rajagopalan *Oxford Handbook of Clinical Medicine*, 6th edn, 2004, Oxford: Oxford University Press.

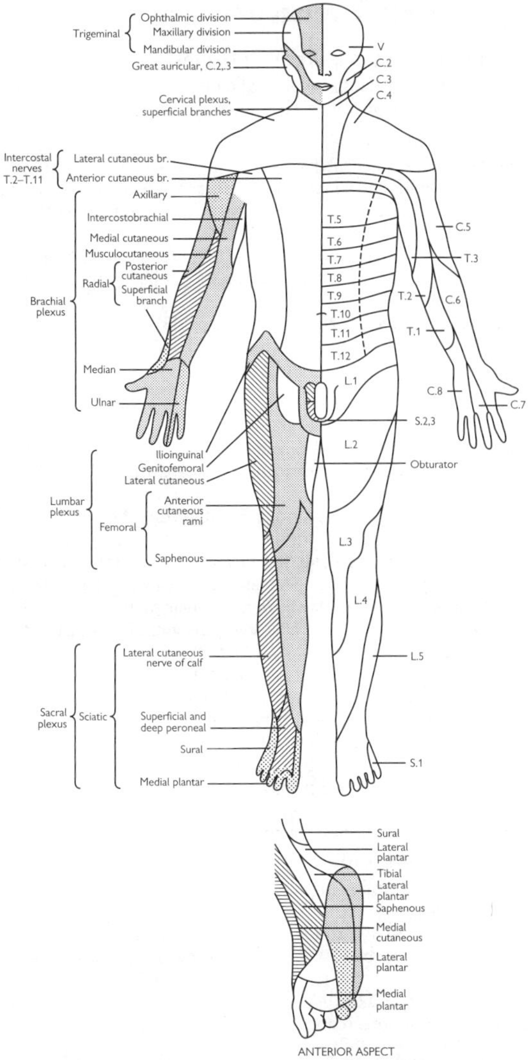

Fig. 4.2 (*Cont.*) Dermatomes, Reproduced with permission from Longmore, Wilkinson, and Rajagopalan *Oxford Handbook of Clinical Medicine*, 6th edn, 2004, Oxford: Oxford University Press.

Scaly or hyperkeratotic red rashes

Erythematous scaly papules or plaques

Scale suggests the pathology involves the epidermis. Scratch the skin with your fingernail to reveal scaling. Consider:

Relatively localized

- Lichen simplex: localized itchy patch. Skin is thickened—see 🕮 p.206.
- Varicose (gravitational, venous stasis): usually not terribly itchy. A single patch may develop over a varicosity—stand the patient up to see the dilated vein—see 🕮 p.204.
- Fungal infection. Usually asymmetrical and often annular. Scale may be lost if topical corticosteroids have been applied. Not terribly itchy—see 🕮 p.156.
- Herald patch of pityriasis rosea—see 🕮 p.143.
- Irritant or allergic contact dermatitis—see 🕮 p.200.
- Bowen's disease: not itchy—see 🕮 p.326.
- Red oozing nipple: atopic eczema or Paget's disease—see 🕮 p.334.

Relatively widespread—see 🕮 Box 4.5

- Scabies: itchy papules, nodules, and excoriations—see 🕮 p.164.
- Eczema: endogenous (symmetrical)—see 🕮 Chapter 10, p.197:
  - Atopic: very itchy.
  - Seborrhoeic: scaly, greasy-looking erythema with relatively little itch. Signs may overlap with those of psoriasis. Look for diffuse scale 'dandruff' in the scalp, flaky eyebrows, central facial erythema (nasolabial folds), flexural erythema, and scaly papules in the centre of the chest and back. May have an annular pattern.
  - Discoid (nummular): generally very itchy and often crusted and weeping.
  - Asteatotic (dry skin): itch is variable. Often limited to the shins.
- Psoriasis (see 🕮 p.177): the amount of itch varies.
- Pityriasis rosea (see 🕮 p.143) or pityriasis versicolor (often pigmented or hypopigmented)—see 🕮 p.160.
- Drug reaction—see 🕮 p.350.
- Secondary syphilis—see 🕮 p.138.
- Photodermatitis: uncommon—see 🕮 p.302.
- Cutaneous T-cell lymphoma: uncommon—see 🕮 p.336.

Scaly annular erythematous lesions

Look for scale either following the erythema or at the expanding edge of the ring. Consider:

- Dermatophyte infection (tinea, ringworm)—see 🕮 p.156. Usually localized. (Scale may be lost if topical corticosteroids have been applied.)
- Pityriasis rosea—see 🕮 p.143.
- Seborrhoeic dermatitis (central trunk, flexures, face, scalp)—see 🕮 p.203.
- Psoriasis—see 🕮 p.177 or, rarely, cutaneous T-cell lymphoma—see 🕮 p.336.
- Subacute cutaneous LE: remember drugs as a cause. Patient is photosensitive, but paradoxically the face is often spared—see 🕮 p.372.
- Annular erythema: uncommon—a few lesions—see 🕮 p.220.

Hyperkeratotic papules and plaques

Rough hyperkeratosis, a sign of a thick horny layer, is not removed as easily as scale by scratching. Is the rash follicular? Consider:

Relatively localized

- Tumours: viral wart, corns (pressure sites), seborrhoeic wart (may be numerous), actinic (solar) keratosis (sun-exposed skin), keratoacanthoma, SCC (sun-exposed skin)—see Chapter 17, p.319.
- Keratosis pilaris: perifollicular rash most often on upper lateral arms and thighs, giving skin a dry rough texture—see Box 31.10, p.555.
- Lichen simplex: itchy nodules or plaques. On legs may resemble lichen planus—see next bullet point—see p.206.
- Hypertrophic lichen planus: itchy purplish nodules or plaques that may become very thickened (hypertrophic) on the leg. Resembles lichen simplex. Look for lichen planus at other sites including buccal mucosa—see p.208.
- Discoid LE: look for scars, follicular plugging, loss of hair—see p.374. May only be 1 or 2 plaques.

More widespread

- Chronic psoriasis: occasionally very hyperkeratotic particularly on palms and soles—see p.177. Reiter's syndrome which is pustular and hyperkeratotic, is probably a variant of psoriasis—see p.194. Usually very symmetrical.
- Follicular eczema.
- Follicular hyperkeratosis: uncommon. May be caused by some inflammatory diseases that target the hair follicle including lichen planus, hereditary conditions, and vitamin A deficiency.

Box 4.5 Erythroderma

⚠ If the patient is red and scaly all over and this has developed suddenly, the patient may be very unwell. Skin failure is a dermatological emergency—see p.102.

Consider:

- Eczema, particularly atopic or seborrhoeic.
- Psoriasis.
- Drug eruption.
- Cutaneous T-cell lymphoma.

Smooth red rashes

Smooth erythematous patches, papules, or plaques

Lack of scale suggests pathology is predominantly dermal but the signs may have been modified by treatment. Consider:

Relatively localized

- Insect bites or papular urticaria (an urticarial reaction to bites).
- Cellulitis: asymmetrical distribution. Hot, tender, erythematous, and swollen. May blister—see 🕮 p.130.
- Acute contact dermatitis may be smooth and oedematous (sometimes with blisters) rather than scaly. Skin may be tender and itchy—see 🕮 p.200.
- Lipodermatosclerosis: tender, indurated erythema on the leg—see 🕮 p.288; Eosinophilic fasciitis—see 🕮 p.391.
- Necrotizing fasciitis: rapidly spreading poorly demarcated purplish erythema in ill patient with high temperature, tachycardia, and low blood pressure—see 🕮 p.118.
- Treated or flexural psoriasis: well-demarcated shiny erythema.
- Treated eczema also loses scale.
- Erythema migrans (not always annular)—see 🕮 p.140.
- Carcinoma erysipeloides (spreading erythema on breast)—see 🕮 p.334.

More generalized

- Urticaria: crops of itchy erythematous papules or plaques (wheals) that may evolve into rings with normal central skin. Wheals last no more than 48h. Skin is normal when wheals fade. May be associated with angio-oedema (deep swelling). No blisters. Stroke the skin with a spatula to test for dermographism (a physical urticaria)—see 🕮 p.214 and p.348.
- Morbilliform or anaphylactoid drug eruption: symmetrical—see 🕮 p.348.
- Viral exanthem: symmetrical.
- DRESS (see 🕮 p.114): papules coalesce into plaques. May have angio-oedema.
- Toxic shock syndrome: may be mild or rapidly fatal—see 🕮 p.95.
- Erythema multiforme (EM): papules that last at least 7 days. May spread into rings with a dusky or blistered centre (target lesions). May have mucosal ulcers—see 🕮 p.105.
- Prodrome of bullous pemphigoid: itchy, erythematous, urticated papules. Look for blisters—see 🕮 p.250.
- Scleroedema (rare): indurated erythematous skin—see 🕮 Box 22.2, p.433.

Smooth annular erythematous lesions

Without scale consider:

- Urticaria: lesions are transient and fade to leave normal skin. Common.
- Basal cell carcinoma (central ulceration): common—see 🕮 p.328.
- Granuloma annulare: fairly common—see 🕮 Box 22.3, p.435.
- Lichen planus (may be a little scale): often on penis or axillary—see 🕮 p.208.
- Sarcoid (may have some scale). Use diascopy to reveal the yellow-brown colour of the 'apple jelly' nodules—see 🕮 p.486. Uncommon.
- Erythema migrans (see 🕮 p.140, Lyme disease): uncommon.

Livedo reticularis: a net-like erythema often on the legs

- Physiological reticulated erythema is continuous and disappears when the skin is warmed. Differentiate from the fixed brownish net-like discoloration that develops after prolonged exposure to external heat—(erythema ab igne)—see 🕮 Fig. 20.5, p.419.
- Discontinuous reticulate erythema that does not disappear on warming. May be purpuric (retiform purpura). Consider:
    - Occlusive vasculopathy caused by cholesterol emboli or thrombi, e.g. in antiphospholipid syndrome—see 🕮 Box 20.8, p.419, p.292, p.294. Look for healed ulcers—scars with a telangiectatic margin.
    - Vasculitis affecting medium and/or large vessels—see 🕮 p.416. Look for purpuric nodules or ulcers with a purpuric rim.

Purpura

Exclude trauma, the commonest cause of purpura. Is the patient taking aspirin, another platelet inhibitor, or an anticoagulant that might potentiate bleeding into the skin? For more discussion of purpura in sick patients see 🕮 p.96.

Flat (macular) purpura

Leakage of red blood cells (RBCs) without inflammation of vessel walls. Consider:

- Legs: non-specific associated with inflammatory rashes, e.g. stasis eczema, psoriasis.
- Forearms: minor trauma to sun-damaged atrophic skin with poorly supported vessels, particularly in elderly patients. Also common in patients with atrophic skin secondary to prolonged treatment with oral or very potent topical corticosteroids.
- Scurvy: perifollicular purpura, corkscrew hairs, poor wound healing—see 🕮 p.475.
- Thrombocytopenia or hyperglobulinaemic purpura—see 🕮 p.498.

Palpable purpura

- Purpuric papules: small vessel cutaneous vasculitis with or without systemic disease—see 🕮 p.404.
- Urticarial vasculitis: erythematous wheals become purpuric and fade to leave bruising—see 🕮 p.409.

Purpura, livedo reticularis, and nodules

- Cholesterol emboli: asymmetrical acral petechiae, subcutaneous nodules, and livedo reticularis—see 🕮 p.418.
- Antiphospholipid syndrome—see 🕮 Box 20.8, p.419.
- Necrotizing vasculitis affecting deeper cutaneous vessels—see 🕮 p.416.
- Extensive irregularly outlined ecchymoses, bullae, and gangrene: disseminated intravascular coagulation with purpura fulminans—see 🕮 p.96.

Telangiectasia (small dilated cutaneous vessels)

- Sun damage (face).
- Rosacea (face).
- Prolonged use of potent topical corticosteroids.
- Diffuse or limited cutaneous systemic sclerosis: matt telangiectasia on face, hands, and/or lips—see 🕮 p.384.
- Hereditary haemorrhagic telangiectasia—see 🕮 Box 24.8, p.483.

Red faces

Although a red face may indicate photosensitivity, always consider other causes:

- ***Seborrhoeic dermatitis:*** scaly, greasy-looking erythema with little itch. Scale and redness tend to involve nasolabial folds, the centre of the forehead, and skin behind ears as well as other sites—see 📖 p.203.
- ***Cellulitis or erysipelas:*** is there fever or malaise? Look for swelling and tenderness as well as erythema. The rash is often asymmetrical.
- ***Contact dermatitis:*** is the skin itchy or scaly? Is the face swollen? Any vesicles? Might this be an acute contact dermatitis (irritant or allergic) to a cosmetic? Remember that the product may have been used for some time before the patient is sensitized—see 📖 p.200.
- ***Acne:*** look for pustules, papules, comedones, nodules, and scars—see 📖 p.224.
- ***Rosacea:*** look for pustules as well as telangiectasia, erythema, and swelling, but some patients have much more of one component than another. Comedones are not a feature of rosacea. See 📖 Box 12.4, p.227 and p.234.
- ***Herpes simplex or herpes zoster:*** any prodrome of tingling or discomfort? Look for vesicles progressing to small pustules. Herpes zoster presents in a dermatomal distribution.
- ***Corticosteroid-induced acneiform rash***: prolonged application of potent topical corticosteroids to the face can produce a telangiectatic rosacea-like eruption with pustules but no comedones.
- ***Angio-oedema:*** usually transient, and swelling is more marked than the erythema. Mucous membranes may be affected—see 📖 p.98.
- ***Photosensitivity:*** what is the distribution of the redness? Check eyelids, under the hair, behind the ears, and under the chin. Compare exposed and covered sites—see Box 4.6 and 📖 p.302 and p.368.
- ***Flushing:*** if repeated, may become fixed. Investigation is only required if flushing is of sudden onset and associated with systemic symptoms—see 📖 Box 24.7, p.482. Ask about triggers. Consider:
  - Blushing: flushing triggered by emotions.
  - Physiological flushing after exercise, heat, hot drinks, alcohol.
  - Menopausal hot flushes (flashes).
  - Rosacea: labile flushing progresses to fixed oedematous erythema, telangiectasia, and pustules—see 📖 p.234.
  - ⚠ Carcinoid syndrome (very rare): look for rosacea-like vascular changes, oedema and induration of face, wheezing, severe diarrhoea, hypotension and tachycardia, features of pellagra (scaly sun-exposed skin, glossitis, angular stomatitis)—see 📖 p.482.
  - Superior vena cava obstruction—face is swollen and red. Look for dilated veins on neck, chest, and arms. Symptoms include dyspnoea, cough, and headache. Associated with malignancy—(bronchial carcinoma, lymphoma)—or, less often, thrombosis, e.g. after pacemaker insertion.

Box 4.6 Is the patient photosensitive?

What should I look for?

The signs will depend on the cause of photosensitivity, but may include erythema, urticaria, papules, blisters, and/or pigmentation. Look for a rash that is maximal on exposed sites and spares covered skin. The skin may be normal between episodes. Chronic sun exposure may induce tolerance, so-called 'hardening', and so, paradoxically, the face may be spared. Drugs are a common cause of photosensitivity—see 🕮 Box 16.5, p.305.

Photosensitive rashes may involve 1 or more of the following sites:

- The prominences of the forehead, the nose, the cheeks, particularly over the cheekbones (malar), and the chin.
- The back of the neck if not covered by hair.
- The helix of the ear if not covered by hair.
- The V on the upper chest where the shirt sits open.
- The extensor surfaces of forearms, the backs of the hands.
- The nails—tender onycholysis with a rim of pigmentation (photo-onycholysis). (Associated with some drug-induced photosensitivity).
- The dorsum of the feet (if exposed).
- Signs of chronic sun damage such as freckling on exposed skin (photoageing) or skin cancer—see 🕮 p.43. Are these signs appropriate for the age and lifestyle of the patient or greater than you would expect?

Is there sparing of covered skin, with a sharp cut-off between involved and uninvolved skin? Check:

- Around the orbit (ask the patient to close his/her eyes to see the eyelids).
- Under the frame of spectacles.
- The upper lip.
- Under the nose.
- Deep wrinkles on face.
- Below the chin.
- Behind the ears.
- Under the hair—on the forehead or at the back of the neck. Is a spared area exposed because the hair has been cut recently?
- Under watch straps.
- The distal phalanges, because the hands often sit with fingers curled.
- Between the fingers.
- Under the shoe.

Red legs and leg ulcers

Red leg(s)

Erythematous

- Cellulitis (unlikely to be bilateral): hot, oedematous, and tender.
- Lipodermatosclerosis: often bilateral. Painful indurated erythema that may simulate cellulitis in acute stages.
- Gravitational eczema: associated with venous stasis and oedema. Stand the patient up to look for varicose veins. Often bilateral.
- Acute allergic or irritant contact dermatitis (may be bilateral): oedematous, erythematous, and may blister—see 📖 Fig. 10.1, p.201. Itchy but also uncomfortable if swollen.
- Deep venous thrombosis: unilateral swelling with erythema and calf tenderness.
- Lymphoedema: initially erythematous and pitting oedema. Later indurated with thick hyperkeratotic skin. Predisposes to cellulitis. See 📖 p.296.
- Erythema nodosum: tender erythematous nodules on shins—see 📖 p.424.
- Necrobiosis lipoidica: well-defined reddish yellow plaques with telangiectasia, atrophic centre (that may ulcerate), and raised erythematous rim—see 📖 p.434. Associated with insulin-dependent diabetes.
- Livedo reticularis: net-like mottled purplish pattern—see 📖 Fig. 3.2, p.41 and p.252. Patients may have leg ulcers and nodular vasculitis or an obstructive vasculopathy—see 📖 p.418, p.292, and p.294. May be purpuric in places (retiform purpura)—see following section. Differentiate from erythema ab igne—fixed brownish reticulate marking where skin has been repeatedly exposed to heat. See 📖 p.418.
- ⚠ Erythromelalgia (erythermalgia, erythralgia): painful burning erythema. May be idiopathic, associated with thrombocythaemia or familial. Involves acral sites—see 📖 p.504.

Purpuric

- A little flat purpura is not uncommon in association with inflammatory rashes on legs, e.g. psoriasis, eczema, simply because of leakage of RBC.
- Capillaritis (pigmented purpura) produces flat purpuric spots (likened to cayenne pepper) and brownish yellow (haemosiderin) pigmentation, but does not signify systemic disease. Capillaritis is most common on legs. The cause is unknown (rarely drugs cause capillaritis). Lymphocytic inflammation around capillaries is associated with extravasation of RBC into the skin.
- Palpable purpura. If purpura is palpable consider small-vessel cutaneous vasculitis (usually bilateral) and exclude systemic disease—see 📖 p.404.
- Retiform purpura (purpura in a livedo pattern): seen with occlusive vasculopathies including cholesterol emboli, antiphospholipid syndrome, deficiency of protein C or protein S, cryoglobulinaemia. See 📖 p.418.

Chronic leg ulcers

The history and examination should help you to pinpoint the cause of the chronic ulcer. More details are given on 📖 p.274.

Consider:

Common

- Venous ulcers: risk factors include deep vein thrombosis (DVT), trauma, operations to hips or knees; obesity and immobility.
- Arterial disease: look for intermittent claudication, rest pain, night pain, pain worse when leg is elevated. Occurs in tobacco smokers.
- Mixed arteriovenous: symptoms of both venous and arterial disease.
- Neuropathic: develop at sites of pressure—painless ulcers. Most common on feet of diabetics.
- Malignancy: don't accept the label 'leg ulcer' without looking under the dressing. BCCs are often misdiagnosed as leg ulcers.
- Trauma: including insect bites and intravenous drug abuse.
- Ecthyma: full-thickness infection of skin, usually by *Staphylococcus aureus* or *Streptococcus pyogenes*, with ulceration and crusting—see 📖 p.129.
- Dermatitis artefacta: deliberate self-harm—see 📖 p.524.
- Drug-related: hydroxyurea, nicorandil.

Less common

- Pyoderma gangrenosum: rapidly growing, painful ulcer with an undermined bluish margin. May be associated with rheumatoid arthritis, inflammatory bowel disease, or myeloproliferative disorders but 50% of patients have no underlying disease—see 📖 p.290.
- Vasculitis: is the rim purpuric? Associated with connective tissue diseases particularly rheumatoid arthritis. See 📖 Box 19.1, p.367.
- Occlusive vasculopathy (see 📖 p.294): suggested by the presence of livedo reticularis. Causes include inherited disorders of coagulation—mutations in protein C, protein S, antithrombin III, fibrinogen, or factor V genes.
- Necrobiosis lipoidica: associated with insulin-dependent diabetes—see 📖 p.434.
- Infection: e.g. deep fungal, treponemal (syphilitic gumma).

Hands, feet, and other extremities

The skin is cool at acral sites such as the hands, feet, ears, and tip of nose. These sites are also exposed to sun and trauma. Conditions that tend to favour acral sites include:

- Scabies: crusting between fingers and burrows on palms. Blisters on palms and soles in children—see 📖 p.164.
- Some infections—see Box 4.7.
- Contact dermatitis (irritant or allergic) is common on hands.
- Chilblains (perniosis): warm erythematous nodules that may become purplish. Itch or cause burning pain. Occur in cold weather in damp temperate climates. Seen most often in the young, especially children, and elderly, but less frequent now homes are centrally heated. Self-limiting. May be associated with acrocyanosis: see later in list.
- Sarcoidosis: may involve the tip of the nose—dusky purplish discoloration and swelling (lupus pernio)—see 📖 p.486.
- Chronic cutaneous LE: hyperkeratotic papules on fingers (chilblain lupus) or photoaggravated disease on the nose—see 📖 p.374.
- Raynaud's phenomenon (sudden pallor followed by cyanosis and finally erythema with swelling and tingling): may affect fingers, toes, nose, and/or earlobes—see 📖 Box 19.18, p.384, p.400.
- Acrocyanosis: persistent dusky mottled discoloration of hands and feet. May be bright red when very cold. Associated with chilblains—see 📖 p.410.
- ⚠ Erythromelalgia (erythermalgia, erythralgia): attacks of painful burning erythema affecting feet, legs, and, less often, hands—see 📖 p.504. May be idiopathic, associated with thrombocythaemia, or familial. Sometimes also associated with acrocyanosis.
- Chemotherapy: induced hand–foot skin reaction—see 📖 p.358.
- EM is associated with erythematous papules and target lesions on palms and soles. Check mucosae—see 📖 p.105.
- Acute GVHD: macular blotchy erythema of palms, soles, and face; a common early sign—see 📖 p.494.
- Fingers are tight and puffy in systemic sclerosis (sclerodactyly): look in hands or fingers for calcinosis and for vascular changes in nail folds. See 📖 p.384.
- Cutaneous vasculitis and obstructive vasculopathy favour cool sites where blood flow is slow—check toes—see 📖 p.406, p.418.
- Cryoglobulinaemia or cryofibrinogenaemia: mottling, retiform purpura, ulceration, or blotchy cyanosis at acral sites exposed to cold—helices of the ears as well as fingers and toes. May be associated with Raynaud's phenomenon and livedo reticularis—see 📖 p.410.
- Cholesterol embolus: blue toe or peripheral gangrene associated with livedo reticularis. May have retiform purpura. Seen when arterial catheterization disrupts an atheromatous plaque or after prolonged anticoagulation when a clot becomes friable—see 📖 p.418.
- Palmoplantar pustulosis: sterile pustules on palms and/or soles—see 📖 p.184 (also see 📖 zinc deficiency, p.475).
- Blisters and erosions on dorsum of hands in porphyria cutanea tarda (trauma and skin is fragile)—see 📖 p.310.

Box 4.7 Infections that may produce acral signs

- Herpes simplex causing a whitlow on a finger—see p.144.
- Orf or milker's nodule on a finger—see p.150.
- Hand–foot–mouth disease associated with infections by coxsackieviruses A10 and A16 and with enterovirus 71. Vesicopustules on hands and feet as well as mucosal ulcers.
- Gianotti–Crosti syndrome (papular acrodermatitis of childhood)—see p.142: flat-topped brownish pink papules or papulovesicles on hands and feet. Most often associated with hepatitis B and Epstein–Barr viral infections in children.
- Purpuric rash in a gloves and socks distribution caused by human parvovirus B19—see p.142.
- Secondary syphilis: copper-coloured macules on palms—see p.138.
- Atypical mycobacterial infection with nodule on finger—see p.136.
- Mycobacterial infections favour the nose and ears: leprosy, cutaneous tuberculosis (TB) (lupus vulgaris)—see p.136.

Flexural rashes

Intertrigo is another name for a flexural rash, but is not a diagnosis. Consider these causes of intertrigo:

Common

- ***Candidiasis:*** look for a bright red erythema and satellite pustules with a collarette of scale. The rash is often asymmetrical and the skin is sore rather than itchy. Candidiasis is more common in obese patients, those with diabetes, and the immunocompromised. Take swabs to exclude streptococcal infection. May complicate an irritant dermatitis—see p.158.
- ***Dermatophyte infection:*** the rash gradually spreads out from the flexure. Look for scale at the edge of the erythematous patch. Tinea cruris (groin) is common. Infection is often asymmetrical. Take a scraping from the scaly margin to confirm the diagnosis—see p.156.
- ***Seborrhoeic dermatitis:*** look for 'dandruff' in the scalp (ill-defined diffuse scaling) and behind the ears or erythematous, greasy scaly plaques in the centre of the face, the centre of the chest, or the centre of the back. The features overlap with those of flexural psoriasis (sebopsoriasis). Look for signs of psoriasis in the nails, e.g. pitting, onycholysis, or subungual hyperkeratosis—see p.203.
- ***Flexural psoriasis:*** presents as a well-demarcated, shiny erythema. Skin is moist rather than scaly. Is there plaque psoriasis on extensors? Check for pitting of the nails or onycholysis and look in the scalp for scaling plaques. Any family history of psoriasis?—see p.182.
- ***Irritant contact dermatitis:*** in obese, sweaty, or incontinent patients—see p.200.
- ***Erythrasma:*** look for symmetrical orange-brown slightly scaly plaques in the flexures. Skin fluoresces coral pink under Wood's light (UVA). Caused by infection with *Corynebacterium minutissimum*. More common in warm humid climates, diabetes, obesity, and old age—see p.124.
- ***Streptococcal infection:*** bright red, painful perianal rash.

Less common

- ***Allergic contact dermatitis:*** e.g. to deodorants, clothing dyes: eczema involves edge of axillae and spares axillary vault—see p.200.
- ***Pseudomonas infection:*** brownish grey scaly rash with painful fissuring. Potentiated by washes with antibacterial lotions—see p.124.
- ***Hidradenitis suppurativa:*** patients present with a history of recurrent 'boils'. Look for comedones, inflamed nodules, pustules, sinuses, and scars—see p.230.
- ***Acanthosis nigricans:*** velvety hyperpigmented thickening of flexural skin associated with skin tags. Seen most often in obese Asian patients with insulin resistance ('pseudoacanthosis nigricans')—see p.432. Presents rarely as a manifestation of underlying malignancy, usually adenocarcinoma of the stomach—see p.502.

Pustules

Pustules are small dome-shaped bumps filled with milky fluid containing neutrophils or, sometimes, eosinophils. Pustules are often caused by bacterial infection of a hair follicle (folliculitis), but may be sterile. Decide if pustules are arising in association with hair follicles (perifollicular pustules). Vesicles (small blisters that contain clear fluid) may evolve into pustules (vesicopustules) or may simulate pustules, when on palms and soles and covered by a thick horny layer. Puncture the vesicle to let out some fluid if you are not sure if it is clear or milky.

Common

- Bacterial folliculitis (usually staphylococcal): may be a secondary bacterial folliculitis in conditions such as atopic eczema—see 📖 p.126.
- Bullous impetigo: superficial vesicles and pustules rapidly rupture leaving golden crusting—see 📖 p.128.
- *Candida*: satellite pustules at the margin of the erythematous flexural rash—see 📖 p.158.
- Irritant or occlusive folliculitis, e.g. with thick applications of greasy emollients—see 📖 Box 6.3, p.127.
- Acne: follicular lesions with comedones, inflammatory papules, pustules, nodules, cysts, and scars. Involves face and may involve trunk—see 📖 p.224.
- Herpes simplex virus including eczema herpeticum; herpes zoster virus infection (dermatomal): vesicles (the primary lesion) evolve into pustules or vesicopustules—see 📖 p.144, p.148.
- Periorifical 'dermatitis': pustulovesicular facial rash most often caused by potent topical corticosteroids—see 📖 p.236.
- Rosacea: look for erythema, telangiectasia, papules, and oedema—see 📖 p.234. Patients do not have comedones. Involves face but spares trunk.
- Steroid-induced acne: look for sterile pustules without comedones.

Less common

- Hidradenitis suppurativa: pustules in flexures with grouped comedones, nodules, scars, and sinuses—see 📖 p.232.
- Chronic palmoplantar pustulosis (sterile non-follicular pustules)—see 📖 p.184.
- Pyoderma gangrenosum may be preceded by a tender pustule—see 📖 p.290.
- Demodicosis in immunocompromised—see 📖 p.168.

Rare

- Bowel-associated dermatosis-arthritis syndrome or Sweet's syndrome (📖 p.480).
- AGEP: sterile non-follicular pustules—see 📖 p.116.
- DRESS: morbilliform rash with 'juicy' papules that may coalesce into plaques. Sometimes sterile pustules or vesicles—see 📖 p.114.
- Pustular psoriasis: waves of non-follicular pustules appear at the edge of erythematous tender plaques or patches. Sick patient with fever and a neutrophilia—see 📖 p.116, p.184.
- Subcorneal pustular dermatosis—see 📖 Box 13.6, p.249.
- Behçet's disease—see 📖 p.264.

Blisters

A blister is a bump, which may be large (bulla) or small (vesicle) that is filled with clear fluid (serum). Blisters may form just below the stratum corneum, within the epidermis or within or below the dermo-epidermal junction—see 🕮 Fig. 13.1, p.241. Causes of blisters include:

Fairly localized blisters

Common

- Physical causes:
  - Friction, pressure, ischaemia, scalds or cold injury, sunlight, radiation.
- Cutaneous infections:
  - Viral: herpes simplex or varicella-zoster (shingles); coxsackievirus A16 (handfoot and mouth disease).
  - Bacterial: bullous impetigo caused by *Staphylococcus aureus*; blisters in association with oedema secondary to streptococcal infection (cellulitis, erysipelas, and necrotizing fasciitis).
  - Fungal: dermatophyte.
- Insect bites and stings.
- Scabies (vesicles or vesicopustules on the palms or soles in infants).
- Contact dermatitis: irritant or allergic, e.g. nickel sensitivity—see 🕮 Fig.10.1, p.200.
- Pompholyx (itching vesicles on hands and feet)—see 🕮 p.205.
- Photosensitivity: drug-induced and phytophotodermatitis—see 🕮 p.200 and Fig. 10.1, p.201.
- Oedema blisters: sudden peripheral oedema in elderly patients with atrophic skin may cause blisters on legs.

Uncommon

- Diabetic blister: on legs.
- Damage to basal cells (lichenoid reaction):
  - EM—see 🕮 Chapter 5, p.105.
  - Fixed drug eruption—see 🕮 Chapter 18, p.354.
- Pseudoporphyria in chronic renal failure—backs of hands—see 🕮 p.312.
- Mastocytoma: a localized increase in mast cells in the skin—seen in infants—see 🕮 Box 31.5, p.547.
- Coma blisters: originally described with barbiturates—see 🕮 p.355.

Rare

- Genetic:
  - Epidermolysis bullosa (EB) simplex.
  - Incontinentia pigmenti—see 🕮 p.518.
  - Acrodermatitis enteropathica—see 🕮 p.475.

More widespread blisters

Common

- Eczema:
  - Contact eczema may generalize after starting in a localized pattern.
  - Atopic eczema (exclude infection if you see blistering in atopic eczema).
- Cutaneous infections:
  - Viral: herpes simplex (may generalize in conditions such as atopic eczema) or varicella-zoster (chickenpox); poxvirus (vaccinia).
  - Bacterial: widespread infection in atopic eczema.
- Miliaria (caused by blockage of eccrine ducts and sweating in a hot humid environment; the itchy vesicles may be superficial or deep).

Uncommon

- Cutaneous infections:
  - Bacterial: staphylococcal scalded skin syndrome caused by a circulating exotoxin produced by *Staphylococcus aureus*—see 🕮 Fig. 6.2, p.123 and p.129.
- Damage to basal cells (lichenoid reaction):
  - SJS—see 🕮 p.110.
  - TEN with full-thickness necrosis of the epidermis—see 🕮 p.110.
  - Lichen planus—see 🕮 p.208.
  - Vesiculobullous cutaneous LE—see 🕮 Box 19.9, p.375.
- Autoimmune blistering diseases:
  - Bullous pemphigoid (most common of the autoimmune blistering diseases in western Europe)—see 🕮 p.250.
  - Pemphigus foliaceus and vulgaris—see 🕮 p.248.
  - Dermatitis herpetiformis—see 🕮 p.254.
- Bullous cutaneous vasculitis (bullae will be haemorrhagic)—see 🕮 p.404.
- Urticaria pigmentosa (increased mast cells in the skin)—see 🕮 Box 31.5, p.547.
- Porphyria cutanea tarda (sporadic more common than inherited):
  - Associated with iron overload (haemachromatosis), alcohol, oestrogens, and hepatitis C—see 🕮 p.310.

Rare

- Autoimmune blistering diseases including:
  - Paraneoplastic pemphigus—see 🕮 Box 13.5, p.249.
  - Mucous membrane (cicatricial) pemphigoid—see 🕮 p.252.
  - Pemphigoid gestationis—see 🕮 p.540.
  - Epidermolysis bullosa acquisita (EBA)—see 🕮 p.252.
  - Linear IgA dermatosis—see 🕮 p.252.
- Genetic:
  - Hailey–Hailey disease ('benign familial pemphigus').
  - EB group of diseases.
  - Bullous ichthyosiform erythroderma.
  - Cutaneous porphyrias associated with subepidermal blistering:
    —variegate porphyria.
    —hereditary coproporphyria.
    —congenital erythropoietic porphyria.

Nodules or induration

Nodules suggest involvement of dermis and, sometimes, subcutaneous tissues. Nodules may be tender or painless. Induration (woody hardness) and thickening of the skin suggest deep involvement with fibrosis.

Nodules

- Cysts: epidermoid ('sebaceous' with a punctum—face, trunk, scalp), pilar (no punctum, scalp), dermoid (congenital and usually in midline on the face), acne (inflammatory on face).
- Thrombophlebitis: tender nodules along a vein.
- Prurigo nodularis: excoriated dome-shaped nodules—see 🕮 p.206.
- Granulomatous: e.g. foreign body with granulomatous reaction, sarcoidosis, rheumatoid nodules—see 🕮 p.366.
- Gouty tophi: hands, elbows, ears—see 🕮 Box 19.2, p.367.
- Calcinosis cutis: hard white nodule that extrudes chalk-like material. Usually hands or pressure sites. May occur in systemic sclerosis—see 🕮 p.386 and Fig 19.11, p.389.
- Tumour (see 🕮 p.42 and Chapter 17, p.319 and Box 4.8). Including:
  - BCC, SCC, melanoma.
  - Lipoma, muscle tumour, neural tumour, vascular tumour.
  - Appendageal tumours.
  - Lymphoma (T-cell or B-cell).
  - Metastatic carcinoma (breast, renal, colon, lung, ovary, gastric).
  - Kaposi's sarcoma.
- Infection including:
  - Furuncle ('boil'): hot, tender, erythematous.
  - Sporotrichosis or atypical mycobacterial infection: nodules spread proximally along a lymphatic.
  - Leprosy, deep fungal infection.
- Xanthoma: elbows, knees, ankles, hands. Yellowish tinge—see 🕮 p.436.
- Panniculitis: e.g. erythema nodosum, traumatic panniculitis, nodular vasculitis—see 🕮 Chapter 21, p.421.
- Perforating disease: rare (see 🕮 p.458, and Box 19.27, p.399). Nodules with a central keratin plug.
- Multicentric reticulohistiocytosis (rare): symmetrical nodules on fingers, characteristic papules around nail folds, destructive arthritis—see 🕮 p.394.

Induration with fibrosis

- Scar or changes after radiotherapy—see 🕮 p.492.
- Lipodermatosclerosis (leg in association with venous stasis)—see 🕮 p.288.
- Morphoea, systemic sclerosis, or drug-induced scleroderma—see 🕮 p.384.
- Chronic GVHD: sclerodermoid form—see 🕮 p.496.
- Scleroedema: associated with infection, diabetes, monoclonal gammopathy. Firm non-pitting oedema of face, neck, upper back—see 🕮 p.384.
- Scleromyxoedema: associated with paraproteinaemia, myeloma, lymphoma and leukaemia—see 🕮 Box 26.7, p.499. Waxy, flesh-coloured papules on face, trunk, and extremities.
- Nephrogenic systemic fibrosis—see 🕮 p.462. Seen in patients with renal failure exposed to contrast medium containing gadolinium. Features similar to scleromyxoedema—see 🕮 Box 26.7, p.499.
- Porphyria cutanea tarda—waxy thickening of sun-exposed skin—see 🕮 p.310.

Box 4.8 Skin checks and skin cancer

Skin cancers are the commonest malignancy. You should carry out a full skin examination when assessing patients. But cutaneous tumours are common and you need to 'get your eye in' so you know when to refer. See 📖 Chapter 17, p.319 for more information. These pointers may be helpful:

- Patients with fair skin who burn in the sun are at greatest risk of skin cancers. Chronic immunosuppression with drugs such as ciclosporin greatly increases the chances of developing skin cancer—see 📖 p.324.
- Most skin cancers grow slowly, an important exception being nodular malignant melanoma.
- BCCs and malignant melanomas are usually painless, but some SCCs may be tender, particularly on the ear.
- Most malignant melanomas arise de novo and not from a pre-existing melanocytic naevus.
- Carry out a skin check in all patients. Examine sun-exposed skin on the face, bald scalp, ears, forearms, and backs of hands. Look at the skin on the back and legs, and check behind the ears.
- Look for signs of chronic sun damage, e.g. mottled pigmentation, telangiectasia, yellowing, wrinkling, and keratoses (see 📖 Box 3.1, p.43). The more sun damage, the greater the likelihood of developing a skin cancer—eventually.
- Remember deeply tanned skin is generally unhappy skin!
- Solar keratoses are common and do not need treatment unless the keratosis is thickened (indurated) when you should suspect a SCC. But solar keratoses do indicate too much sun exposure and you should advise your patient accordingly.
- Put skin on the stretch to see the pearly border of a BCC (the commonest skin cancer).
- Think again before you diagnose melanocytic naevus in an elderly patient. Benign melanocytic naevi, common in youth, gradually regress with age. A pigmented tumour in an elderly patient is much more likely to be a seborrhoeic wart (raised, well-defined margin, 'stuck-on' appearance, rough with a pitted crinkled surface) or a solar lentigo (flat, smooth, even pigmentation), but it just might be a malignant melanoma.
- Use the ABCDEF criteria (see 📖 p.330) to assess the likelihood of any pigmented lesion being a malignant melanoma and remember to look twice at moles that stand out from their neighbours—the 'ugly ducklings'.
- Record your findings including the presence of sun damage and the fact that you carried out a skin check.
- Advise patients how protect their skin from sun damage to minimize the risk of skin cancer. But temper your advice with a little common sense—we all need some sun to lift our spirits and maintain our vitamin D levels!

Eyes, mouth, and genitalia

Causes of a red eye

- Conjunctivitis: redness involves the entire surface of the eye. Examine the conjunctiva, both bulbar and palpebral (lid).
  - If the eye is also sticky, this is likely to be a bacterial or viral conjunctival infection.
- Dry eye. Is the conjunctiva irritated because the eye is dry? Dry eyes burn and feel gritty. Vision may be blurred. Confirm the diagnosis by performing a Schirmer strip test.
- Allergic conjunctivitis: common in atopic eczema.
- Iritis (anterior uveitis): the eye is painful and photophobic. The eye is not sticky. Redness is most marked around the cornea. Small pupil.
  - Iritis occurs in systemic diseases that may also have cutaneous manifestations including sarcoidosis, inflammatory bowel disease, Behçet's disease, herpes virus infection, and Lyme disease.

Causes of oral ulcers

⚠ Biopsy any longstanding unexplained ulcer to exclude malignancy.

Common

- Trauma: check teeth and/or dentures.
- Inflammatory
  - Aphthous ulcers: minor, major or herpetiform—see 📖 p.262.
  - Erosive lichen planus—see 📖 p.266.
- Infections:
  - Herpes simplex, varicella-zoster virus (VZV), hand–foot–mouth disease, *Candida*, syphilis, HIV.
- Drugs:
  - Cytotoxic agents, co-trimoxazole, antithyroid drugs, nicorandil, beta-blockers, clopidogrel, alendronate, protease inhibitors, NSAIDs, anticholinergic bronchodilators, and antihypertensives (captopril, enalapril).
  - Ulcers heal when drug is withdrawn.
- Radiation to head and neck.
- Oral SCC (solitary ulcer, may be asymptomatic).

Uncommon

- Inflammatory:
  - EM, SJS, and TEN—see 📖 p.105, p.106, p.108.
  - GVHD—see 📖 p.492.
  - Eosinophilic ulcer: uncommon benign self-limiting ulcer probably secondary to trauma. Usually a large ulcer on the tongue.
  - LE—see 📖 p.370.
  - Behçet's disease: rare—see 📖 p.264.
- Infection in immunosuppressed patients:
  - TB (prevalence increasing as a complication of HIV infection), fungus (*Cryptococcus*, histoplasmosis, *Aspergillus*), leishmaniasis.

Rare

- Inflammatory:
  - Angina bullosa haemorrhagica (blood-filled blisters that rupture).
  - Immunobullous diseases such as pemphigus vulgaris which may affect oral mucosa before the skin—see 🕮 p.248.
  - Epidermolysis bullosa—see 🕮 p.244.

Causes of genital ulcers

⚠ Biopsy any longstanding unexplained ulcer to exclude malignancy.

- Trauma: including sexual abuse.
- Infections:
  - Herpes simplex virus: may be extensive and chronic in immunosuppressed patients—see 🕮 p.260.
  - EBV—see 🕮 Box 14.2, p.261.
  - Ecthyma gangrenosum caused by *Pseudomonas aeruginosa* in immunosuppressed patients—see 🕮 p.129.
  - Syphilis: *Treponema pallidum.*
  - Chancroid: *Haemophilus ducreyi.*
  - Lymphogranuloma venerum: *Chlamydia trachomatis.*
  - Granuloma inguinale (donovanosis): *Klebsiella granulomatis.*
- Inflammatory:
  - Aphthous ulcers: possibly triggered by local injury or infection including HIV. Most patients also have oral aphthous ulcers—see 🕮 p.262. Genital aphthous ulcers usually measure 1–3cm in diameter and may be quite deep and either round or irregular in outline. Patients usually only have a few genital aphthous ulcers (often just one). Large ulcers may heal with scarring.
  - Erosive lichen planus: check mouth—see 🕮 p.266.
  - EM, SJS, and TEN—see 🕮 p.105, p.106, p.108.
  - Hidradenitis suppuritiva: sinus tracts develop into chronic ulcers—see 🕮 p.230.
  - Crohn's disease—see 🕮 p.472.
  - Pyoderma gangrenosum—see 🕮 p.290.
  - Drugs: including nicorandil.
  - Behçet's disease: rare—see 🕮 p.264.
  - Immunobullous disease such as pemphigoid or pemphigus. The skin is fragile and genital vesicles rupture rapidly to form painful superficial erosions or ulcers (rare) see 🕮 p.248 and p.250.
- Malignancy:
  - Carcinoma: BCC or SCC.
  - Leukaemia or lymphoma.
  - Extramammary Paget's disease.

Change in skin colour

The commonest cause of a change in skin colour is previous inflammation. Ask the patient when the colour change appeared (was it present at birth?) and if anything preceded the change in colour. Examine the skin with a Wood's light to determine if the pigment is epidermal or dermal and to accentuate epidermal changes—see 🕮 p.568.

Acquired hyperpigmentation

Strictly speaking, hyperpigmentation means brown skin, but this list encompasses colours ranging from brown to blue or grey.

Common

- Normal racial variation or sun tan.
- Stasis dermatitis: the pigment is a mix of melanin and haemosiderin.
- Melasma (usually facial): brown colour is caused by melanin—see 🕮 Box 30.1, p.539.
- Postinflammatory hyperpigmentation, particularly in dark skins. Common after acne or lichenoid eruptions such as lichen planus or cutaneous LE. After lichenoid eruptions, the skin has a greyish tinge as the pigment is deep in the dermis—see 🕮 p.208.
- 10% of normal people have 1 or 2 café au lait spots—see 🕮 Box 27.4, p.509.
- Erythema ab igne: repeated local heating of the skin from a hot water bottle or fire causes localized fixed reticulate pigmentation.
- Phytophotodermatitis: linear streaks of brown pigmentation are preceded by erythema and sometimes blisters—see 🕮 Fig. 31.11, p.565.
- Dermatitis neglecta: occasionally patients avoid touching a patch of skin. The unwashed skin builds up brown scale.
- Drugs including minocycline, antimalarials, amiodarone, and heavy metals may give the skin a bluish grey tinge—see 🕮 p.352.

Less common

- Neuropathic itch or chronic rubbing—see 🕮 Box 27.1, p.505.
- Malabsorption, pellagra.
- Cutaneous systemic sclerosis and sclerodermoid chronic GVHD. Skin is thickened, often with perifollicular hypopigmentation—see 🕮 p.384 and Box 26.3, p.497.
- Pseudo-onchronosis secondary to hydroquinone in skin lightening creams (may also cause confetti-like loss of pigment).
- Primary biliary cirrhosis, haemochromatosis.

Rare

- Café au lait spots: neurofibromatosis, McCune–Albright syndrome, multiple mucosal neuromas syndrome—see 🕮 Box 27.4, p.509.
- Widespread freckling in children may be associated with xeroderma pigmentosum, LEOPARD syndrome, Carney complex, and Peutz–Jeghers syndrome—see 🕮 p.563.
- Generalized pigmentation: adrenal insufficiency, Nelson's syndrome, ectopic ACTH-producing tumours, POEMS syndrome in plasma cell disorders—see 🕮 Box 26.6 p.499, p.448.
- Alkaptonuria: blue-black pigment of helices of ear and sclerae.

Hypopigmentation and depigmentation

Hypopigmented skin: loss of pigment is partial. The tone of the skin is creamy rather than absolutely white. Depigmented skin is white and fluoresces a bright white under Wood's light, e.g. vitiligo.

Common

- Pityriasis alba: hypopigmentation on cheeks of children. Subtle scale.
- Pityriasis versicolor: scaly in the active phase but macular postinflammatory hypopigmentation may persist for months until melanocytes are stimulated by sun exposure.
- Idiopathic guttate hypomelanosis: pale macules on sun-damaged forearms of adults.
- Progressive macular hypomelanosis: common in young Afro-Caribbean adults. Progressive symmetrical hypopigmentation in midline of trunk.
- Postinflammatory hypopigmentation: most often in dark skins. Causes include psoriasis, sarcoidosis, leprosy, pinta, and kwashiorkor.
- Vitiligo: smooth depigmented macules or patches—see 📖 p.452.
- Halo naevus: children or young adults. A ring of white skin appears around a melanocytic naevus. The brown 'mole' gradually turns pink and eventually disappears leaving a depigmented macule.
- Scars (may also be hyperpigmentation).
- Chemical (cleaning solutions: contact depigmentation) hypo- and depigmentation on skin exposed to chemical.

Less common

- Tuberous sclerosis: oval or confetti-like hypopigmentation—see 📖 p.512.
- Hydroquinone in skin lightening creams: confetti-like loss of pigment.
- Morphoea or cutaneous systemic sclerosis: perifollicular hypopigmentation in thickened skin. May also be hyperpigmentation—see 📖 p.384, p.390.
- Antiphospholipid syndrome: porcelain white scars with telangiectatic rim (like atrophie blanche)—see 📖 Box 20.8, p.419. Associated with livedo reticularis.
- Naevus depigmentosus: localized hypopigmented skin with discrete, regular, or serrated margins. Stable appearance. Also see 📖 p.569.
- Chronic arsenic ingestion: 'raindrop' hypopigmentation.

Rare

- Extragenital lichen sclerosus—see 📖 p.268. Crinkly, shiny white papules with follicular plugging. Look for genital disease.
- Chronic GVHD—see 📖 Box 26.3, p.497. (Also causes hyperpigmentation.)
- Naevus anaemicus (jagged outline, caused by vasoconstriction)—see 📖 p.520, p.569.
- Cutaneous T-cell lymphoma—see 📖 p.336.
- Pigmentary mosaicism: swirling hypopigmented patches—see 📖 Box 27.10, p.519.
- Focal dermal hypoplasia of Goltz—see 📖 Box 27.11, p.519.
- Albinism: total body depigmentation, light blue iris, nystagmus.
- Waardenburg's syndrome (a form of piebaldism). Autosomal dominant inheritance. Symmetrical patches of hypopigmentation on face, scalp, back, and proximal extremities with a stripe of normal coloured skin down the centre of the back. Also white forelock, neurosensory deafness, widening of the bridge of the nose, and heterochromia of the iris.

Skin of colour

People with black or brown skin may be African, African American, Afro-Caribbean, Indian, or Australasian in origin. Signs in dark skin may be difficult to assess and some conditions are much more common in certain ethnic groups, while others may present differently. Pigmentary disorders may be particularly distressing and disfiguring.

- Traditional medicines, cultural practices, or cosmetics may affect the skin, so ask what the patient is using on the skin.
- Pigmentary demarcation lines may simulate pathology—see 📖 Box 1.4, p.13.
- Benign melanocytic naevi are common in the nail bed of black patients and produce hyperpigmented linear bands of varying width in the nail plate. These may be single or multiple and the number tends to increase with age. Pigment does not extend onto the skin of the surrounding nail fold, although some pigment may be visible beneath the translucent cuticle. If pigment is detected in the nail fold (Hutchinson's sign), arrange a biopsy to exclude malignant melanoma.
- Some black patients have harmless diffuse nail pigmentation.
- Palms and soles are paler than the rest of the skin in dark-skinned patients.
- Palmar creases tend to be hyperpigmented and in black patients may contain punctate conical pits (keratosis punctata).
- Asymptomatic hyperpigmented macules varying in shape and size are common on plantar surfaces in black patients, particularly the ball of the foot and the heel.
- Brown pigmentation of the oral mucosa including the tongue, buccal mucosa, and palate is a normal finding in many black patients.
- Periorbital hyperpigmentation is common in the Indo-Asian population. The colour change may be familial and starts below the eyes around puberty.
- Dermatosis papulosa nigra (1–3mm pigmented, warty papules like small seborrhoeic warts) is common on the cheeks of Africans, African Americans, and dark-skinned South East Asians.
- Redness (erythema) in dark skin may be difficult to assess and the skin may merely appear slightly darker than normal. Ask the patient to show you what is normal or abnormal. Even erythroderma (generalized erythema) may not be obvious. Look for signs of skin failure such as shivering, thirst, and widespread scaling—see 📖 p.100.
- Long-lasting postinflammatory hypopigmentation and/or hyperpigmentation is common after conditions such as acne, psoriasis, or eczema as well as after lichenoid inflammatory conditions such as lichen planus or LE. Ask the patient if anything preceded the colour change.
- Prolonged hypopigmentation may be caused by intralesional corticosteroids or very potent topical corticosteroids, but it is much more common for the colour change to be secondary to the inflammatory skin condition for which the corticosteroids were prescribed.
- Even individuals with dark-coloured skin may be photosensitive, so do not assume anything!

Box 4.9 Presentations more common in black or brown skin

Hair follicles and follicular rashes

- Alopecia related to hair straightening (with chemicals or hot combs) or to tight braiding (traction alopecia) in black patients.
- Pomade acne on the forehead caused by greasy hair oils.
- Acne keloidalis nuchae: firm papules on nape of the neck or scalp, common in black patients with curly hair.
- Pseudofolliculitis barbae: hyperpigmented papules and pustules on neck and cheek where hair is shaved. Triggered by ingrowing hairs.
- Atopic eczema in a follicular pattern is common in black children, as is follicular accentuation in other inflammatory conditions including lichen planus and pityriasis versicolor.
- Disseminated and recurrent infundibulofolliculitis: itchy follicular papules on the chest, back, and buttocks of black patients.

Darker colour (often postinflammatory): also see p.84

- Scaly plaques of psoriasis look blue-black rather than red.
- Lichen planus presents with deeply-coloured purple papules in dark skin. Lichen planus pigmentosa is more common in Asian patients and presents with ashy-grey macules.
- Pseudo-acanthosis nigricans: hyperpigmentation, velvety thickening, and skin tags in the flexures of obese Asian patients. Associated with diabetes and insulin resistance.
- Macular amyloidosis: itching rash with rippled grey-brown pigmentation often on the upper back. More common in Asian patients. See Box 23.3, p.461.
- Acquired onchronosis: hyperpigmentation caused by skin lightening creams containing hydroquinone.
- Suction cups used in the traditional practice of cupping leave circular hyperpigmented macules that may simulate bruising.

Paler colour (often postinflammatory): also see p.85

- Pityriasis alba: pale oval patches with fine scale most often on the face but may involve the trunk. Seen in prepubertal children.
- Trichrome vitiligo, a variant in which the skin has zones of hypo-pigmentation as well as depigmentation and normal pigmentation.
- Leprosy produces anaesthetic macules—see Box 6.8, p.137.
- Dyspigmentation with scarring in plaques of discoid LE—see p.374.
- Confetti-like hypopigmentation on face caused by skin lightening creams containing hydroquinone.

Wounds and scars

- Sickle-cell leg ulcers—see Box 15.2, p.275.
- Keloids (smooth nodular scars that extends beyond the original wound) common on the upper chest, shoulders, and upper back. Avoid taking skin biopsies from these sites in patients with black skin.

Neonates—see p.544

- Mongolian spots (dermal melanocytes). Light blue to slate grey macules, most often lumbosacral. May be multiple. Fade slowly—see Fig. 31.10, p.565. Naevus of Ota affects periorbital skin and sclera.
- Transient neonatal pustular melanosis—see Box 31.4, p.547.
- Infantile acropustulosis—see Box 31.4, p.547. Differentiate from scabies.

Hair: too much or too little

The history and examination in hair problems are described on 🕮 p.24 and p.44. Excess hair may grow anywhere there are hair follicles. Hair loss may be diffuse, localized, complete (bald patches), or partial (thinning). The scalp may be normal or scaly. Decide if alopecia is non-scarring and potentially reversible, or scarring, when loss is irreversible—see 🕮 Box 3.2, p.45.

Hypertrichosis

Definition: excessive hair on any part of the body.

- ***Acquired:*** generalized most often drugs (see 🕮 p.356). Rarely indicates systemic disease including malnutrition (anorexia nervosa, see 🕮 p.474, p.530), advanced HIV infection, porphyria cutanea tarda (see 🕮 p.310), POEMS syndrome (see 🕮 Box 26.6, p.499), and disorders of the CNS. Localized hypertrichosis occurs after chronic cutaneous irritation or inflammation and may develop in association with some tumours (melanocytic naevi, Becker's naevi, plexiform neurofibromas, smooth muscle hamartomas).
- ***Congenital:*** localized hypertrichosis in the midline over the scalp or spine may indicate an underlying neural tube defect, e.g. a hair collar in the scalp or a lumbosacral faun tail—see 🕮 p.548. Hypertrichosis is associated with some rare hereditary diseases including porphyrias, mucopolysaccharidoses, fetal alcohol syndrome, and Cornelia de Lange syndrome.

Hirsutes

- Increased growth of terminal hairs in females in an androgen-dependent pattern (normal male sexual pattern)—face, lips, chest, arms, thighs. Caused by androgen overproduction, androgenic drugs, or increased sensitivity of the hair follicle to androgens. See 🕮 p.440.

Localized non-scarring alopecia

- Alopecia areata: well-defined areas of loss. Scalp is smooth not scaly. You may find exclamation-mark hairs. At first regrowing hair is not pigmented. See 🕮 p.454.
- Tinea capitis (dermatophyte infection, ringworm): scalp is itchy, scaly, and may be inflamed.
- Hair pulling (trichotillomania): short stubby hairs (<2cm). Longer hairs can be pulled out. Common in children.
- Trauma: hair may be pulled out when thick scale is removed in psoriasis or seborrhoeic dermatitis.
- Traction alopecia: affects the margins of the scalp where hair has been pulled back tightly. No scale or exclamation-mark hairs.

Diffuse non-scarring alopecia

- Telogen effluvium (illness in previous 2–3 months?), postpartum.
- Androgenetic alopecia—see 🕮 p.446.
- Thyroid disease or iron deficiency anaemia.
- Drugs—see 🕮 p.356.
- Rare congenital causes of hypotrichosis include ectodermal dysplasias and disorders in which the hair shaft is abnormal and brittle.

Scarring alopecia

Follicles may be replaced by tumour. In inflammatory diseases such as discoid LE, damage to follicular stem cells (see 📖 p.10) probably contributes to permanent hair loss.

More common

- Trauma: including radiotherapy.
- Tumours:
  - Benign: naevus sebaceous: present at birth—see 📖 Fig. 31.2, p.549.
  - Malignant: BCC, SCC, metastatic deposits.
- Discoid LE—see 📖 p.374.
- Acne keloidalis: most often in black men. Firm follicular papules (keloids) at nape of neck and/or occipital scalp. May also have pustules.

Uncommon

- Aplasia cutis: present at birth—see 📖 Box 31.6, p.549.
- Linear morphoea.
- Lichen planopilaris (variant of lichen planus that affects hair follicles).
- Folliculitis decalvans: erythematous perifollicular pustules and scarring. Cause unclear but may involve *Staphylococcus aureus*.
- Dissecting cellulitis of scalp: occurs most often in young black men. Firm deep nodules become fluctuant, discharge malodorous pus, and develop interconnecting sinuses. May be associated with hidradenitis suppurativa and acne conglobata—see 📖 p.230.

Funny nails

As with the skin, the distribution of changes points towards the cause. If many nails are affected (symmetry) the problem is likely to be endogenous, if only 1 nail is affected (asymmetry), the problem is likely to be exogenous. Inflammation of periungual skin in conditions such in eczema leads to secondary changes in the nail plate.

Common or important signs include

- ***Changes in nail colour***—see Box 4.10.
- ***Transverse depressions:*** temporary loss of mitotic activity in proximal nail matrix. Think of trauma if only 1 nail is affected. Some patients damage the nail plate by repeatedly pushing down the cuticle. Beau's lines affect all the nails and indicate slowing of nail growth in the previous 1–2 months, e.g. during a serious illness or chemotherapy—see p.356. Arrest of all nail matrix activity causes nail shedding (onychomadesis).
- ***Nail pitting:*** foci of abnormal keratinization of nail matrix. Psoriasis is the commonest cause of coarse pits. Many fine pits occur in alopecia areata. May see pits in eczema.
- ***Thinning, longitudinal ridging, and fissuring*** (onychorrhexis): diffuse damage to nail matrix. Mild disease is common in the elderly. Also seen with impaired vascular supply, lichen planus, and lichenoid chronic GVHD. May cause permanent loss of the nail plate with a dorsal pterygium (adhesion between the nail fold and nail bed).
- ***Onycholysis:*** the nail plate separates from an abnormal nail bed. If distal and only a few nails, consider fungus, trauma, or subungual tumour. How does the patient manicure the nails? Is something being pushed underneath the nail plate to remove accumulated debris? This will damage the nail bed and worsen onycholysis. Psoriasis may cause proximal oil spots or salmon patches as well as distal onycholysis. Also seen with hyperthyroidism. Drugs, particularly tetracyclines and taxanes, cause painful photo-onycholysis—see Box 16.5, p.305.
- ***Subungual hyperkeratosis and discoloured thickened nail plate:*** fungus, psoriasis. Likely to be fungal infection if only a few nails. The crumbling starts at the free edge of the nail and moves proximally. Exclude psoriasis by looking for nail pitting and/or onycholysis in finger nails—see Box 9.5, p.183.
- ***Splinter haemorrhages:*** indicate damage to nail-bed capillaries. Trauma is likely if only 1 nail is affected and the haemorrhages are distal rather than proximal. Splinter haemorrhages may develop when the nail plate is abnormal, in psoriasis for example. Numerous proximal splinter haemorrhages are more likely to indicate systemic disease such as infective endocarditis.
- ***Nail clubbing:*** is associated with systemic problems including chronic lung disease, cyanotic heart disease, inflammatory bowel disease, and thyroid disease, but may be idiopathic or familial.
- ***Spoon-shaped nails*** (koilonychia): the soft nail plate in iron deficiency becomes concave. Children have a physiological koilonychia.
- ***Abnormalities in nail fold***—see Box 4.11.

Box 4.10 Changes in nail colour

- Dark discoloration of the nail. Longitudinal bands of pigment are common in individuals with dark skin and are caused by melanocytic naevi in the nail matrix.
- Does dark pigment extend onto skin of the proximal or lateral nail fold? The discoloration caused by a subungual haematoma or infection of the nail plate never spreads onto the surrounding skin, but the pigmentation associated with a subungual malignant melanoma may affect adjacent skin (Hutchinson's sign).
- Onycholytic nails become dark green when the space beneath the nail plate is colonized by *Pseudomonas aeruginosa*.
- Drugs such as antimalarials can darken nails—see 🕮 p.356.
- Addison's disease causes darkening of nails.
- Punctate leuconychia: trauma (some fungi cause a white appearance).
- Transverse white lines may occur after trauma, systemic illness, poisoning with arsenic (Mee's lines), or thallium.
- Hypoalbuminaemia e.g. in chronic liver disease, and some drugs cause apparent leuconychia because of changes in the nail bed, but the white discoloration fades with pressure.
- Half and half nails (white proximally and reddish-brown distally) are a rare sign of chronic renal failure.
- Yellow nails. The nails grow slowly and become thick and greenish yellow in the yellow nail syndrome which is associated with lymphatic hyperplasia, peripheral oedema, and pleural effusions (rare).
- Red and white horizontal bands in HIV infection.

Box 4.11 Abnormalities in nail fold

- A boggy, swollen erythematous nail fold: this is most likely to indicate chronic paronychia. The cuticle is missing, low-grade *Candida* infection beneath the nail fold leads to ridging and discoloration of the nail. *Staphylococcus aureus* may cause episodes of tender acute paronychia, when beads of pus exude from the swollen nail fold.
- Dilated nail fold capillaries and periungual erythema are valuable signs of a connective tissue disease—see 🕮 Fig. 19.9, p.380.
- Digital mucous cyst: the smooth swelling in the nail fold produces a vertical furrow in the nail plate.
- Papules in nail fold:
  - Viral warts.
  - Periungual fibroma in tuberous sclerosis.
  - Beaded papules in multicentric reticulohistiocytosis—see 🕮 p.394.
- Pustules around the nail and beneath the nail plate: seen in reactive arthritis (see 🕮 p.194) as well as in acropustulosis and parakeratosis pustulosa (both rare and possible forms of psoriasis)—see 🕮 Box 9.8, p.185.

Chapter 5

Skin failure and emergency dermatology

Contents

This chapter discusses problems that are likely to be referred to the emergency unit. Many, but not all, are life threatening and require immediate intervention and these are highlighted in the text. Also see
Acne fulminans 🕮 p.228
Anticoagulant-induced purpura fulminans 🕮 p.352.

Rash in a patient with a fever

A rash and fever in a sick patient is always worrying but a structured approach to the history and examination will help you to establish the cause. Life-threatening problems include DRESS (a drug reaction with systemic symptoms that may simulate infection), meningococcaemia, toxic epidermal necrolysis (TEN), and toxic shock syndrome (TSS)—see Box 5.1.

What should I ask?

- Document the symptoms—headache, photophobia, arthralgia, myalgia, nausea, diarrhoea, or other systemic symptoms?
- Is fever sustained, is it remittent (elevated each day and returns to baseline but not normal), or is it intermittent (intermittently elevated but returns to normal)?
- When did the rash develop in relation to other symptoms?
- How has the rash evolved?
- Are there mucosal problems such as conjunctivitis, sore throat, mouth ulcers, or genital ulcers?
- Is there a history of contact with an infectious disease?
- Document the travel history (were any preventative measures taken, e.g. vaccines, avoiding mosquito bites?) and sexual history.
- Explore drug history (including use of recreational drugs).
- Any past history of drug reaction, infectious disease, or skin disease?

What should I look for?

- Cutaneous signs:
    - Is the rash morbilliform (measles-like erythematous macules and papules) and is there any desquamation?
    - Does the rash blanch with light pressure, i.e. is the rash erythematous or is it purpuric (non-blanching)? Purpura in a febrile patient raises the possibility of meningococcal septicaemia—see 📖 p.96.
    - Are there erosions (denuded areas where the epidermis has been lost), blisters, or pustules? See Box 5.1.
    - Is the skin scaly or is there superficial peeling (desquamation)?
    - Are palms and soles involved? Is there oedema?
- Examine conjunctiva, buccal mucosa, throat, and tongue.
- Check for lymphadenopathy.
- Is the neck stiff or is there myalgia?
- Examine the joints for warmth, erythema, swelling, or tenderness.
- Examine the cardiovascular, respiratory, gastrointestinal, and neurological systems.

What should I do?

Investigations will be guided by your findings but consider:

- Full blood count and ESR; CRP, clotting screen.
- Liver function and renal function; urinalysis.
- Blood cultures, wound swabs.
- Lumbar puncture.
- Skin biopsy.

Toxic shock syndrome (TSS)

⚠ TSS is a multisystem disease caused by an exotoxin produced by *Staphylococcus aureus*. TSS may be mild or rapidly fatal. Predisposing factors include surgical packing, contraceptive sponges, postpartum infections, and deep abscesses. TSS is also a potentially fatal complication of small burns in young children.

TSS can be produced by other bacterial exotoxins including group A *Streptococcus*, *Pseudomonas*, and *Klebsiella* strains.

Box 5.1 What to look for in TSS

- Sudden onset of high fever >39°C with myalgia, vomiting, diarrhoea, and headache.
- Hypotension.
- Disorientation or altered consciousness.
- Diffuse macular erythematous (not purpuric) rash that starts on trunk and spreads outwards. If you find vesicles or bullae think of SSSS or TEN—see 📖 p.110. If rash is purpuric, consider meningococcaemia—see 📖 p.96.
- Erythema and oedema of palms and soles.
- Erythema of mucous membranes with strawberry tongue and conjunctival hyperaemia. No ulceration, unlike TEN.
- Renal failure, abnormal liver function.
- Lymphopenia is common. Also deranged clotting and low platelets.
- Blood cultures are frequently negative and the diagnosis is clinical.

►► ***Management***
- Resuscitate with IV fluids and vasopressor agents if required.
- Treat the focus of *Staphylococcus aureus* infection with IV antibiotics.
- Remove wound dressings, clean wounds, and remove any potential nidus of infection such as a foreign body.

Skin desquamates, particularly on palms and soles, after 1 to 2 weeks.

Further reading

Fever and erythema Hughey LC. *Semin Cutan Med Surg* 2007; **26:**133–8.

TSS Young AE and Thornton KL. *Arch Dis Child Educ Pract Ed* 2007; **92:**ep97–ep100.

Vasculitis and purpura fulminans

Palpable purpura is the hallmark of a small-vessel cutaneous vasculitis such as Henoch–Schönlein purpura, whereas flat (macular) purpura is associated with non-inflammatory pathology—see 🕮 p.404. In purpura fulminans, fibrin thrombi occlude dermal vessels as well as vessels in the subcutis leading to haemorrhage, ischaemia, and infarction. Purpura fulminans is seen most often in meningococcal septicaemia. See 🕮 Box 5.3, p.97.

Meningococcal septicaemia

⚠ Meningococcal infection may cause devastating septicaemia (acute meningococcaemia) and death within hours of the first symptoms. The non-specific flu-like presentation with fever, vomiting, headache, abdominal pain, and muscle aches may be misleading.

Although 80–90% of patients develop purpura within 12–36h of the onset of infection, this rash may be subtle and lesions few in number. You should examine the skin in a good light.

What should I look for?

- Early: a transient erythematous, maculopapular rash (may simulate TSS—see 🕮 p.95).
- After 12–36h: small purpuric lesions (petechiae) with an irregular outline and (usually) raised centres. You will find petechiae most often on limbs and trunk, but examine head, palms, soles, and mucous membranes. Also look for purpuric lesions in pressure areas, e.g. under the waistband, or at sites of friction.

Box 5.2 ▶▶Immediate management of meningococcal septicaemia

- Consider the diagnosis in any febrile patient with a petechial rash.
- Commence immediate treatment with IV antibiotics, e.g. cefotaxime 2g, without waiting to confirm your suspicions.
- If not in hospital treat with IV or IM benzylpenicillin 1.2g and call an ambulance.
- Secure airway and give high-flow oxygen.
- ***Call the critical care team now.***

Complications

- Disseminated intravascular coagulation (DIC) and purpura fulminans (see Box 5.3). Extensive irregularly outlined haemorrhagic areas (ecchymoses) become bullous and may progress to well-demarcated blue-black gangrene of digits or whole limbs.
- Limb compartment syndrome secondary to thrombosis, venous congestion, and oedema. Muscle infarction and rhabdomyolysis.
- Shock with poor perfusion, hypotension (a late sign in young patients), confusion, and increased respiratory rate.
- Waterhouse–Friderichsen syndrome caused by haemorrhage into the adrenal cortex.
- Coma and multiorgan failure.

Box 5.3 ⚠What is purpura fulminans?

The term purpura fulminans describes a devastating illness that is characterized by rapidly progressive and extensive purpura with dermal vascular thrombosis and haemorrhagic infarction, but without vasculitis (Fig. 5.1). In severe cases, subcutaneous vessels or major veins are thrombosed. Patients have a consumptive coagulopathy. The mortality is high. Survivors may be left with extensive scarring, missing digits, or amputated limbs.

Causes include

- Acute bacterial infection (the most common cause): e.g. *Neisseria meningitidis* or, much less often, beta-haemolytic *Streptococcus, Streptococcus pneumoniae, Staphylococcus aureus,* and other bacteria.
- After infection (usually children 1–3 weeks after varicella or streptococcal infection).
- Congenital deficiency of protein C or protein S (presents in neonates).
- Acquired deficiency of protein C or protein S associated with drugs (warfarin)—see 📖 p.352 or disease (renal dialysis, nephrotic syndrome, cholestasis, bone marrow transplantation).
- Antiphospholipid syndrome—see 📖 Box 20.8, p.419.
- Heparin-induced skin necrosis (antibody-mediated platelet aggregation usually seen at the injection site of subcutaneous heparin). See 📖 p.352.
- Toxins or poisons (spider bites, snake bites).

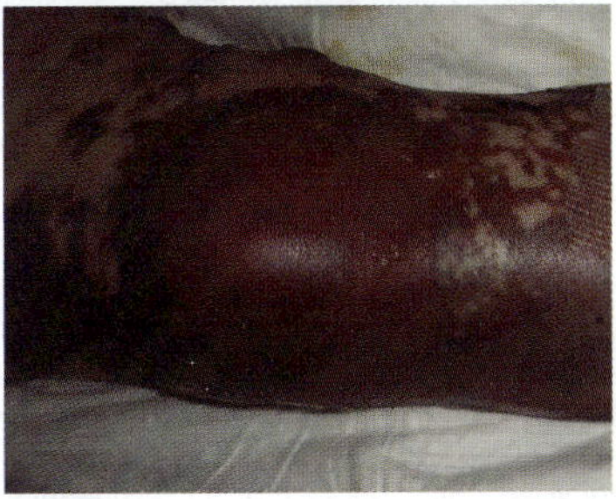

Fig. 5.1 Extensive purpura fulminans.

Further reading

Guidelines for diagnosis and management of DIC: Levi M et al. *Br J Haematol* 2009; **145:**24–33.

Anaphylaxis, angio-oedema, and urticaria

What is anaphylaxis?

⚠ Anaphylaxis is a severe, generalized or systemic hypersensitivity reaction associated with the release of histamine and capillary leak. Anaphylaxis is characterized by rapidly developing, life-threatening airway and/or breathing and/or circulation problems usually associated with urticaria and mucosal swelling (angio-oedema—see later in this section).

Triggers include foods, drugs (see Box 5.4), and venoms (wasp, bee). The reaction develops within minutes of exposure to the trigger, but in many cases no cause can be identified and these cases are not mediated by immunoglobulin E (IgE). See Box 5.5.

What should I look for?

- Sudden onset and rapid progression of symptoms.
- Life-threatening airway and/or breathing and/or circulation problems that may include stridor, hoarse voice, difficulty swallowing, wheeze, cyanosis, tachycardia, hypotension, and decreased level of consciousness.
- Skin and/or mucosal changes (flushing, urticaria, angio-oedema)—these signs may be subtle or absent in up to 20% of reactions.

What is angio-oedema?

Angio-oedema implies oedema of deep dermis, subcutaneous tissues, mucosa, and/or submucosa. Laryngeal oedema, which may cause difficulty swallowing and respiratory obstruction, is life threatening.

Angio-oedema occurs in anaphylactic reactions. ⚠ Rarely, angio-oedema is caused by a deficiency of C1 esterase inhibitor (inherited or acquired). These patients do ***not*** have urticaria and angio-oedema is usually triggered by mucosal trauma such as dental procedures or, in females, sexual intercourse. These patients may also complain of vomiting or abdominal pain. Some will give a family history of angio-oedema.

What is urticaria?

Urticaria (hives, wheals, welts) is a hypersensitivity reaction that may occur on its own or in association with angio-oedema and/or anaphylaxis. Urticaria may be acute or chronic and is often confused with erythema multiforme—see 📖 Box 5.10, p.105. Most patients with urticaria do not develop an anaphylactic reaction. Urticaria is a nuisance, but unless it is associated with airway problems (ask about throat swelling or wheeze), urticaria is not life threatening—see 📖 p.212.

The wheals of urticaria are secondary to dermal oedema. They are raised, smooth, erythematous, and, usually, itchy. They come and go, leaving normal skin, but generally do not last >24h. Some patients will provide a clear history of precipitants such as drugs, latex, or foods (fruit, fish, peanuts), but many, particularly those with chronic urticaria, will not be able to identify the trigger. Many idiopathic cases are not mediated by IgE. Allergy testing in patients with chronic urticaria is unrewarding. Non-sedating antihistamines are the mainstay of treatment—see 📖 p.216.

Box 5.4 Drugs linked to anaphylaxis

Virtually any class of drug can be implicated:
- Antibiotics including penicillin and cephalosporin.
- Aspirin.
- NSAIDs.
- ACE inhibitors.
- Anaesthetic drugs including suxamethonium, vecuronium, and atracurium.
- Contrast media, particularly iodinated media.

Box 5.5 ►► Management of anaphylaxis in adults

Use an ABCDE approach to assess and treat anaphylactic reactions:
- Place the patient in a comfortable position. Conscious patients with breathing difficulty may prefer to sit up.
- Remove the trigger if possible.
- Adrenaline (epinephrine) 0.5mg IM (0.5mL of 1:1000)—repeat after 5min if no better.
- Oxygen: 100% high flow as soon as possible.
- Rapid IV fluid challenge to restore tissue perfusion, e.g. 1L of warmed 0.9% saline infused in 5–10min. Monitor response and give more fluids if necessary, aiming to restore the patient's normal blood pressure.
- If wheeze persists, give bronchodilators.

After initial resuscitation:
- Chlorphenamine 10mg IM or IV slowly.
- Hydrocortisone 200mg IM or IV slowly.
- Ensure the patient is monitored.

⚠ ***Note that patients with angio-oedema secondary to C1 esterase inhibitor deficiency do not have urticaria and will not respond to adrenalin. They should be treated with C1 esterase inhibitor.***

Patients who have had an anaphylactic reaction should be referred to an allergy clinic both for further investigation and for education, as these patients have a substantial risk of further reactions.

Adverse drug reactions should be reported to the Medicines and Healthcare products Regulatory Agency using the yellow card scheme.

For more information about angio-oedema and urticaria see 🕮 p.22, p.212.

Alpha-1-antitrypsin deficiency is a rare cause of angio-oedema—see 🕮 p.428.

Facial swelling in acute contact dermatitis (see 🕮 p.200) or acute dermatomyositis (see 🕮 p.378) may mimic angio-oedema—see 🕮 Fig. 19.8, p.379.

Skin failure

What is skin failure?

Skin failure is the consequence of the sudden onset of a widespread and severe inflammatory dermatosis that impairs the normal physiological functions of the skin. The stratum corneum may be disrupted or the epidermis may be lost completely leaving a denuded dermis.

Skin failure has a number of causes but most often it is either secondary to deterioration of a pre-existing dermatosis or a manifestation of a drug reaction—see Box 5.6. Specific causes are discussed in more detail later in this chapter.

What should I look for?

⚠ Patients with skin failure have an inflammatory skin condition involving at least 90% of the BSA. Skin failure occurs in:

- Generalized scaly erythema (erythroderma, exfoliative dermatitis).
- Generalized erythema with pustules.
- Widespread blistering with or without loss of epidermis.

The other features of skin failure may include:

- Cutaneous pain or widespread itching.
- Impaired temperature regulation: hypo- or hyperthermia. Patients tend to adopt the temperature of their surroundings. Heat is lost because of increased dermal blood flow. Patients feel cold and shiver to raise the temperature.
- Infection (the skin barrier is disrupted).
- Loss of fluid (4 or 5L of fluid are lost each day if 50% of the BSA is involved and the stratum corneum is destroyed).
- Loss of electrolytes and protein.
- Increased energy requirements.
- Oedema (vasodilated cutaneous blood vessels are more permeable).
- High-output cardiac failure (particularly in the elderly).
- Mucosal ulceration in some blistering disorders may complicate the situation and make eating or drinking painful.
- Hair and nails may be lost acutely or 2–3 months later.

The causes of skin failure should be explored and treatment directed towards relieving discomfort—see Boxes 5.6 and 5.7. Although skin failure is not usually acutely life threatening, patients may develop problems such as infection, hypothermia, or cardiac failure. The elderly, patients with extensive skin involvement, and those already taking drugs such as corticosteroids or immunosuppressants are particularly at risk of life-threatening complications.

Box 5.6 Causes of skin failure

- Erythroderma (generalized redness and scale) secondary to eczema, psoriasis, or drugs.
- Cutaneous T-cell lymphoma is a rare cause of erythroderma (red man syndrome).
- SSSS: causes very superficial blistering.
- Generalized pustular psoriasis.
- Widespread blisters with skin loss caused by thermal burns or phototoxicity.
- TEN or SJS caused by drugs.
- Autoimmune bullous disorders such as bullous pemphigoid and pemphigus.
- Inherited group of mechanobullous diseases known as epidermolysis bullosa (rare).

Box 5.7 General approach to the management of acute skin failure

- Search for cause and stop all unnecessary drugs.
- Record the evolution of the skin disease as objectively as possible—photographs may be helpful.
- Nurse patients with blistering disorders or denuded areas on a low-pressure mattress.
- Minimize the risk of infection with reverse barrier nursing.
- Monitor fluid and electrolyte losses.
- Keep the patient (and the room) warm and monitor core body temperature—although the skin may look red and feel hot, this can be misleading and the core temperature may be low. Hyperthermia is less common.
- Take skin swabs every 3–4 days.
- Take blood cultures, monitor for systemic infection, and limit indwelling lines to reduce risk of infection.
- Ensure nutrition is adequate—protein and calorie requirements will increase. High calorific food and protein supplements may be required.
- Be alert for cardiac failure in the elderly with erythroderma.
- Apply bland emollients to soothe red scaly skin, e.g. 50% white soft paraffin (WSP) in liquid paraffin ×3–4/day (you will need 500g tubs).
- Use an emollient as soap substitute.
- Relieve pain.
- Prescribe sedating antihistamines such as hydroxyzine 25–50mg, 4 times a day to relieve intractable irritation.
- Consider low-dose heparin to reduce risk of venous thrombosis—patients may be dehydrated and immobile.
- Contact a dermatologist urgently to discuss diagnosis, investigation, and management.
- The disfigurement caused by widespread skin disease can be very distressing and, as they recover, patients may need psychological support.

Erythroderma

What is erythroderma?

Erythroderma, also known as exfoliative dermatitis, is defined as erythema, with variable amounts of scale, affecting 90% or more of the body surface.

What causes erythroderma?

Search for the cause when you are taking the history, but remember that erythroderma is caused most often by deterioration of a pre-existing skin disorder or by drugs. Erythroderma may develop suddenly, but when associated with a skin problem such as psoriasis, erythroderma may evolve gradually. The prevalence of causes in case series varies, but includes:

- Dermatitis of any type, e.g. atopic, seborrhoeic, contact, stasis, asteatotic (15–40% of cases).
- Psoriasis (8–25% of cases).
- Drugs (10–28% of cases)—numerous drugs have been reported to cause erythroderma. Also see red man syndrome, 📖 p.348.
- Cutaneous T-cell lymphoma or leukaemia (15% of cases).
- Rare skin diseases, e.g. pityriasis rubra pilaris, pemphigus foliaceus, ichthyosiform erythroderma (<1% of cases).

In as many as 30% of patients, erythroderma is classified as 'idiopathic' because no cause is found. Consider performing a skin biopsy before prescribing treatments such as topical or oral corticosteroids, which will reduce inflammation and mask signs. Skin biopsies may not reveal the underlying cause.

What should I look for?

- Itchy, erythematous scaly skin (red man syndrome). See Fig. 5.2.
- Cutaneous oedema.
- Oozing of serous fluid.
- Pustules (suggesting infection or pustular psoriasis).
- Superficial blisters (suggesting acute dermatitis or, much less unlikely, pemphigus foliaceus).
- Keratoderma (thick skin on the palms or soles).
- Ectropion if erythroderma affects face.
- Hair loss.
- Thickened or ridged nails or loss of nails.
- Lymphadenopathy (dermatopathic lymphadenopathy is common in erythroderma and is not caused by lymphoma, but consider a biopsy if the nodes are large and rubbery).
- Evidence of a primary skin disease, e.g. nail pitting suggesting psoriasis, psoriatic plaques on extensor surfaces or in flexures, stasis eczema around a leg ulcer.
- Non-specific symptoms and signs such as fever and malaise.

What should I do?

See Box 5.8 for immediate management.

Box 5.8 Immediate management of erythroderma

- Stop unnecessary systemic drugs.
- Take swabs for culture from oozing skin.
- Apply emollients such as Cetraben® cream or 50% WSP in liquid paraffin (prescribe 500g tubs) ×3–4/day or Emollin® spray.
- Bath or shower daily using a soap substitute such as Epaderm® ointment or Dermol® 500. A bath oil such as Oilatum® can be added to the bath.
- Prescribe a sedating antihistamine, e.g. hydroxyzine 25–50mg ×4/day for severe itching.
- Treat secondary infection with oral antibiotics.
- Check fluid balance and body temperature and monitor for other complications of skin failure—see 📖 Box 5.7, p.101.

⚠Moderately potent topical corticosteroids may be helpful, but do not prescribe very potent topical corticosteroids or oral corticosteroids until the investigation and management have been discussed with a dermatologist. Corticosteroids are helpful in eczema, but can make psoriasis much more unstable and difficult to manage.

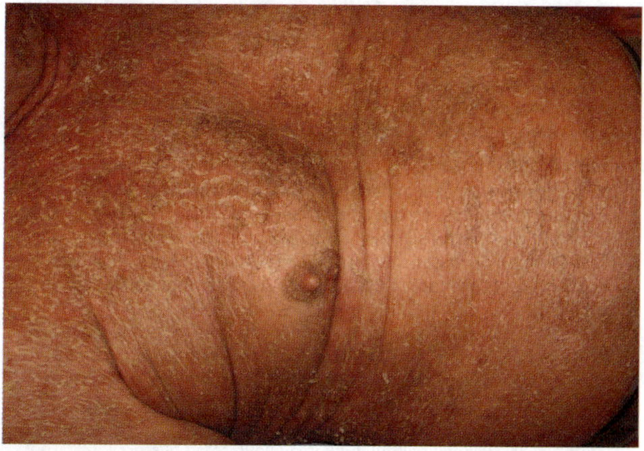

Fig. 5.2 Generalized erythema and scale in this patient with drug-induced erythroderma.

Localized blisters

What is a blister?

- A blister is a bump filled with clear fluid (serum).
- Small blisters, <1 cm in diameter, are called vesicles; blisters >1 cm in diameter are known as bullae.
- Blisters worry both patients and their doctors, but localized blisters are unlikely to be a life-threatening problem. Always find out precisely what the patient or referring doctor means if they use the term blister.
- See 📖 Chapter 13, p.239 for a detailed discussion of blistering diseases.

Localized blistering that may present as an emergency

Acute contact dermatitis (see 📖 Chapter 7, p.200)

The history may suggest the cause. The rash is itchy rather than painful (as it is in cellulitis) and the skin is erythematous and oedematous. Scale takes time to develop and may not be apparent upon presentation if the eruption is acute. A potent topical corticosteroid cream will settle things down promptly. Patch testing is the investigation of choice if you suspect allergy rather than irritancy.

Erythema multiforme (see p.105 and Fig. 5.3, p.108)

Cutaneous infections (see 📖 Chapter 6, p.121 and Chapter 7, p.141)

- Primary herpes simplex infections may be oedematous and painful.
- Herpes zoster.
- Bullous impetigo.
- Blisters in association with cellulitis or erysipelas.
- Blisters associated with dermatophyte infection, usually on the feet.

Physical causes of blisters

- Insect bites: exclude secondary infections and treat with a potent topical corticosteroid cream applied twice daily.
- Sunburn and photosensitivity including phytophotodermatitis (plant-induced photosensitivity) and drug-induced photosensitivity. Treat with a potent topical corticosteroid cream applied twice daily.
- Cold injury.
- Thermal burns: emergency care—remove burned or hot wet clothes (unless stuck to skin), jewellery, etc. Cool the wound with running cold water for 20min—do not use ice, which causes vasoconstriction and more damage. Clinical findings indicate the depth of the burn:
  - Epidermal: painful, red, may be shiny and wet.
  - Superficial dermal: painful, pink, may have small blisters.
  - Mid dermal: may lose sensation, slow capillary refill, dark pink, large blisters.
  - Deep dermal: absent sensation, absent capillary refill, blotchy red, may have blisters.
  - Full thickness: absent capillary refill and sensation, no blisters, thick white leathery appearance. Will heal with scarring.

Refer patients with burns to a plastic surgeon for definitive treatment.

Erythema multiforme (EM)

EM is an acute, self-limited illness triggered by infections, most often by herpes simplex virus. Other causes include orf, histoplasmosis, VZV, and Cytomegalovirus. <10% of cases are caused by drugs. EM resolves within 4 weeks, but some patients have recurrent episodes, usually triggered by herpes simplex infections.

What should I look for?

- Symmetrical, well-defined, round erythematous macules on knees, elbows, and/or palms evolve into papules and target lesions, which may blister, over days. Infrequently the rash is more widespread, 📖 Fig. 5.3, p.108.
- The lesions are at different stages of development (multiform).
- Patients may have a few ulcers on one mucosal surface—usually oral.
- EM is often confused with urticaria (see Box 5.10).

What should I do?

- Take a skin biopsy to confirm the diagnosis.
- Take swabs from oral lesions for viral culture.
- Mouth ulcers: prescribe a mouthwash for pain relief if required—see 📖 Box 14.4, p.263.
- Cutaneous lesions: a potent topical corticosteroid cream applied ×2/day may relieve discomfort but will probably not speed resolution.
- Recurrent disease: consider prophylaxis with aciclovir.

Box 5.9 Clinical criteria for diagnosing EM

- Acute, self-limited illness with duration <4 weeks.
- Symmetrical, discrete, round erythematous papules that persist at the same site for at least 7 days.
- Some papules evolve into target lesions comprising 2 or 3 concentric zones of colour change. A central dusky purple zone is surrounded by an outer red zone and sometimes a white middle zone. The centre may blister or crust after several days.
- No mucosal involvement or mucosal involvement is limited to one mucosal surface.

Box 5.10 Differences between EM and urticaria

- Urticarial lesions persist no more than 48h (usually much less) and then disappear to leave normal skin; EM papules persist for at least 7 days.
- New crops of urticarial lesions continue to appear daily for weeks. All the lesions of EM appear within the first 3 days.
- Urticarial papules may evolve into rings, but the central skin is normal. The central zone in the target lesions of EM is dusky, bullous, or crusted.
- Urticaria, unlike EM, may be associated with angio-oedema (deep swelling) of subcutaneous tissues or mucosa.
- EM, unlike urticaria , may be associated with mucosal ulcers.

Generalized blisters

⚠ Generalized herpes simplex infection (eczema herpeticum)

A generalized infection that is seen most often in children with atopic eczema. Eczema herpeticum is life threatening, particularly in children, when it is generally a primary infection—see 📖 p.144. 20% of children will have localized recurrent infections. Generalized herpes simplex infection may also complicate burns and some rare skin diseases (pemphigus, Darier's disease, ichthyosis).

What should I look for? See Box 5.11.

What should I do? See Box 5.12.

⚠ Staphylococcal scalded skin syndrome (SSSS) (see 📖 p.128)

SSSS occurs most often in infancy or children and less often in the elderly or immunosuppressed. Patients have a localized focus of staphylococcal infection, often in the nasopharynx. The staphylococci release an epidermolytic toxin (ET) that cleaves the skin high in the epidermis.

What should I look for?

- The skin is erythematous and tender. The erythema is accentuated in flexural and periorificial skin—see 📖 Fig. 6.2, p.123.
- The thin-walled blisters rupture rapidly but are extremely superficial and unlike the blisters of TEN do not involve all the epidermis.
- Mucosal surfaces are never involved in SSSS and this, as well as the superficial blistering, helps to distinguish SSSS from toxic epidermal TEN.
- The diffusely erythematous rash in SSSS may resemble TSS in the early stages, before blisters appear, but patients with TSS are more ill with a high fever and hypotension—see 📖 p.95.

►► ***What should I do?***

- Culture swabs from possible foci of infection, e.g. nasopharynx. Culture of skin swabs from the blisters is negative in SSSS because the condition is mediated by a toxin.
- If it is difficult to differentiate SSSS from TEN and if you want a rapid answer, gently peel the roof off a fresh blister, roll the fragment of tissue into a scroll and take the fresh tissue to the pathology laboratory. Ask the pathologist to examine a frozen section. In SSS, you will see the horny layer and very little else, whereas in TEN you will see full-thickness necrotic epidermis.
- Alternatively you can make a Tzank preparation from the base of a fresh blister (see 📖 p.575). In SSSS you will have some keratinocytes in the smear, because the split is high within the epidermis. In TEN the Tzank preparation made from the base of a fresh blister has no keratinocytes, because the whole of the epidermis forms the blister roof.
- Treat with flucloxacillin—the prognosis is generally excellent.

Box 5.11 ⚠ Signs of eczema herpeticum (Fig. 7.3)

- Sudden deterioration of atopic eczema.
- Pain as well as intense itching.
- Malaise, vomiting, anorexia, diarrhoea.
- Fever in variable number of cases.
- Vesicles (the primary lesions), papules, and pustules (older lesions).
- Small punched-out ulcers, sometimes clustered, but these may coalesce into ulcers with irregular outlines.
- Oozing, sometimes haemorrhagic, and crusting.
- Lymphadenopathy.
- Signs may be difficult to differentiate from VZV (see 📖 p.148) or bacterial infection. Secondary bacterial infection may complicate the picture.

Box 5.12 ▶▶ Management of eczema herpeticum

- Take swabs ideally from vesicles for both viral studies (PCR) and bacterial culture—see 📖 p.572.
- A Tzank preparation can be used to confirm the diagnosis—see 📖 p.575.
- Treat with an oral antiviral, e.g. aciclovir, as well as an antibiotic such as flucloxacillin. Severe cases will need IV aciclovir.
- Provide antipyretics, parenteral fluids, and pain relief.
- Eczema: in severe cases all topical corticosteroids should be avoided until infection is controlled. In less severe cases it may be reasonable to treat eczema with a mild topical corticosteroid ointment, once antivirals have been started.
- For less common causes of generalized blisters see Box 5.13.

Box 5.13 Less common causes of generalized blisters that may present as an emergency

- Damage to basal cells (lichenoid reaction):
  - SJS—see 📖 p.108.
  - TEN (full thickness necrosis of epidermis)—see 📖 p.108.
- Autoimmune blistering diseases—see 📖 p.244:
  - Bullous pemphigoid—the commonest.
  - Pemphigus foliaceus.
  - Pemphigus vulgaris.
  - Other rare autoimmune blistering diseases.
- Bullous cutaneous vasculitis (bullae will be haemorrhagic)—see 📖 p.406.

Serious drug reactions

Cutaneous adverse drug reactions are common (2–3% of hospitalized patients). Most drug rashes are morbilliform and settle quickly when the drug is stopped (see 📖 p.348), but rarely a morbilliform rash is the first sign of a much more serious problem such as TEN—see 📖 p.346.

Life-threatening reactions that are discussed in this book include:

- Anaphylaxis, angio-oedema, and serum sickness—see 📖 p.98, p.348.
- Erythroderma—see 📖 p.102.
- SJS—see 📖 Fig. 5.4, p.109, p.110.
- TEN—see 📖 Fig. 5.5, p.109, p.110.
- DRESS—see 📖 p.114.
- Anticoagulant-induced purpura fulminans and skin necrosis—see 📖 p.96.

What should I look for to help me to decide if this adverse drug reaction might be life-threatening?

See 📖 Box 5.14 and p.346, Chapter 18 for information about adverse drug reactions.

Box 5.14 ⚠ Indications of serious drug reactions

- General:
  - Fever >40°C, hypotension, lymphadenopathy.
  - Arthralgia, arthritis.
  - Dyspnoea, wheeze.
- Mucocutaneous
  - Erythroderma (generalized scaly erythema).
  - Swollen face, swelling of tongue, urticaria (anaphylaxis).
  - Skin pain or burning (TEN).
  - Erosions, shearing stress detaches epidermis from dermis, bullae or mucosal erosions (TEN or SJS)—see 📖 Fig. 5.5, p.109.
  - Vasculitis (palpable purpura) or extensive flat purpura.
- Laboratory results:
  - Eosinophilia >1000mm^3, lymphocytosis with abnormal lymphocytes, abnormal liver function tests (LFTs).

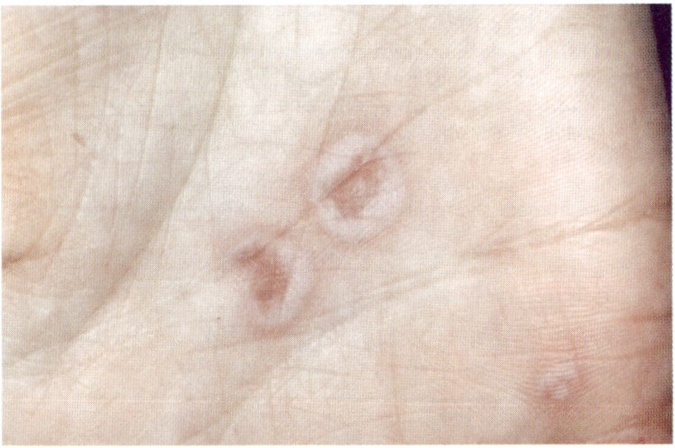

Fig. 5.3 Well-defined target lesions on the palms in EM.

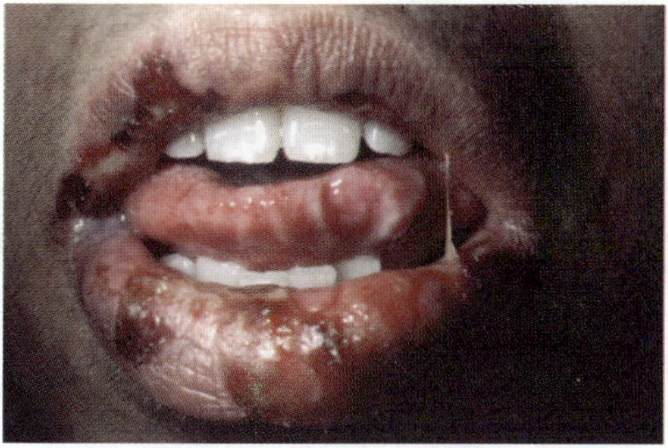

Fig. 5.4 SJS with crusted haemorrhagic lips and extensive mucosal ulceration in the oral cavity.

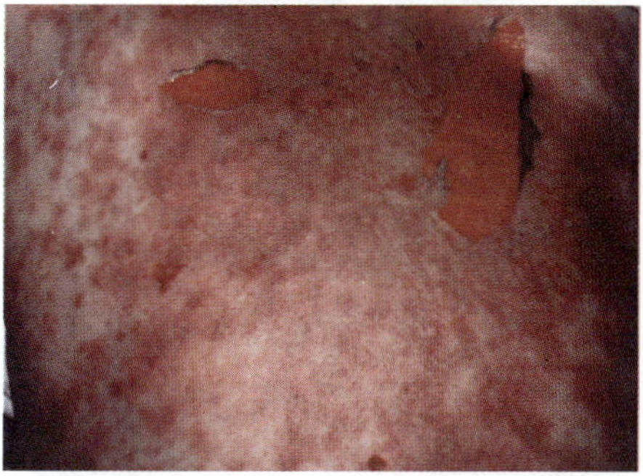

Fig. 5.5 The dusky erythema in TEN progresses to widespread blistering with loss of the full thickness of the epidermis. Even gentle pressure dislodges sheets of necrotic epidermis.

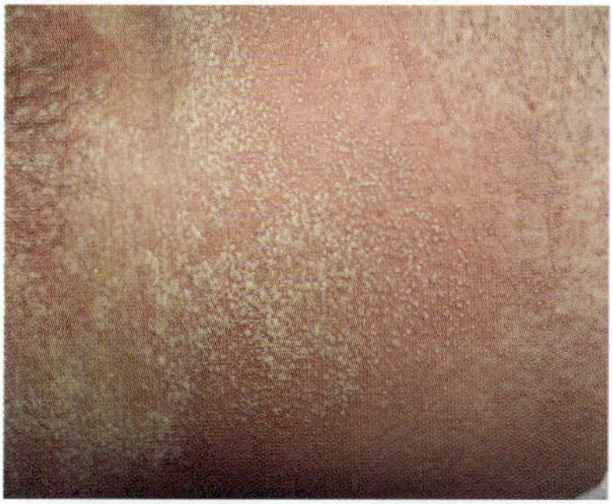

Fig. 5.6 Sheets of sterile non-follicular pustules on an erythematous background in acute generalized exanthematous pustulosis (AGEP). Generalized pustular psoriasis looks similar.

Stevens–Johnson syndrome (SJS) and toxic epidermal necrolysis (TEN)

These serious reactions, with overlapping features (see Box 5.15), are usually caused by drugs—see Box 5.16. They commence about 2–3 weeks after the start of the drug. Patients often have underlying diseases, particularly AIDS.

⚠ If you see any patient with a painful erythematous 'drug rash' and mucosal signs, alarm bells should ring.

SJS

What should I look for?

- Vague upper respiratory tract symptoms (fever, cough, headache, sore throat, rhinorrhoea, and malaise) for 1–3 days prior to onset.
- Symmetrical, poorly defined painful erythematous macules evolving rapidly to papules and target lesions, with 2 or 3 concentric zones of colour change and dark purpuric centres. Large bullae rupture leaving denuded skin but typical SJS affects <10% of BSA—see 📖 Fig 5.3, p.108.
- The rash is usually maximal in 4 days.
- ⚠ Severe mucosal ulceration with involvement of at least 2 mucosal surfaces (lip, oral cavity, conjunctiva, nasal, urethra, vagina, gastrointestinal tract, respiratory tract). The lips become crusted and haemorrhagic. Painful stomatitis interferes with eating and drinking. Purulent conjunctivitis is associated with photophobia.
- Late ocular complications include dry eye, scarring, and loss of vision.

TEN

What should I look for?

- Flu-like symptoms may precede TEN. Fever is higher than in SJS.
- ⚠ Patients may complain of painful skin or a burning discomfort.
- Tender dusky erythema resembling SJS that progresses to widespread subepidermal blistering (the roof of the blisters is formed by dead epidermis). The flaccid thin-walled blisters rupture easily—see 📖 Fig. 5.5, p.109.
- Large sheets of necrotic epidermis that detach leaving a painful denuded oozing dermis involving >30% of BSA.
- Gentle pressure extends blisters and the erythematous epidermis is easily detached from the underlying dermis by lateral pressure (Nikolsky's sign).
- ⚠ Inadvertent shearing pressure when handling the patient may cause further detachment.
- Examine mouth, eyes, and genitalia. Mucosae are usually involved (unlike SSSS). Ulceration causes dysphagia, photophobia, or painful micturition. Epithelia of trachea, bronchi, and gastrointestinal tract may also be involved.
- Sequelae may include scarring, irregular pigmentation, dry eye, corneal scarring, photophobia, visual impairment, phimosis, and vaginal synechiae.

Box 5.15 Classification of SJS and TEN

The features in severe SJS overlap with those of TEN:

- SJS: <10% BSA involved.
- Overlap SJS–TEN: 10–30% BSA involved.
- TEN: >30% BSA involved.

Box 5.16 Causes of SJS and TEN

- Drugs: sulphonamides, NSAIDs, antibiotics—penicillin-related and cephalosporin, anti-epileptics, barbiturates, allopurinol, tetracyclines.
- Viral infections: AIDS, herpes simplex virus, EBV, influenza.
- Bacterial infections: *Mycoplasma pneumoniae*, typhoid, group A streptococci.
- Fungal infections: dermatophyte, histoplasmosis.
- Protozoal infections.
- Malignancy: Hodgkin's lymphoma, leukaemia.
- GVHD.

Box 5.17 TEN: differential diagnosis

No mucosal signs

- TSS (no blisters, but may simulate early TEN)—see 🕮 p.95.
- SSSS (also has blisters)—see 🕮 p.106, and Fig. 6.2, p.123.
- Morbilliform drug rash (no blisters, but may simulate early TEN).
- DRESS: skin may blister—see 🕮 p.114.
- Generalized herpes simplex infection: widespread vesicles—see 🕮 p.106.
- Varicella-zoster infection: widespread vesicles—see 🕮 p.148.

Mucosal involvement

- Acute GVHD.
- Pemphigus vulgaris (may be drug induced).

Management See 🕮 Management in SJS or TEN, p.112.

Further reading

Gueudry J *et al. Arch Dermatol* 2009; **145:**157–62. (ocular complications)
Koh MJA and Tay YK. *Curr Opin Pediatr* 2009; **21:**505–10.

Management in SJS or TEN

►► What should I do?

- Withdraw all drugs started in the last 4 weeks.
- Take a skin biopsy to confirm the diagnosis. Ensure the specimen includes epidermis, which may detach during the procedure. The histology shows full-thickness epidermal necrosis in the roof of blisters.
- Rapid information about the level of the blister to differentiate TEN from SSSS may be obtained by detaching the roof of a blister, rolling this up gently, and freezing in liquid nitrogen. Frozen sections of epidermis can be stained immediately. A Tzank preparation (📖 p.575) can also be used to differentiate TEN from SSSS—see 📖 p.106.
- Calculate the SCORTEN—see Box 5.19.
- ⚠ Involve a multidisciplinary team and remind those caring for the patient that TEN is associated with less oedema, less fluid loss, and less vascular damage than a severe burn. Do not overload with fluids—see Box 5.18.

Box 5.18 Management is essentially supportive

- Admit to ICU, HDU, or burn unit (familiar with TEN).
- Relieve pain.
- Establish peripheral venous access: avoid central venous lines—risk of infection.
- Nutrition: nasogastric (NG) tube (Dobhoff). Avoid total parenteral nutrition (TPN).
- Foley catheter: keep urine output at 40–60mL/h.
- Fluids: do not overload. Pulmonary oedema is a frequent complication because of impaired alveolar barrier.
- Nurse on an air mattress; (air fluidized beds increase transepidermal loss of water and heat) use non-stick sheets and heating blankets; keep room temp at 30–32°C.
- Skin: do not debride (epidermis is a natural dressing). Protect with 50% WSP in liquid paraffin, e.g. Emollin spray® and non-stick dressings, e.g. Mepitel®/Mepilex® or wrap patient with Sofsorb™ impregnated with 0.5% silver nitrate solution.
- Prevent infection: reverse barrier nursing, culture multiple skin sites, sputum, blood, and urine. Repeat every 3 days to guide therapy in the event of sepsis. Avoid prophylactic antibiotics.
- Involve ophthalmologists to advise on care of eyes, e.g. gently separating synechiae to prevent scarring.
- Clean lips and oral mucosae with antiseptic mouth washes.
- Provide local analgesia for oral mucosa.
- IV immunoglobulin, 1g/kg for 4 days, has been recommended but the role is unproven.
- Avoid systemic or potent topical corticosteroids (efficacy unproven, increased risk of infection).
- Prescribe SC heparin for deep vein thrombosis (DVT) prophylaxis.

Box 5.19 Severity of illness score for TEN: SCORTEN (also of use in cases of SJS/TEN overlap)

- The rash is usually maximal in 4 days and skin may start to re-epithelialize within days, but recovery is protracted.
- Sepsis and comorbidities contribute to the high mortality.
- 7 independent risk factors for death have been identified. Allocate 1 point for each risk factor present:
  - Age >40 years.
  - Malignancy.
  - Tachycardia >120bpm.
  - Initial percentage of epidermal detachment above 10%—use the rule of nines to calculate % of BSA affected (see Box 3.5, p.51) or estimate using the patient's palms as a measure. Each palm = 1% of BSA.
  - Serum urea >10 mmol/L.
  - Serum glucose >14 mmol/L.
  - Bicarbonate <20 mmol/L.

Predicted mortality

- 0–1: 3%
- 2: 12%
- 3: 35%
- 4: 58%
- 5 or more: 90%.

Bastuji-Garin S *et al. J Invest Dermatol* 2000; **115:**149–53.

Further reading

Hazin R *et al. Ann Med* 2008; **40:**129–38.

Drug rash, eosinophilia, systemic symptoms (DRESS)

Synonyms: dapsone hypersensitivity syndrome, anticonvulsant hypersensitivity syndrome.

What is DRESS?

DRESS is a life-threatening cutaneous drug reaction with systemic symptoms that is frequently misdiagnosed as infection. Diagnostic criteria are listed in Box 5.20. A latency period of 1–2 months after the drug is started is common, but the presentation is variable (Boxes 5.21 and 5.22).

The course may be protracted with some patients progressing to liver failure. Mortality is 10%.

What should I look for?

- History that a new drug was started within previous 2 months (see Box 5.21).
- Flu-like symptoms such as myalgia, arthralgia, headache, sore throat, abdominal pain.
- Fever.
- Sudden onset of diffuse erythematous scaly rash that is morbilliform with 'juicy' papules that may coalesce into plaques. This sometimes progresses to erythroderma.
- Oedema, particularly of the face (simulates angio-oedema).
- Sometimes pustules or vesicles or purpura.
- Mild cheilitis.
- Lymphadenopathy.

What investigations should I do?

- FBC: eosinophilia common, less often lymphocytosis (sometimes with atypical lymphocytes), thrombocytopenia, neutrophilia, or neutropenia.
- ESR (low normal) and CRP (raised).
- LFTs (raised transaminases and gamma GT): may progress to liver failure.
- Renal function tests and urinalysis: usually normal.
- Skin biopsy: lymphocytic infiltrate with a few eosinophils.
- Blood cultures: no growth.

How should I manage DRESS?

- Stop suspected drugs.
- Manage temperature, fluid balance, etc. as in erythroderma—see 📖 p.103.
- Emollients such as 50% WSP in liquid paraffin to make skin comfortable, e.g. Emollin® spray.
- Potent steroid ointment twice daily.
- Early treatment with oral prednisolone (0.8–1mg/kg body weight) or IV methylprednisolone has been recommended to prevent progression and liver failure.

Box 5.20 ⚠ Diagnostic criteria for DRESS

3 or more of the following:
- Acute drug rash.
- Fever >38°C.
- Lymphadenopathy.
- Systemic involvement: variable but may include hepatitis with raised AST, interstitial nephritis, arthritis, interstitial pneumonitis, and/or carditis.
- Blood anomalies: eosinophilia with or without abnormal lymphocytes.

Box 5.21 Drugs associated with DRESS

Most frequent
- Anticonvulsants
- Dapsone
- Sulphonamides including sulphasalazine.

Others
- Allopurinol
- Antibiotics: vancomycin, minocycline, amoxicillin
- Gold salts
- Sorbinil
- Calcium channel blockers
- Ranitidine
- Thalidomide
- Mexiletine
- Imatinib.

Patch testing may prove drug hypersensitivity, but test 3–6 months after the reaction has settled completely to avoid triggering a relapse.

Box 5.22 Differential diagnosis of DRESS

- Serum sickness or drug-induced vasculitis—see 🕮 p.348, p.352.
- Infection: viral (HHV 6) or bacterial.
- Idiopathic hypereosinophilic syndrome.
- Lymphoma.

Further reading

Eshki M et al. *Arch Dermatol* 2009; **145:**67–72.

Peyrière H et al. *Br J Dermatol* 2006; **155:**422–8.

Pichler WJ. *Ann Intern Med* 2003; **139:**683–93.

Generalized pustules

Introduction

Pustules are a focal accumulation of inflammatory cells and serum in the skin. Pustules may be a manifestation of infection, e.g. staphylococcal folliculitis when pustules are associated with hair follicles, but in most infections, pustules are grouped, localized, and asymmetrical. For causes of widespread symmetrical pustular eruptions in sick patients see Box 5.23.

What should I look for?

- Is the patient ill, e.g. high fever, malaise?
- What is the primary lesion—is it a really a pustule, i.e. a bump filled with creamy fluid, or is it a vesicle, i.e. a bump filled with clear serous fluid that evolves into a pustule (as in VZV infection)?
- Distribution: symmetrical (endogenous cause) or asymmetrical?
- How do pustules evolve? What is the time course?
- Are pustules associated with hair follicles, i.e. is the rash a folliculitis?
- Erythema, oedema, desquamation, or mucosal involvement.

Acute generalized exanthematous pustulosis (AGEP)

>90% of cases are drug-induced. It usually takes 1–3 weeks for the rash to develop, but patients who are sensitized may develop AGEP within a few hours of exposure to the drug—for signs see Box 5.24. May be difficult to distinguish from generalized pustular psoriasis—see later section.

What should I do?

- Reassure patient, medical, and nursing staff that this is a self-limiting condition and is not an infection. Culture blood and skin—these are sterile.
- Skin biopsy (shows subcorneal pustules).
- Stop the causative drug, most often an antibacterial.
- Prescribe emollient, e.g. 50% WSP in liquid paraffin, a mild topical corticosteroid, and a sedating antihistamine to relieve discomfort.

Generalized pustular psoriasis

⚠ Some patients have a history of psoriasis or psoriatic arthritis. Pustular psoriasis may be triggered by irritation of the skin, infections, withdrawal of systemic corticosteroids or drugs (lithium), but it may not be possible to identify the trigger. Lasts longer than AGEP—see earlier in this section and Box 5.25.

What should I do?

- Admit the patient and manage skin failure—see 🕮 Box 5.7, p.101.
- Exclude infection—cultures of blood and skin will be sterile—and reassure patient, medical, and nursing staff that this is not an infection.
- Check FBC, renal function, liver function, and serum calcium.
- Obtain a skin biopsy to confirm the diagnosis (subcorneal pustules).
- Avoid potential irritants. Prescribe an emollient, e.g. 50% WSP in liquid paraffin, a mild topical corticosteroid, and a sedating antihistamine to relieve discomfort.
- Continue to monitor for hypocalcaemia (rare complication).
- Consider acitretin or methotrexate—if not settling, see 🕮 p.594.

Box 5.23 Causes of widespread pustular eruptions

- Eczema herpeticum or varicella: the primary lesion is actually a vesicle, but pustules with crusting may occur as a secondary phenomenon—check for history of atopic eczema—see 🕮 p.106, p.144, p.148.
- Pustular psoriasis: check for a history of psoriasis or arthritis.
- AGEP: ask about drugs started in previous 1–3 weeks.
- Acne fulminans: severe acne flare with haemorrhagic crusted ulcers on trunk and face and systemic symptoms—see 🕮 p.228.
- Subcorneal pustular dermatosis/IgA pemphigus (rare and not usually unwell).

Box 5.24 AGEP—what should I look for? (🕮 Fig 5.6, p.109)

- Sudden onset of an oedematous erythema that burns or itches. Often begins on face, axillae, and groins and spreads within hours.
- This is soon followed by the appearance of hundreds of pinhead-sized, mostly non-follicular, pustules.
- Confluent pustules may produce superficial erosions.
- Some patients have marked facial swelling; a few develop purpura, usually on the legs. May also develop vesicles, bullae, and EM-like lesions.
- <20% have mild mucosal involvement (usually oral).
- Fever >38°C and neutrophilia (blood culture and swabs sterile).
- Spontaneous resolution of pustules in <15 days (more rapid than in pustular psoriasis) followed by desquamation.

Box 5.25 ⚠ Generalized pustular psoriasis—what should I look for?

- Evidence of psoriasis, e.g. nail pitting, psoriatic arthritis, but many patients have no previous history of psoriasis.
- Fever and neutrophilia (swabs and blood cultures sterile).
- Scaly erythematous tender skin.
- Sheets of sterile non-follicular pustules, particularly in the flexures and genital skin arising on a background of tender erythema.
- Pustules may coalesce into lakes of pus.
- Pustule dry and skin desquamates leaving a shiny erythematous surface on which waves of pustules may continue to appear.
- Normal mucosal surfaces.
- The process may continue for weeks (unlike AGEP).
- Complications are those of skin failure—see 🕮 p.100.
- Hypocalcaemia is a rare complication.

Further reading

Sidoroff A *et al.* *J Cutan Pathol* 2001; **28:**113–19.

Necrotizing fasciitis

What is necrotizing fasciitis?

⚠ Necrotizing fasciitis is a ***life-threatening*** soft tissue infection that is characterized by rapidly progressive necrosis that spreads from subcutaneous tissue into deep fascia. The high mortality (at least 25%), is secondary to organ failure and to streptococcal TSS—see 📖 p.95 and Box 5.26.

Consider the diagnosis in any sick patient who is not responding to treatment for 'cellulitis' and has pain that appears out of proportion to the signs. The depth and extent of necrosis may be much greater than the appearance of the skin suggests and, in the early stages, the condition is often misdiagnosed.

What should I look for?

- A history of recent trauma, e.g. insect bite, skin biopsy, chronic leg ulcer, surgery, IV drug abuse. Not all patients have an obvious portal of entry. See Box 5.27 for predisposing factors.
- Ill patient with high temperature, tachycardia, low blood pressure.
- Pain that is out of proportion to the signs in the skin.
- Altered level of consciousness.
- Rapidly spreading poorly demarcated purplish erythema.
- Oedema and tender induration.
- Malodorous serosanguineous exudate ('dishwater' pus).
- Crepitation in soft tissues (gas from aerobic and anaerobic bacteria).
- Blisters.

In the later stages you may see:

- Black necrotic plaques.
- Painless ulcers.
- Vascular occlusion and gangrene.

▶▶ What should I do?

- Request an urgent surgical opinion—immediate deep surgical debridement of all necrotic tissue is absolutely essential. The diagnosis is clinical—do not wait for the results of investigations—see Box 5.29.
- Gram stain and culture any blister fluid or fluid draining from the wound.
- FBC, electrolytes, and renal function.
- Start a combination of IV broad spectrum antibiotics immediately and contact a microbiologist to discuss treatment—see Box 5.28.
- Arrange to take deep tissue at the time of surgery for histological examination and culture for aerobic and anaerobic bacteria.
- Magnetic resonance imaging (MRI) or computed tomography (CT) to identify subcutaneous air and define the extent of involvement.
- Admit to ICU for resuscitation and monitoring.
- Consider IV immunoglobulin for streptococcal TSS.

Box 5.26 Bacteria linked to necrotizing fasciitis

- Group A beta-haemolytic streptococci (50% of these cases occur in young healthy people).
- *Staphylococcus aureus* including meticillin-resistant strains.
- *Clostridium perfringens.*
- Mixed infection with anaerobic and facultative bacteria including streptococci, staphylococci, enterobacteriaceae, and obligate anaerobes (Fournier gangrene is polymicrobial infection of the genitalia).

Box 5.27 What predisposes to necrotizing fasciitis?

- Diabetes
- Surgery and other trauma
- Obesity
- Malignancy
- Alcohol or drug abuse
- AIDS or other immune deficiency
- Malnutrition.

Box 5.28 Antibiotics that may be considered for necrotizing fasciitis

- Empirical therapy with vancomycin and imipenern with cilastatin.
- Penicillin with clindamycin for Gram-positive cocci (clindamycin inhibits toxin production in streptococcal infection).
- Ampicillin and gentamicin for Gram-negative anaerobes.
- Clindamycin or metronidazole for anaerobes.
- Imipenem with cilastatin for aerobes including *Pseudomonas.*

Box 5.29 The finger test

A finger test, performed at the time of surgery, will help to confirm the diagnosis and delineate the extent of necrosis:
- Make a 2cm vertical incision into the skin to the deep fascia.
- Push an index finger (or probe) gently into normal-appearing tissue at the junction of the subcutaneous tissue and fascia.
- If the subcutaneous tissue is easily dissected off the underlying fascia. the finger test is positive. This confirms the diagnosis of necrotizing fasciitis.
- Necrotic tissue or a 'dishwater' pus may be found between the fascial planes.

Further reading

Angoules AG et *al. Injury* 2007; **38**(Suppl 5):S19–26.

Kihiczak GG et *al. J Eur Acad Dermatol Venereol* 2006; **20:**365–9.

Chapter 6

Bacterial and spirochaetal infections

Contents

Relevant pages in other chapters

📖 Chapter 5: Skin failure and emergency dermatology:
Rash in a patient with a fever—see 📖 p.94
Toxic shock syndrome(TSS)—see 📖 p.95
Meningococcal septicaemia—see 📖 p.96
Staphylococcal scalded skin syndrome—see 📖 p.128
Necrotizing fasciitis—see 📖 p.118
Henoch–Schönlein purpura—see 📖 p.408
Septic cutaneous vasculitis—see 📖 p.414

Introduction

Skin flora

Skin creases, surface scale, and deep follicular orifices provide just what is needed for the survival of a wide variety of microflora. Conditions vary—the skin may be dry, greasy, or moist, the temperature warm or cool, the blood supply good or poor, and the surface intact or ulcerated. The environment and the host immune response modify the density and diversity of colonization in individuals.

Resident colonizing species include a mixture of staphylococci, micrococci, and diptheroids, as well as yeasts. These maintain a viable reproducing population on skin and help to defend the skin against pathogens. In some circumstances, overgrowth of the normal skin microflora is linked to problems, e.g. *Propionibacterium acnes* in the hair follicles in acne.

Some people carry *Staphylococcus aureus* in the nostrils, perineum, or axillae—see Box 6.1. Staphylococci also colonize the skin in diseases such as atopic eczema, when large numbers of organisms may be shed with the scale.

Meticillin-resistant *Staphylococcus aureus* (MRSA) may be carried asymptomatically, but is an increasing cause of cutaneous infections (impetigo—Fig. 6.1, folliculitis, 'boils'). MRSA is resistant to the beta-lactam antibiotics including penicillins and cephalosporins—see Box 6.2.

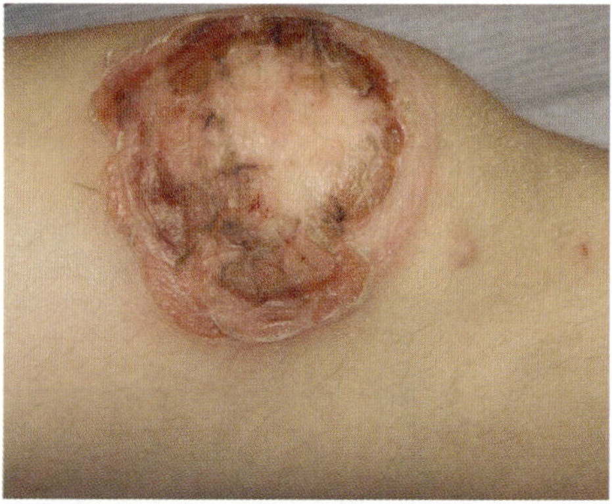

Fig. 6.1 Bullous impetigo with golden crusting. See 📖 p.128.

Box 6.1 Nasal carriage of *Staphylococcus aureus*

- Nasal carriage of *Staphylococcus aureus* is common and some patients carry MRSA in the nose.
- There is no consensus about the best way of dealing with MRSA carriage.
- Mupirocin 2% ointment twice daily inside each nostril for no more than 7 days may eradicate nasal MRSA, but prolonged or repeated use will increase the risk of the emergence of mupirocin-resistant strains.
- Chlorhexidine or neomycin creams may be helpful.

Box 6.2 MRSA and skin infections

- Community-associated and healthcare-associated strains of MRSA cause increasing numbers of skin infections.
- MRSA can survive for long periods in dust, furnishing, and clothing.
- Patients who have received fluoroquinolones are more likely to be colonized with MRSA.
- MRSA is resistant to antibiotics such as penicillins and cephalosporins. Some strains are also resistant to erythromycin and ciprofloxacin.
- Triclosan skin cleanser is effective against skin carriage of MRSA.
- Alcohol-based hand rubs should be used to prevent transfer of MRSA from patient to patient.
- MRSA may be sensitive to drugs such as vancomycin, rifampicin, fusidic acid, tetracyclines, trimethoprim, and clindamycin.
- Some strains of MRSA also produce Panton–Valentine leucocidin (PVL), increasing virulence.

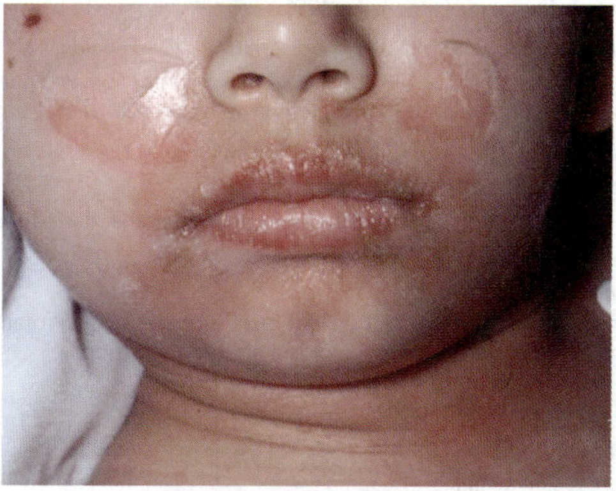

Fig. 6.2 Staphylococcal scalded skin syndrome (SSSS). Tender erythema and superficial desquamation caused by a circulating epidermolytic toxin—see 📖 p.129.

Flexural bacterial infections

Erythrasma

Erythrasma is caused by overgrowth of *Corynebacterium minutissimum*, a skin commensal in the horny layer of the epidermis.

What predisposes to erythrasma?

- Warm humid climates, hyperhidrosis, obesity.
- Diabetes, immunosuppression, old age.

What should I look for?

- One or more asymptomatic, well-demarcated, slightly scaly, reddish brown patches in a moist flexure such as the axilla, under the breasts, in the groin, or between the toes.
- Erythrasma resembles dermatophyte (tinea) infection, but the skin fluoresces a striking coral pink under a Wood's UV light—see 🕮 p.568.

What should I do?

- Prescribe a topical antibiotic such as erythromycin, clindamycin, or tetracycline. Topical miconazole may also be effective.

Pseudomonas and flexures

What should I look for?

- *Pseudomonas* infection of moist toe webs produces superficial erosions with a rather moth-eaten macerated border.
- *Pseudomonas aeruginosa* axillary infections are uncommon, but may be potentiated by washes with antibacterial lotions that reduce colonization with Gram-positive commensals. The brownish-grey scaly rash fissures and is painful, unlike erythrasma.
- ⚠ *Pseudomonas* causes anogenital ecthyma gangrenosum in immunosuppressed patients. If untreated, pustules rapidly become bullous and necrotic—see 🕮 p.129.

What should I do?

- Stop antibacterial lotions in superficial axillary infection. Keep skin dry.
- Biopsy and culture tissue from ecthyma gangrenosum. Treat promptly with IV antibiotics.

Perianal streptococcal dermatitis

Group A beta-haemolytic streptococcus causes perianal dermatitis in prepubertal children and, less often, in adults.

What should I look for?

- A history of an itchy painful perianal rash unresponsive to topical antfungals or topical corticosteroids. Pain on defecation.
- Well-demarcated, bright red perianal erythema.
- Swelling, scale, and fissuring.

What should I do?

- Culture a skin swab.
- Treat with oral antibiotics, e.g. amoxicillin for 10 days.

Folliculitis

What is folliculitis?

Folliculitis is inflammation of hair follicles—Box 6.3. *Staphylococcus aureus* is the commonest cause of a bacterial folliculitis. *Pseudomonas aeruginosa* may cause folliculitis after hot tubs or whirlpools. Superficial bacterial folliculitis is usually self-limiting, but may be recurrent. Deeper folliculitis involving the entire follicle and surrounding tissues (furunculosis) heals with scarring or rarely can progress to cellulitis.

Community-acquired strains of *S. aureus* carrying genes that encode the neutrophil cytotoxin, PVL, cause numerous deep furuncles, abscesses, and cellulitis in healthy young adults and children.

What may predispose to bacterial folliculitis or furunculosis?

(The evidence is inconclusive.)

- Occlusion or maceration.
- Tropical climates.
- Hot tubs or whirlpools (*P. aeruginosa* folliculitis).
- Crowded living conditions, poor hygiene, malnutrition.
- Diabetes, alcoholism, immunodeficiency (AIDS), or oral corticosteroids.
- Blood dyscrasias and disorders of neutrophil function.

What should I look for?

- Superficial folliculitis may be itchy, deep folliculitis is tender.
- Perifollicular erythematous papules or small pustules—the pustule may be pierced by a hair.
- Crusting of follicular openings when pustules rupture.
- Tender inflamed furuncles ('boils') with abscesses in deep infection.
- Furuncles may discharge and heal with scarring.
- If a group of follicles become deeply infected, the tender erythematous nodule is known as a carbuncle. Pus discharges from several points.
- Follicular pustules or papules 8–48h after exposure to hot tub or whirlpool at sites covered by bathing suit (*P. aeruginosa* folliculitis).

What should I do in bacterial folliculitis?

- Remove or minimize precipitating factors.
- Antiseptic washes are all that is needed in most superficial cases.
- If folliculitis does not settle, take swabs for culture from pustules.
- Alcohol-based washes or triclosan are effective against MRSA and strains of *Staphylococcus* producing PVL.
- Topical antibiotics, e.g. 2% mupirocin ointment, clindamycin lotion, or erythromycin lotion may be indicated.
- Deep infection requires oral antistaphylococcal antibiotics.
- Carbuncles should be incised and drained surgically.

How should I manage recurrent bacterial folliculitis?

- Culture swabs from pustules and from potential carrier sites, e.g. nose, axilla, groin, and perineum in the patient and family.
- Exclude diabetes and minimize other predisposing factors.
- Prescribe antimicrobial skin washes or bath additives with triclosan, chlorhexidine, or benzalkonium chloride (Dermol 600®, Oilatum Plus®, or Aquasept®) for staphylococcal folliculitis.
- Treat chronic *S. aureus* carriage with 2% mupirocin ointment.
- 5% benzoyl peroxide gel applied × 2/day may help to prevent recurrent staphylococcal folliculitis.
- Consider oral antibiotics, but check sensitivities.

Box 6.3 Differential diagnosis in patients with folliculitis

Mechanical folliculitis

- Waxing or plucking hairs.
- Ingrowing hairs, e.g. after close shave of curly hair (pseudofolliculitis) or close haircut 'grade 1'.
- Pulling back hair tightly (traction folliculitis).
- Friction caused by tight clothing.

Medicaments

- Topical preparations with high concentrations of tar.
- Occlusion of follicles with ointments.

Infections

- Bacterial: *S. aureus*, *Pseudomonas*.
- Dermatophyte (tinea) scalp: hair is lost, or beard (uncommon).
- Pityrosporum (a commensal yeast) folliculitis on the trunk—see 📖 p.160, p.203.

Inflammatory skin diseases

- Acne: pustules on the face and sometimes trunk—look for comedones, nodules, and scars—see 📖 p.224.
- Rosacea: facial pustules, papules, erythema, but no comedones—see 📖 p.234.
- Demodicosis in immunocompromised—see also 📖 p.168.
- Hidradenitis suppurativa: recurrent furunculosis in groin and/or axilla. Look for groups of comedones, sinuses, and scars—see 📖 p.232.

Non-follicular pustules

- Pustular psoriasis—see 📖 p.116.
- Drug reactions—see 📖 p.116.

Impetigo, toxin-mediated disease, and ecthyma

Impetigo

What is impetigo?

- Impetigo is a superficial skin infection that may develop on normal skin or may complicate eczema (impetiginized eczema).
- Crusted impetigo (impetigo contagiosa) is caused by *Staphylococcus aureus, Streptococcus pyogenes,* or a combination of both.
- Bullous impetigo is mediated by exfoliative toxins released by phage group II *S. aureus*. The toxins disrupt adhesion between the keratinocytes in the superficial epidermis within the area of infection by cleaving a specific desmosomal cadherin, desmoglein 1. This enables *S. aureus* to penetrate the skin barrier, proliferate, and spread under the stratum corneum. Also see SSSS, 📖 p.129.
- Factors that predispose to impetigo include minor trauma including insect bites, eczema, head lice, hot climates, crowded living conditions, poor hygiene, and immunodeficiency.

What should I look for?

- One or more areas of golden, honey-coloured crusting and oozing—Fig. 6.1, p.122.
- Thin-walled flaccid blisters, but these tend to rupture rapidly because the cleavage is in the superficial layers of the epidermis just below the stratum corneum.
- Patients with localized impetigo do not have systemic symptoms.
- Several members of the family may be affected.

What should I do?

- Take skin swabs from crusted skin for culture (in SSSS swabs from the erythema and blisters will be sterile as the signs are causes by the circulating toxin, not local infection)—see 📖 p.129.
- A topical antibiotic such as fusidic acid or mupirocin is sufficient in patients with a small focus of infection. In more widespread or recurrent infections, prescribe an oral antibiotic such as flucloxacillin or erythromycin.
- The focus of infection in SSSS—see 📖 p.129, should be treated with an oral antibiotic.
- An antiseptic wash may be helpful in patients with recurrent impetigo.

Toxin-mediated diseases

- ►► ***SSSS*** (Ritter disease) presents in neonates, young children, adults with renal failure, and the immunosuppressed. Patients have a focus of impetigo caused by the strain of *Staphylococcus* that releases the epidermolytic toxin. This focus may not be apparent. The circulating epidermolytic toxin causes widespread erythema and superficial blistering (see 📖 p.106 and Fig. 6.2, p.123).
- ►► ***TSS*** is a multisystem disease caused by an exotoxin produced most often by *S. aureus*. TSS may be mild or rapidly fatal (see 📖 p.95).

Ecthyma

What is ecthyma?

- A deeper infection than impetigo that is caused by *S. pyogenes* or, less often, *S. aureus*.
- More common in malnourished or immunosuppressed.
- Seen most often on the legs and usually preceded by a minor injury or insect bite.
- Starts as a blister with an erythematous border ('deep impetigo'), but develops into well-circumscribed 'punched-out' ulcer involving the full thickness of the epidermis. May enlarge to a diameter of 2–3cm if untreated. Only a few lesions. Heals slowly with scarring.
- Systemic symptoms are uncommon.

What should I do?

- Take skin swabs for culture and treat with oral antibiotics.

Ecthyma gangrenosum

What is ecthyma gangrenosum?

- ►► This infection caused by *Pseudomonas aeruginosa* is associated with debility and immunosuppression. Ecthyma gangrenosum is usually a manifestation of *Pseudomonas* septicaemia. It may not be possible to demonstrate a bacteraemia in the anogenital form in immunocompromised patients when *Pseudomonas* may enter skin through a wound or hair follicle.
- Starts as a painless erythematous or purpuric macule on limbs or anogenital skin. Develops into a nodule with a central haemorrhagic vesicle that breaks down to form a large necrotic ulcer with a central dark eschar and inflamed border. Several lesions may be present.
- Mortality is 10–20%.
- Differential includes pyoderma gangrenosum, necrotizing vasculitis, cryoglobulinaemia, and septic emboli from other organisms.

What should I do?

- Take a skin biopsy for histology and culture—see 📖 Box 32.2, p.573.
- Culture blood and urine.
- Treat with IV antibiotics.

Erysipelas and cellulitis

What are erysipelas and cellulitis?

These acute infections of dermis and subcutaneous tissue are usually caused by *Streptococcus pyogenes*. Other bacteria such as *Staphylococcus aureus* may be involved, particularly in immunosuppressed patients or those with diabetes. Erysipelas is a superficial form of cellulitis that most often involves the face. Lower limb cellulitis is a common cause of admission.

Recurrent cellulitis (or erysipelas) is common in patients with chronic lymphoedema. Local immune deficiency predisposes to cellulitis, but each episode damages lymphatics, which increases the predisposition to recurrence. Primary lymphoedema of the lower limb, secondary to aplasia or hypoplasia of the lymphatic vessels, may be subclinical and bilateral.

What predisposes to cellulitis?

- Defective skin barrier, e.g. eczema, tinea pedis, leg ulcers, wounds.
- Diabetes or immunosuppression.
- Chronic lymphoedema (local immune deficiency); peripheral vascular disease.
- Previous episodes of cellulitis.

What should I look for?

- Sudden onset of pain.
- Malaise, fever, and rigors may precede the rash, but may not be apparent in the elderly. Systemic symptoms are common in erysipelas.
- Asymmetrical, warm, tender spreading erythema that is particularly well demarcated in erysipelas; swelling sometimes with blisters.
- Examine both the non-cellulitic limb and the affected limb for evidence of chronic lymphoedema, but signs may be subtle (see Box 6.4).

What simulates cellulitis?

- Acute contact dermatitis: the patient usually complains of itch. Early in the presentation, the skin may not be particularly scaly but will be erythematous and oedematous. Blisters are common—see 📖 Fig. 10.1, p.201.
- Dermatitis secondary to venous stasis or asteatotic dermatitis. Typically cellulitis is asymmetrical. Reconsider your diagnosis if the patient seems to have 'cellulitis' affecting both legs. The redness, scaling, and swelling are much more likely to be a manifestation of dermatitis—see 📖 p.204.
- Lipodermatosclerosis, a panniculitis associated with venous stasis (see Box 6.6) and see 📖 p.288 and Fig.15.6, p.289
- Herpes simplex infection, particularly a primary infection—see 📖 p.144.
- Erysipeloid—see 📖 p.132.
- ⚠ Autoinflammatory diseases—see 📖 p.218.

What should I do?

- Superficial skin swabs for culture are not helpful unless there is an open wound or an exudate. Remember no chronic leg ulcer is sterile.
- Take blood for culture if the patient has systemic symptoms. Bacteraemia is common in erysipelas.

- Prescribe antibiotics, initially IV, e.g. ceftriaxone or flucloxacillin and penicillin. Also see Box 6.5.
- Elevate the affected part.

Box 6.4 Signs of chronic lymphoedema

- Firm non-pitting oedema (oedema may pit in the early stages).
- Stemmer sign is present—the thickening of the skin in the interdigital web space between the 2nd and 3rd toes makes it impossible to pick up a fold of skin.
- Papillomatous thickening of the skin surface (elephantiasis nostra).
- Fluid-filled blebs (lymphocoeles).

Box 6.5 Management of recurrent cellulitis in patients with lymphoedema

- Advise on skin care—antiseptics, emollients to prevent cracking of the skin.
- Control limb swelling with compression hosiery.
- Prescribe prophylactic penicillin V 250mg twice daily for at least 6 months.

Box 6.6 Lipodermatosclerosis

Lipodermatosclerosis is a chronic panniculitis (inflammation in fat) associated with venous disease that may be misdiagnosed as cellulitis. Lipodermatosclerosis is not associated with systemic upset and does not respond to antibiotics.

What should I look for?

- Check for a history of venous disease, leg ulcers, or limb swelling.
- Skin in the gaiter area is erythematous, indurated, and tight.
- The skin may be tender but is not hot.
- Look for other signs of venous stasis such as pigmentation.
- You may see varicose veins (stand the patient up).
- Peripheral pulses are normal.
- As the condition progresses, the leg adopts the shape of an inverted champagne bottle with tightening of the tissues above the ankle.
- The other leg may be affected.

What should I do?

- Treat with compression bandaging, but you may have to increase compression gradually because of pain.

Erysipeloid

What is erysipeloid?

This acute infection of skin and soft-tissue is caused by *Erysipelothrix rhusiopathiae*. The organism is inoculated through broken skin, usually on the hand. The infection is seen most often in individuals who are in contact with poultry, fish, crabs, or pigs, e.g. fishermen, butchers, farmers, and vets. The organism remains viable for months in decomposing material and can survive smoking or pickling.

What should I look for?

- Local pain, itching, burning, and swelling, usually on a hand or finger.
- A purplish-red plaque, with demarcated raised borders, that expands peripherally and clears centrally. Occasionally you may find >1 lesion.
- You may see blistering.
- Some patients have regional lymphadenopathy.
- Systemic symptoms such as fever and malaise are uncommon in patients with localized cutaneous disease (unlike erysipelas).
- Rarely erysipeloid presents as a systemic infection. In addition to skin lesions, patients may have septic arthritis, bacterial endocarditis cerebral lesions, or pulmonary involvement. These patients have positive blood cultures.

How can I distinguish erysipeloid from erysipelas or cellulitis?

- The occupational history may provide a clue to the diagnosis.
- Erysipeloid tends to involve the hands or fingers, whereas the face and leg are affected more often by erysipelas or cellulitis.
- Patients with erysipelas or cellulitis are more likely to have systemic symptoms such as fever or rigors.

What should I do?

- The organism is difficult to culture.
- A skin biopsy may help to confirm the diagnosis.
- Incision and drainage are contraindicated as these prolong the course.
- Although localized cutaneous disease is usually self-limiting, prescribe penicillin to prevent progression to systemic disease with the risk of endocarditis.

Cat scratch disease

What is cat scratch disease?

Bartonella henselae, a common infection in cats, causes a localized cutaneous infection in humans. The organism is passed between cats by the bites of cat fleas and is transmitted to humans by cat scratches or the saliva in cat bites. Most patients are under 21 years of age.

What should I look for?

- A history of a cat bite or scratch (90% of patients).
- After 3–10 days an erythematous papule, pustule, vesicle, or nodule develops at the site of the inoculation. It may persist for several months.
- Tender regional lymphadenopathy develops about 2 weeks after the bite or scratch and may persist for 2–4 months. Cat scratch disease is the commonest cause of chronic benign lymphadenopathy in children and adolescents.
- Mild fever.

What should I do?

- The disease is self-limiting, resolving within 2–6 months. No specific treatment is needed.

Bacillary angiomatosis

What is bacillary angiomatosis?

Bacillary angiomatosis is a life-threatening infection caused by *Bartonella henselae* (transmitted to humans by the scratches or saliva of infected cats) or *Bartonella quintana* (transmitted by the human body louse) that presents most often in immunosuppressed patients (HIV, organ transplantation, leukaemia, chemotherapy). Skin, mucosal surfaces, bones, and viscera may be involved by tumour-like vascular masses.

What should I look for?

- Red or purplish cutaneous and/or subcutaneous vascular papules and tender nodules ranging in diameter from a few mm to 10cm. The presentation may simulate Kaposi's sarcoma (KS), but lesions are less common on soles or in the mouth than in KS—see 🕮 p.338.
- Fever, nausea, vomiting, headache, malaise, and weight loss.
- Tender lymphadenopathy which may suppurate.
- Focal bone pain.

What should I do?

- Biopsy the skin and take blood for cultures.
- Treat promptly with erythromycin 500mg × 4/day for up to 4 months in immunocompromised patients.
- Provide analgesia for pain and fever.

Meningococcal infections

Meningococcal disease is caused by *Neisseria meningitidis*, a bacterium that is commonly carried in the nasopharynx. Disruption of nasal mucosal membranes, perhaps by viral infection, may facilitate the development of invasive disease. The severity of disease is related in part to the virulence of the meningococcus and to the potential for release of endotoxin, which plays a key part in the pathogenesis of meningococcal septic shock.

Meningococcal septicaemia

►► Fulminant meningococcal infection can cause septicaemia (acute meningococcaemia) and death within hours of the first symptoms. Early diagnosis may depend on recognition of cutaneous signs that include:

- An erythematous maculopapular rash.
- Petechiae—usually palpable, but they may be sparse in the early stages.
- Purpura fulminans with ecchymoses, large areas of haemorrhage, and haemorrhagic blistering.
- Gangrene and extensive skin infarction.

The condition is discussed on 🕮 p.96.

Chronic meningococcaemia

- This immune complex mediated illness presents with a low-grade relapsing fever that is associated with a vasculitic rash and problems such as arthralgia, pneumonia, or ophthalmitis.
- Several blood cultures may be needed before the diagnosis is confirmed, but chronic meningococcaemia responds rapidly to systemic antibiotics.
- The differential diagnosis encompasses other causes of cutaneous vasculitis including Henoch–Schönlein purpura.

See also 🕮 p.406, p.408.

Mycobacterial infections

Cutaneous TB (Box 6.7)

Cutaneous TB is uncommon. *Mycobacterium tuberculosis* may be inoculated into the skin from an exogenous source or spread to the skin from an underlying infection or from the bloodstream. The presentation is determined by the immune response, as well as the virulence of the mycobacteria. Histology is granulomatous—see 📖 Box 32.5, p.579. *M. tuberculosis* DNA may be detected in skin biopsies using the polymerase chain reaction (PCR). Erythema nodosum is a hypersensitivity reaction to the presence of TB elsewhere, but is not cutaneous TB. See 📖 p.424.

Non-tuberculous (atypical) mycobacterial infection

M. marinum infections are seen in owners of tropical fish (presumably sick fish), who inoculate the bacteria into the skin when cleaning the fish tank. The infection presents as an indolent reddish-brown nodule (fish tank granuloma), usually on a finger or hand, but nodules may spread up the limb along lymphatic channels. Infection is self-limiting after 3–4 months. Antibiotics, e.g. tetracyclines, may be helpful.

M. ulcerans is a tropical infection that causes progressive ulceration with destruction of skin and subcutaneous tissue (Buruli ulcers). *M. chelonae* is a community-acquired infection of skin and soft tissue. The bacteria are found in natural and processed water sources. Cutaneous infection is preceded by trauma such as puncture wounds, subcutaneous injections, lacerations, or fractures. Patients present with non-tender brownish-red erythematous subcutaneous nodules singly or in groups. This infection is more common in immunosuppressed patients, when it may disseminate. Other cutaneous non-tuberculous mycobacteria infections seen in the immunosuppressed include those caused by *M. kansasii* and *M. fortuitum*—see 📖 Box 32.2, p.573 for culture of tissue.

Leprosy (Hansen's disease)

A tropical infection caused by *M. leprae*. Leprosy is likely to be seen more frequently outside the tropics as people migrate to live in other countries. The symptoms and signs are determined predominantly by the host immune response, but the bacteria have a predilection for cool skin, e.g. the nose or ears, and for cutaneous nerves. See Box 6.8.

Patients with tuberculoid leprosy have high cell-mediated immunity and bacilli are difficult to find in the skin lesions. Nerves are damaged early by the immune response. Those with lepromatous disease have more widespread infection, numerous bacilli in the dermis, and poor cell-mediated immunity. Borderline cases have an intermediate immune response. The immune state may downgrade or upgrade.

The diagnosis is confirmed histologically. Drugs such as rifampicin, dapsone, and clofazimine are used in combination according to World Health Organization (WHO) protocols. Surgeons and rehabilitation experts may be involved in the management of deformity or loss of function.

Box 6.7 Spectrum of cutaneous TB

- Chancres (indolent ulcers) after inoculation of skin or mucosae.
- Scrofuloderma: direct extension of TB in underlying lymph nodes, bones, and joints ('the King's evil'). Associated with pulmonary TB.
- Miliary TB: spread by the bloodstream to a variety of organs including skin, where TB presents as papules and pustules or purpura. This form is more common in immunosuppressed patients. Painful eroded papules and plaques may develop on tongue or palate.
- TB abscess (gumma): caused by extension of TB into the skin from an underlying focus, such as the lung or bone.
- Tuberculosis verrucosa cutis: direct inoculation in patients who have some immunity. Hyperkeratotic warty plaques present on knees, elbows, hands, feet, and buttocks.
- Lupus vulgaris: a slow-growing destructive reddish-brown plaque with scarring seen in patients with some immunity. It is difficult to culture bacteria from biopsies of lupus vulgaris.
- Tuberculids: these puzzling conditions occur in patients who have been exposed to TB but do not have clinically obvious infection. The tuberculids include erythema induratum (a nodular vasculitis on the backs of the legs), papulonecrotic tuberculid (crusted papules that heal with scarring), and lichen scrofulosorum (small follicular papules on the trunk). Using PCR, mycobacterial DNA has been detected in biopsies taken from tuberculids.

Box 6.8 Signs in leprosy

Tuberculoid leprosy: mimics sarcoid and mycosis fungoides

- A few well-defined erythematous or hypopigmented macules or plaques with reduced sensation and loss of sweating—skin feels dry and rough.
- Thickened tender regional nerves near the skin lesions, muscle weakness, and muscle atrophy.
- Perforating ulcers at pressure sites secondary to neuropathy.
- Mucous membranes are not affected.

Lepromatous leprosy: mimics mycosis fungoides

- Numerous symmetrical macules, papules, nodules, and plaques. Lesions are hypopigmented and erythematous, but poorly defined.
- Sensation is usually normal in the lesions. Spares warm skin, such as flexures, scalp, palms, soles, midline of back, and chest.
- Thickened skin on the face (leonine) in late disease. Eyebrows and eyelashes lost.
- Bilateral symmetrical peripheral neuropathy: 'glove and stocking'.
- Weakness and atrophy of muscles secondary to neuropathy.
- Ulceration, perforation, and destruction of nasal septum with nasal collapse and deformity (saddle nose).
- Ulceration of nasopharynx, pharynx, palate, and larynx.

Syphilis

Syphilis, a chronic infectious disease caused by *Treponema pallidum*, is increasing in incidence and is a great mimic. The skin is involved at all stages. Patients may not be aware that they have had a primary lesion. Atypical presentations may be a sign of AIDS—see 📖 p.154. Syphilis may be transmitted to the fetus—see Box 6.9.

What should I look for?

Primary syphilis

- A solitary, painless, well-demarcated firm ulcer (chancre), approximately 1cm in diameter, about 3 weeks after sexual contact. The site of presentation—genitalia, anal, oral, face—will depend on the contact.
- Regional lymphadenopathy.
- A depressed atrophic scar when healed (in around 8 weeks).

Secondary syphilis

Presents 1–6 months after the primary infection. The rash settles within 1–3 months.

- Non-itchy symmetrical rash on the face and trunk.
- Initially smooth red macules, then scaly copper-red papules (the rash becomes scalier in late stages and may resemble psoriasis or cutaneous lupus erythematosus).
- Keratotic papules on palms and soles.
- Scaly papules on glans penis or shaft of penis.
- Macerated hypertrophic flat-topped papules (condylomata lata) in moist skin folds–perianal, inframammary, and vulva.
- 'Split papules' at angle of mouth.
- Patchy moth-eaten hair loss, loss of eyebrows and eyelashes.
- Mucous membranes: greyish-white oval patches and erosion on palate, buccal or labial mucosa, tongue.
- Headache, low-grade fever, lymphadenopathy, and arthralgia.

Late (tertiary) syphilis

Some patients with untreated syphilis develop lesions years after the primary infection. Presentations include neurosyphilis (tabes dorsalis, general paralysis) and cardiovascular syphilis (aortitis) and gumma.

Gumma are painless rubbery nodules that ulcerate and scar. They mainly involve skin and bones.

What should I do?

- ***Primary syphilis:*** serology is not positive until 4 weeks after the infection, but spirochaetes can be isolated from the chancre. Refer to genitourinary medicine for investigation, treatment, and contact tracing.
- ***Secondary syphilis:*** serology is positive. A skin biopsy may be helpful.
- ***Tertiary syphilis:*** serology is positive. A skin biopsy may be helpful.
- Discuss investigation with the genitourinary physicians and refer any patient in whom the diagnosis is confirmed to genitourinary medicine for treatment and contact tracing.

Box 6.9 Some late signs of congenital syphilis

Hutchinson's triad

- Interstitial keratitis.
- Abnormalities of the permanent upper central incisors.
- Deafness.

Other signs

- Abnormalities of the 6-year molars (mulberry molars).
- Rhagades (radiating scars around mouth).
- Frontal bossing.
- Depressed saddle nose.
- Shortened maxilla.
- High-arched palate.
- Perforation of the nasal septum and palate by gumma.
- Thickening and anterior bowing of the tibia (sabre shins).
- Thickening of the sternoclavicular portion of clavicle.
- Painless hydroarthrosis of the knees and sometimes elbows (Clutton's joint).
- Hair loss.

Lyme disease

What is Lyme disease?

Lyme disease is an infection caused by spirochaetes of the group *Borrelia burgdorferi sensu lato*. The spirochaetes are transmitted by the bite of *Ixodes scapularis* and related ticks. Birds, mice, deer, voles, and lizards are the main reservoirs of borrelia. Infection is unlikely if the tick is attached for <48h.

Where might you get Lyme disease?

Lyme borreliosis occurs in forested areas throughout most of Europe, but particularly Germany (Black Forest), Austria, Slovenia, and Sweden, as well as the costal areas of the northeast USA, the upper Midwest of the USA, and the west coast of the USA.

How does Lyme disease present?

Erythema migrans is an early sign of localized disease. The rash usually resolves in days to weeks, but may persist for a year.

Disseminated Lyme disease may have cardiac (atrioventricular block, myopericarditis), rheumatological (monoarticular or oligoarticular arthritis) and/or neurological (meningitis, peripheral or cranial neuropathy, myelitis) manifestations. Late persistent manifestations include chronic arthritis, peripheral neuropathy, and acrodermatitis chronica atrophicans (bluish-red atrophic skin on hands, feet, and leg).

What should I look for in early disease?

- Erythema migrans develops 7–10 days after the tick bite.
- The rash may be slightly itchy.
- Flu-like symptoms are common.
- A small erythematous macule or papule appears at the site of the bite.
- Erythema extends over days to weeks to produce either an annular lesion with central clearing or a roundish smooth erythematous patch.
- Erythematous lesions range in size from 10cm to >50cm diameter.
- Warm the skin to make the signs more obvious.

What should I do?

- Take blood for serology.
- Take a skin biopsy.
- Prescribe a 14–21-day course of doxycycline to treat erythema migrans.
- Some authorities recommend prescribing a single 200mg dose of doxycycline within 72h of a tick bite to prevent Lyme borreliosis.

Chapter 7

Viral and fungal infections

Contents

Relevant pages in other chapters

Eczema herpeticum—see 📖 p.106
Herpetic gingivostomatitis—see 📖 p.260
Genital HSV infection—see 📖 p.260

Viral exanthems

- Measles (rubeola): measles is becoming more common in the UK because parents have not immunized their children. The child is irritable with fever, cough, nasal congestion, photophobia, and conjunctivitis. The rash, which is preceded by Koplick's spots on buccal mucosa, develops about 14 days after exposure to the virus, starting on the forehead and then becoming widespread. Erythematous macules evolve into a red-brown maculopapular (morbilliform) eruption that is not itchy. The rash fades after 5 days, when the skin desquamates.
- Rubella: the child is usually well, but may have a mild fever. Erythematous macules and papules appear first on the face and neck and then generalize over 48h. The rash fades within 2–3 days without desquamation.
- Erythema infectiosum (fifth disease, slapped cheek syndrome) is caused by Parvovirus B19 and occurs mainly in young children. Children develop bright erythematous macules on the cheeks and this is followed by a lacy erythematous rash on the proximal limbs that fades within days, but may recur with heat (exercise, bathing). Children are usually well.
- Gianotti–Crosti syndrome (papular acrodermatitis of childhood) is associated with infections with hepatitis B virus or Epstein–Barr virus (EBV). Discrete red-brown papules develop symmetrically first on limbs and buttocks, then the face. The trunk is spared. Papules may be a purpuric. The eruption fades in 3–4 weeks. The child is usually well, but may have a mild fever. Prognosis is good and liver involvement mild.
- Asymmetric periflexural exanthem of childhood. The cause is unknown. The child may have a mild fever and upper respiratory symptoms. The itchy erythematous papular or eczematous rash affects one flexure, often the axilla, from where it extends onto the trunk. It remains strikingly asymmetrical. The rash clears in 6–8 weeks.
- Kawasaki's disease (mucocutaneous lymph node syndrome) mainly affects infants and small children. An infectious trigger is suspected. Children develop a persistent fever. The palms and soles become erythematous (within 5 days) and hands and feet oedematous. Children may also develop a widespread urticated or measles-like (morbilliform) erythematous rash. After 10–15 days, the skin peels (desquamates) around the tips of fingers and toes and sometimes on the palm and wrist. Other signs include conjunctival injection (in 2–4 days), erythematous crusted cracked bleeding lips (may persist for 2–3 weeks), oropharyngeal erythema, strawberry tongue, and cervical lymphadenopathy. ⚠ Cardiovascular disease (pericarditis, myocarditis, endocarditis, coronary arteritis with aneurysms and stenosis) may cause sudden death. Treat early with aspirin and IV immunoglobulin to reduce the risk of coronary artery aneurysms.

Pityriasis rosea

What is pityriasis rosea?

Pityriasis rosea is a common, self-limited rash that presents in adolescents and young adults. It is thought to be caused by a viral infection but this has not been proved. The rash usually clears in around 8 weeks.

What should I look for?

- Some patients have a mild prodrome (headache, fever, malaise).
- A 'herald patch', usually on the trunk, preceding the onset of the rash by hours or a few days.
- A rash on the trunk and proximal extremities, usually sparing face, palms, and soles. Oval to round thin, pink papules and plaques with overlying fine scale or a margin (collarette) of scale—see 🕮 Fig. 18.7 p.363.
- Papules and plaques distributed in a 'Christmas tree' pattern on the back, with long axes aligned along Langer's lines of cleavage.
- Hyperpigmentation may be marked in darkly pigmented skin.
- Atypical presentations include flexural (inverse) pityriasis rosea, vesicular, purpuric, and pustular variants.
- Most patients are asymptomatic. Itching is usually minimal.
- Signs suggesting another diagnosis:
  - Secondary syphilis: copper-coloured macules on palms and soles, split papules at corner of mouth, and condylomata lata, fever, and lymphadenopathy—see 🕮 p.138.
  - Guttate psoriasis: thicker silvery scale and plaques do not follow the 'Christmas tree' pattern. Did a sore throat precede onset of rash? Has the patient a personal or family history of psoriasis? See 🕮 p.182.

What should I look do?

- Check drug history to exclude a drug eruption—see 🕮 p.363.
- Reassure the patient and wait!

Herpes simplex virus

The HSV is a common cause of contagious infections. The virus causes intraepidermal vesiculation and persists in the sensory ganglia of individuals who have been infected. Lesions recur in the same site. HSV-1 causes skin infections and less often genital infection. HSV-2 is the primary cause of genital herpes, a sexually transmitted infection. For oral and genital herpes see 📖 p.260. HSV can trigger EM—see 📖 p.105.

Patterns of HSV-I infection

- Recurrent 'cold sores' common in childhood and adolescence, most often on the lips or face, but any skin surface may be affected. Recurrent infections (see Box 7.1) may cause recurrent EM—see 📖 p.105.
- Herpetic whitlows or 'felons' (painful erythematous vesicular swellings on the tips of fingers) in healthcare workers, e.g. dentists, anaesthetists, nurses on ICU in contact with the lips of patients shedding the virus (many are caused by HSV-2). Also occur in children who suck a digit.
- 'Scrum pox' on the face of rugby players and 'herpes gladiatorium' in wrestlers—caused by direct inoculation into grazed skin (Fig. 7.1).
- Painful gingivostomatitis, lymphadenopathy, and fever in primary HSV-1 infection—see 📖 p.260.
- ⚠ Widespread vesiculation (eczema herpeticum) in patients with atopic eczema, burns, and some rare skin problems. Eczema herpeticum is life threatening, particularly in children—see 📖 p.106.
- Persistent ulcers or systemic infection in the immunosuppressed, Fig. 7.2.

What should I ask?

- Does the patient have warning of the onset? A tingling irritating prodrome of 4–6h is common.
- Does the lesion recur in the same place? This is very suggestive of HSV infection. The differential is fixed drug eruption, another blistering eruption that recurs in the same place, but without a prodrome.
- Does it scar? Uncomplicated cold sores heal without scarring within 7–10 days, but there may be a little residual erythema for some weeks.

What should I look for? (Fig. 7.1)

- Vesicles that rupture and crust within 2–3 days and mild tender lymphadenopathy. See Box 7.2 for signs of eczema herpeticum.

What should I do? (see Box 7.3 for management)

- If you are not sure of the diagnosis, take a swab for virology. The swab must be put into viral culture medium (look in the ward fridge—you may be lucky and find a small bottle of pink fluid, if not contact your laboratory). Use a scalpel to get a little of the blister roof or base as well as blister fluid on the swab. PCR will give you a rapid result.
- A Tzank preparation (smear) for an immediate result—see 📖 Box 7.4, p.146.

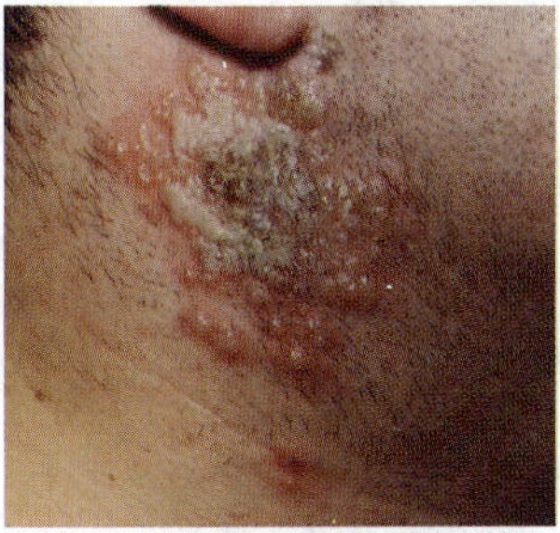

Fig. 7.1 Herpes simplex infection—fresh vesicles are obvious at the periphery of the plaque.

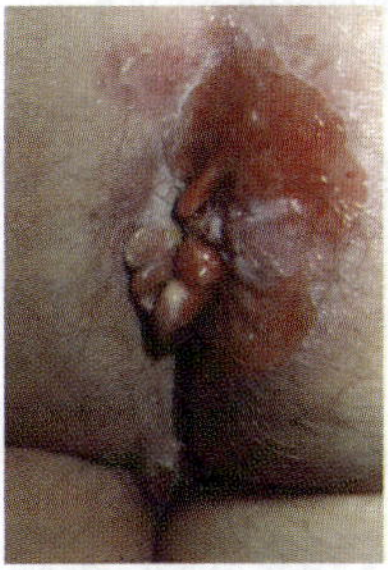

Fig. 7.2 Herpes simplex infection—presenting as a painful ulcer in an immunosuppressed patient.

Box 7.1 Factors that may trigger recurrences of HSV-I infection

- Sunshine
- Menstruation
- Local trauma including dental procedures
- Illness
- Stress.

Box 7.2 ⚠ Signs of eczema herpeticum (Fig. 7.3)

- Sudden deterioration of eczema.
- Pain as well as intense itching.
- Malaise, vomiting, anorexia, diarrhoea.
- Fever in variable number of cases.
- Vesicles (the primary lesions), pustules, and papules; small punched-out ulcers, sometimes clustered, but these may coalesce producing widespread erosions.
- Oozing, sometimes haemorrhagic, and crusting.
- Lymphadenopathy.
- Signs may be difficult to differentiate from VZV or bacterial infection. Secondary bacterial infection may complicate the picture.

Box 7.3 Management of cutaneous HSV infection

- Localized recurrent disease only requires symptomatic treatment.
- Prescribe oral antivirals in patients at risk of developing widespread infection, e.g. immunosuppressed, atopic eczema, Darier's disease—aciclovir 800mg × 5/day, valaciclovir 1g × 3/day, or famciclovir 500mg × 3/day for 7 days. Also see 📖 Box 5.12, p.107.
- Surgery is contraindicated in herpetic whitlows.

Box 7.4 Tzank preparation (smear)

- You will need a glass slide and a No. 10 or 15 scalpel blade.
- De-roof a fresh vesicle and gently scrape the base (you only need tissue fluid and keratinocytes—try not to contaminate the smear with blood).
- Smear the contents of your blade onto a glass slide.
- Air dry, fix with methanol, and stain with Giemsa, toluidine blue, or Wright's stain.
- Examine under a light microscope × 40. Multinucleated giant keratinocytes confirm the diagnosis of HSV or VZV infection.

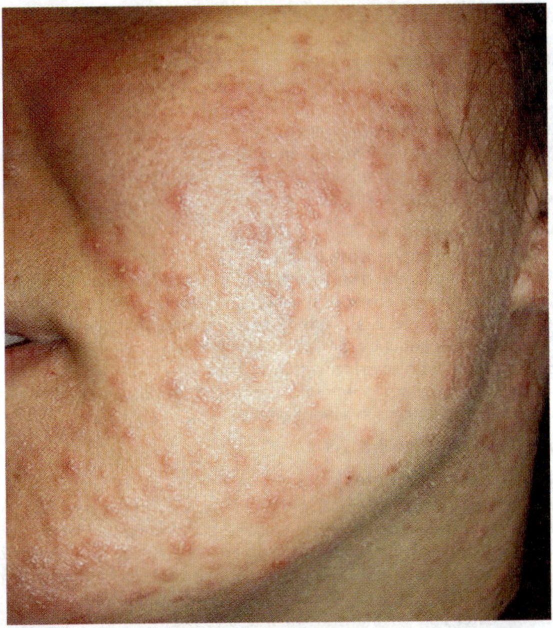

Fig. 7.3 Painful swelling and widespread vesicles in eczema herpeticum.

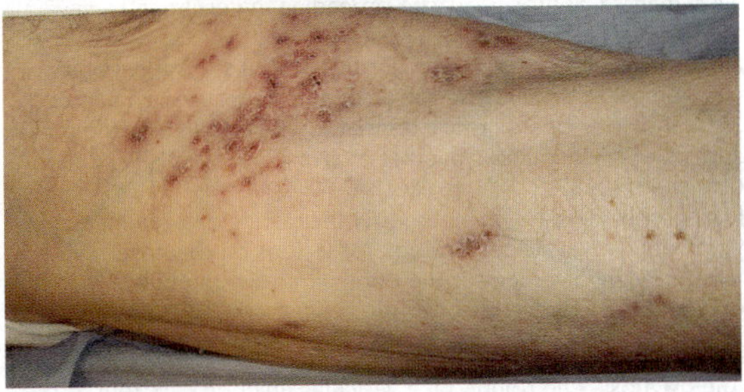

Fig. 7.4 Shingles: dried-up vesicles in the distribution of the L2 and L3 dermatomes.

Further reading

Cernik C *et al. Arch Intern Med* 2008; **168**:1137–44.

Varicella-zoster virus

Varicella (chickenpox)

This contagious infection is spread by mucosal droplets. Patients are infectious from 2 days before until 5 days after the onset of the rash. VZV remains dormant in sensory ganglia after the primary infection. Primary VZV is a more severe infection in adults than children. Complications include pneumonitis and secondary bacterial infection. The live attenuated vaccine prevents severe infection in children.

What should I look for?

- Malaise, cough, coryza, sore throat.
- A rash that affects the trunk more than the limbs or face.
- Crops of itchy erythematous macules and papules that evolve into vesicles (may also be oral). After 2 days, pustules that become crusted.
- Cropping that continues for 4–7 days.
- Healing, often with scarring, within 16 days.
- Haemorrhagic lesions in immunosuppressed patients (may be fatal).
- Respiratory symptoms in severe disease.

What should I do? See Box 7.5.

Herpes zoster (shingles)

Herpes zoster is most common in the elderly. VZV in the sensory ganglia may be reactivated years after the episode of chickenpox. Herpes zoster in a young patient may indicate immunosuppression, e.g. lymphoma. VZV can be passed on to people who have not had varicella by direct contact with the rash. In the elderly, the live attenuated vaccine reduces the incidence of zoster and postherpetic neuralgia (Boxes 7.6 and 7.7).

What should I look for?

- Fever, malaise, and/or headache preceding the eruption by several days.
- Pain, burning, itching, or hypersensitivity often several days before the rash. The pain may simulate renal colic or a myocardial infarction.
- A rash involving one or more dermatomes (it may cross the midline).
- Clusters of erythematous papules evolving into vesicles and then pustules—see 📖 Fig. 7.4, p.147.
- Healing in 10–14 days, sometimes with scarring or pigment change.
- In patients with facial zoster, look for lesions on the nose. These indicate the involvement of the ophthalmic division of the trigeminal nerve and the eye may be infected.

What should I do?

- If the diagnosis is in doubt, take vesicular fluid for PCR (put into viral culture medium) or examine a Tzank preparation (smear)—see 📖 Box 7.4, p.146 and p.575.
- Consider starting antivirals—see Box 7.5.

Further reading

Irving G *et al. Clin J Pain* 2009; **25**:185–92.

Partridge DG and McKendrick MW. *Expert Opin Pharmacother* 2009; **10:**797–812.

Box 7.5 How should I treat VZV infection?

Children with varicella (chickenpox)

- Symptomatic treatment with antipyretics, calamine lotion, and tepid baths, provided immune system is normal.

Adults with varicella (chickenpox) and herpes zoster (shingles)

- Consider antivirals in patients presenting within 24–48h of new vesicles to speed up healing. Treating patients >50 years with antivirals within 7 days of the onset of symptoms of shingles may reduce the duration of post-herpetic neuralgia. Treatment options:
  - Aciclovir 800mg × 5/day, valaciclovir 1g x 3/day, or famciclovir 500mg × 3/day for 7 days.
- Prescribe analgesia.

Immunocompromised or those at risk of severe disease

- Administer varicella zoster Ig within 96h of exposure.
- Treat for 10–14 days starting with IV aciclovir 10mg/kg every 8h for 7 days. Seek advice about treatment in pregnancy.

Box 7.6 Complications of herpes zoster

- Secondary infection with staphylococci or streptococci.
- Ulceration in immunosuppressed patients.
- A generalized eruption in immunosuppressed patients.
- Corneal ulcers, corneal scarring, or blindness if the ophthalmic division of the trigeminal nerve is involved—refer to an ophthalmologist if the eye could be infected.
- Post-herpetic neuralgia.
- Rarely, motor paralysis or encephalitis.

Box 7.7 Post-herpetic neuralgia

This debilitating painful complication is most common in patients aged >50. Pain may persist for many years and is often refractory to treatment. Patients may experience:

- Constant or paroxysmal pain.
- Burning, aching, stabbing, or electric shock pain.
- Allodynia (pain on stimulation of the skin).
- Severe pruritus, with or without pain.

Management—seek the help of a pain clinic.

- Capsaicin cream (pre-treatment with EMLA® may reduce the burning sensation felt when capsaicin is applied).
- Topical anaesthetics: e.g. EMLA®, 5% lidocaine patch.
- Local anaesthetics: SC, IV, epidural, intercostal.
- Other options: amitriptyline, opioid analgesia, gabapentin.

Molluscum contagiosum, orf, and milker's nodule

Molluscum contagiosum

This self-limiting skin infection, common in children, is caused by a pox virus. The virus is transmitted by direct contact, including sexual contact.

What should I look for?

- Translucent, smooth, dome-shaped papules, up to 0.5cm in diameter, with a central umbilicated punctum, from which cheesy material can be expressed.
- Papules may become erythematous and swollen prior to resolution.
- Eczematous patches may develop around mollusca.
- Mollusca may leave small depressed scars.
- Mollusca may be widespread in immunosuppressed or atopic patients. Many mollusca on the face of a young adult may indicate HIV infection.
- A solitary giant molluscum (1–2cm) in an adult may be misdiagnosed as a malignant skin tumour.

What should I do?

- The condition is self-limiting but may persist for 9 months or longer, particularly in atopics. Reassure anxious parents and procrastinate.
- Disrupt papules with a cocktail stick to hasten resolution.
- Removal by curettage, after applying a topical anaesthetic, can be successful in stoical children.
- In adults consider cryosurgery or curettage, but remind patients that mollusca may leave pox-like scars or your surgery may be blamed for the scar.
- Topical hydrogen peroxide cream or topical imiquimod may have a role in persistent disease.

Orf and milker's nodule

Orf is a self-limiting skin infection caused by a parapox virus that is transmitted by direct contact with infected sheep or goats. Milker's nodule is a self-limiting parapox virus infection that simulates orf, but is acquired from cows' udders. Both can trigger EM—see 📖 p.105.

What should I look for?

- A history of contact with infected animals (incubation period may be a few days or several weeks).
- One or more itchy or painful reddish blue papules, usually on a finger—see Box 7.8. Lesions may look very vascular like a pyogenic granuloma.

What should I do?

- No investigations are necessary unless the diagnosis is in doubt, in which case take a skin biopsy for histology or arrange electron microscopy on crust or biopsy material.
- Most lesions resolve spontaneously in 5–7 weeks.
- Treat secondary infection.

Box 7.8 Clinical features in orf and milker's nodule

Lesions progress through a number of stages:

- 0.5–1.5cm macule that evolves into a dome-shaped papule.
- A target-like appearance with a peripheral halo of erythema encircling a white ring that surrounds the central erythematous papule.
- Nodule that may ulcerate and weep.
- Spontaneous healing usually in 6 weeks but may take as long as 6 months.

Other features

- Lymphangitis and/or regional lymphadenopathy.
- Fever.

Human papilloma virus

Human papillomas virus (HPV) infects epithelial cells of skin and mucous membranes; >100 types of HPV have been identified. These cause infections at different sites—see Box 7.9. HPV infections are transmitted by direct contact, which may be sexual, but the incubation time ranges from weeks to more than a year. HPV DNA is widely distributed on the skin in the general population. Infection may be subclinical.

HPV and cancer

HPV-16 and -18 are linked to the development of anogenital and cervical SCCs. Certain HPV types may also play a part in the development of some cutaneous SCCs.

What should I look for?

- Common warts: papules or nodules with a hyperkeratotic surface, often at sites of trauma such as the fingers, elbows, or knees. Warts may coalesce into a plaque (mosaic warts). Warts may be filiform (tiny frond-like projections), often around the mouth. Subungual warts lift the nail plate from the nail bed.
- Plane (flat) warts: flat-topped skin-coloured papules that are more apparent to the patient than the observer. Side-lighting will accentuate the signs. Plane warts are common on the face or other light exposed sites.
- Common and plane warts may appear in lines where the skin has been scratched.
- Deep plantar warts: these are most frequent on weight-bearing skin and may simulate corns (see Box 7.10).
- Anogenital warts: perianal warts may be transmitted sexually or by autoinnoculation of cutaneous warts. Check children for signs that might suggest sexual abuse such as bruising, damage to the hymen, enlargement of the vaginal introitus, or thickening of the anal margin.

What should I do?

- Most viral warts will eventually disappear without treatment, but resolution may take time particularly in immunosuppressed or atopic patients. Procrastinate if at all possible. Explain that when the wart goes, it will not leave a scar. Treatment is difficult but your treatment should not cause more problems than the wart itself—see Box 7.11.
- Immunostimulatory drugs such as oral retinoids or cimetidine have been advocated for widespread warts in adults, but results are variable. Sensitization with topical dephencyprone has also been tried.
- Anogenital warts: refer adults to a genitourinary physician for screening for other sexually transmitted diseases. Women should have cervical smears. Children should see a paediatrician or genitourinary physician (most units will have agreed care paths for children). Topical 5% imiquimod cream or 10% podophylline paint can be very effective.
- Consider HIV in any patient with widespread facial or perianal warts.

Box 7.9 Common mucocutaneous infections and HPV type

- Common warts: HPV-2, -4, -26, -27, -29, -57.
- Plane warts: HPV-3, -10, -28.
- Deep plantar warts: HPV-1, -63.
- Genital and anogenital warts: HPV-6 and -11 (low risk of SCC); HPV-16, -18 (high risk of SCC).
- Oral mucous membranes: HPV-13 and -32.
- Neoplasms in epidermodysplasia verruciformis: HPV-5, -8, and -14 (patients with this autosomal recessive disease have an increased susceptibility to cutaneous HPV infections).

Box 7.10 Is it a plantar wart or a corn?

- Pinch the skin on each side of the wart or corn gently. Plantar warts are tender, unlike corns.
- Paring a wart will reveal bleeding or thrombosed capillaries (black dots), whereas a corn has a uniform glassy appearance without capillaries.

Box 7.11 Treatment of common viral warts and plane warts

- Minimize trauma: e.g. advise patients to stop picking or nibbling at the skin around periungual warts.
- Common warts: regular application of a topical keratolytic containing 10–40% salicylic acid occupies the patient until the wart disappears.
- Duct tape occlusion: apply tape to the wart and leave in place for 6 days at a time for up to 8 weeks (probably a placebo, but painless, unlike cryosurgery, and does prevent trauma).
- Buying warts: another folk remedy, probably best practised by an elderly relative. At least the child profits from the wart!
- Plantar warts: keep flat to minimize discomfort. Pare the warts when the skin is soft after bathing. Most children will not be bothered by a flat plantar wart (parents and teachers may take a different view).
- Cryosurgery is painful and should be reserved for adults unless the child is demanding treatment. Cryosurgery can be a good option for solitary filiform warts which seem less likely to recur than other warts.
- Other surgical options (best for solitary warts) include electro-cautery, hyfrecation, curettage, and laser surgery, but nothing guarantees cure because of latent virus in the skin.
- Intralesional bleomycin 0.5mg/mL is a painful option.
- Plane warts: try 0.025% tretinoin cream or 5% benzoyl peroxide cream x 1/day. Suggest stopping shaving if plane warts are in the beard area.

HIV/AIDS and the skin

More than 40 million people worldwide are infected by the human immunodeficiency viruses HIV-1 or, in a minority, HIV-2. This RNA retrovirus causes the acquired immunodeficiency syndrome (AIDS). HIV binds to CD4 receptors on helper T-lymphocytes, monocytes, macrophages, and neural cells. The virus destroys these CD4 +ve cells or impairs their function causing AIDS. Risk factors—see Box 7.12.

Acute seroconversion

2–8 weeks after exposure to HIV. Most cases are not diagnosed on first presentation. Features include:

- Transient glandular fever-like illness with malaise, fever, headache, sore throat, and lymphadenopathy.
- A generalized erythematous maculopapular rash.
- Ulcers (oral, genital) or candidiasis (oral, vaginal).
- Rarely meningoencephalitis, myelopathy, neuropathy.

Patients may be asymptomatic for 10 or more years after seroconversion, but become progressively more immunodeficient as the CD4 count falls. Severe opportunistic infections are common—Box 7.15. Highly active antiretroviral therapy (HAART) helps HIV-related skin diseases but may trigger inflammatory reactions (immune reconstitution inflammatory syndrome (IRIS)—see Box 7.16).

Cutaneous problems include:

Mucocutaneous infections/infestations

Often florid and atypical. Sometimes a sign of IRIS.

- Viral: herpes simplex (chronic, may disseminate), herpes zoster (severe and recurrent), molluscum contagiosum (facial), warts (facial, perianal), oral hairy leukoplakia often on sides of tongue (EBV).
- Yeasts: recurrent candidiasis (oropharyngeal, vulvovaginitis, cutaneous), pityriasis versicolor. Dermatophyte (tinea): widespread infections.
- Bacterial: staphylococcal folliculitis or furunculosis (📖 p.126), atypical mycobacterial infection (📖 p.136), bacillary angiomatosis (*Bartonella* infections) (📖 p.134). Syphilis: atypical primary, secondary, and late.
- Demodicosis—see 📖 p.168.

Inflammatory dermatoses and other skin problems—Box 7.13

- Seborrhoeic dermatitis: disseminated and atypical.
- Psoriasis: severe, atypical (flexural) and difficult to treat.
- Drug reactions: including SJS and TEN (📖 Box 18.3, p.343).
- Pruritic papular eruption: symmetrical itchy, worst on extremities.
- Eosinophilic pustular folliculitis: itching annular plaques with overlying follicular papules and pustules, usually on face and trunk (see 📖 demodicosis p.168; neuropathic itch 📖 p.504).
- Porphyria cutanea tarda—see 📖 p.310.
- Ichthyosis (scaly skin). Keratoderma (thickened skin on palms and soles).
- Nail disease: hyperpigmentation, yellow nail syndrome.
- Lipodystrophy after treatment with protease inhibitors—see 📖 Box 22.4, p.437.

Cutaneous tumours—see Box 7.14.

Box 7.12 Risk factors for HIV/AIDS

- Sexual partner with HIV infection/AIDS.
- Unprotected homosexual or heterosexual intercourse.
- Multiple sexual partners including one-night stands, holiday sex.
- Sexual partner from country with high prevalence of HIV/AIDS.
- IV drug-abuse: sharing needles.
- Transfusion of blood products between 1977–1985, i.e. prior to screening, but screening may not be rigorous in some parts of the world.
- Other sexually transmitted diseases.

Box 7.13 When should I think of AIDS as a cause of a skin problem?

- Symptoms are more severe than is usual.
- Symptoms are more long-lasting than is usual.
- An inflammatory rash, e.g. psoriasis, which is widespread and affects sites that normally are spared.
- The response to standard treatments is poor.
- Relapses are frequent.

Box 7.14 Cutaneous tumours in HIV/AIDS

- BCC, SCC, and melanoma— see 🕮 p.328, p.330 and Merckel cell cancer (polyoma virus-related).
- Kaposi's sarcoma (herpes virus HHV-8)—see 🕮 p.338.
- Cutaneous lymphoma—see 🕮 p.336.
- Multiple dermatofibromas.

Box 7.15 Non-cutaneous infections in AIDS

- Recurrent bacterial pneumonia; TB.
- Candidiasis: oesophagus, lungs, bronchi.
- *Pneumocystis jiroveci (carinii)* pneumonia (PCP).
- Cytomegalovirus including CMV retinitis.
- Toxoplasmosis, cryptococcal meningitis.
- Progressive multifocal leukoencephalopathy (polyoma JC virus).

Box 7.16 Skin conditions associated with IRIS

Increases in CD4 and CD8 cell counts contribute to inflammation:

- HSV and HZV; warts.
- Kaposi's sarcoma.
- Leprosy.
- Eosinophilic folliculitis.
- Sarcoidosis, SLE.

Dermatophyte infections (ringworm, 'tinea')

Dermatophytes can infect the skin, nails, or hair. Infections are transmitted indirectly through skin scales or shed hair. Fungi can be isolated from contaminated hairbrushes, clothing, carpets, or bed linen. See Boxes 7.17 and 7.18.

What should I look for?

- Asymmetrical, erythematous, scaly well-demarcated patches that may be slightly itchy—Fig. 7.5.
- Lesions expand slowly, often with some central clearing (ring-like). The scale is most marked on the outer edge and is followed by the erythema.
- Infections caused by anthropophilic fungi tend to be less inflamed than those caused by zoophilic fungi (see Box 7.16), which may have raised pustular borders. Check for a history of contact with animals.
- The scale is less obvious in fungal infections that have been misdiagnosed and treated with a topical corticosteroid, but treated patches will become more papular and pustular (tinea incognito). The active spreading edge is still well defined.
- One or more well-defined patches of hair loss and scale. Zoophilic scalp infections are inflamed, swollen, and pustular (kerion). A similar reaction may occur in the beard area. Microsporum-infected hairs fluoresce bright green under Wood's lamp (see 📖 p.568).
- One or more thickened, crumbling discoloured nails. If most of the nails are abnormal consider an alternative diagnosis such as psoriasis.

What should I do?

- Take a skin scraping, scalp brushing, or nail clipping—see 📖 p.574. In children with *Trichophyton tonsurans* infection—take scalp brushings for culture from all the family.
- Treated localized skin infections with a topical antifungal, e.g. terbinafine cream or clotrimazole cream.
- Treat widespread skin infections or infections that have been misdiagnosed and treated with a topical steroid with an oral antifungal, e.g. terbinafine or griseofulvin.
- Treat tinea capitis with an oral antifungal in combination with ketoconazole shampoo. *Microsporum canis* responds to griseofulvin but *T. tonsurans* responds better to oral terbinafine.
- Nail infection is difficult to eradicate and, after longstanding infections, the nail dystrophy may persist. Amorolfine or tioconazole paints may be effective in superficial molds, but dermatophyte infections require an oral antifungal such as terbinafine for 3 months or pulse oral therapy with terbinafine or itraconazole.

Box 7.17 Commonly encountered dermatophytes

Species that infect only humans (anthropophilic) are the most common cause of skin and nail infections:

- *Trichophyton rubrum*: foot, nail, groin, body.
- *Trichophyton interdigitale*: foot, nail, groin.
- *Trichophyton tonsurans*: scalp, body.
- *Trichophyton schoenleinii*: scalp (favus).
- *Epidermophyton floccosum*: foot, nail, groin.

Species of fungus that infect animals (zoophilic) cause a more inflamed rash in humans than the anthropophilic species:

- *Microsporum canis* (cats, dogs): scalp, body.
- *Trichophyton mentagrophytes* (rodents): scalp, body.
- *Trichophyton verrucosum* (cattle): scalp, beard, body.

Ask the patient about contact with animals. Geophilic (soil) species of fungus rarely infect humans.

Box 7.18 Dermatophyte infections at different sites

- Tinea corporis = body—typically occurs in ring-like patterns.
- Tinea cruris = groin—common, usually spares the scrotum. May be unilateral.
- Tinea pedis = foot (athlete's foot)—macerated scale between 4th and 5th toes or diffuse dry scale of soles (moccasin-like).
- Tinea manuum = hand—usually one palm. Dry scale with little inflammation.
- Tinea unguium = nail.
- Tinea capitis = scalp—primarily seen in children. Fungus causes hair loss, unlike psoriasis or eczema. Inflammatory lesions are known as kerions.
- Tinea facei = face—uncommon but may develop a kerion in the beard area.

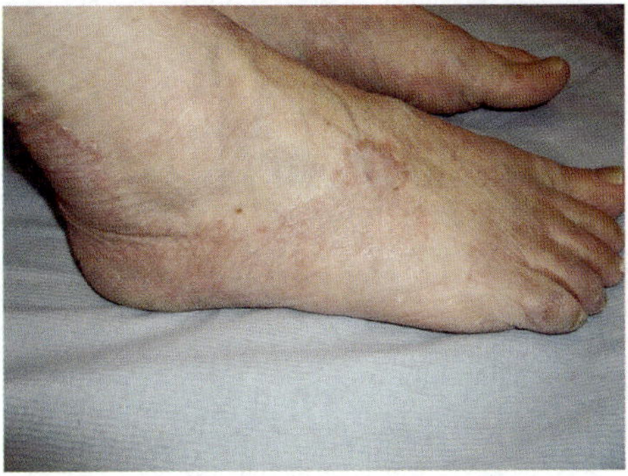

Fig. 7.5 Dermatophyte infection with a clearly demarcated scaly border.

Candida albicans

Candida albicans is a yeast that is a commensal in the mouth and gastro-intestinal tract. *C. albicans* may infect skin or mucosae (mucocutaneous candidiasis) and infection may be the presenting feature of an endocrine disease such as diabetes—see Box 7.19.

Invasive infections and candidaemia occur in immunosuppressed patients. Severe and persistent infections may be linked to a specific T-cell deficiency (chronic mucocutaneous candidiasis).

What should I look for?

- Oral candida (thrush): lacy white lines or whitish plaques on buccal mucosa or tongue. These wipe off with a spatula, leaving an erythematous base (unlike lichen planus—see 🕮 p.266).
- Angular cheilitis: most often in patients with ill-fitting dentures.
- Flexural, including interdigital, candidiasis (candidal intertrigo), erythema with small superficial pustules on adjacent skin (satellite pustules).
- Vulvovaginal: whitish plaques, milky discharge.
- Balanitis.
- Chronic paronychia: boggy swelling of proximal fingernail fold with loss of cuticle and ridging of nail. Plus may exude from under the nail fold. *Candida* may invade the proximal nail plate which becomes friable and discoloured.
- Severe disease: erythematous nodules, pustules, vasculitis.

What should I do?

- Take swabs to confirm the diagnosis if required.
- Minimize risk factors (exclude diabetes) and keep skin dry.
- Prescribe antifungals (Box 7.20). Remember that treatments such as terbinafine and griseofulvin that are used for dermatophyte infections are not effective in yeast infections.

Box 7.19 Risk factors for *Candida* infections

Mucocutaneous candidiasis

- Pregnancy.
- Occlusion and maceration, e.g. in skin folds.
- Wet work or finger sucking—paronychia.
- Prolonged antibiotic therapy.
- Endocrine disease: diabetes, Cushing's syndrome, hypoparathyroidism, hypothyroidism.
- Immune defects and immunosuppressive therapy.
- Iron and zinc deficiency.

Invasive candidiasis

- Neutropenia.
- Prolonged antibiotic therapy.
- Indwelling catheters: urinary or IV.
- Gastrointestinal surgery.
- IV drug abuse.

Box 7.20 Treatment options for candidiasis

- Skin: imidazole creams.
- Oral: miconazole oral gel or nystatin suspension or amphotericin lozenges.
- Vulvovaginal: itraconazole vaginal pessaries (200mg × 2/day for 1 day) and antifungal creams.
- Severe disease requires systemic therapy with oral antifungal tablets.

Pityriasis versicolor

This infection, common in young adults, is caused by malassezia yeasts. These skin commensals proliferate in the stratum corneum producing azelaic acid, which inhibits melanogenesis and prevents the skin in lesions from tanning (for risk factors see 📖 Box 7.21).

What should I look for?

- Asymptomatic lesions predominantly on the trunk (Fig. 7.6).
- Brownish-red or pale (hypopigmented) macules of varying size, with a dusting of fine scale. Scrape the skin gently to see the scale.
- Lesions that appear darker than surrounding untanned skin initially, but after sun exposure appear paler than adjacent skin because the uninvolved skin tans.
- Pale lesions may be misdiagnosed as vitiligo, but vitiligo is not scaly and pigment loss in vitiligo is complete (depigmentation) not partial.
- Malassezia yeasts (also known as pityrosporum yeasts) may cause folliculitis on the trunk in patients with seborrhoeic dermatitis—see 📖 p.203.

What should I do?

- Examine under Wood's light: infected skin fluoresces yellow—see 📖 p.568.
- Take scrapes for microscopy: look for hyphae and spores ('spaghetti and meat-balls') to confirm the diagnosis.
- Prescribe an antifungal—see Box 7.22.
- Explain that once the scale has gone so has the infection, but pale skin will continue to look paler than surrounding skin until exposed to sunlight.
- Warn that relapses are frequent (a sign of youth?).

Box 7.21 Risk factors for pityriasis versicolor

- Warm humid climates when disease may be very extensive.
- Sweating.
- Systemic corticosteroids.
- Cushing's syndrome.
- Immunosuppression associated with transplantation, but not AIDS.

Box 7.22 Treatment options for pityriasis versicolor

- A topical imidazole, e.g. 2% miconazole nitrate or 1% clotrimazole cream for localized disease of a few lesions only.
- 2% ketoconazole shampoo (preferable to 2.5% selenium sulphide) as a body wash daily for 5 days. Leave in contact with the skin for 5min. This can be very drying and the patient may need a moisturizer.
- Oral itraconazole 200mg/day for 7 days is an option for patients with widespread disease.
- Relapses are frequent after any of these treatments.

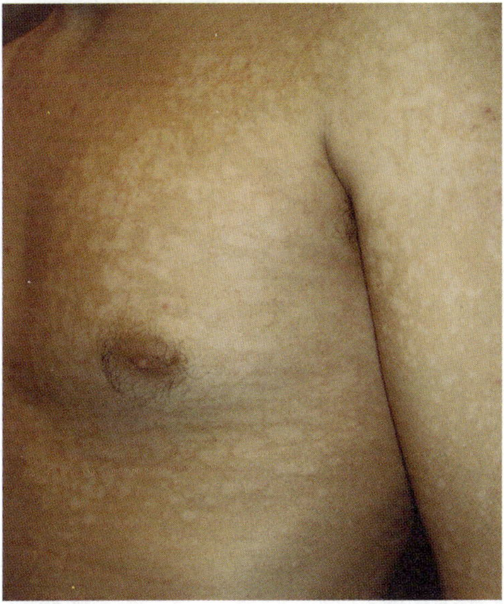

Fig. 7.6 Pityriasis versicolor with widespread scaly pale macules. Uninvolved skin has tanned.

Chapter 8

Infestations and parasites

Contents

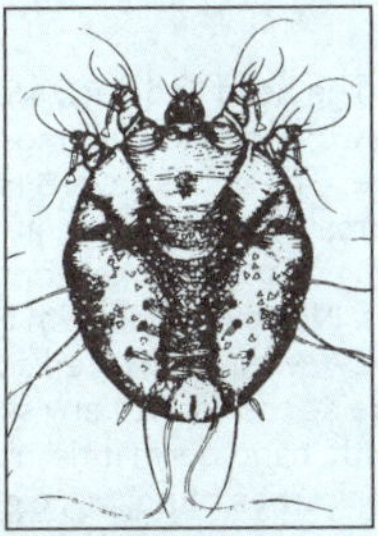

Fig. 8.1 Female scabies mite. Reproduced with permission from Eddleston M *et al. Oxford Handbook of Tropical Medicine*, 3rd edn, 2008. Oxford: Oxford University Press.

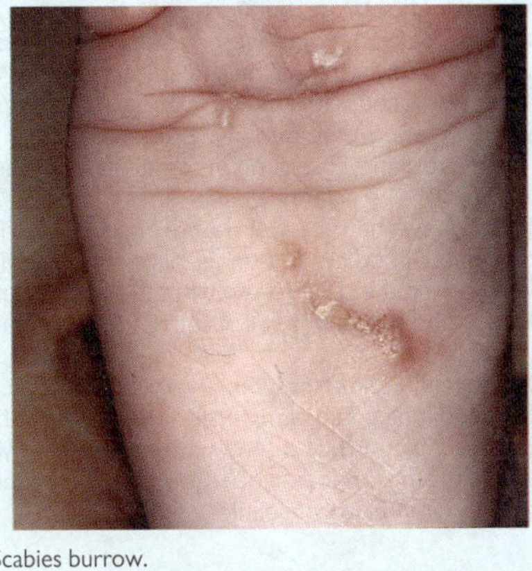

Fig. 8.2 Scabies burrow.

Scabies

Scabies is a common contagious infestation in which allergy to the saliva, eggs, and excrement of the mite, *Sarcoptes scabiei* var. *hominis*, causes extraordinarily intense itching. The mite burrows into the epidermis and once the female (0.4mm long) is fertilized (the male dies after mating), she begins to lay eggs. These hatch in 3–4 days and within 10–15 days reach adulthood. Although the patient may have only 10–12 adult mites, the itch is widespread, severe, and distressing. Overwhelming infestation in a debilitated, old, or immunosuppressed patient (>1000 mites per person) is known as crusted (Norwegian) scabies—see Box 8.1, Fig. 8.1.

The mites cannot jump. Scabies is transmitted by skin-to-skin contact, e.g. sharing a bed, holding hands, sexual intercourse. The good news is that scabies can be cured—so it is a rewarding diagnosis to make.

What should I ask?

- Where is the itch? The head and neck are usually spared except in the very young, the very old, or the immunosuppressed.
- What is the itch like? The itch is severe (some patients liken the itch to pain) and made worse by warmth, e.g. at night.
- Is anyone else itching? Carers, family contacts, including grandparents, and sexual contacts. Not everyone with an infestation will be itchy. Sensitization takes 2–6 weeks. Crusted scabies may not be very itchy.
- Is a close contact being treated for any skin complaint (scabies is often missed)? Granny with 'hand dermatitis' may be the index case.
- Enquire about other causes of itching, e.g. drugs (see 📖 p.60).
- What treatment has been provided? Treatment fails if all those infested (i.e. all close contacts) have not been treated at the same time.

What should I do?

Search for proof—most signs are secondary to scratching (papules, erythema, and excoriation), but look for:

- Burrows—see Box 8.2; finger web crusting; nodules on the penis.
- Blisters or pustules on the palms and soles in infants.
- Mites either visualized with the dermatoscope as a tiny dark triangle just beyond the end of the burrow, extracted from a burrow using a needle (very satisfying), or found in scrapings from the roof of the burrow (you may see eggs as well as mites). Inspect your catch under a light microscope—the mite will walk around, don't lose it.
- Numerous mites in crusts and under nails in Norwegian scabies.
- Consider showing the mite to the patient—can be very therapeutic.
- If you cannot find mites, but still suspect scabies, either treat the patient and all close contacts for scabies—see Box 8.3—or (preferred option) reduce inflammation with a very potent topical steroid cream, prescribe a sedating antihistamine, add in an oral antibiotic (if required for secondary infection), and renew the search next week … setting aside sufficient time to do a proper job. Ask the patient to bring close contacts with him/her to the clinic.

Box 8.1 Crusted 'Norwegian' scabies

- The same mite as in ordinary scabies, but many more of them.
- Occurs in debilitated or immunosuppressed patients.
- Itching is often less marked than in normal scabies.
- The hands, elbows, knees, and ankles develop extensive thick crusts.
- The face, scalp, and nail beds are often involved.
- All the skin may be red and scaly.
- Crusts contain hundreds of live mites that can survive for a few days.
- Large number of mites may be found beneath the nails.
- This form of scabies is extremely contagious.

Box 8.2 Scabies burrows—see Fig. 8.2

Comma-shaped lines a few millimetres long are diagnostic. The narrow superficial curved lines are visible in the horny layer of the epidermis, but may be difficult to find if the skin is eczematous, scratched, and crusted.

Inspect finger webs, flexural aspect of wrists, elbows, and axillary folds, breasts (in women), genitalia (in men), and the medial and lateral borders of the feet.

In infants and young children you may also find burrows on head and neck as well as palms and soles, often in association with blisters.

The mite is visible to the naked eye as a pin-point dark dot just beyond the end of the burrow. With a dermatoscope you will see a small dark triangle. Sometimes a vesicle forms near the end of burrows—the mite is just beyond the vesicle.

Linear burrows on the creases of palms and soles may be followed by a V-shaped pattern of scale and inflammation that has been likened to the wake of a moving ship. The wake and associated burrow make a Y-shaped sign that points to the mite.

Box 8.3 Management of scabies

Treat all members of the household and all close contacts (including sexual partners) at the same time, even if they do not have symptoms.

Norwegian (crusted) scabies—treat all those in the nursing home or hospital ward if the patient has been there >24h as well as other contacts. Use 2 treatments 3 days apart.

Apply 5% permethrin cream to the whole body, except the head, including the fingers, toes, and the skin under the nails. In a child <2 years or elderly or immunosuppressed patients also apply the cream to scalp, face, and ears. Leave the cream on for 8–12h. Repeat treatment after 7 days.

Although the mites die rapidly once off the body, patients should either wash all clothes, bed linen, and towels in a hot wash or place these items in a plastic bag for at least 72h.

Itching may persist for 2–3 weeks after treatment. Prescribe calamine oily lotion or a moderately potent topical corticosteroid ointment. A sedating oral antihistamine (e.g. hydroxyzine 25–50mg at night) will help to relieve itch.

Ivermectin 200mcg/kg in a single dose repeated in 7–14 days has been recommended for severe scabies, e.g. Norwegian scabies.

Lice

Lice suck blood. Itching, which may take 1–3 weeks to develop, is secondary to allergy to the lice, not to bites. Heavy and longstanding infestation causes fatigue (incessant itching), anaemia (feeling lousy), and underperformance (nit-wit). For treatment see Boxes 8.4, 8.5, 8.6.

Head louse (*Pediculus humanus capitis*)

- Head lice are almost ubiquitous in school-age children in the UK and sometimes infest their parents (and grandparents!) too. The elongated grey-brown lice, which are as fond of clean as dirty hair, are adapted to swing from hair to hair.
- Egg cases are cemented firmly to the base of hair shafts, but you will see them more easily once the louse has hatched, when they become white and the growing hair carries the empty case (nit) away from the surface of the scalp. Scalp scale, dandruff, or hair casts (pseudonits) may resemble nits, but are easily removed from the hair, unlike nits which are firmly attached to the hair shaft.
- You may see elongated lice (2–4mm) moving in the scalp (look behind the ears or at the nape of the neck) or you may find lice if you comb the hair over a piece of paper.
- Heavy infestations may become secondarily infected with bacteria.

Pubic (crab) louse (*Pthirus pubis*)

- Pubic lice are transmitted by close contact, including sexual contact.
- The lice infest short, coarse body hair—pubic, perianal, axillary, moustache, beard, eyelash, eyebrow.
- The translucent lice, 2mm long, may be visible crawling through the hair or you may see the nits (empty egg cases) glued to the hair shafts. Look for louse droppings (dark brown or black powder) in underwear.
- Bites produce bluish macules (maculae cerulea) that may be mistaken for bruises.

Body louse (*Pediculus humanus humanus*)

- Infestations cause severe itching, especially at night.
- Look for bite reactions—small erythematous papules or wheals where the skin is covered by clothing—as well as evidence of scratching.
- Secondary infection is common.
- Check the seams of clothing worn next to the skin for lice (2–4mm) and eggs.

Box 8.4 Treatment of head lice

- 0.5% malathion lotion is applied until hair is thoroughly wet down to the roots. The hair is allowed to dry and the lotion left on the hair for 8–10h.
- 2 treatments a week apart may be useful as eggs take a week to hatch.
- Head lice are becoming resistant to many insecticides.
- Regular wet combing ('bug-busting') with a fine-toothed nit comb for 30min repeated every 4 days for 2 weeks may reduce the population of lice, but is considerably less effective than an insecticide.

Box 8.5 Treatment of pubic lice

Aqueous 0.5% malathion lotion or 5% permethrin cream—wash off after 12h and repeat application after 7 days.

Box 8.6 Treatment of body lice

- Launder clothing and bedding. The lice are killed by extremes of temperature.
- Treat secondary cutaneous infection.
- Prescribe sedating antihistamines for itching.

Female *Pediculosis capitis*

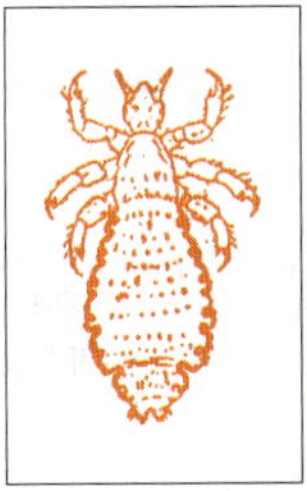

3mm length

Fig. 8.3 Headlouse, adapted to swing through hair. Reproduced with permission from Eddleston M *et al. Oxford Handbook of Tropical Medicine*, 3rd edn, 2008. Oxford: Oxford University Press.

Female *Phthirus pubis* with ovum within

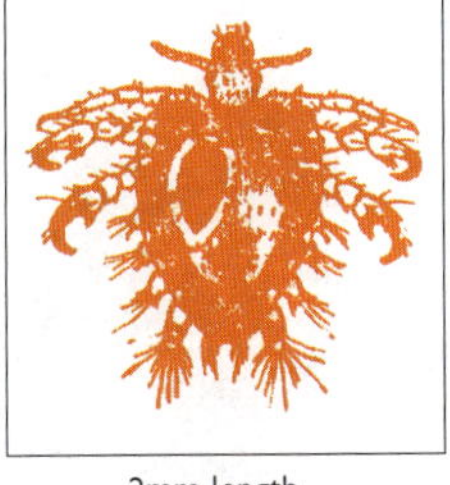

2mm length

Fig. 8.4 Crab louse. Reproduced with permission from Eddleston M *et al. Oxford Handbook of Tropical Medicine*, 3rd edn, 2008. Oxford: Oxford University Press.

Demodicosis and other mites

Demodex are mites, 0.1–0.4 mm long, that live in or near normal hair follicles (*Demodex folliculorum)* and the ducts of sebaceous glands (*Demodex brevis*) predominantly on the scalp, eyelashes, external ear canals, forehead, sides of nose, and cheeks. The tiny mites come out of follicles at night to walk around slowly (8–16cm/h) on the surface of the skin. They mate in the follicular openings.

Demodex are rare in children <5 years old.

Demodex are probably not pathogenic in immunocompetent humans. Increased numbers of mites are found in some papulo-pustular follicular eruptions such as rosacea, but their role in pathogenesis is controversial.

However, demodex infestation in immunocompromised patients with conditions such as HIV or acute lymphoblastic leukaemia may cause inflamed papular eruptions (demodicosis).

What should I look for?

- Scaly erythematous papules or papulopustular lesions on face associated with variable swelling.
- No response to treatments for rosacea, e.g. oral tetracycline, topical metronidazole.
- Erythematous papules or papulopustular lesions on scalp or chest.
- Blepharitis and pustules around the eyelids.
- Groups or clusters of erythematous papules, sometimes in annular patterns.
- Minimal itch.

What should I do?

- Take a skin scraping. Large numbers of mites will be visible in scale suspended in KOH—see 📖 p.574.
- Treat with 5% permethrin cream applied once a day for 3–5 days.
- Severe infestations can be treated with oral ivermectin.

Other mites—see Boxes 8.7 and 8.8.

Box 8.7 Harvest mites

- The larvae of these minute mites (*Trombicula autumnalis*) are found in grassy meadows, cornfields, and other herbage. The larvae are active during the day and can be a problem in dry sunny weather, especially in late summer and early autumn.
- The reddish larvae (0.2mm long) are just visible to the naked eye.
- The larvae congregate to feed on warm-blooded animals—including humans. The larva hooks onto the exposed skin and repeatedly sucks blood from the same site for 3 or 4 days, before dropping off the skin onto the ground to complete its life cycle.
- Bites cause intense irritation.
- Look for erythematous papules, 'heat spots', usually on the legs.
- Larvae are easily killed with an insecticide.
- Relieve irritation with a moderately potent topical corticosteroid cream.
- Local names for the larvae include:
  - Harvest bugs
  - Velvet mites
  - Harvesters
  - Berry bugs
  - Bracken bugs
  - Chiggers
  - Orange-tawneys (in Ireland).
- The adult mites are harmless.
- The larvae of some related tropical species transmit a *Rickettsia* organism to humans causing scrub typhus (mite typhus).

Box 8.8 Bird mite dermatitis (gamasoidosis, acariasis)

- Pigeons are a well-known host for the blood-sucking bird mite, *Dermanyssus gallinae* (the chicken mite). The mites are found where pigeons build their nests and can survive for 4–6 months without feeding on blood. The female measures 0.7mm × 0.4mm, and the male 0.6mm × 0.3mm.
- Humans working in buildings near the nesting sites of pigeons (window ledges, air conditioners), or patients lying beside open windows, may become infested with mites looking for a meal. Bites may be painful and the rash is extremely itchy.
- Look for an intensely itchy papulovesicular rash on exposed surfaces of skin. The 1–2mm papules erupt in clusters or lines. The eruption resembles scabies, but you will not find burrows.
- The mites move extremely rapidly and leave the host once they have fed, so may be difficult to find. They hide in shady cracks and crevices during the day but emerge at night to 'bite and run'.
- The solution—get rid of the nests and the pigeons!
- Note: the mites infest other birds … and pet gerbils.

Fleas and bugs

Fleas are small (1.5–3.3mm), dark-coloured wingless insects adapted to feeding on the blood of warm-blooded vertebrates including dogs, cats, pigs, chickens, and, unfortunately, humans. Most often humans are bitten by animal fleas (usually cat or dog fleas), but these fleas do not live on humans and need access to their animal host to reproduce. Nowadays human fleas are found most often on farms. They live on pigs, which have similar skin to humans.

Fleas have extraordinarily hard shiny bodies that are virtually impossible to crush between the fingers or with a hard instrument. They are prodigious jumpers—their muscular legs can launch them vertically up to 18cm and horizontally up to 33cm (Fig. 8.5).

Bed bugs are an increasing problem—see Box 8.10.

Papular urticaria

This eruption, frequent in children, is caused by allergy to bites, usually those of cat fleas. The flea lays eggs on the cat, but these fall off into the bedding (or the sofa) where they pupate and then hatch in about 1 month. If the cat is not available, the flea is happy to bite another warm-blooded creature. Bites cause few symptoms, unless the patient is allergic to the flea's saliva. Fleas can survive for a year between meals and pupae can remain dormant for 2 years or more. Presentation may be particularly dramatic if the house has been empty for a while, no cats have been in residence, and the fleas are hungry.

What should I look for?

- Clusters of itchy papules on ankle and legs (the fleas jump up from the carpet to the nearest exposed skin). In crawling infants the eruption may be more widespread.

What should I do?

- Try to convince the patient (or parent) that the problem lies with the cat (dog) and fleas. Explain that cat fleas are virtually impossible to eradicate, even though the pet has been treated, because the fleas are not living on the cat.
- Prescribe an antihistamine and a moderately potent topical steroid cream such as clobetasone butyrate to be applied to bites ×2/day.
- Reassure everyone that the allergy will gradually become less of a problem.
- Recommend treating carpets, furnishings, pet bedding (and the cat) with appropriate insecticides and vacuuming frequently (but dispose of the vacuum bag afterwards).
- Recommend washing pet bedding every week and consider moving the pet's bed to an area without carpets.

Human fleas (*Pulex irritans*)

- Itching dark red papules clustered in small groups ('breakfast, lunch, and tea') round the waist or abdomen suggest the bites of human fleas.
- Hunt for the flea(s) to prove the diagnosis—see Box 8.9.

Box 8.9 Tracking down human fleas

Heavy infestation is no longer common. Most patients will have acquired just 1 or 2 human fleas. The fleas are found in the seams of clothing worn next to the skin, not on the patient, but they are difficult to see and even more difficult to catch and kill.

The following technique has proved successful. Advise the patient to:

- Prepare for action by dampening a bar of soap, which will be used to catch the flea(s).
- Stand fully clothed in a well-lit, pale-coloured bath tub (empty!).
- Take off each item of clothing, turn inside out, and shake thoroughly over the bath tub, paying particular attention to clothing next to the skin and the seams of the clothing.
- The flea or fleas will drop onto the shiny surface of the bath tub, where they are easy to see.
- Capture the flea using the sticky bar of soap (don't try to squash the flea—they are remarkably resilient and they jump).
- Drown the flea by putting the bar of soap into water.

Heavy infestation of the home by human fleas will need professional treatment.

Box 8.10 Bed bugs

- Bed bugs thrive where standards of hygiene are poor and laundering is infrequent. The reddish brown bugs are 5mm long.
- The bugs feed on human blood at night. Bites irritate and some people develop very brisk inflammatory reactions.
- The bed bugs hide in a dark crevice during the day, e.g. in the mattress, within the bed frame, or in the bed headboard, behind loose wallpaper or skirting boards, within paintings.
- You will not see bedbugs during the day.
- Look for spots of blood on bedding or brown excrement on bedding or close to where the bedbugs are living.
- Launder infested bedding in a hot wash.
- Contact a pest control expert—heavily infested furnishings may have to be destroyed.

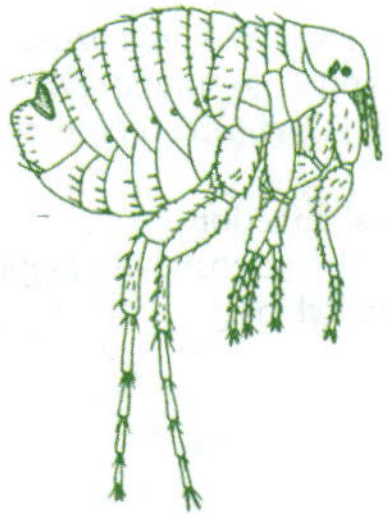

Fig. 8.5 The flea. Reproduced with permission from Collier J *et al. Oxford Handbook of Clinical Specialties* 8th edn, 2009. Oxford: Oxford University Press.

Cutaneous larva migrans (creeping eruption)

This parasitic skin disease is caused by hookworm larvae that usually infect domestic animals—see Box 8.11. In their animal hosts, the larvae penetrate the skin to reach the blood and lymphatic systems. They mature in the intestine. Eggs are excreted in faeces and take about 7 days to hatch. The larvae are found on beaches and moist soils that have been contaminated with animal faeces.

Cutaneous larva migrans presents in individuals whose skin has come into direct contact with the larvae, e.g. walking barefoot or lying on sandy beaches. The larvae tunnel through the stratum corneum into the epidermis, but are unable to reach the dermis in humans because they cannot penetrate the basement membrane. The disease is self-limiting as humans are a 'dead-end' host.

Cutaneous larva migrans is usually acquired in tropical and subtropical regions, including the USA (south-eastern Atlantic and Gulf coastal regions), South America, South-East Asia, and East and West Africa.

What should I look for?

- The larvae migrate through the superficial epidermis producing itchy erythematous linear or serpiginous tracks (creeping eruption) (Fig. 8.6).
- Tracks are often found on the feet, but may be found on any skin surface that has been in direct contact with larvae.
- The track elongates 1–2cm per day.
- Sometimes blisters develop around or within the tracks.
- Most patients have 1 or 2 tracks, but heavy infestations are associated with numerous itchy erythematous tracks, crusting, and secondary bacterial infection.

What should I do?

- The diagnosis is based on the history and clinical findings.
- A skin biopsy is not helpful as it is difficult to predict exactly where to find the larva, which is somewhere just ahead of the leading edge of the track.
- Antihelminth treatment options include:
  - Ivermectin: single dose of 12mg or 200mcg/kg (available on a named patient basis).
  - Albendazole: single dose of 400 mg or 400mg/day for 3–5 days for widespread infection (available on a named patient basis).
  - Topical 10–15% tiabendazole solution: applied ×4/day for 1 week under an occlusive dressing (no commercial preparation available in the UK).
- Treat secondary bacterial infection.
- Prescribe a potent topical corticosteroid (apply ×2/day) to reduce inflammation and relieve itching.

Box 8.11 Main causes of cutaneous larva migrans

- *Uncinaria stenocephala*: dog hookworm found in Europe.
- *Ancylostoma braziliense*: hookworm of wild and domestic dogs and cats found in central and southern USA, Central and South America, and the Caribbean.
- *Ancylostoma ceylonicum*: dog and cat hookworm found in Asia.
- *Ancylostoma caninum*: common dog and cat hookworm found in Australia.
- *Bunostomum phlebotomum*: cattle hookworm.

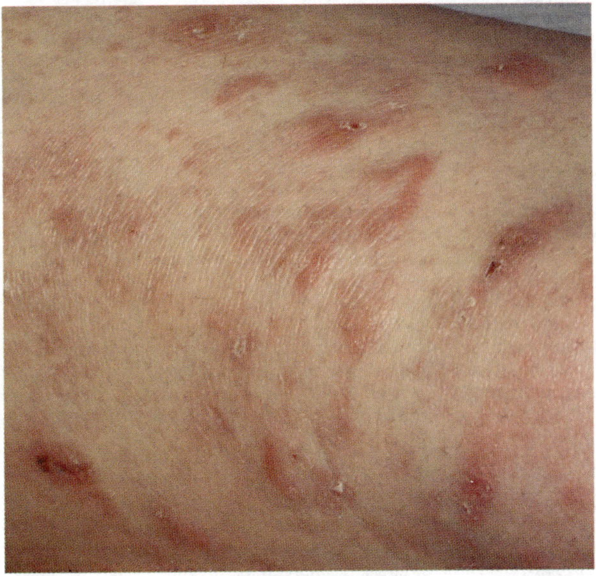

Fig. 8.6 Itchy serpiginous tracks in cutaneous larva migrans.

Cutaneous leishmaniasis

Synonyms include: tropical sore, oriental sore, Baghdad sore, bouton d'orient, Delhi boil, Aleppo boil, Chicleros ulcer.

Leishmaniasis is a vector-borne disease caused by obligate intramacrophage protozoa that belong to the genus *Leishmania*. 21 species of *Leishmania* can infect humans. The disease is endemic in tropical, sub-tropical, and southern European countries including Central and South America, Asia, the Middle East, the Mediterranean, and East and North Africa. The animal reservoir hosts for the parasites include rodents, bats, wolves, and foxes. Bites of female sandflies transmit the parasite to humans.

Cutaneous leishmaniasis is the commonest type of leishmaniasis—see Box 8.12. The presentation is determined by the infectivity and virulence of the parasite and the host response—some species induce a brisk inflammatory response, while others produce more indolent disease.

What should I look for?

- A history of travel to an endemic region: the average incubation time is about 2 months but cutaneous leishmaniasis may not present for more than a year after the sandfly bite.
- A history of sandfly bites (patients may not be aware of bites).
- Lesions on nocturnally exposed skin: face, neck, arms.
- One or more painless brownish nodules that may resemble bites, but usually do not itch, and slowly enlarge into plaques or warty lesions (Old World disease) or boil-like erythematous nodules that crust centrally and ulcerate in 1–3 months. Ulcers may expand to a diameter of 3–6 cm (New World disease).
- Satellite nodules may develop around the primary nodule. Nodules may spread along lymphatics ('sporotrichoid spread').
- Other members of the family may also have lesions, suggesting that the infection was acquired by bites at the same time.

What should I do?

- Take 1 or 2 full-thickness 4 mm punch skin biopsies from the raised edge of a lesion or a nodule for histological examination. Histology is granulomatous, but even with a Giemsa stain, amastigote parasites may be difficult to find. Parasite DNA can be detected in lesional material by PCR and this has replaced culture in many centres.
- Make a smear from a slit skin scrape, tissue or aspirate—see Box 8.13—the amastigote parasites are easier to find in a smear than in a biopsy.
- Culture material: first you will need to obtain culture medium.
- Serological testing is usually unhelpful because antibody levels are low.
- Discuss management with an expert. Most lesions will heal without treatment in 3–18 months, but leave a depressed scar which may be very disfiguring. Patients with New World leishmaniasis are at risk of developing mucosal disease. Intralesional, IM, or IV pentavalent antimony (sodium stibogluconate) is still the mainstay of treatment.

Box 8.12 Clinical types of leishmaniasis

Cutaneous leishmaniasis: commonest form—Old World: caused *by L. tropica, L. major, L. aethiopica.* New World: *L. mexicana* species complex, *Viannia* subgenus, *L. major*-like organisms and *L. chagasi.*

Leishmaniasis recidivans: a chronic destructive central facial lesion that enlarges over many years—seen in Iran and Iraq. Caused by *L. tropica.*

Mucosal leishmaniasis: deep destructive mucosal ulceration (nose, pharynx, palate, lip) occurs 1–5 years after cutaneous disease has healed. Occurs in South and Central America. Caused by *Viannia* subgenus (mainly *L.* [*V.*] *brasiliensis*, also *L.* [*V.*] *panamensis*, *L.* [*V.*] *guyanensis*, *L. amazonensis*).

Visceral leishmaniasis (kala-azar, black sickness): caused by *L. donovani* complex, *L. tropica*, and *L. amazonensis* occurs in South America, Asia, the Mediterranean, and Africa. Patients are systemically unwell with a fever, sweats, weight loss, and massive splenomegaly. The skin is hyperpigmented. Intercurrent infections are common. Mortality untreated is >80%. Visceral leishmaniasis may be an opportunistic infection in patients with HIV-1. Depigmented macules, nodules and malar erythema are found in ***post kala-azar dermal leishmaniasis***.

Box 8.13 Investigations in cutaneous leishmaniasis (talk to an expert first)

PCR Tissue the size of a rice grain should be placed in 300 microlitres of PCR buffer (Qiagen ATL).

Scrape Pinch the skin around a nodule to exclude blood, slit the skin of a nodule with a scalpel blade to a depth of 1–2mm. Scrape the walls of the incision and smear the fluid thinly onto a clean microscope slide (the smear should not contain blood). Label (identify the patient and the sampling technique), air dry, and fix in methanol for 1min before staining.

Impression smear If you have taken a punch biopsy, remove excess blood by gently blotting on a towel and then firmly press the cut surface of the tissue onto a clean glass slide several times. Label, air dry, and fix in methanol for 1min before staining.

Aspirate smears Sample 3 different areas from a nodule or the edge of a lesion.

Attach a 0.5mm needle firmly to an empty 1–3mL syringe. Apply negative pressure and advance the needle slowly in a straight line (to avoid blood contamination) along the edge of an ulcer or into the centre of a solid lesion. Withdraw in a straight line, but be careful not to draw any air into the syringe.

Disconect the needle, draw air into the syringe, re-attach the needle, and blow out the contents rapidly onto a clean, polished, and alcohol-free microscope slide. Spread the aspirate gently on the slide using the tip of the needle. Label, air dry, and fix in methanol for 1min before staining.

Further reading

Murray HW *et al. Lancet* 2005; **366:**1561–77.

Chapter 9
Psoriasis

Contents

Relevant pages in other chapters

SAPHO syndrome—see 📖 p.228
Napkin psoriasis—see 📖 Box 31.12, p.557

What is psoriasis?

Derived from the Greek psor = itch or psorin = to have the itch.

Introduction

Psoriasis is a chronic inflammatory skin disease characterized by scaly erythematous papules and plaques. Prevalence varies in different ethnic groups, but psoriasis affects around 2% of the population in Northern Europe. People of any age may be affected and the incidence is similar in men and women. 75% of cases occur before the age of 46, but some studies have suggested that there are 2 peaks of onset, between 16–22 years and between 57–60 years. The disease remits spontaneously in 1/3 of patients, sometimes for 50 years, but the course is not predictable.

Pathogenesis

The epidermis in psoriatic plaques is hyperproliferative and the dermis contains tortuous, dilated small blood vessels as well as an inflammatory infiltrate of CD4 +ve and CD8 +ve T-cells. Neutrophils are present in some forms of psoriasis. Dendritic cells also contribute to the pathogenesis.

It has been hypothesized that antigen penetrating a defective epidermal barrier stimulates an immune response, but although innate and adaptive immunity seem to be activated, no antigen has been identified. Cytokines released by epidermal keratinocytes and activated T-cells drive new vessel formation and proliferation of keratinocytes and T-cells. TH-1 cytokines (interferon gamma, interleukin-2 (IL-2), and interleukin-12) as well as tumour necrosis factor alpha (TNFα), a pro-inflammatory cytokine, are present in psoriatic plaques. Interleukin-22 and -23 (which activate TH17 cells) may also have a role in pathogenesis.

Genetic factors

Susceptibility to psoriasis is inherited—about 30% of patients with psoriasis vulgaris have an affected first-degree relative. Linkage studies have shown that the genetics of psoriasis is complex—see Box 9.1. Environmental factors may trigger psoriasis in genetically predisposed individuals—see 🕮 Box 9.3, p.181.

Psoriasis is more than skin deep

Patients with psoriasis have an increased risk of developing 2 more inflammatory diseases that are immunologically mediated—seronegative arthritis (psoriatic arthritis—see 🕮 p.192) and Crohn's disease.

Case–control studies have also shown an increased prevalence of the metabolic syndrome (see Box 9.2) in patients with psoriasis, possibly related to chronic inflammation and circulating inflammatory cytokines including TNFα. The psychosocial burden of psoriasis is considerable. Anxiety and depression are common and patients tend to smoke and to drink too much alcohol. Treat the whole patient, remembering potential comorbidities such as cardiovascular disease, hypertension, obesity, and type 2 diabetes.

Box 9.1 Genetics: psoriasis susceptibility loci

Psoriasis risk genes or genes that modify severity of disease may include:
- Genes for factors that control inflammation.
- Genes involved in keratinocyte signalling.
- Genes regulating vascular growth.

At least 9 chromosomal loci, PSORS1–9, have been linked to psoriasis, but no single psoriasis gene has been identified. Loci of particular interest include:
- PSORS1: the major genetic determinant of psoriasis. Located in the MHC on chromosome 6p close to HLA-Cw6. Strongly linked to guttate psoriasis. Hla-Cw6 is a marker for early-onset psoriasis.
- PSORS4: within the epidermal differentiation complex on chromosome 1q.
- PSORS8: overlaps with the Crohn's disease locus on chromosome 16q. The frequency of Crohn's disease in patients with psoriasis is increased.

Box 9.2 Components of metabolic syndrome

- Elevated waist circumference: men >102cm; women >88cm.
- Elevated triglycerides.
- Reduced high density lipoprotein (HDL) cholesterol.
- Elevated blood pressure >130/85mmHg.
- Elevated fasting glucose.

Metabolic syndrome is defined as the presence of 3 or more of these criteria. The syndrome produces a prothrombotic and proinflammatory state.

Further reading

Di Cesare A *et al. J Invest Dermatol* 2009; **129:**1339–50.
Griffiths CEM and Barker JNWM. *Lancet* 2007; **370:**263–71.
Nijsten T and Wakkee M. *J Invest Dermatol* 2009; **129:**1601–3.

The history in psoriasis

The diagnosis may be obvious to you (and the patient) from the appearance of the skin, but listen to the patient's story to help you to assess the impact of the psoriasis and to plan management.

What should I ask?

- Invite the patient to tell you about his/her skin condition and then ask specific questions, taking a history as described in 📖 Chapter 2, p.18, p.20, and p.32.
- Inquire about symptoms—in psoriasis these may include itch, bleeding from the skin, scaling, showers of 'dandruff', or pain (fissures on palms and soles may be very uncomfortable).
- Find out what helps or exacerbates the rash—see Box 9.3.
- Explore quality of life—how does psoriasis affect daily activities, work, or school? Is the patient prepared to go swimming or wear clothing that reveals the affected skin? How does the attitude of other people affect the patient?
- Psoriasis fluctuates in severity. How bad is the rash today? Ask the patient to rate the severity on a scale of 0 to 10 (worst possible).

Treatments/drug history

- What treatments are being used now or have been used in the past? How effective are these—why were they stopped?
- Patients may have been treated with UVB or PUVA photochemotherapy. Was burning a problem? Did the psoriasis respond? How quickly did psoriasis recur? How long was each course and how many courses has the patient had?
- Is the patient taking drugs that might worsen psoriasis? See Box 9.3.

Family history

Does anyone else in the family have a skin disease? Patients who have relatives with severe psoriasis may be particularly concerned about their own prognosis and the risk of their children developing psoriasis.

Past medical history

- Has the patient had any previous skin problems?
- Is there a history of skin cancer? (A risk after excessive PUVA.)
- Is there a history of arthritis? See 📖 p.192.
- Remember that psoriasis is associated with the metabolic syndrome. Document cardiovascular risk factors—hyperlipidaemia, smoking, obesity, hypertension, and diabetes.
- Is there a history of depression?
- How much alcohol does the patient drink?
- Does the patient have HIV? HIV/AIDS may trigger severe psoriasis.

Measuring the impact of the psoriasis

Ask the patient to complete the DLQI (Dermatology Life Quality Index) to obtain a validated measure of the impact of the skin disease—see 📖 p.32.

Box 9.3 Environmental factors that may trigger or exacerbate psoriasis

- Infections: beta haemolytic streptococcal tonsillitis or pharyngitis, HIV.
- Drugs: beta-blockers, antimalarials, lithium, interferon alpha (IFNα), alcohol. Rebound is common after systemic steroids.
- Trauma to the skin (Köbner phenomenon).
- Hormones: may improve or deteriorate in pregnancy.
- Stress or emotional upset.
- Sunlight: usually makes psoriasis better, but in 10% of patients exacerbates psoriasis.

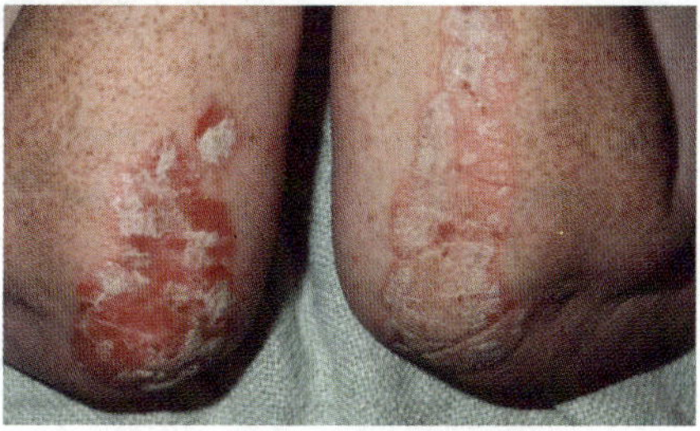

Fig. 9.1 Symmetrical plaque psoriasis on extensor surfaces.

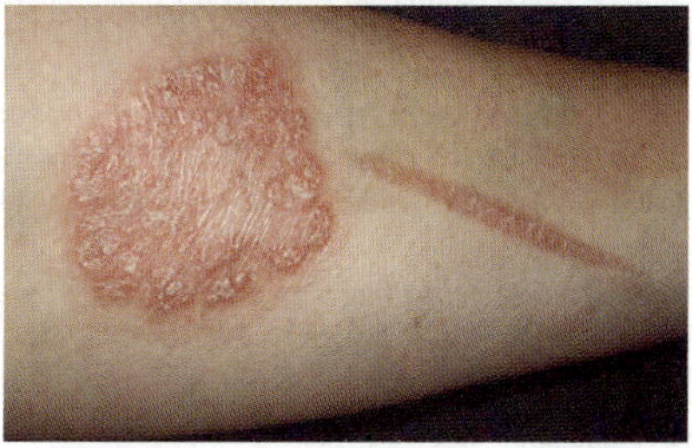

Fig. 9.2 Köbner phenomenon—psoriasis appearing in a scratch.

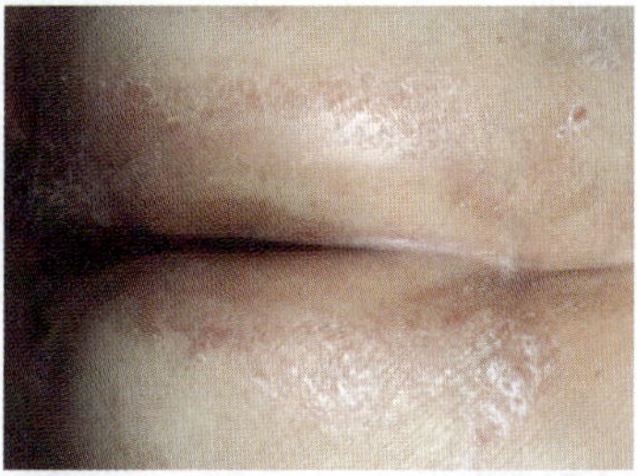

Fig. 9.3 Shiny well-demarcated erythema in flexural psoriasis. Scaling is lost in the moist flexure.

Common clinical patterns

Psoriasis vulgaris (plaque psoriasis)

This is the most common pattern of psoriasis (Box 9.4). Onset may be gradual or sudden. Disease may be limited to a few sites or widespread. Measure the extent of disease and assess severity—see 🕮 PASI, p.186.

What should I look for?

- Well-defined pinkish scaly plaques of variable size, thickness, and shape in a symmetrical pattern, predominantly on extensor surfaces. Examine elbows and knees, the hairline (psoriasis is uncommon on the face but often involves the scalp margin), and the trunk 🕮 Fig. 9.1, p.181.
- Silvery scaling over the surface of the plaques: this may be thick in untreated disease or minimal if the patient is applying a treatment such as a topical corticosteroid.
- Bleeding points where scale has been scratched off.
- Plaques in the scalp: ask about 'dandruff', palpate to find the plaques. Scalp psoriasis is not obvious on inspection because hair is retained.
- The Köbner phenomenon: new psoriasis appearing at sites of cutaneous trauma including excoriations or surgical scars (Fig. 9.2).
- Post-inflammatory hypo- or hyperpigmentation: e.g. when psoriasis has improved after treatment or a sunny holiday.
- Nail involvement (50% of patients)—see Box 9.5, Fig. 9.4, and Fig. 9.5.
- Flexural psoriasis—see later in this section (🕮 Fig. 9.3, p.181).

Guttate psoriasis (gutta is Latin for droplet)

An acute form triggered by infection with group B haemolytic *Streptococcus* (usually tonsillitis or pharyngitis), that presents in children and adolescents. The rash erupts 2–3 weeks after the infection.

Guttate psoriasis usually resolves within 3 or 4 months, but some patients will progress to psoriasis vulgaris. Guttate psoriasis may recur after subsequent streptococcal infections.

What should I look for?

- A history of an infection preceding the eruption by 2–4 weeks.
- A history of the sudden onset of a widespread rash.
- Teardrop-sized erythematous scaly papules, mainly on the trunk.

Flexural psoriasis and sebopsoriasis

Psoriasis in moist flexural sites is not scaly and is often misdiagnosed as fungal infection, but symmetry suggests psoriasis (🕮 Fig. 9.3, p.181).

What should I look for?

- Well-defined, shiny, erythematous, minimally raised plaques in flexures including inframammary skin, umbilicus, axillae, groins, and natal cleft.
- Ill-defined erythematous greasy, slightly scaly skin in the central face (nasolabial folds), eyebrows, behind and within ears, and the scalp resembling seborrhoeic dermatitis (sebopsoriasis).
- Nail signs may help to confirm the diagnosis of psoriasis—see Box 9.5.

Box 9.4 Clinical patterns of psoriasis

Patients may have >1 pattern of psoriasis:

- Psoriasis vulgaris (large plaque and/or small plaque) on extensor surfaces.
- Guttate psoriasis (sudden onset of widespread scaly papules triggered by a streptococcal tonsillitis or pharyngitis).
- Flexural (inverse) psoriasis, also known as sebopsoriasis, may be difficult to distinguish from seborrhoeic dermatitis—see 📖 p.203.
- Palmoplantar pustulosis; generalized pustular psoriasis.
- Erythrodermic psoriasis.
- Nail psoriasis: may be the only sign of psoriasis.
- Napkin psoriasis—📖 Box 31.12, p.557.

Box 9.5 The nails in psoriasis

Nail signs may help to confirm the diagnosis of psoriasis. Signs depend on the location of the pathology—nail matrix or nail bed.

- Pits: usually small and shallow and scattered irregularly (likened to the surface of a thimble) but may be deep—best seen with magnification and side lighting. Psoriasis of the proximal matrix leads to a defective nail plate which partially desquamates leaving a depression on the surface of the nail (equivalent to scale on the surface of the skin)—Fig. 9.4.
- Onycholysis (separation of the free edge of the nail plate from the nail bed): the nail appears yellowish-white with a proximal brownish-red margin—Fig. 9.5. Oval spots of salmon-coloured discoloration (oil spots). Both caused by psoriasis of the nail bed.
- Thickening and crumbling of the whole nail plate: caused by psoriasis of the entire nail matrix. (Asymmetrical nail dystrophy suggests fungal infection. In psoriasis, most nails are affected.)
- Subungual hyperkeratosis: caused by psoriasis of the nail bed.
- Splinter haemorrhages in fingernails.
- Soft tissue swelling of proximal nail fold with chronic paronychia and horizontal ridging of nail plate.
- Acral pustulosis/parakeratosis pustulosa—see 📖 Box 9.8, p.185, p.194.

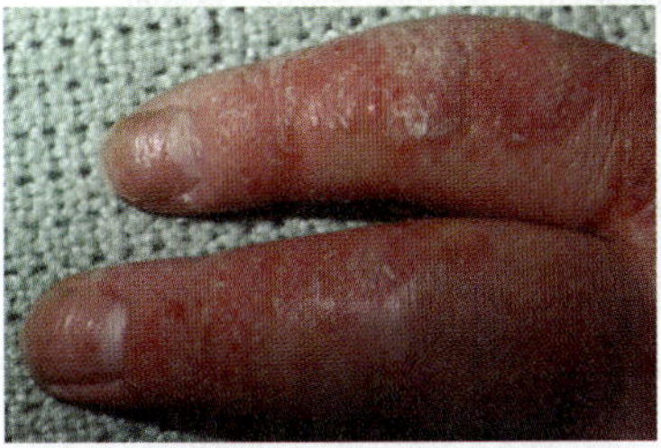

Fig. 9.4 Nail pitting and psoriatic arthropathy.

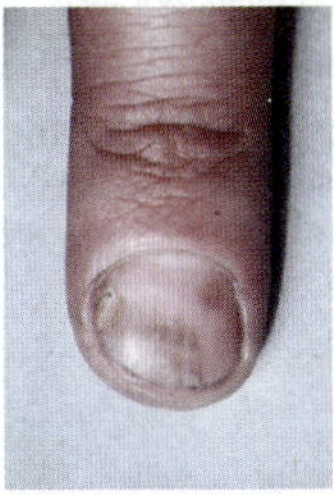

Fig. 9.5 Onycholysis.

Erythrodermic and pustular psoriasis

Erythrodermic psoriasis

Erythroderma is defined as redness and scaling affecting 90% of the BSA. Plaque psoriasis may evolve into erythroderma suddenly or gradually. Topical treatments that irritate the skin may precipitate erythroderma as may some systemic drugs. Psoriasis may also flare after withdrawal of systemic corticosteroids. Less often, patients with no past history of psoriasis will present erythrodermic.

What should I do?

- Ask if the patient has any history of previous skin diseases (conditions such as atopic eczema may become erythrodermic) or has started any new drugs.
- Check the nails for signs of psoriasis.
- Seek expert help—erythroderma is a form of skin failure. The principles of management are discussed on 🕮 p.103.
- ⚠The skin is easily irritated—prescribe a bland emollient.
- Once the condition is stable, you may be able to introduce specific treatments e.g. UVB, tar, methotrexate.

Palmoplantar pustulosis

Palmoplantar pustulosis is a chronic condition affecting palms and soles (Box 9.6) that is seen most often in middle-aged women who smoke cigarettes, but stopping smoking does not alleviate the problem. Genetic studies have shown that palmoplantar pustulosis is not linked to the same loci as psoriasis vulgaris. Most patients do not have any other psoriasis. For management see Box 9.7.

Palmoplantar pustulosis is clinically and histologically identical to early keratoderma blenorrhagicum—see 🕮 p.194. Palmoplantar pustulosis also seems to have been triggered in some patients by treatment with anti-TNF drugs—see 🕮 p.362.

Generalized pustular psoriasis

This rare life-threatening presentation is often misdiagnosed as infection because patients have a fever, neutrophilia, and widespread superficial (subcorneal) pustules on a background of erythema. The clinical features are outlined in 🕮 Box 5.25, p.117. ⚠Pustular psoriasis may be precipitated by withdrawal of oral or very potent topical corticosteroids.

What should I do? See 🕮 p.116.

Acropustulosis and parakeratosis pustulosa

Rarely pustulosis may affect one or more digits in the absence of other forms of psoriasis—see Box 9.8 and 🕮 p.194.

Box 9.6 Palmoplantar pustulosis: what should I look for?

- Well-defined erythematous scaly plaques on palms and/or soles are studded with pustules and/or vesicopustules.
- Dried-up pustules appear as yellowish-brown, slightly scaly papules.
- The condition may be unilateral.
- Hyperkeratosis and fissuring complicate the picture.
- The condition may resemble infected chronic dermatitis, particularly if the vesicopustules and hyperkeratosis dominate the picture (vesicles without pustules suggest eczema).

Box 9.7 Palmoplantar pustulosis: what should I do?

- The diagnosis is clinical—a skin biopsy is not usually required.
- Take skin scrapes to exclude fungal infection, particularly if unilateral.
- If hyperkeratosis with vesicopustules dominates the picture, it may be difficult to decide if the patient has infected dermatitis or psoriasis. Patch test to exclude an allergic contact dermatitis if any doubt.
- Greasy emollients and soap substitutes reduce the tendency to fissuring.
- Potent or highly potent topical corticosteroid ointments applied twice daily will control inflammation and pustules in many patients. Skin on palms and soles is thick so steroids can be used for a considerable time before producing atrophy. However, disease tends to be chronic and the use of topical corticosteroids must be monitored. If disease is not well controlled after 8–12 weeks, an alternative therapy should be considered.
- Keratolytics such as salicylic acid are combined with a topical corticosteroid in some proprietary preparations. These may control hyperkeratotic disease.
- Topical vitamin D_3 analogues or 0.1% tacrolimus ointment may be helpful.
- Deep fissures—close with quick-drying glues such as superglue.
- Localized UV light treatment can be helpful (topical PUVA).
- Acitretin 20–30mg/day achieves control in some patients.

Box 9.8 What are acropustulosis and parakeratosis pustulosa?

- ***Acrodermatitis continua/acrodermatitis of Hallopeau:*** affects 1 or more digits. Sterile pustules form beneath and around the nail plate which is lifted off by crust and lakes of pus. Nail loss may be permanent and associated with resorptive osteolysis. Very potent topical steroids or oral retinoids are indicated.
- ***Parakeratosis pustulosa:*** affects a single digit in young children. The skin is erythematous and scaly. Pustules or vesicles may be present early, but do not persist and the changes look eczematous. The nail plate lifts up and becomes thickened. The condition is chronic but self-limiting. Topical steroids may be helpful. It is uncertain whether this condition is a form of eczema or psoriasis.

Assessing severity

Severity is a function of both the extent of the disease (impairment) and the impact on quality of life (disability). Impact should be assessed with a tool such as the DLQI—see 📖 p.32.

Severity may be measured using a global rating—see Box 9.9—or with a disease-specific tool such as the Psoriasis Area and Severity Index (PASI).

Box 9.9 Global assessment

- Mild = <5% BSA.
- Moderate = 5–10% BSA.
- Severe = >10% BSA.

Measure BSA using the patient's hand. The palm and palmar surface of the digits = 1% of the BSA. But a simple assessment of area of involvement does not take into account other problems such as itch, scale, redness, or thickness of plaques.

What is the PASI? See Fig. 9.6

The PASI is a tool that was devised for assessing chronic plaque psoriasis. The PASI is a widely used outcome measure in clinical trials—a PASI 50 means that the patient shows a 50% improvement from the baseline PASI.

The PASI can be used in your practice to record the progress of patients with chronic plaque psoriasis. It is less useful in other forms of disease such as palmoplantar pustulosis.

How do I interpret the PASI?

- Higher scores indicate more severe psoriasis.
- Although the PASI ranges from 0 (no psoriasis) to 72 (100% coverage in the worst possible psoriasis), in practice a PASI of 12 or more indicates severe chronic plaque psoriasis and a PASI of <7 indicates mild chronic-plaque psoriasis.

How is the PASI calculated? See Fig. 9.6

- The body is divided into 4 anatomical regions (head, upper limbs, trunk, lower limbs).
- Redness (erythema), thickness (infiltration), and scaling in the psoriatic plaques in each region are each scored on a 5-point scale (0 = none, 1 = slight; 2 = moderate; 3 = severe; 4 = very severe).
- The area of skin affected in each region is estimated and given a numerical value.
- The final calculation uses a simple formula to adjust the score for each region according to the proportion that the skin in each region is of all the skin.
- The PASI will only take you a few minutes to complete once you have had some practice. PASI scoring sheets which will take you through the calculation are widely available.
- Although the PASI is subjective, with experience results are reproducible.

Score for symptom and area for head, trunk, upper and lower limbs

Score	0	1	2	3	4	5	6
Erythema Infiltration Desquamation	None	Slight	Moderate	Severe	Very severe		
Area %	0	<10	10<30	30<50	50<70	70<90	90–100

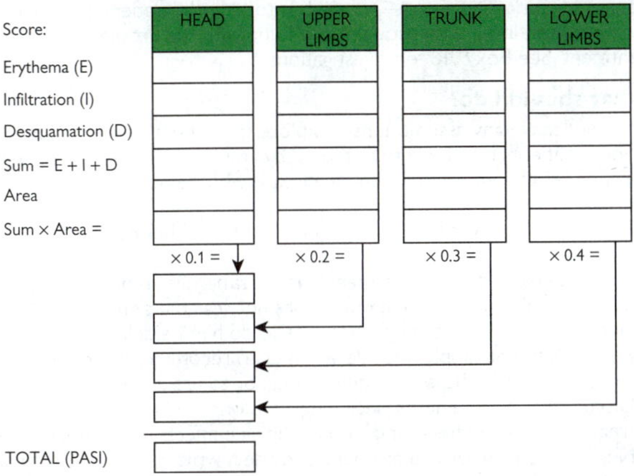

Fig. 9.6 Psoriasis area and severity index (PASI). Adapted with permission of Salford Royal Hospital NHS Trust © 2002.

Further reading

Feldman SR and Krueger G. *Ann Rheum Dis* 2005; **64**(Suppl II):ii65–ii68.

Schmitt J and Wozel G. *Dermatology* 2005; **210:**194–9.

Approach to management

Most psoriasis is not life threatening, but living with psoriasis can ruin lives. You are breaking bad news when you explain to someone that he/she has psoriasis. Treatments offer control rather than cure—psoriasis remits despite treatment, not because of treatment.

Your assessment should have provided insight into the impact of the disease, the efficacy of previous treatments, and the extent of disease. Managing psoriasis is an art—your job is to help the patient to find a balance between living with psoriasis and living with the problems caused by treatment. See Box 9.10 for investigations.

What should I do?

- Do not make any assumptions—explore the patient's expectations. Some patients may be very bothered by limited skin disease. You will also meet patients with extensive disease who do not want systemic drugs.
- Explain what is possible—treatments can control but not cure psoriasis.
- Does the patient want treatment? No treatment is an option—psoriasis may scar the mind but it does not scar the skin.
- Find out what the patient can manage to do him/herself.
- Keep treatment simple. Decide whether to recommend topical treatments, UV light, or a systemic drug, or to use a combination.
- Discuss the likely benefits (including how long it will take before treatment has an effect) and explain the side effects of treatments.
- Negotiate a plan for management, provide a written management plan, and agree follow-up arrangements.
- Provide information about psoriasis, including patient support groups such as the Psoriasis Association (UK).
- Advise on life style to minimize cardiovascular risk.

Topical treatment See 📖 p.190.

Ultraviolet light

Patients with widespread psoriasis, including guttate psoriasis, may benefit from a 6–8-week course of phototherapy with UVB (broadband 311–313nm or narrow band 311nm). UVB may be combined with topical vitamin D_3 analogues, tazarotene, or systemic treatments (methotrexate, retinoids). Sunbeds emit UVA, which is much less effective than UVB.

Systemic treatments

PUVA photochemotherapy (oral psoralen plus UVA 320–400nm) is more carcinogenic than UVB.

Methotrexate (weekly dose), oral retinoids (acitretin), and ciclosporin are the most widely used systemic drugs in extensive disease. Other options include fumaric acid esters, mycophenolate mofetil, hydroxycarbamide, and leflunomide—see 📖 Chapter 33, p.594.

The new biological agents (e.g. anti-TNFα) have revolutionized treatment of severe psoriasis unresponsive to other treatments.

Box 9.10 Investigations in psoriasis

- Diagnosis is not usually a problem and skin biopsies are seldom required.
- If disease is asymmetrical, take skin scrapings or nail clippings for fungal culture.
- If the patient is obese and at risk of the metabolic syndrome, check fasting glucose, cholesterol, and triglycerides.

Screening prior to systemic treatment

If you are considering prescribing systemic treatments check:

- FBC.
- Liver function and renal function.
- Pro-collagen peptide 3 (prior to methotrexate).
- Fasting cholesterol and triglycerides (prior to oral retinoids).

Further reading

Menter A and Griffiths CE. *Lancet* 2007; **370:**272–84.

Topical treatments

General principles

- Topical treatment is a reasonable option for limited disease.
- Discuss the likely outcome—control not cure. Explain that you are not aiming to get rid of the psoriasis, but to make the condition tolerable.
- Patients need time (and may need help) to apply treatments. If time is a problem, suggest concentrating on the most troublesome area.
- Demonstrate how to apply the treatment—ideally you will have a specialist nurse to help you.
- Select the right base (usually the one the patient prefers) for each treatment—ointment, cream, lotion, gel, or foam.
- Keep the treatment plan simple—the patient is much more likely to adhere to treatment—and prescribe enough of the preparations.
- In patients with extensive disease, topical treatments can be combined with UV light or with systemic treatment.

Emollients

- Emollient creams (moisturizers) reduce scale and may relieve itch partially, but are less effective in psoriasis than eczema.

Vitamin D_3 analogues: most suitable for limited plaque psoriasis

- Vitamin D_3 analogues (e.g. calcitriol, calcipotriol, tacalcitol) are effective if applied $\times 1$–2/day for at least 3 months. Patients like these preparations because they are colourless and odourless.
- Plaques eventually become erythematous smooth patches, but do not disappear.
- Vitamin D_3 analogues may be used for short periods in combination with a potent topical corticosteroid to reduce the likelihood of irritation (combination preparations are available).
- Vitamin D_3 analogues are not suitable for extensive psoriasis because treatment has to be limited to the affected skin and patients should not use more than 100g per week because of the risk of hypercalcaemia.
- Some vitamin D_3 analogues may irritate and are not suitable for the face or flexures.

Tar lotion: suitable for limited or widespread plaque psoriasis

- 1% coal tar lotion (Exorex® lotion) applied $\times 1$–2/day is as effective as a topical vitamin D_3 analogue for trunk and limbs and easier to use in widespread psoriasis because application does not have to be limited to affected skin.
- The lotion can be applied quickly all over the skin.
- Coal tar lotion may irritate and is not suitable for the face or flexures.
- Patients may not like the smell, but this is reduced by applying an emollient on top of the lotion.
- 10% liquor picis carbonis (LPC) in emulsifying ointment is also suitable for home use, but it is messier to use than coal tar lotion.

Topical corticosteroids: most suitable for limited plaque psoriasis

- Potent and highly potent corticosteroid creams or ointments are clean and easy to use.
- Applied ×1–2/day daily, corticosteroids are very effective and work quickly.
- If used for prolonged periods corticosteroids cause skin atrophy. Large amounts used for prolonged periods may also cause adrenal suppression.
- Psoriasis tends to rebound when corticosteroids are stopped abruptly.
- Patients should be reviewed 8-weekly if using potent topical corticosteroids and usage kept to a minimum (<50g/week).

Topical retinoids: most suitable for limited plaque psoriasis

- Topical retinoid (tazarotene) may reduce thickness, scaling, and erythema if applied ×1/day for 3 months, but can be irritant.

Facial and flexural psoriasis

- Calcineurin inhibitor (tacrolimus, pimecrolimus) ointments can be useful in facial and flexural psoriasis (sebopsoriasis).
- Moderately potent topical corticosteroids are suitable for facial and flexural psoriasis, including sebopsoriasis. Apply ×1–2/day. For flexures the corticosteroid is usually combined with an antifungal agent such as miconazole. Stronger topical corticosteroids are more effective, but very likely to cause atrophy in thin flexural skin.
- Some vitamin D_3, analogues are suitable for the face or flexures, but others irritate the skin.

Scalp

- Mild scale: control with potent or highly potent steroid lotions or foams applied at night or use a vitamin D_3 analogue scalp preparation. Advise the patient not to let the preparation drip onto the neck or forehead (risk of atrophy).
- Thick scale: remove with keratolytic scalp compound e.g. Cocois®, Sebco® (coal tar solution and salicylic acid in coconut oil with applicator nozzle). Apply to scalp (part the hair) once weekly. If severe use daily for first 3–7 days. Leave on overnight and shampoo off next morning.
- Tar shampoos may be helpful.

Inpatients

- Dithranol (anthralin) and crude coal tar preparations, once the mainstay of topical treatment, are no longer first-line therapies. They are messy and difficult to use. They tend to be reserved for inpatients or for day care often combined with UVB.

Psoriatic arthritis

4–30% of patients with psoriasis have an associated arthritis. 70% of these patients develop psoriasis before arthritis, 10–15% arthritis before psoriasis, and in the rest the 2 occur within 1 year of each other. See Box 9.11 for classification criteria.

Joint involvement is classified into 5 major clinical subtypes which overlap. Most patients present with monoarthritis or oligoarthritis, but more joints tend to be involved in long-standing disease. Erosive and deforming arthritis occurs in 40–60% of patients. Simultaneous flares in skin and joint disease have been reported, but there is conflicting evidence about whether severity of psoriasis is related to severity of arthritis.

What should I look for?

- A history of joint stiffness in the mornings that lasts >30min suggesting inflammatory disease.
- Symmetrical polyarthritis that may be indistinguishable from rheumatoid arthritis (rheumatoid factor negative, no rheumatoid nodules). Look for boggy soft tissue swelling in the small joints of hands suggesting synovitis.
- Asymmetric oligoarthritis with <5 small or large joints affected in an asymmetrical pattern. Look for effusions in large joints, e.g. knees.
- Distal interphalangeal (DIP) inflammation usually with psoriatic nail changes.
- Involvement of spine (spondylitis) and sacroiliac joints (sacroilietis). This pattern is associated with the MHC class I molecule HLA-B27 like the other seronegative spondyloarthropathies (see 📖 Reactive arthritis 📖 p.194 and 📖 SAPHO syndrome, p.228).
- Arthritis mutilans = destruction of the small joints of the hand, especially the DIP joints. This is associated with prolonged disease.
- Dactylitis, i.e. swelling of a whole digit producing a sausage-like appearance (seen in 1/3 of patients). Probably a combination of tenosynovitis and synovitis or diffuse digital oedema (Fig. 9.4).
- Enthesopathy, i.e. pain at sites where ligaments, tendons, fascia, and joint capsule are inserted into bone, e.g. at the heel (plantar fasciitis), elbow (golfer's elbow or tennis elbow), and the Achilles tendon.

What should I do?

- Investigations—see Box 9.12.
- Early treatment prevents joint destruction, deformity and loss of function.
- Refer to a rheumatologist if symptoms not controlled by anti-inflammatory agents, or evidence of synovitis, joint effusion, or deformity.
- Management options—see Box 9.13.

Box 9.11 CASPAR criteria for classifying psoriatic arthritis

These criteria were developed in 2006 for classification in research rather than for diagnostic purposes. Sensitivity 91%, specificity 98%.

Inflammatory musculoskeletal disease with features such as erythema, warmth and swelling of joints; morning and rest stiffness; painful joints, spine, and/or enthesium.

Plus at least 3 points from the following features:

- Current psoriasis (score = 2).
- A past history of psoriasis (unless psoriasis is present) (score = 1).
- A family history of psoriasis (unless psoriasis is present or there is a history of psoriasis) (score = 1).
- Nail changes (score = 1).
- Dactylitis (score = 1).
- Juxta-articular new bone formation on radiographs (score =1).
- Negative rheumatoid factor (score = 1).

Box 9.12 Investigations in suspected psoriatic arthritis

- FBC: normocytic anaemia; leucocytosis in acute inflammatory arthritis.
- CRP: raised in acute inflammatory arthritis.
- ESR or plasma viscosity: raised in acute inflammatory arthritis.
- Renal function, LFTs (raised alkaline phosphatase in inflammation; ensure otherwise normal LFT and electrolytes prior to prescribing disease modifying antirheumatic drugs such as methotrexate).
- Rheumatoid factor: usually negative in psoriatic arthritis.
- Radiographs of affected joints or lumbar spine and sacroiliac joints if low back pain sounds inflammatory, i.e. stiffness improving with exercise and not relieved by rest.

Box 9.13 Management of psoriatic arthritis

- Early treatment prevents joint destruction, deformity, and loss of function. Patients benefit from a multidisciplinary approach involving physiotherapists, occupational therapists and podiatrists, as well as rheumatologists and orthopaedic surgeons.
- Pharmacological:
  - Mono- or oligoarticular disease may be managed with NSAIDs or intra-articular steroids (warn patients about potential flare of psoriasis as effect of intra-articular steroid wears off).
  - More severe erosive or polyarticular disease is treated with disease-modifying antirheumatic drugs such as methotrexate, sulfasalazine, or leflunomide. Anti-TNF biologic agents may be indicated in severe disease unresponsive to other treatments.
- Patients with severe skin and joint disease requiring systemic therapy may be managed best by rheumatologists working with dermatologists in a combined clinic.
- Surgical: timely fusion of unstable joints prevents arthritis mutilans.

Reactive arthritis

What is reactive arthritis?

Reactive arthritis is a seronegative, HLA-B27-linked, spondyloarthropathy that shares features with the other arthropathies in this group including psoriatic arthritis—see 🕮 p.192. Typically patients (usually men aged 20–40) have a mono- or oligoarthritis affecting the lower limbs. Mucocutaneous signs are common.

Arthritis develops several days to several weeks after an extra-articular infection. Viable pathogen is not detected in the joint itself (though intra-articular bacteria or bacterial fragments have been identified). The common causes of reactive arthritis are genitourinary infections (e.g. *Chlamydia* trachomatis) and gastrointestinal infections (e.g. *Yersinia, Shigella, Salmonella,* and *Campylobacter*). HIV infection is another cause.

The triad of arthritis, a sterile (aseptic) urethritis, and conjunctivitis in a patient with dysentery was described by Reiter in 1916. The term Reiter's syndrome is still used sometimes to describe this triad in patients with reactive arthritis.

What mucocutaneous signs should I look for?

- Keratoderma blenorrhagicum—a pustular rash on palms and soles—clinically and pathologically indistinguishable from palmoplantar pustulosis. However, pustules are followed by gross conical hyperkeratosis, which are not usually seen in palmoplantar pustulosis or psoriasis—see 🕮 p.184.
- Nail changes tend to be more pustular than in psoriasis and include:
  - Onycholysis, ridging, and splitting.
  - Brownish-red or greenish-yellow discoloration of the nails.
  - Small yellow pustules under the nail often near the lunula.
  - Subungual hyperkeratosis.
  - Nail pitting.
- Erythematous macules at the urethral meatus and on the glans penis. These may coalesce into a circinate scaly erythematous patch (circinate balanitis)—see Fig. 9.7.
- Flaccid pustular lesions that develop thick horny scale.
- Well-demarcated erythematous scaly psoriasiform plaques on the scrotum, buttocks, trunk, and limbs.
- Thick psoriasiform scale in the scalp.
- Asymptomatic superficial erosions in oral mucosa.
- Patches of denuded papillae on the tongue.
- Bilateral mucopurulent conjunctivitis, acute anterior uveitis (photophobia, redness, watering, pain, decreased visual acuity), keratitis (corneal inflammation).

What should I do for cutaneous disease?

Manage as you would psoriasis or palmoplantar pustulosis—see 🕮 Box 9.7, p.185. Treatment options include moderately potent topical corticosteroids and oral retinoids.

The condition is self limiting, but relapses are common.

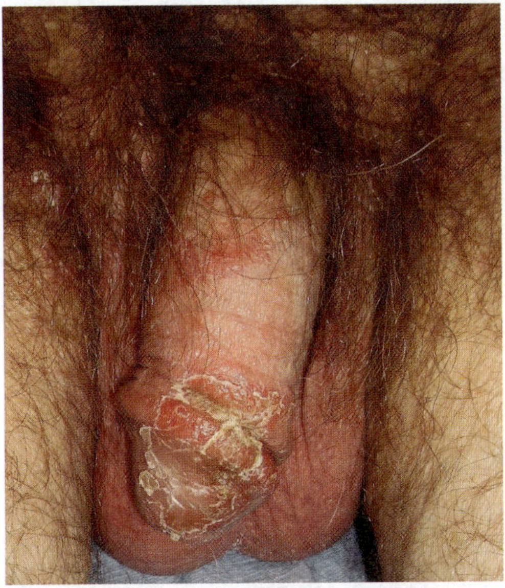

Fig. 9.7 Well-demarcated erythematous scaly patch on penis.

Chapter 10

Eczema and lichen planus

Contents

Relevant pages in other chapters

Childhood eczema is discussed in 📖 Chapter 31, p.554, p.556, p.558, p.560
Use of emollients and topical corticosteroids—📖 p.584, p.586
Soaks and wet dressings—📖 p.592

What is eczema (dermatitis)?

The word eczema, derived from the Greek 'to break out or boil over' refers to the vesicles (bubbles) seen in acute eczema. Dermatitis means inflammation of skin. The terms tend to be used synonymously.

Eczema is a cutaneous reaction pattern that is poorly understood and this is reflected by the confusing terminology used to describe different patterns of eczema—see Box 10.1. Oedema within and between keratinocytes (spongiosis) may produce weeping with thin-walled vesicles (intra-epidermal) that soon rupture.

Eczema may be endogenous, the commonest form being atopic eczema, or exogenous, but the barrier function of the epidermis is abnormal in most forms of eczema so the skin is easily irritated.

What should I look for?

Eczema is itchy. Patients with acutely inflamed eczema may also be very uncomfortable. Endogenous disease tends to be symmetrical, whereas the distribution of a contact dermatitis is determined by the site of the contact. Signs depend on whether acute, subacute, or chronic, but include combinations of:

- Erythema: often ill defined—see 🕮 Fig. 31.8, p.561 (compare with psoriasis which is well defined—see 🕮 Fig. 9.1, p.181).
- Scaling, i.e. epidermal pathology: may not be present in the early stages of acute contact eczema in which skin is erythematous and oedematous—see 🕮 Fig. 10.1, p.201 and Figs. 10.2 and 10.3, p.204.
- Scratch marks (excoriations).
- Papules, oedema, and/or vesicles (occasionally bullae) in acute eczema.
- Exudation of serous fluid (weeping) and crusting in acute eczema (crusting may be a sign of secondary bacterial infection as may pustules).
- Thickening of the skin with increased skin markings (lichenification) secondary to endless rubbing in chronic eczema—see 🕮 Fig. 31.9, p.561.
- Prurigo (itchy erythematous nodules): secondary to chronic rubbing—see 🕮 Fig.10.6, p.207.
- Hyperkeratosis in chronic eczema.
- Hyperpigmentation secondary to chronic rubbing.
- Postinflammatory hypo- or hyperpigmentation in dark skins.

What should I do?

- Generally a skin biopsy is not required—the histology will not tell you the cause of the eczema and the diagnosis is clinical.
- Take skin swabs from crusted weeping eczema for bacterial culture.
- In vesicular rashes, exclude herpesvirus infection. Eczema herpeticum may complicate atopic eczema—see 🕮 p.106.
- Skin scrapes to exclude fungal (dermatophyte) infection in asymmetrical scaly rashes.
- Patch test if you suspect allergic contact dermatitis—see 🕮 p.200.
- Topical treatments—see 🕮 Chapter 33, p.582.

Common patterns of eczema

Eczema is a cutaneous reaction pattern that is poorly understood and this is reflected by the complexity of the terminology applied to eczematous conditions (see Box 10.1). The name may imply cause (contact dermatitis), links with other diseases (atopic eczema), the appearance of the skin (discoid eczema, pompholyx, asteatotic eczema), or the distribution (varicose eczema, seborrhoeic eczema).

Patients may have >1 type of eczema—for example, the abnormal skin barrier function in atopic eczema predisposes to irritant contact dermatitis; environmental irritants such as soap exacerbate asteatotic eczema; and allergic contact dermatitis may be superimposed on varicose eczema.

Box 10.1 Patterns of eczema (dermatitis)

Endogenous

- Atopic
- Seborrhoeic
- Discoid (nummular)
- Pompholyx (dyshidrotic)
- Varicose (gravitational, venous stasis)
- Asteatotic
- Prurigo nodularis
- Lichen simplex.

Exogenous

- Irritant contact
- Allergic contact
- Photodermatitis
- Drug-induced eczema.

Contact dermatitis

What is contact dermatitis?

Contact dermatitis is caused by exposure of the skin either to an irritant or an allergen. Irritant contact dermatitis is more common than allergic contact dermititis. Impaired skin barrier function facilitates the penetration of irritants and contact allergens into the epidermis, e.g. in atopic individuals, neonates, or the elderly. Hands and forearms are often affected by contact dermatitis. Individuals at risk of occupational contact dermatitis include hairdressers, nurses, housewives, caterers, and builders (Fig. 10.1).

Irritant contact dermatitis

Urine and faeces are irritants—the buttocks and perineum may be affected in incontinent patients. Detergents, alkalis, solvents, and cutting oils are also potential irritants. Some plants contain light-sensitizing furocoumarin chemicals that are phototoxic in the presence of sunlight—see 🕮 Box 16.6, p.305.

Allergic contact dermatitis

The pathogenesis is a delayed (type 4) cell-mediated allergic reaction—see Box 10.2. The patient has to be sensitized by prior exposure before developing an allergic reaction that is characterized by itching, erythema, vesiculation, and scaling. For common cutaneous allergens—see Box 10.3.

Always consider patch testing in chronic hand dermatitis, facial dermatitis, pruritus ani (when many over-the-counter medicaments may have been used), and dermatitis associated with chronic leg ulcers. Patch tests are applied on day 0, are removed and read on day 2 and usually read again on day 4 or 5. A positive result is indicated by an eczematous reaction.

What should I ask?

- Take a history as recommended in 🕮 Chapter 2 p.22. Ask about occupation and hobbies; is the patient an obsessive handwasher?—see 🕮 p.542.
- Find out what the patient puts on the skin—cosmetics, perfumes, hair dyes, over-the-counter medicaments, etc. Remember that the patient may become allergic to a product that has been used for some time.
- Explore what provokes the rash. Does the problem improve when the patient is not in contact with the preparation, e.g. weekends, holidays?
- Has the patient a history of atopic eczema (irritant contact dermatitis is more common than allergic contact dermatitis in atopics).

What should I do?

- Exclude secondary infection, particularly in genital dermatitis.
- Minimize contact with irritants, e.g. by avoiding soap and using gloves, and prescribe emollients. This may be sufficient to alleviate the problem, but the patient may have to consider a different occupation.
- Reduce inflammation with a potent corticosteroid ointment. A short course of prednisolone may be needed in severe blistering reactions.
- Refer for patch testing if you suspect an allergic contact dermatitis.
- If the patient is allergic to something, any contact with that allergen will produce a reaction and complete avoidance is essential. An inevitable consequence of this diagnosis may be change of occupation.

Box 10.2 Pathogenesis of allergic contact dermatitis

- Abnormalities in skin barrier function may facilitate penetrance of allergen and make some patients more prone to developing an allergic contact dermatitis—see Box 1.2, p.6.
- Antigen penetrates the stratum cornea and enters the epidermis.
- Antigen is taken up by dendritic Langerhans cells within the epidermis and processed into small peptides. Peptides bound to class II MHC proteins are expressed on the surface of Langerhans cells. (Dermal dendritic cells may also process and present antigens.)
- Langerhans cells bearing antigen migrate from the skin via lymphatics to the pancortical area of the draining lymph node where they activate CD4+ T-lymphocytes.
- IL-1 released by Langerhans cells triggers T-cells to release IL-2 and proliferate with the generation of allergen-specific memory T-cells. These will recognize the antigen on re-exposure and migrate to the challenge site to produce cytokines and cytotoxic damage to the skin. This results in itch, erythema, and oedema.

Box 10.3 Some common cutaneous allergens

- Nickel: in cheap jewellery and jean studs.
- Chrome: in cement.
- Fragrance mix: in perfumed cosmetics, soaps, household furniture spray polishes, etc.
- Rubber hardeners (mercapto-mix) and accelerators (thiuram-mix).
- Epoxy resin: in quick-setting adhesive mixtures.
- Colophony: adhesive in adhesive plaster.
- Paraphenylene diamine (PPD): in dark dyes.
- Parabens mix: preservative in many creams and lotions.
- Wool alcohols: lanolin in many creams.
- Medicaments such as benzocaine, neomycin, quinoline-mix, and hydrocortisone.
- Primin: in *Primula obconica*, a flowering house plant.

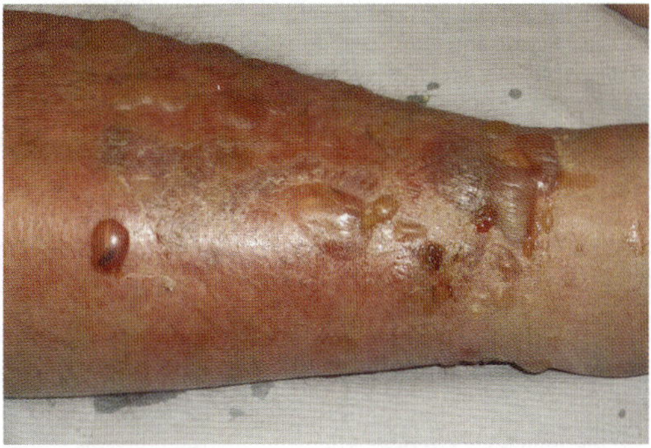

Fig. 10.1 Acute contact dermatitis simulating cellulitis with erythema and blistering.

Atopic eczema and seborrhoeic dermatitis in adults

Adult atopic eczema (dermatitis)

Atopic eczema is common in childhood. Eczema in 50–60% of children clears by puberty, but in others the disease is persistent or recurrent in adult life. In any adult with an eczematous rash, ask about personal or family history of atopic disease—infantile eczema, bronchial asthma, and/or allergic rhinitis. See 📖 Chapter 31, p.554–560 for more detailed discussion of the cause and management of atopic eczema in children.

What should I look for?

- Dry scaly skin.
- A symmetrical erythematous scaly rash, worse in flexures.
- Intense itch with excoriations, nodules (prurigo nodularis—see 📖 Fig. 10.6, p.207), and/or thickened (lichenified) skin secondary to scratching and rubbing—see 📖 Fig. 31.9, p.561.
- Crusting, weeping, or vesicles suggesting secondary infection (bacterial or herpesvirus). Widespread vesicles and a fever suggest eczema herpeticum, an emergency, most often seen in children—see 📖 p.106.
- Atopic individuals have skin that is easily irritated and adults may also have an irritant contact dermatitis, often on hands or face.
- Erythroderma in severe disease—see 📖 p.102.
- Thin skin (bruising, telangiectasia, striae) secondary to prolonged use of potent topical corticosteroids.

What should I do?

- Skin swabs for bacterial and viral culture if signs suggest infection.
- Soap substitutes (containing antibacterials) and emollients control dryness and reduce bacterial colonization of skin. Even though the patient may have a long history of eczema, it is worth finding out exactly how the skin is being managed and explaining how to use emollients and to avoid irritants such as soap or shower gels—see 📖 p.30, p.584 and p.592.
- Prescribe a moderate or potent topical corticosteroid ointment to use once or twice daily. 0.1% tacrolimus ointment is an alternative, but tacrolimus should not be used on infected skin.
- Oral antibiotics or antivirals to control infection if required.
- A sedating antihistamine may relieve irritation, e.g. hydroxyzine.
- A short course of oral prednisolone (30mg/day tailing off over 2–3 weeks) may be required for severe acute flares.
- Consider referral for patch tests to exclude an allergic contact dermatitis, particularly in patients with facial eczema or patients with no previous history of eczema.
- Consider skin biopsy to exclude cutaneous T-cell lymphoma if the patient does not have a personal or family history of atopic disease and this is a new presentation.
- Courses of phototherapy or steroid-sparing agents (e.g. azathioprine, ciclosporin) may be indicated in severe chronic disease.
- Wet dressings can help—see 📖 Box 33.4, p.593.

Adult seborrhoeic dermatitis (eczema)

The pathogenesis is poorly understood, but malassezia (pityrosporum) yeasts that are skin commensals are found in large numbers in involved skin. Reaction to the yeasts may play some part in the pathogenesis.

Adult seborrhoeic dermatitis is chronic and recurrent. Parkinson's disease and epilepsy predispose to seborrhoeic dermatitis. Patients with HIV/AIDS may have very severe disease. Although seborrhoeic dermatitis is not particularly itchy, it is disfiguring. Infantile seborrhoeic dermatitis is unrelated to the disease in adults—see 🕮 p.554.

What should I look for?

One or more sites may be affected.:

- Poorly-defined scalp erythema and fine white scale (dandruff). Hair is retained.
- Poorly defined greasy scaly erythema affecting nasolabial folds and central forehead.
- Fine scaling in eyebrows, behind ears, and within ears (otitis externa), and/or blepharitis.
- Orangish ill-defined erythema with fine scale in flexures—axillae, groins, umbilicus. May resemble flexural psoriasis—see 🕮 Fig. 9.3, p.181.
- Greasy scaly erythematous papules in central chest and central back. May have an annular configuration.
- Follicular papules or pustules over the back and sometimes the chest (pityrosporum folliculitis—see 🕮 Box 6.3, p.127).
- Normal nails—pitting suggests psoriasis.
- Erythroderma in severe disease—see 🕮 p.102.

What should I do?

It may be difficult to differentiate seborrhoeic dermatitis from flexural psoriasis (sebopsoriasis) but do not worry, the approach to management is similar. Consider HIV/AIDS in any patient with severe disease unresponsive to treatment. Your treatment should tackle inflammation, scaling, and the overgrowth of yeasts. Treatment options include:

- A creamy emollient to use as a soap substitute and skin moisturizer.
- 1% hydrocortisone ointment combined with an imidazole, e.g. Canesten HC®, Daktacort® applied ×2/day to the face and flexures—combinations of corticosteroid with antifungal are more effective than corticosteroid alone.
- A stronger topical corticosteroid may be needed for a short time in the flexures, e.g. Trimovate® cream.
- Topical 0.1% tacrolimus ointment ×2/day is an alternative to a mild corticosteroid for facial or flexural seborrhoeic dermatitis.
- Ketoconazole shampoo for the scalp and as a body wash (useful in pityrosporum folliculitis)—perhaps ×2–3/week. The shampoo is drying and can irritate the skin—the patient may also need to use a moisturizer.
- Alternative shampoos include preparations with tar or salicylic acid, e.g. Capasal®, Polytar®, T-Gel®.
- A potent steroid lotion applied overnight may control scalp disease, e.g. Betnovate® scalp application or Diprosalic® scalp application.

Other common types of eczema

Asteatotic eczema

This pattern of mildly itchy eczema, common in the elderly, is often precipitated by admission to hospital. Old skin is dried out by enthusiastic washing with soap, low humidity, and central heating.

What should I look for?

- The rash usually starts on the shins, but may spread in a patchy fashion to the thighs and trunk—also see 📖 p.534.
- A network of shallow erythematous fissures in the epidermis giving the skin the appearance of 'crazy paving' (eczema craquelé) (Fig. 10.2).

What should I do?

- Soap substitutes and emollients may be sufficient to settle irritation.
- Prescribe a mild topical corticosteroid ointment to use twice daily.

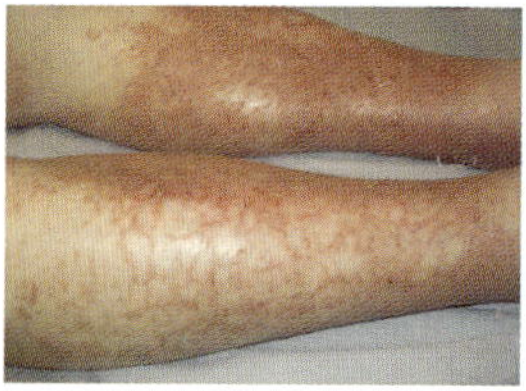

Fig. 10.2 Asteatotic eczema with a 'crazy paving' pattern of superficial cracking (eczema craquelé).

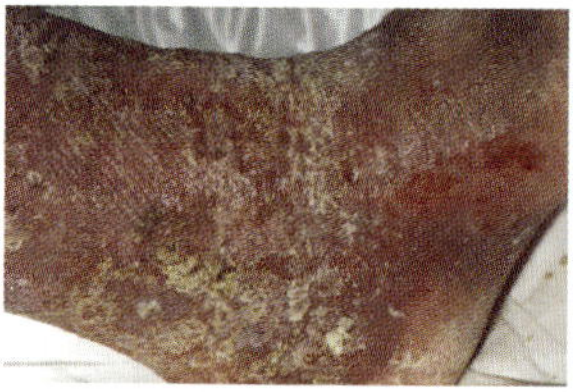

Fig. 10.3 Venous (stasis) eczema with erythema and scale in the gaiter area.

Varicose (stasis) eczema

What should I look for?

- Itching, erythema, scaling, and crusting (not pain) in the gaiter area.
- Signs of stasis-hyperpigmentation, oedema, atrophie blanche (see 📖 Box 15.5, p.279), or venous leg ulcers—see Fig. 10.3.
- The differential diagnosis includes cellulitis and contact dermatitis.

What should I do?

- Check the foot pulses and measure the ankle–brachial pressure index (ABPI) to exclude arterial disease—see 📖 p.280.
- Control oedema—ankle exercises, elevation, compression.
- Prescribe emollients and a moderately potent corticosteroid ointment.
- Refer for patch testing if the rash does not settle promptly—patients with chronic leg ulcers become sensitized to constituents in topical preparations.

Discoid (nummular = coin-shaped) eczema

The pathogenesis is uncertain, but this chronic eczema is common in middle age. Atopic eczema may present in a discoid pattern in children. Differential diagnosis includes psoriasis and fungal infection.

What should look for?

- A number of well-defined, extremely itchy, 'juicy' round or oval erythematous papules and plaques that may be scaly or vesicular (Fig. 10.4). (Vesicles are not seen in psoriasis.)
- Golden crusting is often a sign of secondary staphylococcal infection.
- The distribution tends to be symmetrical on limbs and trunk.
- Check the nails—they are normal in discoid eczema, unlike psoriasis.

What should I do?

- Take skin scrapings to exclude fungal (dermatophyte) infection.
- You may wish to take swabs for bacterial infection.
- Prescribe a soap substitute, an emollient, and a potent or very potent corticosteroid ointment to be applied ×2/day. Mild corticosteroid ointments are not sufficient to control irritation and inflammation.
- Treat infection with oral antibiotics.
- A sedating antihistamine in the evenings may relieve irritation at night.

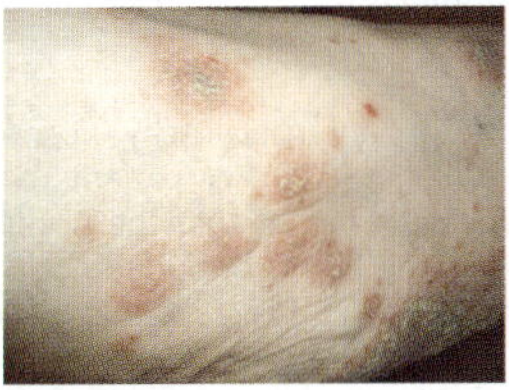

Fig. 10.4 Crusted itchy plaques in discoid eczema.

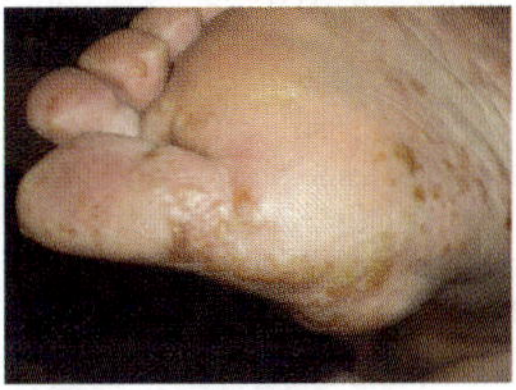

Fig. 10.5 Blisters in pompholyx eczema.

Pompholyx (cheiropompholyx; dyshidrotic eczema)

Pompholyx (Greek for bubble) is a common recurring endogenous dermatitis that usually occurs in people aged 20–40 years.

What should I look for?

- An itchy rash on the sides of the fingers and centre of palms and soles.
- Erythema and pinhead-size vesicles (not pustules) that may evolve into bullae (Fig.10.5).
- Peeling as the rash settles over 3–4 weeks.
- Exacerbations in hot weather.

What should I do?

- Exclude tinea pedis which sometimes precipitates pompholyx.
- Sooth weeping eczematous skin with 0.01% potassium permanganate soaks (make a solution of rosé wine colour) or 0.65% aluminium acetate solution (Burrow's solution)—see 🕮 p.592.
- Prescribe a potent corticosteroid lotion or cream to be applied ×2/day.
- Consider referral for patch tests—usually negative.

Chronic scratching and rubbing

Lichen simplex chronicus

A localized area of skin becomes thickened and leathery (lichenified) because of chronic rubbing—sometimes a stress-related habit—see Box 10.4. Lichen simplex favours sites such as the calf, the nape of the neck, the vulva, and perianal skin.

What should I do?

- Take scrapes from scaly lesions to exclude dermatophyte infection and swab genital skin to exclude candidiasis.
- Non-genital skin: apply a very potent corticosteroid ointment ×2/day or use under an occlusive hydrocolloid dressing, e.g. Duoderm®. The dressing protects the itchy skin from fingernails and can stay in place for 4 or 5 days, after which corticosteroid ointment is reapplied under a fresh dressing. Continue treatment until the skin has flattened and itch has settled—see 📖 p.590.
- Genital skin: treat with a potent corticosteroid–imidazole ointment for 1–2 weeks and then step down to a weaker corticosteroid–imidazole combination to reduce the risk of atrophy. Use aqueous cream as a soap substitute.
- Consider patch testing in genital lichen simplex.

Prurigo nodularis

A chronic form of eczema characterized by intensely itchy nodules. Pathogenesis is poorly understood—Box 10.4, but 80% of patients have a personal or family history atopy. Patients often insist that the nodules appear before the skin becomes itchy, but if the skin is occluded nodules flatten.

What should I look for?

- Middle-aged or older patient with excoriated firm erythematous nodules, 1–2cm diameter, usually symmetrically distributed on the extensor aspects of the limbs and the upper back. Numbers vary from a few to hundreds—Fig.10.6.
- Postinflammatory hyperpigmentation or scarring—Fig. 10.7.
- Normal skin in the centre of the back (difficult to scratch).

What should I do?

- Explain that it is difficult to find the cause of the itching… and to treat.
- Try to convince the patient that the changes are secondary to scratching.
- Exclude systemic causes of itching—renal failure, chronic liver disease, malignancies, psychological or psychiatric conditions, HIV.
- Exclude scabies.
- Attempt to break the itch–scratch cycle with a very potent corticosteroid ointment applied under occlusion—see 📖 p.590.
- Consider a course of UV light (UVB).
- Consider sedating antihistamines or a small dose of amitriptyline (10mg) at night.

Quantifying itch See 📖 p.32.

Box 10.4 What is itch?

- Itch is the commonest symptom in skin disorders but the neurophysiology is poorly understood and itch may be very difficult to control.
- The sensation of itch is transmitted by itch-dedicated afferent C neurons that are distinct from pain fibres.
- Itch causes a characteristic pattern of focal functional changes in the brain that is different from the changes seen in association with pain.
- Keratinocytes express neuropeptide mediators and receptors associated with itch. The epidermis with the associated fine intraepidermal C-neuron filaments is the 'itch receptor'.
- Visual, auditory, and other stimuli that activate the reticular system lead to inhibition of itch pathways, so itch is less troublesome during waking hours than at night.
- Histamine and other mast cell mediators mediate itch by activating C neurons.
- Keratinocytes also release neurotrophins that may predispose to itch by causing proliferation of unmyelinated afferent nerve terminals, sensitization of afferent nerve terminals, and increased expression of neuropeptides.
- Sensory neuropathy may cause localized itch often associated with burning, tingling, stinging, hypoaesthesia, or hyperalgesia (neuropathic itch)—see 📖 p.504.
- Localized itch, pain, or burning without any objective changes in the skin may be associated with psychological factors or stress—see 📖 p.526, and Box 28.1, p.525.

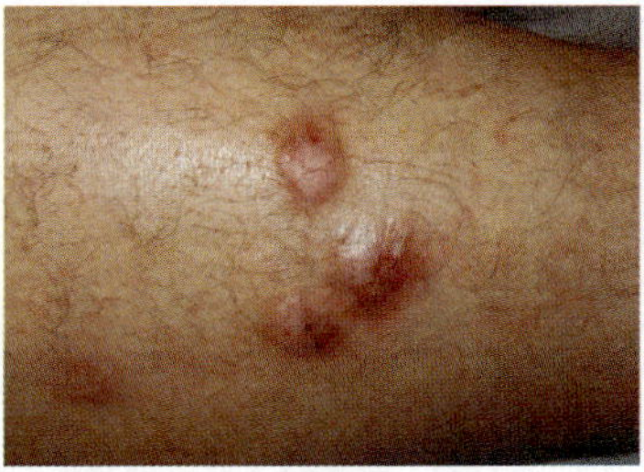

Fig. 10.6 Itchy nodules of prurigo nodularis.

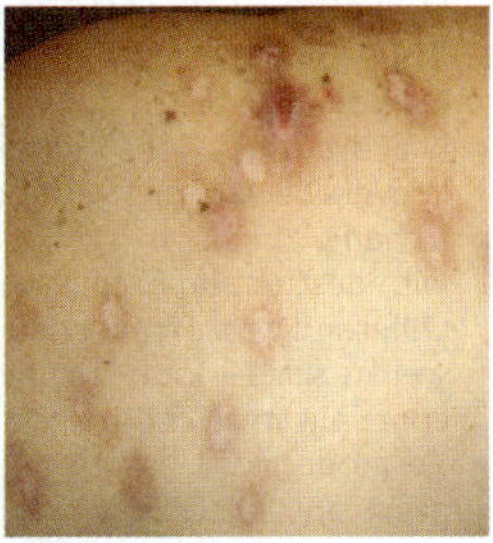

Fig. 10.7 Scarring secondary to picking and scratching in longstanding prurigo nodularis.

Lichen planus

Lichen planus (LP) is a chronic inflammatory condition of unknown cause that may affect skin and/or mucosal surfaces—see 📖 p.266.

A band-like 'lichenoid' infiltrate of lymphocytes hugs the basal layer of the epidermis or epithelium. Apoptotic basal keratinocytes release melanin into the dermis, where it is taken up by macrophages.

The prevalence of autoimmune conditions such as alopecia areata, vitiligo, and ulcerative colitis is increased in LP. Some studies suggest an increased prevalence of infections with hepatitis B or C virus. LP can also be drug-induced—see 📖 p.350.

Many variants of cutaneous LP have been described. Itching is a common complaint. Lichen nitidus may be a variant of LP—see Box 10.5. See Box 10.6 for management.

What should I look for?

- Flat-topped, smooth, shiny polygonal purplish-red itchy papules (lichenoid papules) in a symmetrical distribution often involving flexural aspects of wrists, but the rash may be localized or generalized. Unlike eczema, the skin is not particularly scaly (Fig. 10.8).
- Look closely to see the lacy white streaks (Wickham's striae) that overlie the surface of the papules.
- The Köbner phenomenon (papules in areas of trauma such as scratch marks).
- Lacy white streaks on buccal mucosa (cannot be scraped off, unlike mucosal candidiasis) and other oral and/or genital mucosal signs—see 📖 p.266.
- Hypertrophic LP: itchy hyperkeratotic purplish nodules on shins resembling lichen simplex.
- Annular LP: often flexural. Look in axillae and on shaft of penis.
- Photoexacerbated LP: differentiate from cutaneous LE by checking ANA (often negative in cutaneous LE) and taking a skin biopsy—see 📖 Box 16.5, p.305.
- Nail dystrophy: longitudinal ridging, atrophy of the nail plate, irreversible scarring with pterygium, and loss of nails.
- Lichen planopilaris (LPP): patchy inflammation around hair follicles with destruction of follicles and eventually a scarring alopecia. Differentiate from cutaneous discoid LE. LPP may affect body hair as well as scalp—look for tiny purplish follicular papules many of which contain a small central horn plugging the ostium of the follicle.
- Keratoderma: LP causing a well-demarcated thickening of skin on palms and soles. Look around the edges of the inflamed skin to see the characteristic shiny papules.
- Painful erosive disease on the soles.
- LP pigmentosa (ashy dermatosis): seen in patients with dark skins, usually from the Indian subcontinent. The disease causes longstanding disfiguring macular greyish hyperpigmentation. Inflammation is minimal and treatments ineffective.
- Bullous LP: rarely these patients have autoantibodies to the bullous pemphigoid antigen BP 180 (LP pemphigoides).

Box 10.5 What is lichen nitidus?

Lichen nitidus is an uncommon self-limiting eruption of unknown cause that occurs in children and adults. It is characterized by:

- Asymptomatic or mild itch.
- Shiny, discrete, flat-topped pin-head sized papules (not follicular).
- Predilection for flexural surfaces of upper extremities, anterior trunk, genitalia, and dorsa of hands.
- Rash may be generalized.
- Mucosal surfaces are not involved (unlike LP).
- Displays the Köbner phenomenon.
- Clears within a few years.
- Generally no treatment is needed except reassurance.

Box 10.6 Cutaneous LP: what should I do?

- Take a careful history to ensure this is not a lichenoid drug reaction—see 📖 Box 16.5, p.305, p.350.
- Confirm the diagnosis with a skin biopsy.
- The disease is generally self-limiting.
- Asymptomatic LP does not require treatment but most patients are itchy.
- A potent or very potent topical corticosteroid ointment or cream ×2/day may reduce inflammation and itch.
- Topical 0.1% tacrolimus ointment ×2/day is worth trying if LP is unresponsive to topical corticosteroids.
- A sedating antihistamine may relieve night-time itch.
- Localized hypertrophic skin disease—apply very potent corticosteroids under occlusion (see 📖 p.590) or use intralesional corticosteroids.
- Severe cutaneous LP: short courses of oral corticosteroids will control itching, but unfortunately disease usually recurs on stopping corticosteroids. Other therapies that have been tried include UVB, oral retinoids, and oral ciclosporin.

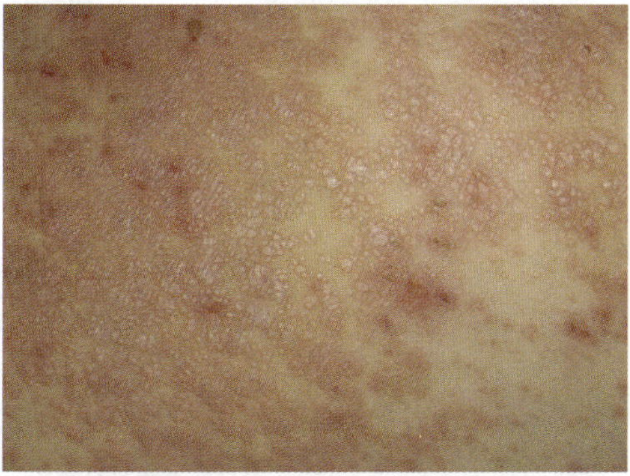

Fig. 10.8 Purplish (violaceous) smooth shiny flat-topped papules of LP.

Chapter 11

Urticaria and erythema

Contents

Ordinary urticaria

What is ordinary urticaria?

Urticaria erupts spontaneously and the smooth erythematous itchy swellings (wheals) persist for 2–24h before fading to leave normal skin (📖 Fig. 11.1, p.215). Some patients have wheals every day; in others the course is episodic. The condition may persist for a few weeks (acute ordinary urticaria) or may last for months or even years (chronic ordinary urticaria). Sometimes patients have angio-oedema in addition to urticaria (see 📖 p.98 and Box 11.1).

Acute urticaria may be precipitated by insect bites, drugs, e.g. penicillin, infections, contact with latex, and food allergies (see 📖 p.98).

In most patients with chronic urticaria, the cause is not identified, but about 30% of these patients have histamine-releasing autoantibodies (routine tests for these autoantibodies are not available). Helminth infections should be considered as a cause of chronic urticaria and urticaria is also common in SLE. Thyroid autoimmunity is more prevalent in chronic ordinary urticaria than in controls. Children and adolescents with severe ordinary urticaria have an increased prevalence of coeliac disease.

The diagnosis depends on the clinical findings.

What should I ask?

- Exclude a physical urticaria by enquiring about precipitating factors (pressure, sun, heat, cold) and how long it takes urticaria to appear. Physical urticaria may complicate ordinary urticaria. Patients who are dermographic may have noticed that wheals appear immediately when skin is rubbed or scratched—wheals last no more than an hour (Box 11.1).
- What are the symptoms—itch, burning, pain?
- How long do the marks last? Delayed pressure urticaria may last up to 72h. Urticarial vasculitis is also long-lasting—see 📖 p.409.
- Is urticaria precipitated by contact with latex or foods, e.g. fish, nuts?
- What does the skin look like when the urticaria fades? The skin should appear normal in ordinary urticaria. Urticarial vasculitis leaves bruising.
- Ask about wheezing and angio-oedema: lip swelling, difficulty swallowing during episodes—see 📖 p.98.
- Is the patient taking any drugs that may cause or worsen urticaria: opiates (direct mast cell-releasing agents), salicylates, non-steroidal anti-inflammatories, ACE inhibitors?—see 📖 p.348.
- Has the patient symptoms suggesting an underlying systemic disease, e.g. fever, arthralgia, myalgia, diarrhoea, weight loss?
- Is there a family history of urticaria?—see 📖 p.218.

What should I do?—see 📖 Management, p.216

- Check skin surface—smooth not scaly in urticaria (Fig. 11.1).
- Confirm that the rash is erythematous (does it blanch?).
- Stroke the skin with a spatula to see if the patient is dermographic (a wheal and flare appears within 10min at the site of the pressure).
- Check that the skin looks normal where wheals have faded.
- Are lips or tongue swollen?

Box 11.1 Clinical classification of the urticarias

Urticaria (hives, wheals, wheals, welts) is a hypersensitivity reaction that may occur on its own or in association with angio-oedema and/or anaphylaxis. The underlying mechanism may be immunological or non-immunological, but the end result is generally the same—mast cell degranulation with release of histamine and other inflammatory mediators, increased capillary permeability, and transient leakage of fluid into the dermis causing swelling.

Ordinary urticaria

- Acute (up to 6 weeks of continuous activity).
- Chronic (6 weeks or more of continuous activity).
- Episodic (acute intermittent or recurrent activity).

Physical urticarias—see 📖 p.218

(Reproducibly induced by the same physical stimulus.)

- Mechanical:
  - Delayed pressure urticaria (swelling may last up to 48h).
  - Symptomatic dermographism.
  - Vibratory angio-oedema.
- Thermal:
  - Cholinergic urticaria (mediated by acetylcholine liberated from sympathetic nerves).
  - Cold contact urticaria.
  - Localized heat urticaria.
- Other:
  - Aquagenic urticaria.
  - Solar urticaria.
  - Exercise-induced anaphylaxis.

Angio-oedema without wheals—see 📖 p.98

- Idiopathic.
- Drug-induced.
- C1 esterase inhibitor deficiency.

Contact urticaria (contact with allergens or chemicals e.g. latex).

Urticarial vasculitis (long-lasting wheals with bruising—vasculitis on skin biopsy. May be a sign of SLE)—see 📖 p.409.

Autoinflammatory diseases—see 📖 p.218

- Hereditary:
  - Cryopyrin-associated periodic syndromes (*CIAS1* mutations) cause familial cold urticaria.
- Acquired:
  - Schnitzler syndrome (non-itchy urticaria, intermittent fever, bone pain, arthritis or arthralgia, raised erythrocyte sedimentation rate (ESR), IgM gammopathy, neutrophils in skin biopsy). Possibly a variant of urticarial vasculitis.

From Grattan CE and Humphreys F. *Br J Dermatol* 2007 **157:**1116–23.

Physical urticarias

Each physical urticaria is induced reproducibly by the same physical stimulus and may coexist with ordinary urticaria. Consider challenge testing to prove the diagnosis, but testing is not without risk in severely affected patients who may develop systemic symptoms including hypotension, wheezing, and anaphylaxis.

Symptomatic dermographism

Dermographism is the most common physical urticaria. An itchy wheal develops within 10min of rubbing the skin lightly and lasts about 1h. Patients may have normal looking skin and you will need to stroke the skin with a spatula to elicit dermographism (Fig. 11.2).

Cold contact urticaria

Itchy wheals appear within minutes if skin is exposed to cold. Angio-oedema and hypotension may complicate the picture and can be life threatening. Common triggers include cold winds and swimming in cold water.

Diagnosis is confirmed by an ice cube test—an ice cube in a polythene bag (the skin must remain dry to exclude aquagenic urticaria) is held against the forearm skin for 20min. Wheals develop rapidly when the skin re-warms.

Cold urticaria is occasionally associated with cryoglobulins, cold agglutinins, or cryofibrinogens—see 🕮 p.410. Familial cold urticaria is one of the rare autosomal dominant hereditary fever syndromes caused by mutations in the *CIAS1* gene—see 🕮 p.219.

Delayed pressure urticaria

Sustained pressure causes itchy or painful wheals after a delay of between 30min and 6h. Swellings last up to 72h. Pressure urticaria may affect any site including the soles or the palms (after carrying a heavy bag).

Solar urticaria

Itchy wheals develop within 10min of exposure of the skin to UV or visible radiation. Solar urticaria occurs in erythropoietic protoporphyria, but this is a rare cause. See 🕮 p.313.

Cholinergic urticaria

Stimuli that increase the core temperature such as anxiety, exertion, hot baths, or sexual activity precipitate a transient, itching, stinging erythematous rash within 15min. Each small urticated papule is surrounded by a wide erythematous flare and flares coalesce so that the rash resembles a flush. The rash can usually be provoked by asking the patient to exercise hard enough to induce sweating. Urticaria is caused by the release of acetylcholine from sympathetic nerves in the skin.

Other physical urticarias

Water (aquagenic urticaria), heat (heat contact urticaria), or vibration (vibratory angio-oedema) trigger localized itchy urticarial reactions at the site of application of the stimulus.

Urticaria appears within 10min and resolves within 2h.

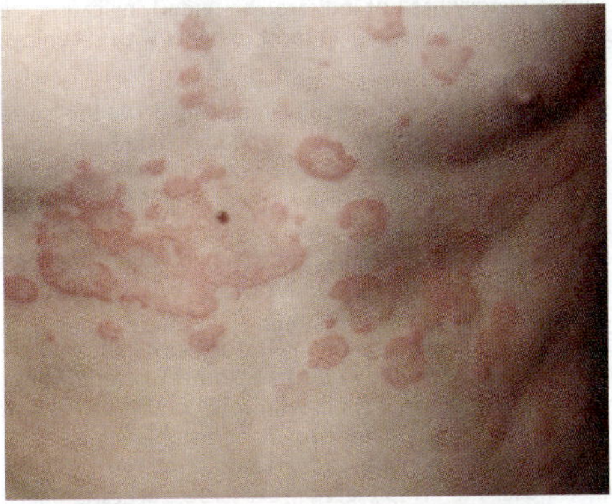

Fig. 11.1 Widespread ordinary urticaria. The smooth erythematous papules and plaques may expand into annular shapes.

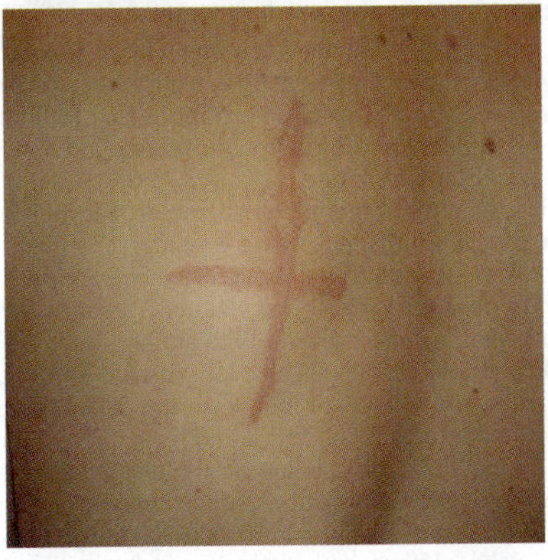

Fig. 11.2 Stroking the skin elicits wheals in patients who are dermographic.

Management of urticaria

What should I do?

Investigations

Investigations should be guided by the history and clinical findings—see Box 11.2. If the history has not indicated an underlying cause, it is unlikely that investigations will be helpful in most patients with chronic urticaria.

General measures

- Explain the disease and the difficulty in pinning down the cause.
- Reassure the patient that urticaria can be controlled—but that it may persist for some time. 50% of patients with chronic ordinary urticaria are clear within 6 months but urticaria with angio-oedema may persist for years, as may physical urticarias.
- Offer written information about urticaria (patient information sheets are available on the website of the British Association of Dermatologists—see 📖 Resources, p.602).
- Discuss how to minimize aggravating factors such as alcohol, overheating, pressure on the skin (tight clothes), or other physical triggers if relevant. Warn patients with cold contact urticaria about the risk of immersion in cold water provoking anaphylaxis.
- Advise dermographic patients to try not to scratch.
- Minimize exposure to drugs that may exacerbate urticaria—see Box 11.3.
- Prescribe a soothing antipruritic topical preparation such as oily calamine lotion or aqueous cream with 1% menthol.

Specific measures

- Prescribe a non-sedating H1 antihistamine such as fexofenadine, cetirizine (works quickly but sedating in high doses), or desloratadine. Patients may need to try several preparations before finding the optimal antihistamine and the optimal dose. Around 40% of patients respond to antihistamines alone.
- Suggest taking the antihistamine so that the drug level is highest before the urticaria usually erupts, e.g. in the evenings if urticaria is worst at night. The dose may need to be above the manufacturer's recommended dose, provided potential benefits outweigh risks.
- Reassure that prolonged treatment with antihistamines is safe.
- A sedating H1 antihistamine, e.g. chlorphenamine 4–12mg, hydroxyzine 10–50mg, can be added at night, but warn the patient that he/she may feel drowsy the next morning. This could pose a risk if driving.
- The addition of an H2 antihistamine or antileukotriene may be helpful.
- Oral corticosteroids should not be used in chronic urticaria, but may shorten the duration of severe acute urticaria (prednisolone 20–30mg a day for 3 days in adults) and may be required in delayed pressure urticaria.
- Topical corticosteroids are not recommended for urticaria.
- Cholinergic urticaria may improve with anticholinergics and anxiolytics as well as antihistamines.

Box 11.2 Investigations

Acute urticaria

Skin-prick testing (not patch testing) or specific IgE quantification may be indicated if you suspect immediate reactions to latex or foods such as nuts or fish.

Chronic ordinary urticaria

- Investigation is usually unrewarding, but reassures the patient.
- FBC (eosinophilia may indicate bowel helminth infection).
- ESR (raised in hereditary fever syndromes).
- Thyroid autoantibodies and/or thyroid function tests.
- Skin biopsy if you suspect an urticarial vasculitis—see 🕮 p.409.

Box 11.3 Triggers for ordinary urticaria

Infections and infestations

- Viral infections, e.g. hepatitis, infectious mononucleosis, seroconversion rash of HIV infection.
- Bacterial infections.
- Mycoplasma infection.
- Intestinal parasites including helminth infection.

Chemicals and venoms

- Drugs: opiates are direct mast cell-releasing agents. Salicylates, non-steroidal anti-inflammatories, and ACE inhibitors may aggravate urticaria—see 🕮 p.348.
- Foods, most often fish, nuts, or fruit.
- Insect bites and venoms.
- The role of food additives in urticaria is unclear.

Systemic disease

- Connective tissue disorders such as SLE.
- Thyroid disease.
- Coeliac disease in children and adolescents.
- Lymphoma.
- Cancer.
- Hypereosinophilic syndrome—rare.
- Hereditary auto inflammatory diseases—rare (see 🕮 p.218).

⚠ Autoinflammatory diseases

These rare inherited diseases are characterized by unexplained bouts of fever and inflammation mainly involving the abdomen, musculoskeletal system, and skin. Symptoms are intermittent without true periodicity and with a variable frequency (weekly to yearly). Amyloidosis is a life-threatening complication. Genetic basis—Box 11.4.

The autoinflammatory diseases also include the dominantly inherited pyogenic arthritis, pyoderma gangrenosum, and acne syndrome (PAPA)—see 📖 p.228.

Familial Mediterranean fever (FMF) (autosomal recessive)

The most frequent type affecting populations of Mediterranean descent. FMF is characterized by episodic fever, serositis (peritonitis, pleuritis, scrotitis, pericarditis), and large-joint arthritis. Attacks can last hours to days. An erysipelas-like erythema of the legs or foot occurs in about 46% of patients. Other cutaneous signs may include urticaria, dermographism, and angio-oedema.

Colchicine is used for long-term prophylaxis.

TNF receptor superfamily 1A-associated periodic fever syndrome (TRAPS; familial Hibernian fever) (autosomal dominant or sporadic)

Attacks last longer than in FMF, usually 5 days to 3 weeks. Patients may have myalgia, thoracic and scrotal pain, arthritis, orbital oedema, and conjunctivitis. Skin is affected in 75% of cases and may present as a pseudocellulitis—a warm, erythematous plaque of variable size on the limbs or torso—or urticaria-like patches and plaques.

Colchicine is ineffective. Corticosteroids are the mainstay of treatment. Etanercept, which inhibits the action of TNFα, may be helpful.

Hyperimmunoglobulin D syndrome (HIDS) (autosomal recessive)

High serum levels of IgD distinguish HIDS from FMF. The disease begins in infancy and is characterized by attacks lasting 7 days and recurring every 4–8 weeks with fever, abdominal pain, diarrhoea, vomiting, arthritis, and cervical lymphadenopathy. Cutaneous signs include erythematous macules, papules, nodules, and urticarial lesions.

Corticosteroids are helpful. Anti-TNF agents may be effective.

Cryopyrinopathies

This group of diseases is characterized by cold-induced urticaria—see 📖 p.214. They respond to anakinra, an interleukin-1 receptor antagonist.

Three separate entities have been described:

- ***Familial cold urticaria (familial cold autoinflammatory syndrome)*** (autosomal dominant): the mildest, urticaria with delayed onset after exposure to cold.
- ***Muckle–Wells syndrome*** (autosomal dominant): urticaria, renal amyloidosis, and sensorineural deafness, sometimes conjuctivitis and arthritis.
- ***Chronic infantile neurological cutaneous and articular syndrome (CINCA) also known as NOMID (neonatal-onset multisystem inflammatory disease)*** (sporadic or autosomal dominant): neonatal onset of a chronic urticarial eruption associated with neurological disease (meningoencephalitis, seizures, motor deficit, learning difficulties), hepatosplenomegaly and articular disease with a disabling and deforming arthropathy. The facial appearance is characteristic.

Box 11.4 Genetic basis of the autoinflammatory diseases

Most are due to mutations in genes that encode the pyrin and TNF receptor superfamilies of molecules and cause dysfunction of innate immunity. Mutations may lead to persistence of leucocytes that would ordinarily undergo apoptosis so that relatively mild inflammatory stimuli are amplified. The interleukin 1beta pathway is activated.

- FMF: mutations in the *MEFV* gene that encodes pyrin. Pyrin and related proteins are involved in regulation of apoptosis, inflammation and processing of cytokines.
- TRAPS: mutations in the *TNFRSF1A* gene that encodes the 55kDa TNF receptor TNFR1.
- HIDS: mutations in the *MVK* gene cause deficiency of the enzyme mevalonate kinase—involved in cholesterol and haem metabolism.
- PAPA: mutations in the PSTPIP1/CD2BP gene that encodes a protein that interacts with pyrin—see 📖 p.228.
- Cold-induced autoinflammatory syndrome: mutations in the *CIAS1* gene that encodes cryopyrin.

Further reading

Farasat S *et al. Arch Dermatol* 2008; **144:**392–402.

Erythema annulare centrifugum

What is erythema annulare centrifugum (EAC)?

This curious but uncommon condition is thought to be a 'hypersensitivity reaction', perhaps to drugs or infection, but in most cases the trigger is not identified. Small dermal blood vessels are cuffed by clusters of lymphocytes. EAC is more common in adults than children. Do not confuse this with all the other erythemas (see Box 11.5).

What should I look for?

- A history of recurring red marks that slowly expand by 2–3mm a day into annular or arcuate shapes that clear centrally and then fade over days to weeks to leave normal skin.
- The speed of evolution contrasts with the waves of rapidly expanding (1cm/day) erythematous concentric bands of erythema gyratum repens, a rare manifestation of internal malignancy (see 📖 p.502).
- EAC tends to recur in the same place, usually on the trunk or proximal limbs.
- A seasonal EAC that recurs annually has been described—Fig. 11.3.
- Sometimes patients complain the rash is itchy.
- 1 or more erythematous macules, papules, well-defined annular (ring-shaped) lesions or arcuate shapes. Lesions reach a maximum of 10cm diameter.
- The trailing inner edge of the erythematous rings may be finely scaly in superficial EAC. Tinea corporis ('ringworm') is more scaly and the scale is on the outer margin of the ring rather than the inner edge.
- Sometimes EAC is oedematous and vesicular.

What should I do?

- Look for possible triggers—drugs, infections.
- Take a skin scrape for mycological culture to exclude fungal infection.
- Consider taking a skin biopsy if the diagnosis is in doubt.
- In widespread annular erythematous rashes check the ANA and ENA to exclude subacute cutaneous LE—see 📖 p.372.
- Explain that you are unlikely to be able to find the cause of the rash—'another of life's great mysteries'—but that it won't do the patient any harm. Most cases pursue a fluctuating course over many years, but eventually regress spontaneously.
- Prescribe a moderately potent topical corticosteroid ointment to relieve irritation. Corticosteroids will have no impact on the course of the disease.

Box 11.5 'Erythemas'

Many skin conditions have descriptive names that include the word erythema. These are considered separately in different sections of the book.

Erythema migrans—see 📖 p.140.
Erythema nodosum—see 📖 p.424.
Erythema multiforme—see 📖 p.105.
Erythema marginatum—evanescent erythematous macules that spread into patches or may be polycyclic. Associated with acute rheumatic fever (fever, carditis, migratory polyarthritis) caused by group A β-haemolytic streptococcal infection.
Erythema induratum—see 📖 p.426.
Erythema gyratum repens—see 📖 p.502.
Erythema ab igne—see 📖 p.418, and Fig. 20.5, p.419.

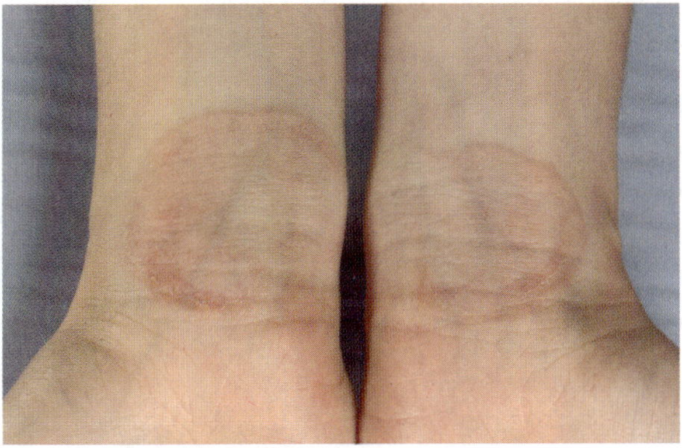

Fig. 11.3 Erythema annulare centrifugum was seasonal in this patient, appearing every summer. The scale follows the expanding erythematous ring.

Chapter 12

Pustular rashes

Contents

Relevant pages in other chapters

Generalized pustules: pustular psoriasis and acute generalized exanthematous pustulosis (AGEP)—see 📖 p.116.
Folliculitis—see 📖 p.126.
Palmoplantar pustulosis—see 📖 p.184.
Reactive arthritis—see 📖 p.194.
Behçet's disease—see 📖 p.264.
Neutrophilic dermatoses—see 📖 p.480.

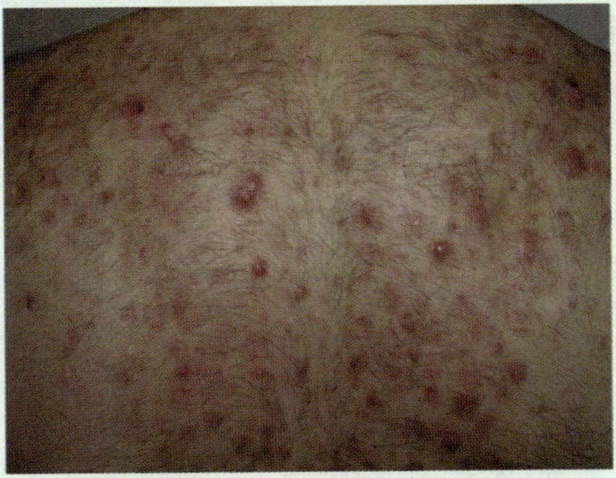

Fig. 12.1 Acne with papules, pustules, and nodules. Reproduced with permission from Warrell D *et al.* (eds) *Oxford Textbook of Medicine*, 5th edn, Layton A. Sebaceous and sweat gland disorders 2010. Oxford: Oxford University Press.

Acne: presentation

Acne is a disfiguring disorder of the pilosebaceous unit, usually starting between the ages of 12–14, that is experienced to some extent by almost all teenagers. Acne may persist into adult life and we seem to be seeing more acne in older women. Pathogenesis is multifactorial—see Box 12.1.

What should I ask?

- When did the acne start? How bad is it today?
- What impact is the acne having on the patient's life? (see 📖 p.32). Acne may have a major psychosocial impact eroding self-confidence and causing depression or even suicide.
- What treatment has the patient used and for how long? Most acne treatments take up to 4 months to have a maximal effect.
- How are topical preparations such as benzoyl peroxide or topical retinoids being applied—all over the face or trunk (as they should be) or just on 'spots'? Any adverse effects such as irritation of the skin?
- Oral antibiotics—most patients will need prolonged treatment for several years. What does the patient mean by 'taking a course'?
- What else is being applied to the skin—greasy cosmetics or pomades?
- What is the patient's occupation? Is he or she in a hot or humid environment, working with tars or oils, or wearing a cap that occludes the forehead?
- Is trauma irritating hair follicles, e.g. a chin strap, plucking hairs?
- Is the patient taking drugs that might exacerbate acne? See Box 12.3.
- Refractory severe acne—see 📖 Box 12.5, p.227.

What should I look for? (Figs. 12.1 and 12.2)

- Acne affects the face and/or upper trunk. If the acne is in an unusual or asymmetrical distribution could this be related to an external factor?
- Acne is characterized by the presence of >1 type of lesion: pustules, papules, comedones (blackhead = open comedone; whitehead = closed comedone), nodules, cysts, and scars (deep 'ice-pick' or flat).
- Record the types of lesions that are present so you can monitor the outcome of treatment.
- Do comedones predominate? Suggests exposure to tar or chlorinated hydrocarbons. Could this be pomade acne on the forehead?
- Are there signs of virilization such as hirsutes? (Check for cliteromegaly if you suspect virilization—see 📖 p.440, p.442.)
- Even mild acne may cause acne keloids or, in dark skins, long-lasting hyperpigmentation. Prolonged courses of minocycline may cause hyperpigmentation in scars.
- See Box 12.2 for clinical variants.

Box 12.1 Pathogenesis of acne

The pathogenesis is not fully understood, but a number of factors play a part in triggering chronic inflammation around pilosebaceous units:

- Sebum excretion is increased (but may remain high when acne has cleared).
- Androgens stimulate sebum secretion by the sebaceous glands.
- Occlusion of follicular ducts by hyperkeratinization (may be exacerbated by application of some greasy topical preparations or tar).
- Bacterial colonization of follicular ducts by *Propionibacterium acnes*, a skin commensal. *P. acnes* breaks down triglycerides releasing free fatty acids that trigger dermal inflammation. *P. acnes* may also activate Toll-like receptors on keratinocytes which induce inflammation.
- Increased fibroblast growth factor receptor-2 (FGFR2) signalling (mutations in FGFR2 leading to increased signalling cause acne in Apert's syndrome). Androgens upregulate signalling.
- Genes—about 50% of patients have a family history of acne.

Further reading

Melnik BC *et al. J Invest Dermatol*, 2009, **129**:1868–77.

Box 12.2 Variants of acne

- Acne 'excoriée de la jeune fille': young girls with mild acne, but obsessional picking scars the skin. Difficult to manage. Even mild disease may need systemic treatment.
- Neonatal and infantile acne: usually face. May persist until age 3 or 4.
- Acne conglobata: severe acne with grouped comedones, deep nodules, and abscesses with sinuses oozing pus—see 🕮 p.230.
- Acne fulminans: nodulocystic acne, fever, and joint pains—see 🕮 p.228.
- Synovitis, acne, pustulosis, hyperostosis, osteitis (SAPHO) syndrome—see 🕮 p.228.
- PAPA syndrome—rare autosomal dominant autoinflammatory disease—see 🕮 p.218 and p.228.

Box 12.3 Drugs that cause or exacerbate acne (see 🕮 p.362)

- Antiepileptics
- Corticosteroids
- Testosterone, anabolic steroids (athletes, body builders)
- Lithium
- Iodides, bromides
- Isoniazid, rifampicin
- Epidermal growth factor receptor inhibitors (used for the treatment of some cancers).

Acne: management

What should I do?

- Provide written information about acne—reassure that the skin is not dirty, that diet is not relevant, and that you can do something.
- Explain that all treatments take 3–4 months to have a maximal effect and that acne may get a little worse before it gets better. Treatment may have to be continued for months or even years.
- If acne is not responding to treatment (and the patient is following your advice), have you made the right diagnosis? Is there an underlying systemic disease? See Boxes 12.4 and 12.5.

Mild acne

Start with 1 or more topical preparations (some can be prescribed in combinations). Explain the preparation should be applied to all the skin not just the spots. Continue treatment for at least 4 months and usually longer. Topical preparations (cream, gel, or lotion) include:

- Antibiotics, e.g. erythromycin or clindamycin lotion.
- Benzoyl peroxide 2.5%, 5%, or 10% (start with a low %, bleaches clothing) with a topical retinoid (avoid in pregnancy), e.g. tretinoin, isotretinoin or 0.1% adapalene (a retinoid-like drug). These preparations are irritants and may cause postinflammatory hyperpigmentation in dark skin. Build up the contact time gradually, washing the preparations off after 30–60min in the first instance.

Moderate acne

- Oral antibiotics for a 4-month course in the first instance, e.g. oxytetracycline 500mg twice daily, lymecycline 408mg/day or erythromycin 500mg twice daily combined with topical benzoyl peroxide to reduce incidence of bacterial resistance to antibiotics. Do not combine with a topical antibiotic. Tetracyclines should not be used in children aged <12.
- Females: oral contraceptive with antiandrogen activity such as co-cyprindiol (takes 6 months to have maximal effect). Avoid contraceptive pills containing norethisterone, which has androgenic properties.

Severe acne or acne with a major psychosocial impact (Fig. 12.2)

- Refer to a specialist. The oral retinoid, isotretinoin, may be the best option. Isotretinoin is teratogenic and has other adverse effects including mucosal dryness and, rarely, depression. Contraception is essential in women of child-bearing age during treatment and for 1 month after stopping isotretinoin.
- Cysts: intralesional triamcinolone (0.1mL of 2.5–10mg/mL solution).

Scars

- Shallow scars become less obvious with time. Refer for advice on cosmetic camouflage.
- Surgical approaches (chemical peels, lasers, dermabrasion) may improve the appearance of deep scars, but are not available through the NHS and are not indicated until acne has been controlled.

Box 12.4 What is this pustular rash?

Papulopustular facial eruption but no comedones

- Is this rosacea (Fig 12.3)? Usually older patients—see 📖 p.234.
- Is the patient being treated with a systemic corticosteroid?
- Is this perioral dermatitis secondary to application of a topical corticosteroid? See 📖 p.236.
- Could this be a bacterial folliculitis or fungal folliculitis, demodicosis or a pseudofolliculitis? See 📖 p.126, p.168.

Superficial small follicular pustules on back

- Is this pityrosporum folliculitis?—see 📖 p.203.
- ⚠ Could this be Behçet's disease? (rare)—see 📖 p.264.

Box 12.5 Why is severe acne not improving?

In patients with severe acne that is refractory to treatment take the history again. Has anything been applied to the skin or is the patient taking drugs such as anabolic steroids? Also consider:

- Polycystic ovary syndrome (obese female, oligomenorrhoea and/or infertility, hirsutism)—see 📖 p.442.
- Congenital adrenal hyperplasia (rare and caused by 21-hydroxylase deficiency)—see 📖 p.440.
- An androgen-secreting tumour (adrenals, ovaries, or testes).
- XYY syndrome (tall male).
- Apert's syndrome (low IQ, acrocephalosyndactyly).

Further reading

Thiboutot D *et al. J Am Acad Dermatol* 2009; **60:**S1–50.
Purdy S and de Berker D. *BMJ* 2006; **333**:949–53.
Strauss JS *et al. J Am Acad Dermatol* 2007; **56:**651–63.

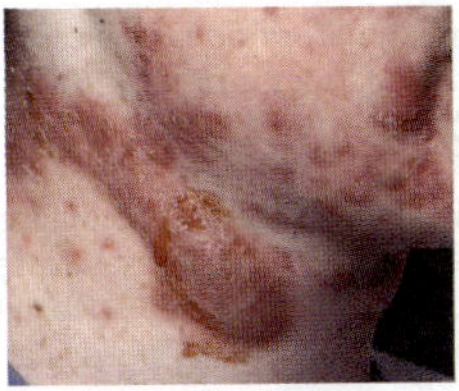

Fig. 12.2 Isotretinoin is indicated in severe cystic acne.

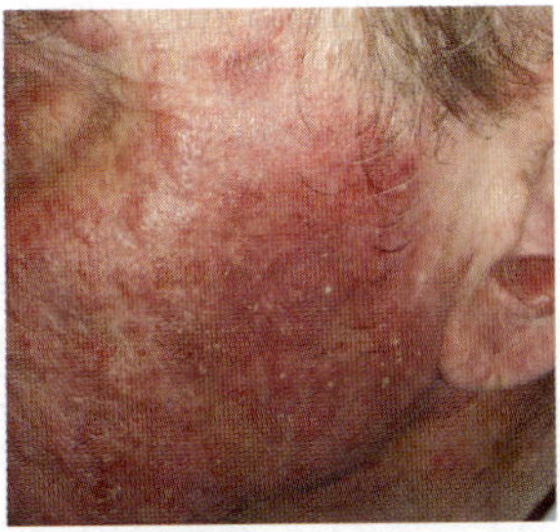

Fig. 12.3 Rosacea: erythema, papules and pustules, but no comedones.

Acne with arthritis

⚠ Acne fulminans

This emergency affects adolescent boys who have previously had mild to moderate acne—see Boxes 12.6 and 12.7. Haemorrhagic, crusted ulcerative skin lesions erupt on the back, chest, arms, and face. Systemic symptoms include fever, malaise, weight loss, myalgia, and arthralgia. Patients may have hepatosplenomegaly or erythema nodosum.

Radiographs show lytic bone lesions most often affecting sternum and clavicle, but osteolytic lesions have been seen in the hips, ankles, and humerus. Osteolytic lesions are sterile. Sternoclavicular hyperostosis and sacroilietis have also been described. Periosteal formation of new bone, sclerosis, and thickening occur late. Bony changes are transient and the prognosis is good. Findings may be consistent with SAPHO syndrome.

Acne conglobata

Seronegative spondyloarthropathy and SAPHO syndrome have also been described in patients with acne conglobata—see 📖 p.230.

What is SAPHO syndrome?

SAPHO syndrome may account for 4% of all patients with seronegative spondyloarthropathies. Inflammatory bowel disease is frequently associated with SAPHO. The syndrome is characterized by:

- Intermittent predominantly axial **S**ynovitis (sternum, clavicles, ribs, spine, pelvis).
- Aseptic **O**steitis and **H**yperostosis. Bony pain is common.
- CT scans show lytic bone lesions—these are sterile.
- Chronic (or relapsing) sterile pustular **A**cneiform eruptions or palmoplantar **P**ustulosis—see Box 12.8 for other skin diseases.
- Leucocytosis and anaemia.

Treatment is unsatisfactory. Tetracycline antibiotics or isotretinoin may control acne. Topical steroids and acitretin may control palmoplantar pustulosis. NSAIDs, prednisolone, and methotrexate have been used for synovitis. Infliximab (anti-TNF) and bisphosphonates (suppress osteoclasts) have also been recommended.

⚠ PAPA syndrome

This very rare autosomal dominant autoinflammatory disease is caused by mutations in the *PSTPIP1/CD2BP1* gene that encodes a protein that interacts with pyrin. PAPA, like FMF, is associated with decreased apoptosis and high levels of IL-1β—see 📖 p.218.

Patients have a severe destructive sterile arthritis (often precipitated by minor trauma) as well as scarring cystic acne, sterile abscesses (often at injection sites), and pyoderma gangrenosum-like ulcers—see 📖 p.290.

Treatments include corticosteroids, etanercept, infliximab, and anakinra.

Box 12.6 ⚠ What is acne fulminans?

Acne fulminans is a severe variant of cystic acne characterized by:

- Sudden onset of inflamed, crusted haemorrhagic plaques and ulcers on face, trunk, and arms (usually in an adolescent boy who has had mild to moderate acne).
- Systemic symptoms that may include fever, malaise, weight loss, myalgia, synovitis, and arthralgia.

Box 12.7 Acne fulminans: what should I do?

►►Seek help from a dermatologist—acne fulminans is an emergency that needs immediate treatment.

Investigation

- Take skin swabs to exclude secondary staphylococcal infection.
- Check FBC (leucocytosis, anaemia), ESR (raised), and CRP (raised).
- Bone scans in areas of pain show increased uptake of radionuclide (not always required).

Immediate treatment

- Patients may need to be admitted if very uncomfortable.
- Apply a potent topical corticosteroid ×2/day to exuberant granulating ulcers.
- Use antiseptic washes to prevent secondary infection.
- Prescribe NSAID for arthralgia and myalgia.
- Start oral prednisolone 0.5–1.0mg/kg per day immediately and continue for 4–8 weeks to control inflammation and prevent relapse.

Long-term treatment

- After 2–6 weeks of oral steroids, when the ulcerated lesions are beginning to settle, start isotretinoin, initially in a low dose (0.25–0.5 mg/kg per day) to prevent a flare.
- After 4–6 weeks, provided acne has not deteriorated, gradually increase the dose of isotretinoin to 1.0mg/kg per day. Continue treatment for about 6 months.
- Tail off prednisolone once the patient is established on treatment with isotretinoin.

Box 12.8 Skin diseases associated with SAPHO syndrome

- Acne fulminans.
- Acne conglobata and hidradenitis suppurativa.
- Palmoplantar pustulosis, generalized pustular psoriasis, and plaque psoriasis.
- Other neutrophilic dermatoses including pyoderma gangrenosum, Sweet's syndrome, and subcorneal pustular dermatosis.

Further reading

Editorial. *Joint Bone Spine* 2007; **74:**123–6.

Follicular occlusion diseases: signs

Acne conglobata, hidradenitis suppurativa, and dissecting cellulitis of the scalp are diseases of adults in which follicular occlusion seems to play a part in pathogenesis. The conditions may coexist. Pilonidal cyst is another member of the 'folliculitis occlusion tetrad'.

Seronegative spondyloarthropathy has been described in association with both acne conglobata and hidradenitis suppurativa, as has pyoderma gangrenosum—see 🕮 p.290. ⚠ Rarely SCC may complicate chronic disease.

Acne conglobata

What should I look for? (see also Fig. 12.4)

- Open comedones (blackheads) clustered into groups on face and trunk. Papules, pustules, and nodules typical of acne.
- Numerous fluctuant abscesses ('cysts') draining pus on the face, chest, and upper back, but also sometimes affecting buttocks, groins, and axillae, when signs overlap with those of hidradenitis suppurativa.
- Interconnecting sinus tracts linking adjacent abscesses.
- Large bowl-like scars, hypertrophic scars, or keloids.

Hidradenitis suppurativa

Hidradenitis suppurativa (acne inversa) is a chronic debilitating inflammation of the flexures that is often misdiagnosed as staphylococcal furunculosis. The pathogenesis is uncertain, but follicular plugging may cause dilatation and rupture of the follicle with secondary inflammation of apocrine glands. Hidradenitis is associated with the polycystic ovary syndrome and insulin resistance. It is also more common in Crohn's disease, but cutaneous Crohn's disease may simulate hidradenitis—see 🕮 p.472.

What should I look for? (see also Fig.12.5 and Fig. 12.6)

- Recurrent 'boils' in axillae, breasts, groins, vulva, or perianal skin. Women tend to have involvement of the front of the body (groin, breasts) and men the back of the body (buttocks, perianal area).
- Signs of insulin resistance—skin tags, acanthosis nigricans around neck or flexures, and obesity (friction and sweating in flexures probably exacerbate follicular occlusion and the tendency to hidradenitis).
- Grouped open comedones (blackheads) in affected skin suggest hidradenitis. Look for these in patients with recurrent flexural 'boils'.
- Tender subcutaneous nodules, abscesses, scars, and sinuses in flexures.

Dissecting cellulitis of the scalp

This rare condition also known as 'perifolliculitis capitis abscedens et suffodiens' is more common in black patients.

What should I look for?

- A history of recurrent and chronic painful abscesses in the scalp.
- Tender subcutaneous fluctuant scalp nodules, some of which drain pus, and intercommunicating sinuses.
- Patchy scarring with loss of hair (scarring alopecia).

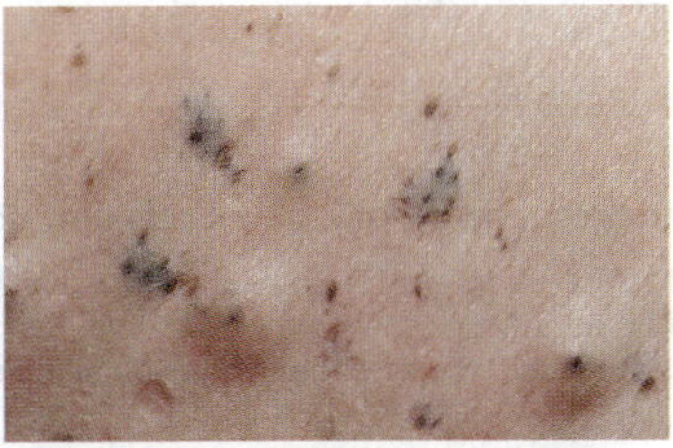

Fig. 12.4 Grouped comedones in acne conglobata.

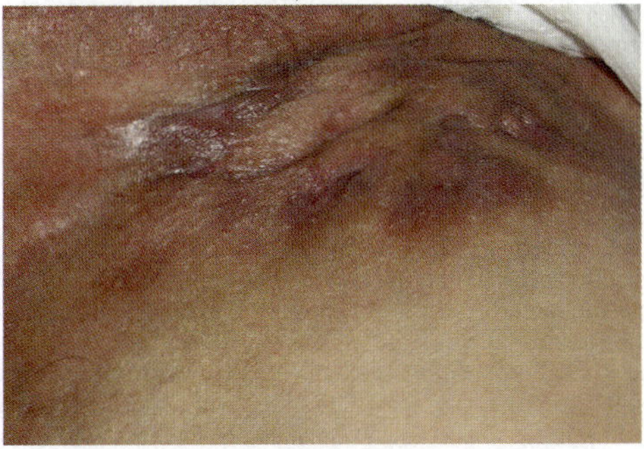

Fig. 12.5 Hidradenitis suppurativa with tender subcutaneous nodules, scars and sinuses in the groin.

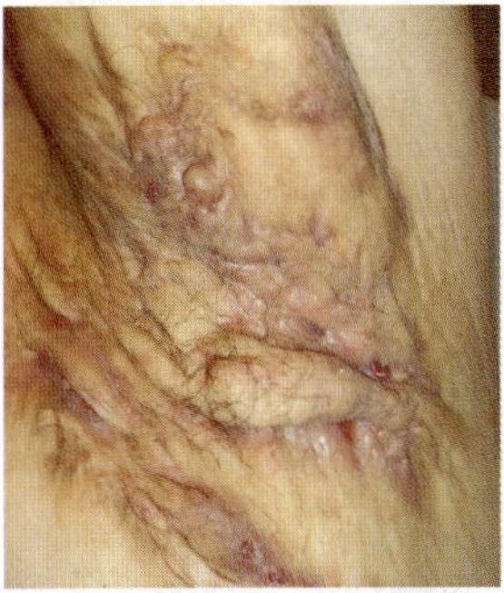

Fig. 12.6 Axillary hidradenitis suppurativa with considerable scarring and deformity.

Follicular occlusion diseases: management

Box 12.9 Management of follicular occlusion diseases

Management is difficult and at best control will be limited. Cultures of skin swabs may be negative or show a mixed growth, but *Staphylococcus aureus* may play some part in the pathogenesis of inflammation.

Acne conglobata

- Minimize exacerbating factors—e.g. drugs that may cause acne.
- The response to standard acne treatments with topical and oral antibiotics and topical retinoids is usually disappointing.
- Isotretinoin is worth trying but the disease can be very resistant.
- Intralesional steroids may reduce inflammation in large cysts.
- Cysts may be drained surgically.

Hidradenitis suppurativa

- Weight loss, if the patient is obese, and the patient should stop smoking (some evidence nicotine exacerbates disease).
- Cool loose-fitting cotton clothing will reduce friction and sweating.
- Minimize follicular irritation by avoiding shaving and depilation.
- Topical antibacterial soaps and antiseptics may be helpful (no evidence for efficacy).
- Topical clindamycin lotion applied ×2/day can control mild disease.
- Prolonged treatment (at least 6 months) with an oral tetracycline or erythromycin (as for acne) can be effective. Patients who do not respond may be treated with rifampicin 300mg ×2/day in combination with clindamycin 300mg ×2/day for 10 weeks.
- Anecdotal reports of other therapies that may be helpful include antiandrogens (cyproterone acetate, finasteride), retinoids, and dapsone as well as anti-TNF drugs, e.g. infliximab and etanercept.
- In severe disease, a multidisciplinary approach is needed. Surgery may be indicated to remove scarred sinus tracts or to marsupialize recurrent lesions. Carbon dioxide laser surgery has been helpful. Leaving wounds to heal by secondary intention has been advocated, but grafts or flaps may be needed. Recurrence is common, particularly after incision and drainage of abscesses, which is not recommended.

Dissecting cellulitis of the scalp

- Prolonged treatment with tetracycline antibiotics, as for acne, may be helpful. Combinations of rifampicin and clindamycin can be tried as in hidradenitis.
- Isotretinoin has been tried (0.5–1.0 mg/kg) with limited success.
- Dapsone (50–100mg/day) has been used in combination with isotretinoin.

Further reading

Gener G *et al. Dermatol* 2009; **219:**148–54.
Lam J *et al. Pediatr Dermatol* 2007; **24:**465–73.
Lee RA *et al. Adv Dermatol* 2007; **23:**289–306.

Rosacea

Rosacea is common in the 3rd and 4th decades. The pathogenesis is uncertain, but genetic factors play a part. Rosacea has a particularly high prevalence in Ireland (Celts with fair skin).

What should I ask?

- Patients will often have had a long-standing tendency to flush or blush easily, but now the face is permanently red (also see 🕮 p.482).
- What makes the redness worse? The skin is easily irritated by topical products. Alcohol, spicy foods, sudden temperature change, and hot drinks can all precipitate reddening. Sunlight may also exacerbate rosacea. The role of demodex is uncertain—see 🕮 p.168.
- What does the patient notice? Crops of red bumps (papules), 'yellow-heads' (pustules)? Is the skin rough or scaly? (scale is seen more often in seborrhoeic dermatitis than rosacea, but the conditions may overlap) (Fig. 12.3).
- What medicaments is the patient using and for how long have they been used? Topical corticosteroids can cause a rosacea-like rash (perioral dermatitis—see 🕮 p.236). Oral corticosteroids also cause a pustular acne-like rash and redness.
- Patients may have noticed enlargement of the nose.
- Eye symptoms are common, e.g. burning, itching, redness, grittiness.

What should I look for?

Not all signs are present in every patient, for example, some may have a very erythematous papular rash, others a more pustular eruption.

Look for:

- A rash affecting the central face usually in a symmetrical pattern, but on occasion rosacea can be strikingly asymmetrical.
- Erythema and telangiectasia (Fig. 12.3).
- Dome-shaped erythematous papules and pustules without comedones (Fig. 12.3). Comedones suggest acne (see 🕮 p.224) not rosacea. Facial angiofibromas in tuberous sclerosis may be misdiagnosed as rosacea (see 🕮 p.512).
- Brownish yellow papules suggest granulomatous rosacea—see Box 12.11.
- Greasy skin but little scale. Scale suggests dermatitis (seborrhoeic or contact) or, if in a limited area, fungal infection. (Also see demodicosis 🕮 p.168.)
- Facial swelling (lymphoedema).
- A bulbous nose (rhinophyma) because of hypertrophic sebaceous glands and an overgrowth of the soft tissues.
- Ocular rosacea—conjunctivitis, blepharitis, chalazion, or hordeolum (stye).
- An absence of pustules on the trunk. Rosacea, unlike acne, does not affect the back or chest.

Management—See Box 12.10.

Box 12.10 Rosacea: what should I do?

- Soap substitutes minimize irritation of the skin.
- A hat and sun-block creams will prevent photoexacerbation.
- Mild inflammatory disease may be controlled by topical 0.75% metronidazole cream or 15% azelaic acid gel applied ×2/day for 3–4 months.
- Topical pimecrolimus or tacrolimus may also have a role in mild disease.
- An oral antibiotic (oxytetracycline 500 mg ×2/day, lymecycline 408mg/day or erythromycin 500mg ×2/day) taken for 4 months will control papulopustular disease, but has little impact on redness. The dose of antibiotic can be reduced once the disease is under control.
- Oral isotretinoin may reduce sebaceous gland overgrowth.
- Rhinophyma can be pared down electrosurgically.
- Cosmetic camouflage or laser surgery may reduce redness.

Box 12.11 What is granulomatous rosacea?

Granulomatous rosacea is characterized by:

- Features of rosacea, but brownish yellow or red papules predominate.
- A skin biopsy will show granulomatous inflammation around hair follicles without necrosis.
- The condition usually responds to oral antibiotics, e.g. minocycline 100mg/day, lymecycline 408mg/day taken for 4–6 months.
- Isotretinoin is an alternative treatment.

Acne agminata (lupus miliaris disseminatus faciei) is probably a variant of granulomatous rosacea:

- Patients present with clusters of reddish-brown or yellow papules, 1–3mm in diameter, distributed symmetrically around the eyes, including the eyelids, and sometimes elsewhere in the central face. Some patients have nodules in the axillae. Lesions last months, may become pustular and crusted, and eventually heal with pitted scarring.
- The histology shows superficial granulomatous inflammation with caseation necrosis, possibly a reaction to damaged pilosebaceous units. Acne agminata has no relationship to TB.
- The disease tends to regress spontaneously in 1–2 years.
- Tetracycline antibiotics, in acne doses, are usually effective in about 6 months.
- Isotretinon and dapsone have also been effective.

Further reading

Wilkin J *et al. J Am Acad Dermatol* 2002; **46:**584–7.

Perioral dermatitis (periorificial dermatitis)

Perioral dermatitis is an inflammatory condition that occurs in children and in adults, usually young and middle-aged women. The cause is unknown, but exogenous factors such as potent topical corticosteroids—see 📖 p.588, inhaled corticosteroids, irritant cosmetics, and occlusive emollients may play some part in the pathogenesis.

The name is misleading. Perioral skin is affected more often than other sites, but the condition may affect periocular and perinasal skin. It has also been reported on the trunk. Nor is perioral dermatitis a typical dermatitis—it is more akin to rosacea. Dermatitis is treated with topical corticosteroid, yet topical corticosteroids are one of the commonest causes of perioral dermatitis.

What should I look for?

- A history of a rash that burns rather than itches.
- Explore what has been applied to the skin. Many (but not all) patients with perioral dermatitis will have been applying a potent topical corticosteroid to their face prior to the onset of eruption. The corticosteroid relieves burning and causes transient vasoconstriction, which reduces the redness, so the patient continues to apply the cream in the mistaken belief that the corticosteroid is helping.
- Clusters of tiny (<2mm diameter) erythematous papules and vesicopustules (the tiny vesicles rapidly evolve into pustules) around the mouth (Fig. 12.7).
- The background skin is erythematous and may be scaly.
- The rash tends to spare the vermillion border of the lips.
- Periocular (usually below the eye) and perinasal lesions are probably more common in children than adults.

What should I do?

- Try to identify the underlying cause—most often applications of potent topical corticosteroid to the face—and advise avoidance of any potential skin irritant.
- Convince the patient that the topical corticosteroid (or other preparation) is the cause of the problem—this may be difficult. (Try to avoid blaming the doctor who prescribed the strong corticosteroid—it is quite possible that the patient has not followed the doctor's instructions or has obtained the corticosteroid from a well-meaning friend or relation.)
- Warn the patient that the skin is going to look worse before it gets better, and to resist the temptation to restart the topical corticosteroid (the redness and irritation will be more obvious when the corticosteroid is withdrawn).
- Prescribe topical or oral therapy—see Box 12.12.
- Reassure the patient—the prognosis is good and the rash generally clears in 8–12 weeks.

Box 12.12 Treatment of perioral dermatitis

- Withdraw potential skin irritants and potent corticosteroid preparations.
- Topical 1% pimecrolimus or 0.1% tacrolimus ointment may be effective in mild cases. Apply ×2/day for 4 weeks.
- An oral tetracycline (e.g. oxytetracycline 250–500mg ×2/day) will be required for 6–8 weeks in more severe cases.
- Avoid tetracyclines in children <12 years (they stain teeth) and use erythromycin instead, but this is not as effective as tetracycline.
- Prescribe a weak topical corticosteroid (1% hydrocortisone ointment) in combination with miconazole for any underlying eczematous skin problem (possibly seborrhoeic dermatitis) if required.

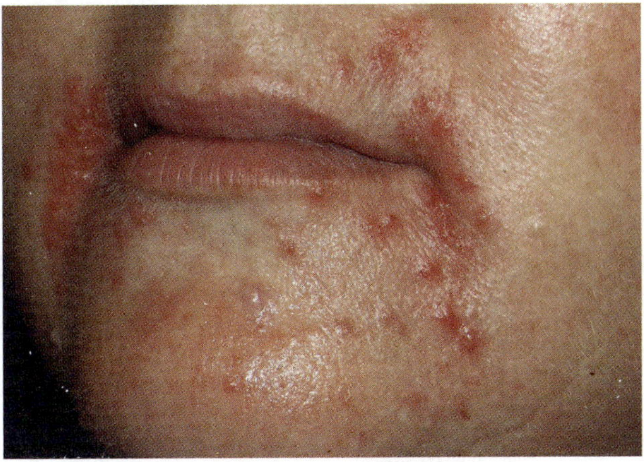

Fig. 12.7 Perioral dermatitis caused by very potent topical corticosteroid.

Chapter 13
Blisters

Contents

Relevant pages in other chapters

Causes of blisters—see 🕮 p.78
Emergency dermatology—see 🕮 p.104, p.106, and p.108
Photosensitivity—see 🕮 p.302 and p.304
Blisters in infants and children—see 🕮 p.546

Introduction to blisters

What is a blister?

- A blister is a bump filled with clear fluid (serum).
- Small blisters, <0.5 cm in diameter, are called vesicles.
- Larger blisters, >0.5 cm in diameter, are known as bullae.

Why does the skin blister?

Blisters form because adhesion fails either between the keratinocytes just below the stratum corneum (subcorneal blisters), within the epidermis (intraepidermal blisters), or within or below the dermo-epidermal junction (subepidermal blisters). See Fig. 13.1.

Always exclude the common (and often more easily treated) secondary causes of blisters such as trauma, eczema, insect bites, or infection before you diagnose a primary bullous disease.

Common secondary causes of blisters are discussed in more detail elsewhere in the book. See 📖 p.78 for the causes of blisters.

It is beyond the scope of this book to discuss the inherited epidermolysis bullosa (EB) group of disorders.

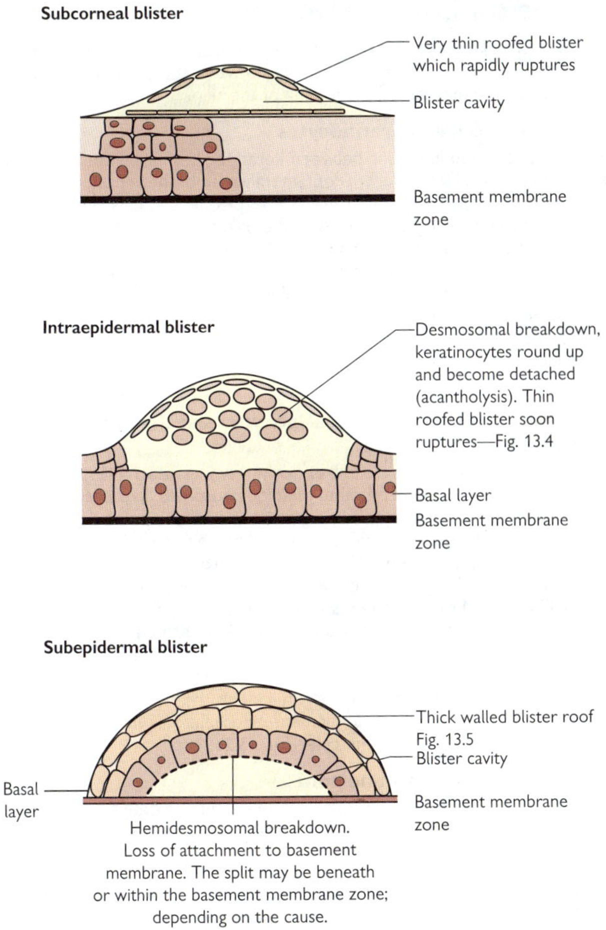

Fig. 13.1 Level of splits in blisters.

Adhesion in the epidermis

In order to make sense of the primary bullous diseases, it will help to have some understanding of the interactions between the structural proteins that provide the mechanical scaffolding of the skin.

Adhesion between keratinocytes

The main adhesion junctions between keratinocytes in the epidermis are the desmosomes. Desmosomes contain transmembrane adhesion proteins (desmosomal cadherins) and cytoplasmic plaque proteins. Interactions between the extracellular portions of the transmembrane cadherins hold the keratinocytes together. The cytoplasmic portion of the cadherin inserts into the desmosomal plaque, where it interacts with plaque proteins such as desmoplakin or plakoglobin. These plaque proteins link to keratins in the intermediate filament cytoskeleton which are themselves linked to the nucleus. Thus the whole network is stable and signals can be transduced from the external surface of the cell through the desmosome to the nucleus—see Fig. 13.2a.

Adhesion between basal keratinocytes and the basement membrane

Hemidesmosomes at the base of basal keratinocytes attach these keratinocytes to the basement membrane. Hemidesmosomes, like desmosomes, contain transmembrane adhesion proteins as well as cytoplasmic plaque proteins. Transmembrane hemidesmosomal proteins such as bullous pemphigoid antigen 2 (collagen XVII) (BP180) and $\alpha6\beta4$ integrin extend into the basement membrane zone, where they interact with proteins such as laminins in anchoring filaments to bind the epidermis to the basement membrane. The cytoplasmic portions of these transmembrane hemidesmosomal proteins interact with cytoplasmic plaque proteins in the hemidesmosome such as plectin and bullous pemphigoid antigen 1 (BP320). As in desmosomes, these plaque proteins link the hemidesmosomes to the keratins of the intermediate filament cytoskeleton, which are, in turn, connected to the nucleus of the cell—Fig. 13.2b.

The basement membrane zone

The surface area of the basement membrane interface between epidermis and dermis is increased and adhesion enhanced by downward projections from the epidermis (epidermal rete pegs) that interdigitate with upward projections from the dermis (dermal papillae).

Interactions between laminins, collagens, and non-collagenous proteins in the basement membrane zone promote adhesion. The lamina lucida (electron-lucent zone) of the basement membrane, containing laminins, lies immediately beneath the basal keratinocytes. Laminins attach to collagen IV in the underlying lamina densa. Fine anchoring filaments (laminin-332, laminin-311) bound to extracellular domains of the hemidesmosomal protein, $\alpha6\beta4$ integrin, extend across the lamina lucida into the lamina densa, where the filaments link to anchoring fibrils (collagen VII). The anchoring fibrils fasten the lamina densa to the underlying collagen bundles of the papillary dermis—Fig. 13.2b.

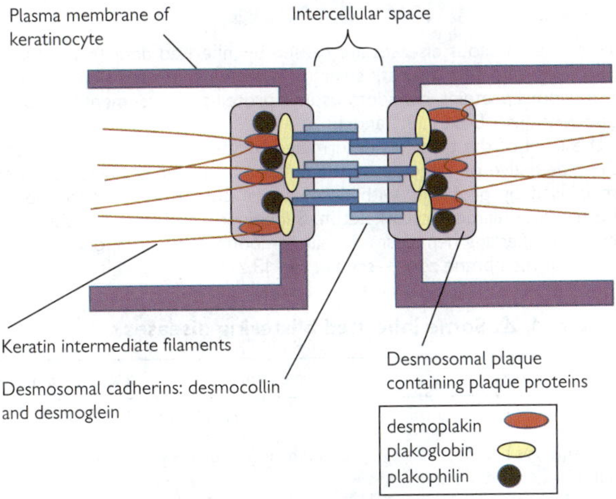

Fig. 13.2a Model of a desmosome, the main adhesion junction providing adhesion between keratinocytes.

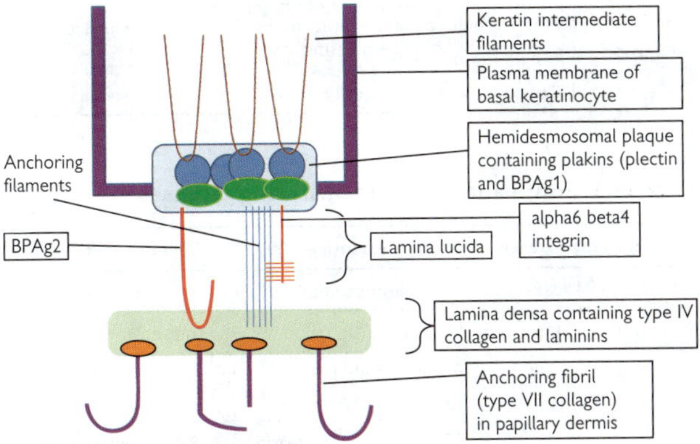

Fig. 13.2b Model of the basement membrane zone showing attachment of the hemidesmosome of a basal keratinocyte to the underlying papillary dermis.

Primary bullous diseases

The primary bullous diseases are caused by inherited defects in, or autoantibodies directed against, structural proteins in the skin—keratins, desmosomal proteins, hemidesmosomal proteins, or basement membrane zone proteins—Boxes 13.1 and 13.2.

The level of the blister is determined by the structural protein that is either defective or targeted by the autoantibody. Intraepidermal blisters are caused by problems with desmosomal components or the keratin intermediate filament cytoskeleton. Subepidermal blisters are caused by problems affecting hemidesmosomal components or components of the basement membrane zone—see 📖 Fig. 13.2.

Box 13.1 ⚠ Some inherited blistering diseases

Genetic disease	Defective protein	Level of split
Epidermolysis bullosa simplex	Keratin 5 or 14 (cytoskeleton)	Intraepidermal
Epidermolysis bullosa simplex with muscular dystrophy	Plectin (hemidesmosome)	Intraepidermal
Junctional epidermolysis bullosa	Laminin 332 or BPA2 (anchoring filament or hemidesmosome)	Lamina lucida
Junctional epidermolysis bullosa with pyloric atresia	$\alpha6\beta4$ integrin (hemidesmosome)	Lamina lucida
Epidermolysis bullosa dystrophica	Type VII collagen	Sublamina densa

Box 13.2 Some autoimmune blistering diseases

Autoimmune disease	Major autoantigen (s)	Level of split
Pemphigus foliaceus	Dg 1 (desmosome)	Intraepidermal
Pemphigus vulgaris	Dg 1 and 3 (desmosome)	Intraepidermal
Bullous pemphigoid	BP230 and BP180 (hemidesmosome)	Subepidermal
Cicatricial pemphigoid (mucous membrane pemphigoid)	BP180 and $\alpha6\beta4$ integrin (hemidesmosome), laminins 332, 311 (anchoring filaments), and type VII collagen (anchoring fibrils)	Subepidermal
Epidermolysis bullosa acquisita	Type VII collagen (anchoring fibrils)	Subepidermal

Dg = Desmoglein

Further reading

Diaz LA and Giudice GJ. *Arch Dermatol* 2000; **136:**106–12.
Fassihi H *et al. Clin Exp Dermatol* 2006; **31:**252–9.
Hertl M *et al. J Clin Invest* 2006; **116:**1159–66.
Mihai S and Sitaru C. *J Cell Mol Med* 2007; **11:**462–81.

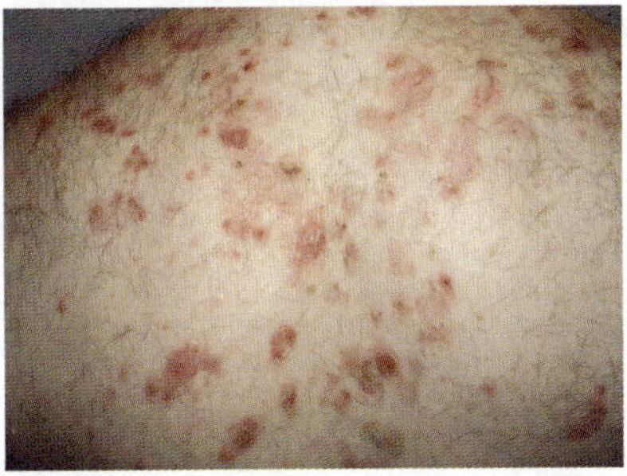

Fig. 13.3 Erythematous crusted papules on the trunk in pemphigus foliaceus resembling seborrhoeic dermatitis. The split is so superficial that blisters are uncommon.

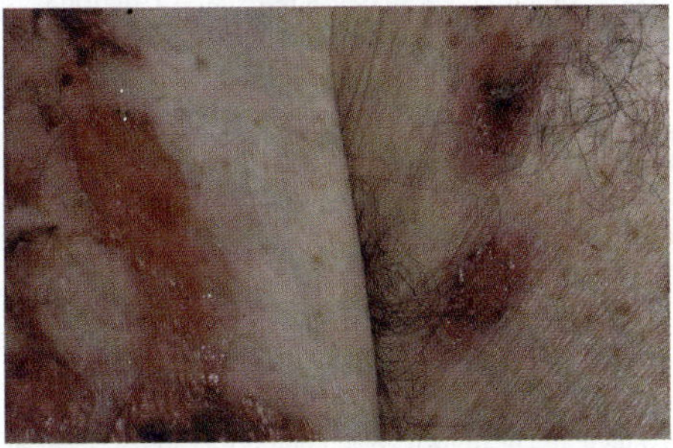

Fig. 13.4 Typical erosions in pemphigus vulgaris—the intraepidermal blisters rupture easily.

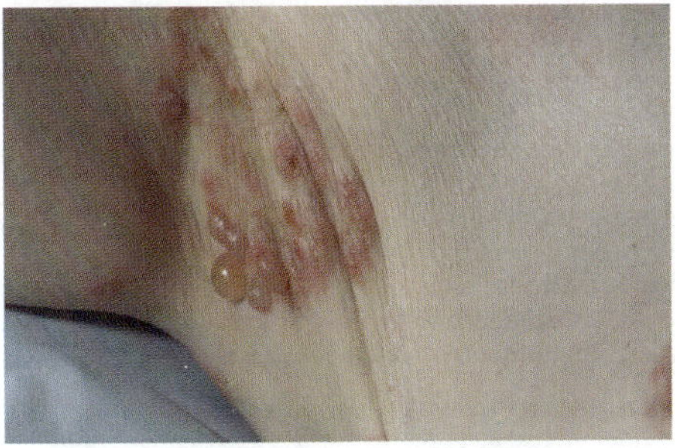

Fig. 13.5 Tense blisters, erosions, and urticated erythema (erythema without scale) in bullous pemphigoid.

The approach to the patient

Blisters worry patients (and their doctors). ⚠ Extensive blistering with disruption of the epidermal barrier is potentially life threatening and should be treated as a medical emergency (see 📖 p.106, 108).

What should I ask a patient with blisters?

Take a full dermatological history (see 📖 p.18 and p.78). Ask:

- If a rash precedes blistering?
- When blistering started?
- Does the skin seem fragile or photosensitive?
- Are there mucosal symptoms—oral, conjunctival, or genital discomfort?
- What drugs or topical preparations are being used?
- If there are symptoms suggesting systemic disease?
- Does anyone else in the family have a blistering condition?

What should I look for in a patient with blisters?

- Is the patient ill, suggesting a systemic cause such as infection or drug?
- What is the distribution of the blistering?
    - Localized and asymmetrical (suggesting an exogenous cause), e.g. at sites of pressure or in streaks suggesting a reaction to something that has been in contact with the skin.
    - Generalized and symmetrical (suggesting endogenous disease).
    - On sun-exposed skin suggesting photosensitivity.
- What precedes the blister—e.g. are there itchy erythematous urticated papules or plaques (sometimes seen in bullous pemphigoid)?
- Are the blisters intraepidermal or subepidermal?
    - Blisters that form within the epidermis have a thin roof and rupture easily leaving oozing crusted erosions or scaling—see Figs. 13.3 and 13.4
    - Blisters that form at or below the basement membrane of the dermo-epidermal junction are tense, may contain blood, and are less likely to rupture, as the roof is formed by the whole of the epidermis—Fig. 13.5.
- Are there ulcers? These form when epidermis and superficial papillary dermis are lost. Ulcers suggest deep subepidermal blistering or secondary infection.
- Are blisters umbilicated, i.e. do they have a central depression? Seen in some viral infections.
- Are there pustules? A secondary finding in a primary vesiculobullous disease.
- Are there mucosal blisters, erosions, or scarring? Check eyes, mouth, and genitalia—see 📖 p.48.
- What is left when the blisters have healed—scars, postinflammatory hyper- or hypopigmentation?
- Are there milia? These pinhead-sized firm white papules are tiny intradermal cysts that are left when some subepidermal blisters heal. Milia suggest that blistering was subepidermal.

Investigations See Boxes 13.3. and 13.4.

Box 13.3 Investigations in patients with blisters

- Exclude infection by taking skin swabs from erosions for microbiological and/or viral culture—see 🕮 p.572.
- Take a 4mm punch biopsy that includes a small early intact blister to show the level at which the blister has arisen. If the biopsy is taken from an old or ruptured blister, the roof may be lost and the floor may be re-epithelializing, making it difficult to decide if the blister is intraepidermal or subepidermal.
- Take a 3–4mm punch biopsy from perilesional skin for direct immunofluorescence microscopy to look for deposits of immunoglobulin and complement within the epidermis or at the basement membrane zone. Either snap freeze the specimen in liquid nitrogen or fix in Michel's medium.
- Take a blood sample for indirect immunofluorescence microscopy to look for circulating autoantibodies to antigens in the epidermis or the basement membrane zone.
- In patients with a history of skin fragility, blistering at sites of trauma, or photosensitivity, check for porphyrins in urine, stool, and blood. Wrap the specimen pots in tinfoil to prevent exposure to UV light—see 🕮 Box 16.4, p.303.

Box 13.4 Indirect immunofluorescence on salt-split skin

In subepidermal blistering diseases, the autoantigen may be associated with the hemidesmosomes of the basal keratinocytes or a component of the basement membrane or dermis. Indirect immunofluorescence studies on intact skin will produce a bright linear subepidermal band that does not differentiate between these autoantigens. Salt-split skin helps to localize the autoantigen in subepidermal blistering diseases.

- The lamina lucida is the weakest part of the basement membrane. Skin that it stressed mechanically by suction or exposure to salt will always split through the lamina lucida.
- A biopsy of normal skin is immersed in 1 M saline for 3 days and the artificially split skin is used as the substrate in an indirect immunofluorescence reaction.
- The patient's serum containing the autoantibody is incubated with skin that has been fractured through the lamina lucida and antibody binding detected in the usual way.
- Autoantibodies that bind to antigens associated with the hemidesmosomes of basal keratinocytes (e.g. in bullous pemphigoid) will bind to the epidermal side (roof) of the artificial split whereas autoantibodies that bind to antigens associated with the lamina densa or dermis (e.g. in epidermolysis bullosa acquisita or bullous SLE) will bind to the dermal side (base) of the split.

Pemphigus

From the Greek 'pemphix' meaning bubble or blister.

Pemphigus is a group of rare intra-epidermal autoimmune blistering diseases that can be life threatening. Widespread superficial blisters and painful erosions are caused by circulating autoantibodies that disrupt the desmosomal attachments between keratinocytes—see Box 13.5.

What should I look for?

Pemphigus vulgaris—see Fig. 13.4

- Slow-healing irregularly-shaped erosions in oral mucous membranes—it is rare to see intact bullae in the mouth. Painful oral ulceration may precede skin involvement by months and make eating very difficult.
- Involvement of conjunctiva, nasal mucosa, pharynx, larynx, oesophagus, urethra, vulva and/or cervix.
- Flaccid blisters and painful slow-healing cutaneous erosions affecting scalp, face, axillae, upper trunk, groins, and pressure points. Sometimes these are heaped up and vegetating in flexures (pemphigus vegetans).
- Nikolsky sign—applying a firm sliding pressure to the skin with your finger will produce an erosion, because the epidermis separates from the dermis. This test is painful and rarely necessary.

Pemphigus foliaceus—see Fig. 13.3

- A slowly extending rash on scalp, face, chest, and upper back.
- Scaly erythematous papules that may resemble seborrhoeic dermatitis.
- Flaccid vesicles that rupture easily leaving crusted painful shallow erosions that may be malodorous.
- Mucosae are not affected.

What should I do?

- Check the drug history—Box 13.6.
- Take biopsies of fresh lesions for histology and perilesional skin for direct immunofluorescence microscopy and blood for indirect immunofluorescence microscopy.
- Check FBC, and renal and liver function.
- Take skin swabs from erosions and prevent sepsis by cleansing eroded skin and mucous membranes—see 📖 p.592.
- Potent topical corticosteroids may be sufficient to control mild localized pemphigus but most patients require oral treatment with systemic corticosteroids (prednisolone 40–60mg/day). Side effects, including septicaemia, are a major cause of death.
- Topical steroids may help to suppress oral ulcers in pemphigus vulgaris.
- Painful oral ulceration and oral candida can be relieved with mouthwashes containing nystatin and 2% lidocaine.
- Other immunosuppressive agents that have been used include azathioprine, cyclophosphamide, and mycophenolate mofetil.
- Plasmapheresis, IV immunoglobulin and, more recently, rituximab have been used with some success in resistant cases.

Box 13.5 The antigens, histology, and immunohistology in pemphigus

Pemphigus vulgaris

- The antigen in pemphigus foliaceus is the desmosomal cadherin, desmoglein 3, which is expressed in mucosa and predominantly in the lower part of the epidermis.
- A biopsy taken from an early lesion will show intraepidermal spongiosis (oedema between keratinocytes), sometimes with eosinophils (eosinophilic spongiosis).
- Biopsy from intact vesicles will show splitting just above the basal layer of the epidermis forming intraepidermal blisters. Keratinocytes round up and separate from each other (acantholysis), but the basal keratinocytes remain attached to the basement membrane by hemidesmosomes. Their appearance has been likened to a row of tombstones, because the cells stand up in a row without their lateral attachments to each other.
- Direct and indirect immunofluorescence microscopy—IgG and C3 between keratinocytes.

Pemphigus foliaceus

- The antigen in pemphigus foliaceus is the desmosomal cadherin, desmoglein1, which is expressed most strongly in the upper parts of the epidermis and is absent in mucosa.
- The split is high in the epidermis, just below the stratum corneum, but splitting can be difficult to find. The blister may contain a few neutrophils and some acantholytic keratinocytes.
- Direct and indirect immunofluorescence microscopy—IgG and C3 between keratinocytes.

Box 13.6 ⚠ Rare variants of pemphigus

- ***Drug-induced pemphigus:*** sulphydryl drugs such as captopril, enalapril, and D-penicillinamine may trigger pemphigus, most often pemphigus foliaceus.
- ***Endemic or Brazilian pemphigus foliaceus*** (fogo selvagem = 'wild fire' in Portuguese): clustered in certain states in Brazil and precipitated by an environmental factor, possibly a biting insect.
- ***Paraneoplastic pemphigus***: associated with B-cell lymphoma, thymoma, and Castleman's disease (a rare lymphoproliferative disorder). Some cases have been linked to treatment with fludarabine—see 📖 p.498.
- ***IgA pemphigus*** (very rare!) with features that overlap those of subcorneal pustular dermatosis (Sneddon–Wilkinson disease).

Further reading

Harman KE *et al.* 2003. Evidence-based guidelines, prepared on behalf of the British Association of Dermatologists, which include an overview of epidemiological aspects, diagnosis, and investigation of pemphigus vulgaris. Available at: http://www.bad.org.uk/healthcare/guidelines.

Pemphigoid

From the Greek meaning 'resembling pemphigus'.

Bullous pemphigoid

Bullous pemphigoid (BP) is the commonest of the autoimmune blistering diseases seen in the West. It presents most often in elderly patients but can affect younger adults and, rarely, children.

Autoantibodies to collagen XVII, a transmembrane component of the hemidesmosomes, appear to initiate disease—see Box 13.7. The course is punctuated by exacerbations and partial remissions, but the disease may remit in 5–10 years.

What should I look for?

- Evidence of a common cause of blisters, e.g. eczema or infection—see 📖 p.78.
- Itchy urticated papules or plaques (this itchy rash may be present for up to a year before the blisters appear).
- Numerous tense blisters, 1–3cm in diameter, on inflamed or normal-appearing skin. Blistering in bullous pemphigoid tends to predominate on the lower trunk, flexural surfaces of limbs, axillae, and groins—see 📖 Fig. 13.5, p.245.
- Crusted erosions.
- Healing without scarring, provided that blisters have not been scratched or become secondarily infected.
- Oral blisters or erosions (present in about 1/3 of patients).
- Check the eyes—conjunctiva are not affected in BP.

What should I do?

- Take a skin biopsy for histology and direct immunofluorescence microscopy—see Box 13.8.
- Take blood for indirect immunofluorescence microscopy.
- Aspirate fluid from any large uncomfortable blisters.
- Take swabs from eroded skin to exclude infection.
- Treatments include:
  - Skin care to prevent infection—see 📖 p.592.
  - Very potent topical corticosteroid, e.g. 0.05% clobetasol propionate cream applied liberally ×2/day to all erythematous, eroded, and blistering skin.
  - Oral corticosteroids 20–60mg/day (and bone protection).
  - Oral tetracyclines, erythromycin, or nicotinamide as steroid-sparing agents.
  - Immunosuppressive drugs such as azathioprine and methotrexate as steroid-sparing agents if disease proves difficult to control.

Rare variants of pemphigoid

- Pemphigoid gestationis occurs in pregnancy or the puerperium—see 📖 p.540.
- Mucous membrane (cicatricial) pemphigoid—see 📖 p.252.

Box 13.7 Antigens in bullous pemphigoid

- The 230kDa ***bullous pemphigoid antigen 1*** (BPAg1, BP230) is a member of the plakin protein family, a group of intracellular proteins that link the intermediate filament cytoskeleton to adhesion plaques such as hemidesmosomes and desmosomes in plasma membranes. BPAg1 is not exposed on the cell surface and the antibodies to BPAg1 may only develop after keratinocyte injury, but probably enhance the immune response.
- The 180kDa ***bullous pemphigoid antigen 2*** (BPAg2, BP180) also called collagen XVII, is a transmembrane protein in the hemidesmosomes that anchors basal keratinocytes to the basement membrane. BPAg2 extends from the cytoplasm of basal keratinocytes into the lamina densa of the basement membrane zone. The autoantibodies bind to epitopes in the NC16A domain which is part of the molecule that is outside the basal keratinocyte but close to the keratinocyte plasma membrane. Autoantibodies to collagen XVII may initiate disease.

Box 13.8 Histology and immunohistology in bullous pemphigoid

- A biopsy taken from an early urticated erythematous lesion will show subepidermal oedema with an eosinophilic infiltrate in the papillary dermis. The amount of inflammation varies.
- Blistering is subepidermal and blisters usually contain eosinophils.
- Direct and indirect immunofluorescence microscopy show a linear band of IgG and/or C3 at the dermo-epidermal junction.
- The autoantibodies are directed against antigens that are associated with hemidesmosomes and localize to the epidermal side (roof) of salt split skin (see 📖 Box 13.4, p.247).

Further reading

Wojnarowska F *et al.* 2002. Evidence-based guidelines, prepared on behalf of the British Association of Dermatologists; include an overview of epidemiological aspects, diagnosis, and investigation of pemphigoid. Available at: http://www.bad.org.uk/healthcare/guidelines.

Rare subepidermal blistering diseases

⚠ Mucous membrane pemphigoid

Mucous membrane (cicatricial) pemphigoid is a rare variant of pemphigoid that is characterized by painful subepithelial blistering, ulceration, and scarring—see Box 13.9. This chronic, disabling form of pemphigoid is difficult to control. Corticosteroids, dapsone, and other immunosuppressants may be used in treatment.

What should I look for?

- Scattered tense blisters or ulcers on the scalp, face, or upper trunk—these heal with scarring.
- Oral blisters or ulcers (particularly affecting the gingiva or buccal mucosa).
- Conjunctival inflammation, blisters, or erosions.
- Adhesions between the surfaces of bulbar and palpebral conjunctiva (best seen by gently pulling down the lower eyelid and asking the patient to look to the left and then to the right)—see 🕮 p.49.
- Involvement of other mucosal surfaces—nasopharynx, larynx, oesophagus, genitalia, and/or rectum.

⚠ Epidermolysis bullosa aquisita (EBA)

EBA is a very rare mechanobullous subepidermal blistering disease that is associated with autoantibodies to type VII collagen—see Box 13.10. It is sometimes associated with inflammatory bowel disease or rheumatoid arthritis. Patients are usually aged 40–60. Corticosteroids, dapsone, other immunosuppressants, IV immunoglobulins, plasmapheresis, and rituximab have been used in treatment with variable success.

What should I look for?

- Sudden onset of skin fragility or blistering in areas exposed to trauma—knuckles, elbows, knees, sacrum, and toes (may resemble porphyria cutanea tarda but patients are not photosensitive nor do they have hypertrichosis—see 🕮 p.310).
- Tense blisters and ulcers affecting skin exposed to trauma.
- Blisters may be haemorrhagic and underlying skin inflamed or scarred.
- Healing with scarring and milia (tiny subepidermal white firm cysts).
- Nail dystrophy or loss of nails; scarring alopecia.
- Less often:
    - Bullous pemphigoid-like with no predilection for sites exposed to trauma, tense bullae on erythematous skin, and minimal scarring.
    - Predominantly mucosal involvement. Ulcers and scars may affect conjunctiva, oral mucosa, upper oesophagus, anus, trachea, and/or vagina.

⚠ Other rare subepidermal blistering diseases

- Linear IgA disease—affects children (also known as chronic bullous disease of childhood) and adults.
- Bullous LE—see 🕮 Box 19.9, p.375.
- Dermatitis herpetiformis—see 🕮 p.254.

Box 13.9 Antigens in mucous membrane pemphigoid

- The 180kDa bullous pemphigoid antigen 2 (BPAg2, BP180) is also involved in mucous membrane pemphigoid, but the predominant epitope site is in the C-terminal portion, much deeper within the epidermal basement membrane zone than in bullous pemphigoid.
- Mucous membrane pemphigoid sera also have autoantibodies to laminin 332 and sometimes to laminin 311 as well as type VII collagen.
- Binding to these deeper antigens may be relevant to the scarring pathology that is a feature of this form of pemphigoid.

Box 13.10 Antigens in EBA

- Type VII collagen, a component of the anchoring fibrils that fasten the lamina densa of the basement membrane to the underlying papillary dermis, is the antigen in EBA.
- Blistering is subepidermal.
- Direct and indirect immunofluorescence microscopy shows a linear band of IgG and/or C3 at the dermo-epidermal junction.
- The autoantibodies are directed against antigens that are associated with anchoring fibrils and localize to the dermal side (base) of salt-split skin (see 🕮 Box 13.4, p.247).

Dermatitis herpetiformis

This uncommon blistering disease presents at any age and is associated with a gluten-sensitive enteropathy—see 📖 coeliac disease, p.476. Epidermal transglutaminase appears to be the dominant autoantigen in dermatitis herpetiformis, but the pathogenesis of the rash is uncertain. Patients also have circulating antibodies that bind to tissue transglutaminase in reticulin fibres such as endomysium—a component of smooth muscle.

Patients with dermatitis herpetiformis have an increased incidence of other autoimmune diseases including thyroid disease, pernicious anaemia, type 1 diabetes, and SLE.

Patients also have an increased risk of intestinal lymphoma.

What should I look for?

- Sudden onset of an extremely itchy rash exacerbated by oral gluten.
- Symptoms suggesting coeliac disease—fatigue, 'irritable bowel' symptoms, diarrhoea—but the patchy enteropathy is often sub-clinical.
- A family history of dermatitis herpetiformis or coeliac disease (10% of patients).
- Clusters of excoriated papules in a symmetrical distribution on extensor surfaces—elbows, knees, buttocks, shoulders. It is unusual to see intact vesicles because the rash is so itchy ('herpetiformis' because vesicles erupt in groups like herpes simplex)—Fig. 13.6.
- Excoriated papules on the scalp or chin.
- Purpura on fingers suggesting vasculitis.
- Another cause of itching such as eczema or scabies (burrows on sides of fingers, wrists, sides of feet, genitalia)—***very*** much more likely than dermatitis herpetiformis! (see 📖 p.60).

What should I do?

- FBC, iron, vitamin B_{12}, and folate.
- LFT, serum calcium.
- Autoantibody screen including IgA anti-endomysial antibodies.
- Take a biopsy of an intact vesicle or non-excoriated papule for histology—see Box 13.11.
- Take a 4mm punch biopsy from uninvolved buttock skin for direct immunofluorescence microscopy (you may have to repeat the test on another skin biopsy before a positive result is obtained, but you should not diagnose dermatitis herpetiformis without a positive result).
- Arrange investigation of the small intestine if diagnosis is confirmed.
- Treat with dapsone (1–2mg/kg/day)—the itching will subside within 48–72h of taking dapsone. Dapsone has no effect on the enteropathy.
- Arrange for the patient to see a dietician—a strict gluten-free diet will control the enteropathy and, eventually, the rash (may take 2 years). Dapsone requirements will fall slowly if the patient adheres to the diet.
- Encourage the patient to stick to the diet—a strict gluten-free diet will protect against the increased risk of lymphoma in dermatitis herpetiformis.

Box 13.11 Histology and immunohistology in dermatitis herpetiformis

- A skin biopsy taken from an early lesion will show small collections of neutrophils (microabscesses) at the tips of oedematous dermal papillae.
- In older lesions you may see small subepidermal vesicles containing neutrophils and some eosinophils.
- Direct immunofluorescence microscopy of biopsies taken from uninvolved skin show granular deposits of IgA at the basement membrane zone in the tips of the dermal papillae.

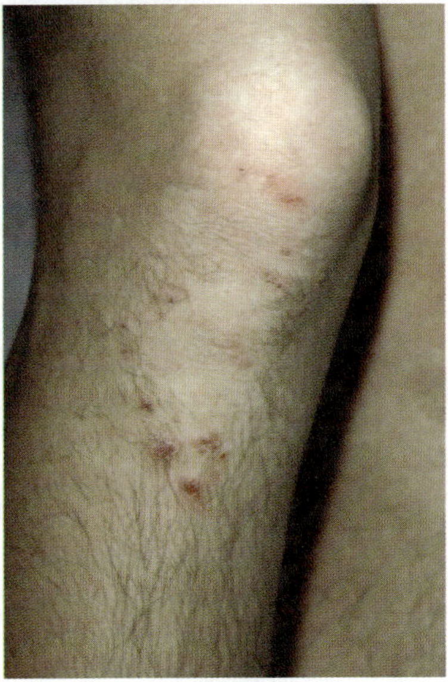

Fig. 13.6 Dermatitis herpetiformis: the itchy vesicles on extensor surfaces soon rupture leaving small erosions and excoriated papules.

Chapter 14

Oral and genital mucosae

Contents

Relevant pages in other chapters

Examination of mucosae is discussed in detail in Chapter 3, 🕮 p.48. Also see Chapter 4, 🕮 p.82.

Oral and genital ulcers

Inflammation of the oral mucosa (stomatitis) may be caused by drugs, infections, skin diseases, or systemic diseases. Pain or burning are common presenting symptom and ulcers a frequent secondary finding. >1 mucosal surface may be affected, so in any patient with stomatitis it is important to ask about the eyes and genital symptoms.

Patients may be reluctant to volunteer anogenital symptoms. Genital ulceration may be secondary to trauma, infection, or inflammatory disease. *Pseudomonas aeruginosa* causes anogenital ecthyma in immunosuppressed patients—see 📖 p.129. Disease may be localized or generalized, so examine skin and other mucosal surfaces. SCC may present as an 'ulcer'. Take a biopsy from any persistent ulcer (Box 14.1).

Causes of oral and genital ulcers are discussed on 📖 p.82.

Box 14.1 ⚠When to biopsy

- Persistent ulcer (>2 weeks) of unknown cause.
- Ulcer unresponsive to treatment.
- Ulcer that persists despite removal of known precipitant.

Herpes simplex virus

Herpetic gingivostomatitis

Primary infections with HSV (usually type 1, occasionally type 2) may be asymptomatic, but can cause a painful ulcerative gingivostomatitis (most often in children) that resolves in 10–14 days. Recurrent herpes labialis is caused by reactivation of the latent virus—see 📖 p.144. A tingling, burning, or itching prodrome is common. EM may be caused by herpes infections and may recur—see 📖 p.105.

What should I look for in primary infections?

- Malaise, headache, and fever; cervical lymphadenopathy.
- Well-defined vesicles, 2mm in diameter, on the dorsum of the tongue and the hard palate, but vesicles may be scattered over the entire oral mucosa. Vesicles rupture rapidly to form very painful shallow ulcers with a yellowish-grey floor and erythematous margins.
- Inflamed gingival margins.

What should I do?

Management is symptomatic with fluids and pain relief. Oral aciclovir, 200mg ×5/day for 5 days, is helpful in primary attacks if vesicles are still present (within the first 3 days). Recurrent herpes labialis does not usually need treatment with aciclovir.

Genital HSV infection

Genital infections are usually caused by HSV-2 and only occasionally by HSV-1. Primary attacks are more severe and long-lasting than subsequent attacks. Prevalence is highest in individuals adopting high-risk sexual behaviour, but viral carriage is often asymptomatic. Genital HSV increases the risk of acquiring and/or transmitting HIV.

What should I look for?

- Genital pain, itching, and/or burning.
- Erythematous vesicles, but these rapidly rupture forming painful ulcers.
- Dysuria leading to urinary retention.

What should I do?

- Consider other causes of ulcers including EBV infection—see Box 14.2.
- Take swabs for bacterial and viral culture—use viral culture medium.
- Biopsy may be indicated if diagnosis is uncertain.
- Prescribe oral analgesia and topical 2% lidocaine gel.
- Encourage high fluid intake.
- Recommend warm baths (easier to urinate in a bath).
- Prescribe oral antivirals in primary disease.
- Oral prophylaxis with antivirals in severe recurrent disease.
- Genital HSV infection can be transmitted to the fetus or neonate. Prophylactic aciclovir from 36 weeks of gestation reduces the risk of HSV recurrence or HSV viral shedding at delivery.
- Refer for screening for other sexually transmitted diseases.

Box 14.2 Epstein–Barr virus (EBV) infection causing vulval ulcers

Clinical

- Age 10–30 years.
- Genital contact is not a prerequisite for EBV genital ulcers.
- Prodrome: fever and lymphadenopathy.
- Deep, painful, single or multiple vulval ulcers, 0.5–2cm in diameter.
- Irregular erythematous edges.
- Ulcer base: clean, seropurulent, or granulating.
- Heal within 2 weeks.

Investigations

- Monospot (heterophile antibody) test falsely negative during first 2 weeks of symptoms.
- Request IgM antiviral capsid antigen antibodies if you suspect EBV.

Management

- Avoid irritants and use aqueous cream as a soap substitute.
- Warm baths.
- Zinc oxide ointment.
- Pain relief.

Further reading

Sen P and Barton SE. *BMJ* 2007; **334:**1048–52.

Aphthous ulcers (canker sores)

These painful ulcers affect around 20% of the population and may occur in association with systemic disease—see Box 14.3—but most patients are healthy. Aphthous ulcers may be precipitated by stress, trauma, menstruation, or stopping smoking. Genetic factors may also be important.

Aphthous ulceration is divided into minor, major, and herpetiform subtypes. The diagnosis is clinical and management symptomatic—see Box 14.4.

Minor aphthous ulcers (80% of cases)

Ulcers start in childhood or adolescence, are <10mm diameter, and heal in 7–14 days. Crops of ulcers recur every 1–4 months. Ulcers become less frequent with age.

What should I look for?

- 1–5 shallow round or oval ulcers (<10mm diameter) on non-keratinized mucosa—floor of mouth, buccal or labial mucosa (vesicles in herpes simplex rupture to form ulcers most often on the dorsum of the tongue and the hard palate).
- Erythematous haloes.
- Grey-white slough on the base of the ulcer.
- Exclude other mucosal involvement, e.g. genital ulcers, ocular inflammation.

Major aphthous ulcers (10% of cases)

Ulcers usually start in childhood or adolescence, may be as much as 3cm in diameter and heal over months, often with scarring. Ulcers recur at shorter intervals than minor aphthae. Major aphthae may be a sign of Behçet's disease—see 📖 p.264.

What should I look for?

- Crops of 1–6 large ulcers (>10mm diameter) with a firm raised margin in any part of the mouth.
- Considerable pain.
- Scarring and fibrosis (60%).
- Other mucosal involvement, e.g. genital ulcers, ocular inflammation.
- Palpate solitary longstanding non-healing ulcers to check for induration and if indurated consider biopsy to exclude oral cancer.

Herpetiform ulcers (10% of cases)

These tend to occur in patients in their 3rd decade. The ulcers, which resemble ulcers caused by herpesvirus, usually heal within 2 weeks and do not recur more frequently than monthly.

What should I look for?

- Many (up to 100) tiny ulcers (1–2mm diameter) anywhere in the mouth.
- Scarring and fibrosis (30%).

Box 14.3 Diseases associated with aphthous ulcers

- Iron, folate, or vitamin B_{12} deficiency.
- Malabsorption: gluten sensitive enteropathy, Crohn's disease, ulcerative colitis—see 📖 p.472.
- Behçet's disease—see 📖 p.264.
- HIV infection—see 📖 p.154.
- Reiter's syndrome—see 📖 p.194.
- Sweet's syndrome—see 📖 p.480.
- Aplastic anaemia, neutropenia, and other immunodeficiencies.

Box 14.4 Management of aphthous ulcers

- Eliminate predisposing factors and investigate for underlying systemic disease as indicated by the history and examination.
- Topical corticosteroids speed ulcer healing, e.g.:
  - Hydrocortisone 2.5mg oral pellets placed on or held next to the ulcer ×3–4/day.
  - Soluble betamethasone tablets 0.5mg dissolved in 15–20mL of water and held in the mouth for 3min ×4/day—emphasize that this is to be used as a mouthwash and that the solution should not be swallowed.
  - Beclometasone dipropionate 50 or 100 inhaler sprayed onto the affected areas and held in the mouth for as long as possible ×4–6/day.
- Antiseptic mouthwashes:
  - Chlorhexidine.
- Soothing oral preparations with local anaesthetic, e.g.:
  - 30mL nystatin sugar-free mix plus 20mL lidocaine injection 2% plus 10mL of a suspending agent such as mucilage.
  - Prescribe 5mL of this mixture to be rinsed around the mouth before meals.
- Major aphthous stomatitis may require treatment with systemic corticosteroids, prolonged courses of low-dose oral tetracyclines (e.g. minocycline 100mg/day or lymecycline 408mg/day for 6 months) or, rarely, thalidomide.

Further reading

Scully C and Felix DH. *Br Dent J* 2005; **199:**339–43.
Scully C and Shotts R. *BMJ* 2000; **321:**162–5.

Behçet's disease

Behçet's disease, named after the Turkish dermatologist who described it in 1936, is rare, chronic, multisystem, and relapsing. The pathogenesis is not understood, but involves an immune complex-mediated vasculitis. The disease most commonly affects populations along the 'silk route' in Turkey, Iran, and Japan, but is seen worldwide. Behçet's disease is associated with HLA-B51. Diagnosis is based on clinical criteria—see Box 14.5.

What should I look for?

Mucocutaneous lesions

- Oral ulceration (all patients): recurrent and painful, small ulcers heal without scarring but larger ulcers may scar.
- Genital ulceration (85% of patients): usually scrotal or labial, may affect vagina and cervix, usually leaves scars.
- Papulo-pustular lesions (85% of patients): resembling acne or folliculitis, appear as papules on an erythematous base and develop into a pustule over 24–48h. Most common on the trunk.
- Erythema nodosum-like lesions (50% of patients) on the legs, leaving residual pigmentation.
- Superficial thrombophlebitis (25% of patients): erythematous, tender, subcutaneous nodules in a linear distribution which may be confused with erythema nodosum.
- Extragenital ulceration: uncommon but may occur at any site.
- A history of pustules developing at sites of needle-prick (pathergy): e.g. after venepuncture.

Eye disease (50% of patients)

- Chronic, relapsing anterior and posterior uveitis are a major cause of morbidity and may result in retinal haemorrhage, papilloedema, and macular disease with loss of visual acuity and the threat of blindness.

Musculoskeletal disease (50% of patients)

- Most often a non-deforming, non-erosive peripheral oligoarthritis lasting a few weeks.
- Some patients have chronic arthritis, osteonecrosis, and myositis.

Neurological disease (5% of patients)

- Pyramidal, cerebellar, and sensory signs, sphincter disturbance, behavioural changes, and dural sinus thrombosis.
- Peripheral nerve lesions are unusual.

Vascular disease (5% of patients)

- Large-vessel vasculitis can result in thrombosis and occlusion.

Other systems (rare)

- Gastrointestinal mucosal ulceration, splenomegaly, glomerulonephritis, and cardiac involvement have been reported.

Box 14.5 Criteria for the diagnosis of Behçet's disease

Recurrent oral ulceration	Minor aphthous, major aphthous, or herpetiform ulceration observed by a physician or patient that recurred at least 3 times in one 12-month period.
Plus 2 of the following:	
Genital ulcers	Aphthous ulceration. Includes anal ulcers/swollen testicles or epididymitis observed by physician or patient.
Eye inflammation	Anterior uveitis, posterior uveitis, or cells in vitreous on slit lamp examination; or retinal vasculitis observed by ophthalmologist.
Cutaneous lesions	Erythema nodosum observed by physician or patient, folliculitis or papulo-pustular lesions; or acneiform nodules observed by physician in post-adolescent patients not receiving corticosteroids.
Positive pathergy test	Read by physician at 24–48h.

Findings applicable only in absence of other clinical explanations.

Reference: see International Study Group for Behçet's disease. *Br J Rheumatol* 1992; **31:**299–308.

What should I do?

Investigations

- The pathergy test: hyper-reactivity of the skin to needle prick (skin prick of the forearm results in a papule or pustule in 24–48h). Test positivity varies (approximately 60%) and is highest in Japan and Mediterranean countries, but is highly specific for Behçet's disease.
- Biopsy: papulopustular lesions or pathergy reactions.
- Genital ulcers: exclude infection, e.g. herpesvirus, EBV—see 🕮 p.260.
- FBC may show anaemia of chronic disease and leucocytosis.
- Inflammatory markers are not good indicators of disease activity.
- ANA, RF, and ANCA are negative.

Treatment

- A very potent topical corticosteroid ointment (clobetasol propionate) and topical 2% lidocaine gel may relieve pain in oral and genital ulcers.
- The use of systemic corticosteroids is controversial.
- Other immunosuppressives that have been used include azathioprine, ciclosporin, methotrexate, and cyclophosphamide.
- Thalidomide can be effective for aphthous ulcers but is teratogenic and is difficult to obtain. Irreversible painful peripheral neuropathy is another potential adverse effect.
- Colchicine may reduce arthralgia and mucocutaneous lesions.
- IFNα may have a role in oral and genital ulcers.
- Anti-TNF biologic agents or the interleukin-1 receptor antagonist, anakinra, may be effective.

Mucosal lichen planus

Lichen planus (LP) is a chronic inflammatory condition of unknown cause that may affect mucosal surfaces and/or skin—see 📖 p.208. A band-like 'lichenoid' infiltrate of lymphocytes hugs the basal layer of the epidermis or epithelium.

LP can be drug-induced—see 📖 p.350. Infrequently oral LP is caused by allergies to metals or flavourings in foods.

What should I look for?

- Asymptomatic lacy white streaks (Wickham's striae), white papules, and plaques on buccal mucosa, tongue, or genitalia (vulva, glans penis, shaft of penis). These cannot be scraped off, unlike mucosal candidiasis (Fig. 14.1).
- Erosive mucosal disease: glazed erythema, erosions with white lacy border, painful oral ulcers. May also have erosive genital disease—vulvovaginal-gingival syndrome, peno-gingival syndrome.
- Gingivitis (erythematous erosions, patchy hypopigmentation).
- Genital lesions may become hypertrophic.
- Annular LP on shaft of penis may be associated with flexural annular LP, e.g. in axillae.
- Erosive vulvovaginal LP (vulvar vestibule and vagina) with itch, dysuria, and/or dyspareunia. Associated with oral disease especially gingival LP.
- Scarring in chronic erosive vulvovaginal disease with atrophy and fusion of labia and narrowing of vaginal introitus.
- SCC is a rare complication in chronic erosive disease and may be asymptomatic—check for mucosal thickening, a nodule or a persistent ulcer.
- Cutaneous disease: flat-topped, shiny polygonal purplish papules. Seen more often in oral and penile LP than vulval LP—see 📖 p.208.
- Rarely LP affects the oesophagus, larynx, bladder, and/or anus.

What should I do?

- A biopsy may be required to confirm the diagnosis.
- Take swabs for culture from painful erosions.
- Withdraw any potentially causative systemic drugs.
- Oral LP: consider patch testing to exclude allergy to metals or oral flavourings (rarely positive).
- ⚠ Erosive mucosal disease may be chronic and persistent: patients should be counselled about the risk of SCC and reviewed regularly.

Differential diagnosis

- Chronic cutaneous GVHD shares many clinical and histological features with LP—see 📖 p.496, and Fig. 26.2, p.491.
- Oral discoid LE (see 📖 p.374) can look similar to oral LP.
- Vulval LP may simulate lichen sclerosus—see 📖 p.268.

Box 14.6 Management of mucosal lichen planus

- Asymptomatic mucosal disease does not require treatment.
- Potent or very potent corticosteroid ointments ×1 or 2/day.
- Analgesia with topical 2% lidocaine gel as in aphthous stomatitis if symptomatic—see 🕮 Box 14.4, p.263.
- Topical 0.1% tacrolimus ointment ×2/daily is worth trying in severe disease unresponsive to corticosteroids, but monitor erosive disease carefully because of the risk of malignancy.
- Genital LP: aqueous cream as a soap substitute.
- Very severe cutaneous or mucosal LP: short courses of oral corticosteroids to control itching or pain, but unfortunately disease recurs on stopping corticosteroids. Other therapies that have been tried include UVB, oral retinoids, and ciclosporin.

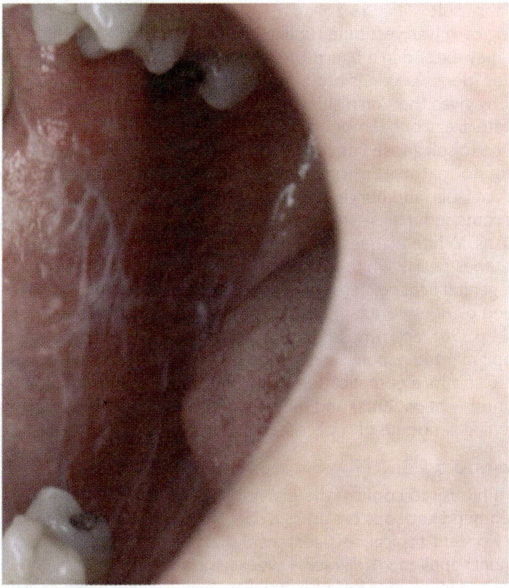

Fig. 14.1 Oral LP with lacy white streaks on the buccal mucosa.

Further reading

Scully C and Carrozzo M. *Br J Oral Maxillofac Surg* 2008; **46:**15–21.

Lichen sclerosus

This chronic inflammatory disease with a predilection for genital skin has two peaks of onset—childhood and postmenopausal. The cause is uncertain but a lymphocyte-mediated autoimmune pathogenesis is suspected. Lichen sclerosus may occur in association with morphoea (📖 p.390) (with which extra-genital lichen sclerosus shows considerable clinical and histological overlap), LP, and vitiligo.

Lichen sclerosus is most common in adult females. It may be asymptomatic, but usually presents with itch, pain, and/or dyspareunia. Perianal involvement with painful anal fissures may lead to constipation in young girls. Uncircumcised males may be affected. Lichen sclerosus of the foreskin (balanitis zerotica obliterans) is a major cause of circumcision.

What should I look for?

- Pearly white papules and plaques on labia minora, clitoris, and interlabial sulci—Fig. 14.2.
- Sparing of vulvar vestibule (unlike LP).
- Signs may extend in a figure-of-eight configuration to perianal skin in females (perianal skin is not affected in males).
- Atrophy gives the skin a shiny crinkled appearance—Fig. 14.2.
- Discrete areas of haemorrhage (ecchymoses) within the white plaques (may be misdiagnosed as sexual abuse in young girls)—Fig. 14.2.
- Loss of normal anatomy in chronic disease—resorption of labia minora, fusion of labia, and burying of clitoris.
- Uncircumcised males—thickening and tightening of foreskin causing phimosis. White plaques on glans penis, sometimes with scarring. Sometimes pearly white papules on shaft of penis.
- Extra-genital lichen sclerosus is uncommon—the hypopigmented crinkled plaques contain follicular plugs (unlike morphoea—see 📖 p.390), ecchymoses, and, rarely, haemorrhagic blisters. Hypopigmented papules are sometimes seen in children.
- ⚠ SCC is a rare complication in chronic genital disease in adults (around 5% of patients) and may be asymptomatic—check for mucosal thickening, a nodule or a persistent ulcer.

What should I do?

- Take a biopsy to confirm the diagnosis.
- Recommend aqueous cream as a soap substitute for genital use.
- A very potent topical corticosteroid (0.05% clobetasol propionate ointment) applied x 1/day for 4 weeks and then with gradually decreasing frequency for a further 8 weeks usually controls disease and may even reverse the early changes (may also be effective in children).
- Counsel about the small risk of SCC, teach self-examination, and recommend annual reviews.

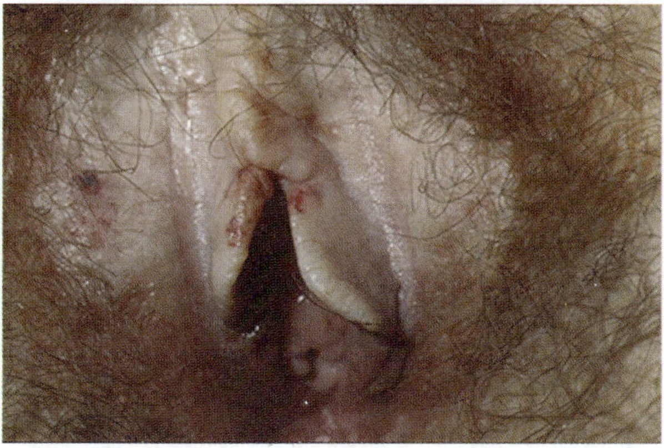

Fig. 14.2 Typical lichen sclerosus with pallor and haemorrhage (courtesy of Dr Susan Cooper, Oxford).

Further reading

Cooper SM *et al. Arch Dermatol* 2004; **140:**702–6.

Neill SM *et al. Br J Dermatol* 2002; **147:**640–9.

Chapter 15

Leg ulcers and lymphoedema

Contents

Introduction

You are likely to come across a patient with a chronic leg ulcer at some stage in most branches of adult medicine. 1–2% of people will develop a leg ulcer during their life and chronic ulcers cause morbidity and disability, particularly in the elderly.

Traditionally, nurses care for leg ulcers and doctors are asked to see the patient when complications ensue or the ulcer is not healing as expected. Many doctors feel poorly trained to deal with such patients, particularly because they have no experience of what is a 'normal' leg ulcer.

Learn from the expertise of the wound-care nurses and take an interest in your patients' leg ulcers. Ulcers may be associated with systemic disease as well as vascular problems, infections, and malignancy—you may be surprised what you find underneath the dressings!

The history

Take a full dermatological history (see 📖 p.18, p.20) asking questions that will help you to pinpoint the likely cause of the ulcer as well as factors that may delay healing—see Boxes 15.1–15.3.

What should I ask?

- When the ulcer developed and how it progressed? What preceded ulceration, e.g. trauma, pressure, tender pustule (may indicate pyoderma gangrenosum) or blister?
- Explore concerns (patients may fear that they are going to lose the leg).
- Pain: character, how much, what makes it worse or better? See 📖 p.284.
- Does the patient sleep in a bed or in a chair at night?
- How much elevation is tolerated?
- Impact of ulcer on quality of life? Use the DLQI (see 📖 p.32).
- Mobility: how much exercise?
- Weight: obesity is common in venous disease.
- Problems with skin around ulcer: redness, pain, itch?
- Swelling of limb: does it improve after elevation, e.g. overnight?
- Present management:
  - Dressings and bandages: how often is the ulcer dressed?
  - Any compression? How much elevation?
  - Pain relief: how much, how often is it taken?
- Number of previous episodes of ulceration?
- Any cellulitis?
- Previous treatments for ulcer:
  - Dressings or bandages?
  - Topical treatments?
  - Surgical interventions, e.g. angioplasty, skin graft?
- Past medical history and functional Inquiry including:
  - Skin cancers and sun exposure? See 📖 p.26
  - Hypertension, claudication, angina, myocardial infarction?
  - Cerebrovascular accident?
  - Diabetes, peripheral neuropathy?
  - Obesity?
  - Hypercholesterolemia?
  - DVT or pulmonary emboli?
  - Varicose veins: varicosities in pregnancy, varicose vein surgery?
  - Major orthopaedic intervention, long bone fracture?
  - Rheumatoid arthritis?
- Family history of varicose veins, leg ulcers, DVT, or pulmonary emboli?
- Social history: carers, home environment; job: prolonged standing?
- Drug history: e.g. nicorandil, prednisolone, hydroxycarbamide?
- Allergies: 'reactions' to dressings or bandages. Patch tested?
- Smoker?

Further reading

Sarkar PK and Ballantyne S. *Postgrad Med J* 2000; **76:**674–82.

Box 15.1 Common causes of leg and foot ulcers—see Figs. 15.1–15.4

- ***Valvular incompetence*** with venous reflux leads to venous hypertension and finally to ulcers (70%). Older patients, most often women. Pain and swelling; PMH of DVT, trauma, operations to hips or knees; obesity and immobility; personal and family history of varicose veins.
- ***Arterial disease*** (5–10%). Intermittent claudication, rest pain, night pain, pain worse when leg is elevated. Smokers.
- ***Mixed arteriovenous*** (15%): symptoms of both venous and arterial disease.
- ***Neuropathic:*** sites of pressure—often asymptomatic. Blood on the floor may be the first indication of trouble to the patient. Most common on feet of diabetics when also associated with small-vessel disease—see p.506.

Box 15.2 Other causes of leg ulcers

- ***Malignancy:*** BCC commonest. Misdiagnosed as an 'ulcer'—see p.328.
- ***Pyoderma gangrenosum:*** rapidly growing, very painful ulcer. Often preceded by a tender pustule. Associated with rheumatoid arthritis, inflammatory bowel disease, and myeloproliferative disorders but 50% of patients have no underlying disease. See Fig. 15.5, p.277 and p.290.
- ***Vasculitic:*** associated with connective tissue diseases particularly rheumatoid arthritis, when immobility and coexisting arteriovenous disease often contribute to ulceration. See p.366.
- ***Occlusive vasculopathy*** e.g. livedoid 'vasculitis' with atrophie blanche, sickle cell disease, thalassaemia, thrombocythaemia, hypertensive ulcer (Martorell's)—see Box 15.4, p.278 calciphylaxis, cryoglobulinaemia, antiphospholipid syndrome—see p.418.
- ***Inherited disorders of coagulation***: mutations in protein C, protein S, antithrombin III, fibrinogen, or factor V genes.
- ***Necrobiosis lipoidica:*** associated with insulin-dependent diabetes.
- ***Infection:*** fungal, treponemal.
- ***Drug-related***: hydroxyurea, nicorandil.
- ***Trauma*** including IV drug abuse.
- ***Dermatitis artefacta:*** deliberate self-harm.

Box 15.3 Factors that may delay healing

- ***Oedema***: gravitational, congestive cardiac failure.
- ***Immobility***: contributes to poor calf muscle pump and oedema.
- ***Anaemia or malnutrition***: vitamin C deficiency may be a particular problem in the elderly.
- ***Corticosteroids*** (the impact of other immunosuppressive drugs is less certain).
- ***Repetitive trauma*** including poor dressing technique.
- ***Heavy colonization with bacteria*** (suggested by increasing malodour, increasing pain, and heavy exudate). Paradoxically some bacteria may promote healing, but the role played by bacteria is not fully understood.

Preparing to examine the ulcer

The leg ulcer is likely to be hidden away under dressings and bandages. Many doctors are reluctant to remove bandages, perhaps for fear of what they might find underneath, but more often because they are pressed for time or feel ill-prepared to re-dress the leg, a task that may not be as easy as it is as it sounds without the help of a skilled nurse. But it is important to inspect the limb beneath the bandages—try not to be put off.

Explain to the patient what you wish to do and why. Ask if any preparation is required before the dressing is removed. Is analgesia required?

Try to find out what dressings or bandages are being used.

Discuss your plans with the nurses, arrange a suitable time, help the nurses to set up a dressing trolley… and take the plunge.

What do I need?

- Plastic gloves (do not need to be sterile) and a plastic apron.
- A trolley with:
  - Gauze swabs, scissors, plastic forceps, and a sinus probe (if the ulcer might be deeply penetrating).
  - A bag for disposing of contaminated dressings.
- Water for washing the leg and the ulcer—a bucket may be useful.
- Clingfilm to cover the ulcer—exposing the ulcer to air may be painful.
- A sphygmomanometer, stethoscope, and Doppler ultrasound probe for checking the ankle brachial pressure index (ABPI)—see 📖 Box 15.6, p.281.
- A tendon hammer, tuning fork (128-Hz) and disposable neurological pin if you suspect a neuropathic ulcer. (Ideally a Semmes–Weinstein 10-g monofilament for evaluation of sensation if you know how to use it.)
- A tape measure.
- An acetate sheet (or the transparent cover of a dressing pack) and pen for tracing the ulcer.
- A digital camera.
- 50% liquid paraffin in WSP or a bland ointment such as Hydromol® to moisturize the skin.
- Dressings and bandages (see 📖 p.286) including a viscose stockinette® bandage long enough to run from toe to just below knee to hold the dressing in place.
- Surgical adhesive tape for securing the end of the bandage—avoid safety pins.

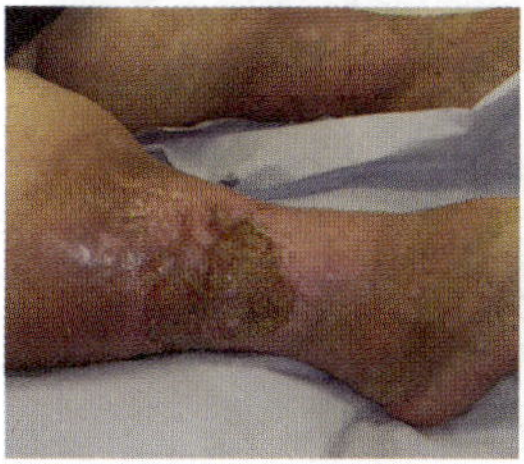

Fig. 15.1 Venous ulcer in gaiter area in an obese woman.

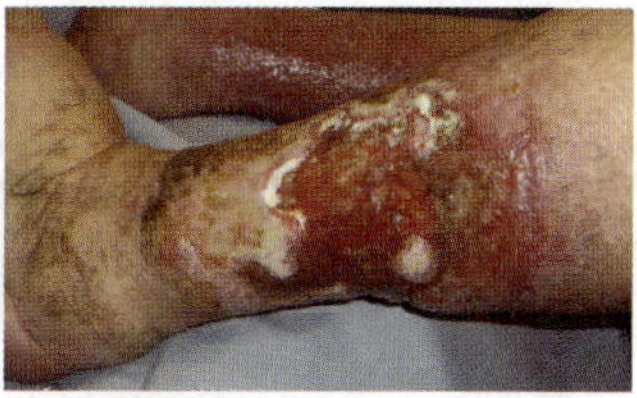

Fig. 15.2 Ulceration in a patient with a combination of venous disease and lymphoedema (thick swollen folds of skin around the ankle, hyperkeratosis, and swelling of the dorsum of the foot as well as the leg).

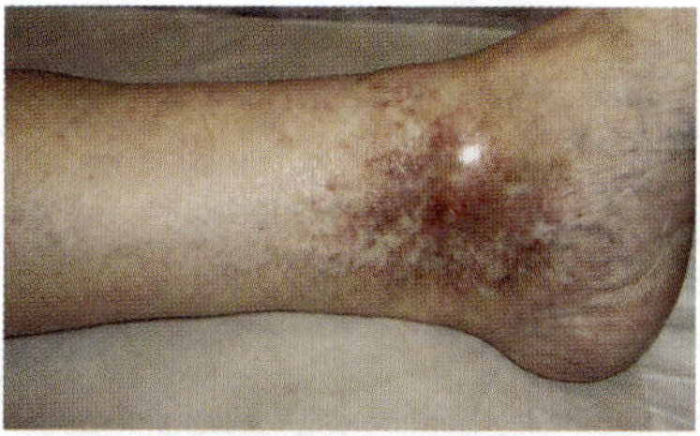

Fig. 15.3 Atrophie blanche (shiny white stellate scar with peripheral telangiectasia) in venous disease. Atrophie blanche may also be seen in occlusive vasculopathies such as livedoid vasculopathy or antiphospholipid syndrome (see 🕮 p.294, p.418).

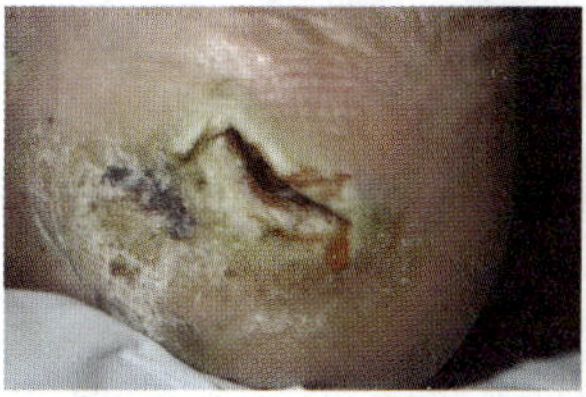

Fig. 15.4 Deeply penetrating neuropathic ulcer with surrounding callus and underlying osteomyelitis.

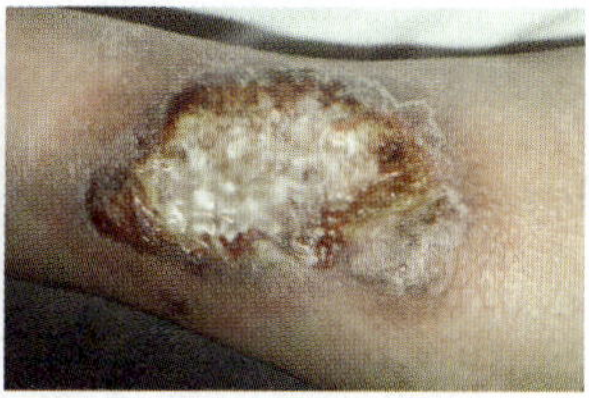

Fig. 15.5 Typical pyoderma gangrenosum with a purplish undermined border.

The examination

What should I do?

- Lie the patient comfortably on an examination couch.
- Adjust the lighting so you can see the legs and the ulcer.
- Protect bedding beneath the legs with incontinence pads.
- Carry out a full physical examination that includes palpation of the abdomen to look for masses that might be causing external venous compression.
- Check the blood pressure—see Box 15.4.
- Remove bandages to expose the leg.
- Gently peel off dressings so that the ulcer is exposed. You may need to soak the dressing with normal saline prior to removal if it has stuck to the wound.
- Note the colour and quantity of exudate on the dressing. Heavy exudate suggests heavy bacterial colonization. Green dressings indicate the presence of *Pseudomonas*.
- Remove loose crust, scab, or adherent dressing and gently wash the ulcer with water so you can see the base and the wound edges.
- If the ulcer is painful when exposed to air, cover temporarily with clingfilm or a moist gauze swab.
- Assess the ulcer—site, wound edge, and wound bed (slough, granulation tissue, necrotic base)—see Box 15.5.
- Measure the ulcer (maximum diameters or trace onto acetate sheet).
- Probe to assess amount of undermining and depth of the ulcer.
- Record the appearance of the ulcer with photographs if possible.
- Examine the surrounding skin looking for signs of venous or arterial disease—see Box 15.5.
- Look for cellulitis—heat, swelling, tender erythema (this may be difficult to differentiate from lipodermatosclerosis—see 📖 p.288).
- Assess the peripheral circulation including the ABPI—see 📖 Box 15.6, p.281.
- Assess joint mobility at ankles and feet.

Box 15.4 ☛ Hypertensive ulcer (Martorell's ulcer)

- The existence of this entity is controversial and these ulcers must be rare.
- Painful ulceration may be secondary to a thrombo-occlusive vasculopathy of cutaneous arterioles in longstanding hypertension.
- Patients present with an extremely painful superficial ulcer with an erythematous or purpuric rim, usually on the anterolateral aspect of the shin. Ulcers start as purpuric lesions which soon become necrotic. Management involves control of hypertension, pain relief, and compression bandaging.

Box 15.5 Signs in different types of ulcer

Venous (Figs. 15.1 and 15.2)

- Gaiter area, just above the medial malleolus or (less often) lateral malleolus. Sloping, poorly defined wound edge and a shallow, but large ulcer that may extend circumferentially around the limb. Pitting oedema.
- Varicose veins (assess standing): gently press any swelling to confirm it is a varicosity. The vein will empty and refill when you let go. Varicosities of the short saphenous vein are seen posterolaterally below the knee; varicosities of the long saphenous vein run more medially along the whole length of the limb.
- Venous flare (dilated superficial venules at the ankle), brownish pigmentation (haemosiderin and melanin), eczema in gaiter area. Sometimes these signs are localized to skin over varicosities—stand the patient up to see the varicosities.
- Scar at sites of previous ulcer, atrophie blanche (Fig. 15.3).
- Lipodermatosclerosis: erythematous tender tight indurated skin above the medial malleolus that may simulate cellulitis—see 🕮 Fig. 15.6, p.289.

Arterial

- Peripheral on borders or sides of feet. Elsewhere initiated by trauma.
- Round ulcer, sharply demarcated with a punched-out appearance. Tendon may be exposed at base.
- Cool, shiny pale or dusky skin with loss of hair. Peripheral gangrene. Reduced peripheral pulses, delayed capillary refill—see 🕮 p.280 for assessment of circulation.

Mixed arteriovenous: reduced peripheral circulation and evidence of venous disease.

Neuropathic (Fig. 15.4)

- Pressure sites on foot, most often under second metatarsal head. Surrounded by callus. Look for limited joint mobility or deformity (Charcot joints are caused by impaired joint position sense and sensation).
- Check footwear for source of pressure or trauma. Osteomyelitis complicates deep neuropathic ulcers.
- Dry skin may indicate autonomic dysfunction.
- Assess vibration sense (128-Hz tuning fork to apex of great toe), pinprick (just proximal to great toenail), temperature (on dorsum of foot with tuning fork placed in iced water or warm water), sensation with 10g monofilament (if you can), and Achilles tendon reflex.

Pyoderma gangrenosum: bluish, undermined wound edge, base with slough—see 🕮 Box 15.11, p.291, and Fig. 15.5.

Vasculitis: purpuric wound edges. Palpable purpura, nodules, livedo—see 🕮 p.406, 410.

Occlusive vasculopathy: livedo, atrophie blanche—see 🕮 p.292, p.294, p.418, and Box 15.4.

Lymphoedema: see 🕮 p.296.

Malignancy: BCCs or SCCs may be misdiagnosed as 'leg ulcers'. Rarely SCC arises within a chronic ulcer.

Assessing peripheral circulation

What should I do?

- Compare the signs in the legs.
- Check peripheral pulses (dorsalis pedis, posterior tibial, popliteal, femoral).
- Listen for bruits in the femoral arteries.
- Peripheral perfusion: push on the nailbed until it turns white. Let go and colour should return (capillary refill) in <2s—not a very reliable test.
- Buerger's test. Soles should be pink with patient supine. Elevate both legs to 45° for 1–2min. Compare the soles. Marked pallor suggests ischaemia. Sit the patient up and lower the legs over the side of the bed. Colour will return to the legs but an ischaemic limb will become blue and then very red. Post-hypoxic vasodilatation causes hyperaemia.
- Assess the peripheral arterial circulation by measuring the ABPI using a handheld Doppler ultrasound probe—see Box 15.6.
- Pulse oximetry has been recommended as an alternative to the Doppler ABPI for assessing peripheral circulation, particularly if the leg is very oedematous, but not all vascular surgeons agree that relying on pulse oximetry is safe practice. More work is needed in this area.
- Consider referral to vascular surgeons for lower limb venous duplex scans to detect venous reflux in superficial and deep venous systems.
- Refer to vascular surgeons for arterial colour duplex scan if ABPI is <0.8—►► refer urgently if the ABPI is 0.5 or less.

Box 15.6 How to measure the ABPI

- Seek for permission for what you are going to do—'I would like to compare the blood pressures in your arm and in your leg. We will both be able to hear your pulse because I am going to use this Doppler machine'. Warn that the cuff may feel uncomfortable for a short time when it is tightened on the leg.
- The patient should lie relatively flat for 20–30min before you commence measurements. Ensure the patient is comfortable in that position.
- Apply a sphygmanometer cuff to the arm.
- Inflate the cuff while feeling radial pulse to get a rough idea of the systolic pressure.
- Apply ultrasound gel to the skin over the brachial pulse.
- Angle the Doppler probe at 45–60° and find the brachial pulse (adjust the position and angle of the probe until the sound is maximal).
- Inflate the cuff until the sound disappears.
- Slowly release the pressure and record the pressure at which the sound of the brachial pulse reappears.
- Repeat in the other arm and take the higher of the 2 readings.
- Place clingfilm around the leg covering the surface of the ulcer.
- Place the cuff around the leg just above the medial malleolus.
- Palpate the dorsalis pedis pulse between the 1st and 2nd metatarsals. Apply ultrasound gel to the skin over the pulse and find the dorsalis pedis pulse using the probe. Angle the probe at 45–60° to the foot.
- Inflate the cuff until the sound disappears, deflate slowly, and record the pressure at which the sound reappears.
- If possible repeat at the posterior tibial pulse and take the higher of the 2 readings—but some patients do find the tight cuff uncomfortable.
- Repeat in the other leg.
- Calculate the ABPI in each leg: ABPI = highest ankle pressure/highest brachial pressure.

Box 15.7 Interpretation of the ABPI

- ABPI: 0.9–1.0 Safe to apply high compression.
- ABPI: 0.8. Excludes significant arterial disease. Probably safe to apply compression—start slowly.
- ABPI: 0.6–0.8 = moderate arterial disease. Very gentle compression may be tolerated if required to control venous incompetence and oedema, but bandages should only be applied by an expert and the patient should be monitored. Pulse oximeter may be used to check immediate impact of compression.
- ABPI: <0.5 = severe arterial disease. Do not use compression—refer for an urgent vascular opinion.

⚠ ***Warning*** The arteries are calcified and cannot be compressed in some elderly patients and in some diabetics. In this situation the ABPI is falsely high. If the results do not fit with your clinical findings, review the patient and the test.

Investigations

Investigations should be directed towards determining the underlying cause of ulceration and excluding factors that may delay healing.

Blood tests

- FBC, iron studies.
- ESR, CRP.
- Serum albumin (low in malnutrition) and vitamin C if indicated (may be deficient in elderly patients with a poor diet).
- Random glucose.
- Clotting screen including lupus anticoagulant, anticardiolipin antibody, factor V Leiden, protein C, and protein S levels if multiple DVTs or a family history of DVTs and leg ulcers.
- If signs suggest vasculitis—ANA, RF, hepatitis serology, and complement 4 (low C4 with raised RF may indicate type II or III mixed cryoglobulinaemia—see 📖 p.410). Check ANCA if indications of a systemic vasculitis.
- Cryoglobulins (keep the sample at 37° in a thermos flask—it may be easiest to send the patient to the laboratory)—check if you suspect ulceration is secondary to Type I cryoglobulinaemia associated with a paraprotein e.g. myeloma, lymphoma—see 📖 p.410.

Microbiology

Surface ulcer swabs for microbiological culture are of limited value—ulcers are always colonized with some bacteria.

Only take swabs if you suspect heavy colonization (increasing pain, malodour, and large amounts of exudate) or if you detect signs of cellulitis—warmth, extending tender erythema, oedema—see 📖 p.130.

Ulcer biopsy

The histology of biopsies from the edge of most ulcers, including pyoderma gangrenosum and many vasculitic ulcers, is not diagnostic. Biopsies may be indicated to exclude malignancy or for culture. To exclude fungal or treponemal infection, take a deep biopsy that extends into the base of the ulcer. Send for histological examination as well as culture.

Radiology

Radiograph, MRI, or CT may be used in chronic deep penetrating ulcers to exclude osteomyelitis, e.g. neuropathic foot ulcers in diabetics.

Patch tests

Patients with leg ulcers may be sensitized to topical medicaments, including topical corticosteroids, neomycin, and balsam of Peru (a fragrance in many creams), as well as constituents of dressings or bandages. The resulting allergic contact dermatitis can delay wound healing. All patients with chronic varicose eczema or chronic leg ulcers should be patch tested.

Pain and leg ulcers

Severe pain is common in patients with arterial ulcers, but do not underestimate the pain suffered by patients with venous ulcers. The pathogenesis of pain is complex. Local dehydration caused by dressings, cutaneous ischaemia, and bacterial infection may play a part. Chronic pain demoralizes patients, limiting physical activity, but elderly patients may be reluctant to report pain—Box 15.8.

What should I ask?

- Where is the pain? Ask the patient to point. Ensure the pain is caused by the ulcer—arthritis of back, hip, or knee may cause leg pain.
- What is the pain like? See Box 15.8.
- How bad is the pain? Obtain a measure of the overall intensity of the pain by asking the patient to grade pain (mild, moderate, or severe) or rate pain on a scale of 0 (no pain) to 10 (most severe).
- When did the pain start and how long does the pain last?
- Has the pain changed? Worsening may indicate ischaemia or cellulitis.
- What causes the pain? Typically arterial ulcers cause severe pain at night but many patients with venous ulcers also have pain that interferes with sleeping. Standing and walking cause pain in venous as well as arterial ulcers. Dressing changes may be very painful.
- What relieves the pain—elevation? Compression?
- What is the impact of the pain?
- What analgesia is being taken and how often?
- Is the patient depressed or socially isolated?

What should I do?

- Ensure skin is not inflamed and there is no evidence of infection.
- Review dressings. Most 'non'-adherent dressings are drying, adhere to wounds (despite the name), and cause pain; hydrogels and hydrocolloids relieve pain.
- Review dressing technique—use warm water for washing ulcer, leave ulcer uncovered for the minimum amount of time.
- Ensure that bandages are not compromising the vascular supply. Check with pulse oximeter if any doubt—see 📖 p.280.
- Prescribe analgesia to be taken prior to dressing changes.
- A bed-cradle may help to relieve night pain as may elevating the head of the bed by 4–6 inches in patients with arterial disease.
- Elevation and compression bandages may alleviate much of the pain associated with venous ulcers, but not all patients tolerate this treatment and some have neuropathic pain that does not respond to compression.
- Advise patients to avoid standing for prolonged periods.
- Refer for vascular opinion if the Doppler ABPI is reduced below 0.8.
- Prescribe analgesics according to a pain ladder—see 📖 p.285.
- Reassure the patient that analgesia taken for pain is rarely addictive and ensure the patient understands the importance of taking analgesia regularly to prevent the onset of pain.

Box 15.8 Descriptors from short form McGill Pain Questionnaire (SF-MPQ)

Pain is a complex sensation difficult to describe. Physical, psychological, and social factors influence the perception of pain. Patients may have a mix of nociceptive and neuropathic pain. The SF-MPQ has 15 descriptors (11 sensory; 4 affective). Patients are asked to rate the intensity of each descriptor. Nociceptive pain associated with venous and arterial ulcers is usually throbbing or aching. Shooting, stabbing, or sharp pain suggests a neuropathic component. Burning may indicate damage to the skin.

Sensory descriptors: throbbing, shooting, stabbing, sharp, cramping, gnawing, hot/burning, aching, heavy, tender, splitting.

Affective descriptors: tiring/exhausting, sickening, fearful, punishing/cruel.

Melzack R. *Pain* 1987 **30:**191–7.

Pain ladder

Nociceptive pain

Mild pain: paracetamol 0.5–1g 4-hourly (max. = 4g a day).

Moderate pain

- Try increasing strengths of codeine with paracetamol.
- Co-codamol weak (8mg codeine phosphate plus 500mg paracetamol) 1–2 tablets 4-hourly (max. = 8 tablets/day).
- Co-codamol medium (15mg codeine phosphate plus 500mg paracetamol) 1–2 tablets 4-hourly (max. = 8 tablets/day).
- Co-codamol strong (30mg codeine phosphate plus 500mg paracetamol) 1–2 tablets 4-hourly (max. = 8 tablets/day).
- If not controlled try dihydrocodeine, 30mg every 4–6 hours (max. = 240mg/day). Stimulant laxatives may be required with these drugs.

Severe pain

- Day pain: short-acting morphine, e.g. Oramorph® oral solution 10mg 4-hourly (5mg in elderly) and increase dose by 50% incrementally as necessary.
- Night pain: twice 4-hourly dose, i.e. 10 or 20mg nocte. Incident or breakthrough pain 5–10mg morphine prn, i.e. the 4-hourly dose.
- An antiemetic may be used in conjunction with these initially, but if still nauseated after 3 days, the dose should be reduced.
- Once pain control is stable, change from short-acting morphine to slow release, e.g. MST Continus®. Divide total dose into 2 portions for 12-hourly administration. Ensure that patient has an 'escape' dose of short-acting morphine for break-through pain. The escape dose should be 1/6 of the daily morphine dose in mg.

⚠ *Avoid NSAIDs in the elderly (frequently recommended as an adjunct to paracetamol.). Adverse effects include gastrointestinal bleeding, duodenal or gastric ulceration, and renal failure.*

Neuropathic pain: antidepressants e.g. amitriptyline 25–50mg/day may be helpful. Increase the dose gradually. Antiepileptic drugs, e.g. gabapentin, are also effective in some cases. Neuropathic pain is difficult to alleviate.

Management of ulcers

General advice

Correct factors such as iron or vitamin C deficiency, congestive cardiac failure, oedema, and pain (see 📖 p.284). Wash ulcers and surrounding skin with tap water. Pick off loose scale and moisturize the skin with 50% WSP in liquid paraffin or Hydromol® ointment. (Ointments are less likely to sensitize than creams.) Clean and dry skin between toes and trim or file nails (a chiropodist may help).

Wound care

Reduce bacterial contamination with antiseptic soaks or wet dressings—see 📖 p.592.

Moist wounds heal more quickly than those exposed to air, but too much moisture irritates the skin and macerates the wound edges which become friable and break down. Protect the edges of ulcers with zinc oxide paste or Cavilon® (expensive). The choice of dressing depends on type of ulcer and state of the wound (see Box 15.9).

Venous ulcers

- Graduated compression bandaging promotes healing. Bandages should extend from base of toes to below the knee. Experts apply bandages with an even tension so that pressure steadily reduces from the ankle to the calf—see Box 15.10. ⚠ ***Check the ABPI before compressing the limb—see 📖 Box 15.6, p.281.***
- Avoid prolonged standing (stand on tiptoes at intervals to activate leg muscle pump) or sitting with the feet dependent (elevate legs with feet at level of heart and dorsiflex feet regularly to activate the muscle pump).
- Encourage mobility and weight loss.
- Once ulcer has healed, ensure that the patient has compression hosiery (ideally class II). The patient may need help to put on stockings.
- Aspirin and pentoxifylline have been advocated to promote healing of venous ulcers, but their role is unproven.

Arterial ulcers

- Keep the limb warm. Advise patients to stop smoking and control other risk factors for arterial disease such as hypertension or diabetes.
- Encourage regular graded exercise to promote circulation.
- Protect bony prominences and pressure areas (heels) with padding.

Surgical interventions

In venous ulcers, once oedema is controlled, skin grafts (pinch, punch, or split-thickness) may hasten the re-epithelialization of ulcers with healthy granulating bases. Skin grafting may also have a role in arterial ulcers once underlying vascular problems have been corrected. Consider involving a plastic surgeon.

In arterial ulcers, vascular surgeons may be able to improve the blood supply with balloon angioplasty or femoropopliteal bypass graft.

Box 15.9 Primary dressings and topical treatments

Pain Non-adherent dressings: Mepitel®/Mepilex® (also useful as blister dressings).

Hydrating dressings (also encourage granulation tissue)—hydrogels, e.g. Granugel®, Actiform® cool or hydrocolloids, e.g. Granuflex®, Aquacel®. May over-hydrate.

Dressings containing silver or metronidazole to reduce bacterial colonization. Iodine dressings are an alternative but may be painful.

Topical steroid for short periods, e.g. Trimovate® cream (not evidence-based).

Moderate exudate Alginates, e.g. Sorbsan® or cellulose dressings e.g. Aquacel®.

Heavy exudate Foams, e.g. Allevyn® or alginates, e.g. Kaltostat®, Sorbsan®, Sorbalgon®—will fill deep holes.

Odour Reduce bacterial load with topical metronidazole, (eliminates anaerobes) or dressings containing silver, e.g. Aquacel Ag®.

Absorb odour with Clinisorb® (cheap) or Carboflex® (expensive).

Bacterial colonization Dressings containing iodine e.g. Iodoflex® (may be painful) or silver, e.g. Aquacel Ag®, honey, topical metronidazole.

Adherent slough/necrotic tissue Larvae (maggots) remove necrotic tissue but do not damage healthy tissue. Sterile maggots may be ordered from the Biosurgical Research Unit, Princes of Wales Hospital, Bridgend, Wales CF31 1RQ.

Surgical debridement—cut away necrotic tissue.

Autolysis promoted by softening tissues with hydrating dressings e.g. hydrogels, hydrocolloids.

Change dressings if wound leaks, smells, or is painful. Dressings should always be changed within 7 days.

Box 15.10 Compression bandages for venous ulcers

Apply bandages evenly from toe to below the knee without ridges or folds. Applied correctly, pressure steadily reduces from about 40mmHg at the ankle to 15–20mmHg at the calf. Do not tape anything directly to the skin.

Mobile patients

Tubifast® (elasticated viscose stockinette) and Soffban® with Actico® short stretch (inelastic) bandages or long stretch (elastic) bandages.

3-layer or 4-layer systems of bandages (bulky and patients may not be able to wear usual shoes).

Immobile patients

Long stretch (elastic) bandages, e.g. Tensopress®, Setopress®, or short stretch (see above).

Shaped Tubigrip® (elasticated tubular bandage) provides some compression but is not available in the community. Some graduated compression can be provided by placing a layer of unshaped Tubigrip® (elasticated tubular bandage) size D from toe to mid calf with a second layer size E from ankle to knee. Always use Tubifast® under Tubigrip® (elasticated tubular bandage).

Hosiery (2-layer) designed for patients with ulcers made by Activa and Medi.

Venous eczema

Paste bandage: Ichthopaste® or Zipzoc® (also consider applying a topical steroid such as eumovate ointment) under compression—see 📖 Box 33.3, p.591.

Tubigrip® (elasticated tubular bandage): see earlier. Easy to remove if topical treatment is required.

Note: There are many equivalent products. Determine what is available locally before you choose dressings or bandages.

Further reading

Fonder MA et *al. J Am Acad Dermatol* 2008; **58:**185–206.

Lipodermatosclerosis (sclerosing panniculitis)

- Lipodermatosclerosis is a complication of venous stasis that is seen more often in women than in men. Chronic inflammation causes fibrosis with progressive induration.
- ⚠ The diagnosis is clinical, but frequently pain and erythema in acute lipodermatosclerosis are misdiagnosed and mistreated as cellulitis—see 📖 p.130.

What should I ask?

- Look for a history of longstanding painful 'cellulitis' that has not responded to repeated courses of antibiotics.
- Ask about factors suggesting venous insufficiency, e.g. chronic swelling, previous DVT, varicose veins, orthopaedic procedures—see 📖 p.274.
- What factors improve or exacerbate the pain? Pain in lipodermatosclerosis is worse on standing and may be relieved by elevation.

What should I look for?

- Acute lipodermatosclerosis: a well-defined, very tender, indurated, erythematous plaque in the gaiter area, usually on the medial side of the leg, with little or no swelling—see Fig.15.6.
- Chronic lipodermatosclerosis: a well-defined, slightly tender, indurated 'woody' plaque. Fibrosis tethers subcutaneous tissues (sclerosing panniculitis). Eventually the leg adopts the shape of an inverted champagne bottle.
- Signs of venous insufficiency including a venous eczema, venous flare, pigmentation and ulceration in the gaiter area—see 📖 Box 15.5, p.279.
- An absence of signs suggesting cellulitis: spreading erythema (the erythema is localized in lipodermatosclerosis), acute swelling (the skin is usually tight in lipodermatosclerosis), lymphangitis, systemic flu-like symptoms.

What should I do?

- Explain that lipodermatosclerosis is caused by venous disease and is not an infection. Stop antibiotics.
- Provide pain relief—see 📖 p.284.
- Control venous hypertension with compression (first exclude peripheral arterial disease). 30–40mmHg of pressure at the ankle may not be tolerated in acute lipodermatosclerosis. Start with less pressure and try to increase compression gradually.
- Advise about weight loss (if indicated), elevation, and exercise as for patients with venous leg ulcers—see 📖 p.286.
- The role of systemic treatments such as prednisolone (to reduce acute inflammation) or fibrinolytic agents is unproven.

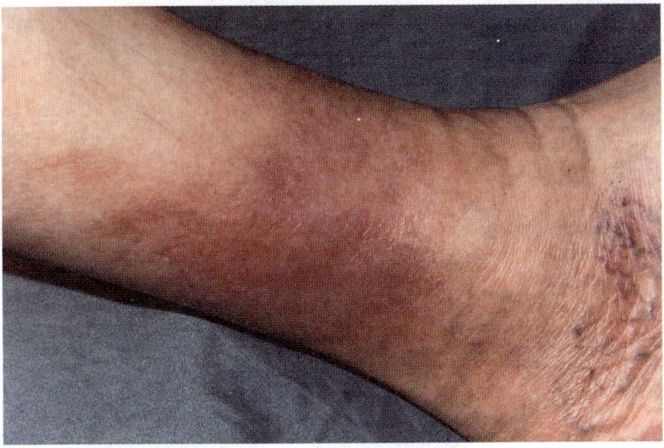

Fig. 15.6 Tender indurated lipodermatosclerosis simulating cellulitis.

Pyoderma gangrenosum

⚠ Pyoderma gangrenosum is neutrophilic dermatosis characterized by acutely painful, rapidly enlarging, deep ulcers—see Box 15.11. Pyoderma gangrenosum is neither an infection nor gangrenous, but is probably an inappropriate reaction to an unidentified stimulus. Clearance of inflammatory cells may be impaired by abnormalities in, for example, neutrophil chemokines, integrins, or T-cells.

Ulcers can occur at any site, including the genitalia, but pyoderma gangrenosum usually presents on the leg. It is seen most often in middle-aged adults, but can affect any age. About 50% of patients have an underlying disease—see Box 15.12. The diagnosis is clinical and may be difficult.

What should I ask? (📖 p.274)

- How did the ulcer start? (Was minor trauma involved?)
- Is the ulcer painful? How quickly is it enlarging?
- Has the patient another reason to have an ulcer (venous disease, arterial disease, infection)?
- Has the patient any systemic disease that might predispose to pyoderma gangrenosum? See Box 15.12.

What should I look for? (Fig. 15.5)

- Look for signs suggesting pyoderma gangrenosum—see Box 15.11.
- Rule out common causes of ulceration, but venous or arterial disease may coexist with pyoderma gangrenosum making the diagnosis difficult—see Box 15.13.

What should I do?

- Check FBC, ESR, CRP, protein electrophoresis and immunoglobulin (20% have a benign monoclonal gammopathy), RF, antiphospholipid antibodies.
- Take a biopsy from ulcer edge for histology (may be suggestive but is not diagnostic—see Box 15.13); culture (bacteria, fungi such as sporotrichosis)—see 📖 Box 32.2, p.573.
- Prescribe analgesia.
- Dressings such as hydrocolloids or alignates may relieve pain.
- Try gentle compression to control oedema (if tolerated).
- ⚠ Avoid surgery as trauma will exacerbate ulceration.
- Pustules, bullae, or small ulcers—try a very potent topical corticosteroid ointment or 0.1% tacrolimus ointment to control pain, inflammation, and ulceration, but watch for secondary infection, e.g. with *Pseudomonas aeruginosa*.
- ►► Large ulcers—prompt treatment with prednisolone 40–60mg/day or pulse IV methylprednisolone is essential to minimize scarring. Steroid-sparing agents that may be tried include minocycline, ciclosporin and dapsone.
- Infliximab may be effective, particularly in patients with Crohn's disease.

Further reading

Hoffman MD. *Clinics Dermatol* 2007; **25:**131–8.

Box 15.11 Clinical features of pyoderma gangrenosum

Direct the history and examination towards eliminating more common causes of ulceration and establishing if the patient has features that suggest pyoderma gangrenosum.

Major features (Fig. 15.5, p.277)

- Very painful necrotic cutaneous ulcer (pain is out of proportion to the appearance of the ulcer) with a purulent discharge.
- Rapid progression of ulcer—may enlarge by 2cm/day.
- Irregular, violaceous, and undermined border—you may be able to insert a probe several millimetres under the edge.
- Rapid response to corticosteroids—sometimes one has to resort to a clinical trial if the diagnosis is not clear cut.

Other suggestive features

- The ulcer was preceded by a sterile pustule or, less often, an erythematous nodule or a blister.
- History that minor trauma initiates ulcers, i.e. pathergy.
- Base with much slough or haemorrhagic base.
- Cribriform scarring (uneven sieve-like with perforations).
- Histology: follicular or perifollicular inflammation, intradermal abscesses, and/or sterile dermal neutrophilia without vasculitis. Findings are not specific.

Box 15.12 Systemic diseases and pyoderma gangrenosum

50% of patients with pyoderma gangrenosum have an underlying condition:

- Arthritis of various types, seropositive and seronegative.
- Inflammatory bowel disease: pyoderma gangrenosum may be peri-stomal—see 🕮 Box 24.2, p.473.
- Myeloproliferative disorders including leukaemia, myeloid metaplasia, and other pre-leukaemias—pyoderma gangrenosum is often bullous (signs overlap with Sweet's syndrome—see 🕮 p.480).
- ⚠ PAPA syndrome (pyogenic arthritis, pyoderma gangrenosum, and acne)—vanishingly rare! See 🕮 p.228.

Box 15.13 Differential diagnosis

- Venous or arterial insufficiency.
- Infection: deep fungal, atypical mycobacterial.
- Vasculitis or occlusive vasculopathy—see 🕮 p.290, p.292, and p.418.
- Wegener's granulomatosis: ulcers affecting the limbs, perineum, or face may resemble pyoderma gangrenosum.
- Cutaneous malignancy.
- Bite of brown recluse spider.
- Dermatitis artefacta: well defined, angular ulcers without undermined edges—see 🕮 p.524.

Calcific uraemic arteriolopathy (calciphylaxis)

This life-threatening condition occurs most often in patients with chronic renal failure on dialysis. Calcium deposited in the media of small cutaneous arteries leads to thrombosis and ischaemic necrosis with refractory ulcers often involving lower extremity, abdomen, or buttocks. Deposition of metals (iron, aluminium) may play a part in the pathogenesisis of endothelial injury and vascular calcification. Secondary infection may lead to fatal sepsis and mortality is high (80%).

The incidence is increasing and calciphylaxis may be seen in other situations—see Box 15.14—when it may be confused with cutaneous vasculitis or pyoderma gangrenosum. Rarely patients may have systemic problems such as proximal myopathy, aortic valve involvement, or pulmonary calciphylaxis.

What should I look for?

- A history of underlying risk factors—see Box 15.14.
- Sudden onset of painful mottled erythema on thigh or leg evolving to indurated plaques which eventually become necrotic and ulcerate. Initially may be misdiagnosed as cellulitis—see Fig. 15.7, p.295.
- Livedo reticularis: mottled reddish-purple reticulated discoloration reflecting sluggish vascular flow in the superficial dermis—see 📖 p.294 and p.418.
- Ischaemic necrosis with black eschars—see Fig. 15.7, p.295.
- Other cutaneous signs may include:
  - Pathergy: minor trauma triggers ulceration.
  - Recurrent digital ischaemia with gangrene, necrosis of penis.
  - Subcutaneous nodules on breasts and abdomen.

What should I do?

- Check for cutaneous infection—take skin swabs (but surface swabs from ulcers are generally not very informative).
- Exclude peripheral vascular disease by clinical examination.
- Check renal function, serum calcium, serum phosphate, parathyroid hormone (PTH) level, and alkaline phosphatase.
- Check fasting glucose.
- Exclude other causes of an occlusive vasculopathy—check FBC and coagulation profile including lupus anticoagulant, anticardiolipin antibody, protein C, and protein S—see 📖 p.418.
- Exclude cutaneous vasculitis—check complement (C3, C4), cryoglobulins, hepatitis B and C serologies.
- Consider taking a deep elliptical skin biopsy to demonstrate the calcification in small arteries, vascular thrombosis, and intimal hyperplasia (endarteritis obliterans)... but the biopsy may not heal.
- Plain X-ray of the leg may demonstrate the extent of calcification.
- Management is difficult and requires a multidisciplinary approach—see Box 15.15.

Box 15.14 Risk factors for calciphylaxis

Major risk factors
- End-stage renal disease.
- Elevated calcium-phosphate product.
- Hyperparathyroidism—primary and secondary.

Non-uraemic risk factors
- Female gender.
- Obesity.
- Diabetes.
- Autoimmune diseases such as SLE, rheumatoid arthritis, and antiphospholipid syndrome.
- Protein C and protein S deficiency.
- Malignancy.
- Alcoholic liver disease.
- Warfarin.

Box 15.15 Management of calciphylaxis

- Pain relief and supportive care.
- Optimize wound dressings.
- Avoid compression which may exacerbate cutaneous ischaemia and pain.
- Treat cutaneous infections promptly with oral antibiotics, e.g. flucloxacillin.
- Attempt to normalize calcium and phosphate levels—discuss management with the renal physicians. The evidence base for management is weak but strategies may include:
  - Discontinuing oral calcium supplements.
  - Lowering calcium concentration in dialysate.
  - More frequent dialysis.
  - Bisphosphonates such as IV pamindronate and oral etidronate.
  - Cinacalcet to downregulate PTH levels and correct elevated calcium-phosphate products.
  - Parathyroidectomy.
  - Hyperbaric oxygen.
- Control blood glucose.
- ⚠ Avoid aggressive debridement as this is likely to trigger further ulceration.
- Avoid immunosuppressive drugs which increase the risk of infection.
- The role of anticoagulation is controversial.

Further reading

Amuluru L *et al. J Am Acad Dermatol* 2009; **61**:73–9.

Lee JL *et al. Autoimmun Rev* 2008; **7**:638–43.

Livedoid vasculopathy

Synonyms: segmental hyalinizing vasculitis, livedo reticularis with summer/winter ulceration, livedoid vasculitis.

This thrombo-occlusive vasculopathy affects young to middle-aged women. Hyaline thrombi occlude small vessels in the upper and mid-dermis. The cause is unknown, but fibrinolytic and coagulation systems are usually normal. Ulceration may be chronic and recurrent.

What should I look for?

- Focal purpuric lesions on the leg, usually around the ankle.
- Small, excruciatingly painful ulcers surrounded by a purpuric rim.
- Porcelain-white, stellate scars with a rim of telangiectasia (atrophie blanche)—see Fig. 15.8.
- Livedo reticularis: mottled reddish-purple reticulated discoloration reflecting sluggish vascular flow in the superficial dermis—see 📖 p.418 and Fig. 20.4, p.419.
- Net-like hyperpigmentation on the leg at the site of previous livedo (differentiate from erythema ab igne, a reticulated brown staining that can develop if skin is exposed chronically to heat from a radiator, open fire, or hot-water bottle—see 📖 Fig. 20.5, p.419).

What should I do?

- Investigations:
  - FBC to exclude thrombocythaemia.
  - Clotting screen including antiphospholipid antibodies, protein S and C.
  - A deep biopsy is needed to demonstrate hyaline thrombi.
- Control pain—see 📖 p.284.
- Try antiplatelet therapy, antithrombotic regimens, or fibrinolytic agents but treatment is difficult and there is no consensus about the best approach.
- Treatment with immunosuppression is ineffective.

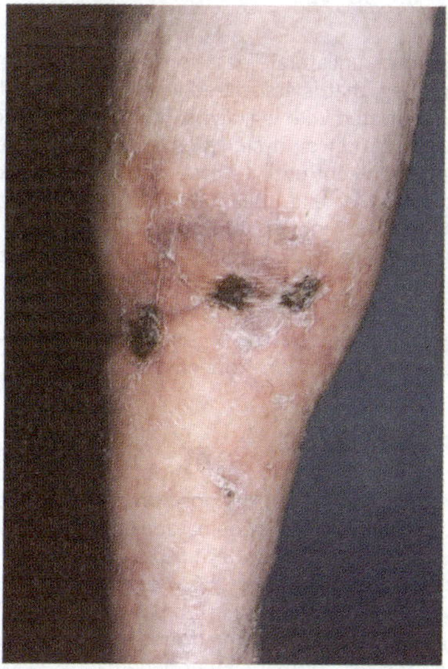

Fig. 15.7 Calciphylaxis: mottled erythema (livedo reticularis) and painful ulceration in a patient with diabetes.

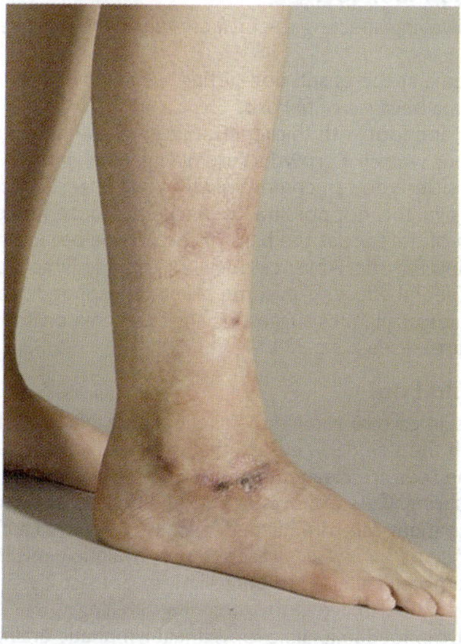

Fig. 15.8 Livedoid vasculopathy: atrophie blanche with painful ulceration around the ankles.

Lymphoedema

Lymphoedema causes unilateral (occasionally bilateral) chronic swelling, most often of the leg, that is associated with recurrent cellulitis and may occasionally be associated with leg ulcers. Primary lymphoedema is caused by inherited malformation or dysfunction in the lymphatic system. Lymphoedema may not present until adolescence or adulthood. Mutations in genes such as the vascular endothelial growth factor receptor-3 (*VEGFR3*) gene play a part in pathogenesis.

Secondary lymphoedema is caused by lymphatic obstruction or damage to the lymphatic system, e.g. by radiotherapy, lymph node dissection or cellulitis. Sirolimus is a rare cause of secondary lymphoedema.

Distinguish lymphoedema of the leg from lipoedema—see Box 15.16 and Table 15.1. Rarely pretibial myxoedema simulates lymphoedema—see 🕮 Fig. 22.4, p.439.

What should I ask?

- Where is the swelling, when it commenced, and how it progressed?
- Does the swelling change with the position of the limb, e.g. overnight? Unlike venous swelling, lymphoedema does not reduce with elevation.
- Any episodes of cellulitis? Flu-like symptoms with fevers, rigors, or vomiting precede blotchy redness. How often are these episodes?
- Any pain? (Usually not a problem in lymphoedema.)
- Any family history of lymphoedema (found in 20% of cases of lymphoedema. Suggests primary lymphoedema.)
- Past history of malignancy or surgery, including lymph node dissection.

What should I look for?

- Persistent swelling affecting the foot as well as the leg (see 🕮 Fig.15.2, p.227).
- Pitting oedema at the onset; non-pitting 'woody' swelling in chronic lymphoedema because of fibrosis.
- A warm leg and foot with thickening, fissuring, and hyperkeratosis and papillomatous wart-like growths resembling 'elephant skin'.
- Bleb-like vesicles you can compress with your finger (lymphoceles).
- Stemmer's sign. It is not possible to pinch up a loose fold of skin on the dorsum of the foot at the base of the 2nd toe because the skin is thickened and fibrotic. Absence does not exclude lymphoedema.
- Ascites or pleural effusions in some primary lymphoedemas.
- Bluish nodules or plaques suggesting angiosarcoma or Kaposi's sarcoma (rare)—see 🕮 p.338.

What should I do?

- Advise on skin care to reduce the likelihood of infection. The patient should wash the skin daily, ensure that folds of skin and the skin between the toes are cleaned and dried, and use an emollient to prevent fissuring. Cuts or abrasions should be kept scrupulously clean.
- Ensure the patient can trim his/her toenails or refer to a chiropodist.
- If cellulitis occurs >×2/year, prescribe prophylactic penicillin V 500mg daily (clindamycin if allergic to penicillin) for at least 2 years to prevent further lymphatic damage with worsening swelling.
- Refer to a lymphoedema clinic for manual lymphatic drainage, advice about exercise, and compression bandaging.

Box 15.16 Swelling of the leg: differential diagnosis

Unilateral

- Deep venous thrombosis.
- Ruptured Baker's cyst.
- Cellulitis.
- Chronic venous insufficiency.
- Lymphoedema, e.g. pelvic tumour or lymphatic damage.
- Immobility.

Bilateral

- Congestive cardiac failure, renal failure, or nephrotic syndrome.
- Liver failure and hypoalbuminaemia.
- Malnutrition.
- Drugs, NSAIDs, calcium channel blockers.
- Lipoedema.
- Immobility, e.g. sitting in a wheelchair.

What is lipoedema?

Lipoedema, also known as painful fat syndrome, affects women and starts around puberty. It may be familial (40% of cases). Nodules containing 'wet' fat are deposited in subcutaneous tissues on the buttocks, hips, thighs, and legs. The feet are not affected. Treatment is unsatisfactory. Dieting does not alter lipoedema—the trunk may become slim but the legs remain large. Exercise and surgical support stockings may help.

Table 15.1 Lipoedema or lymphoedema?

Lipoedema	*Lymphoedema*
• Swelling is bilateral.	• Swelling is usually unilateral.
• The legs are painful and skin is tender.	• Lymphoedema is usually painless.
• The fat on the ankles creates a ring of fatty tissue that overhangs normal looking feet. Fat is deposited on buttocks and lower limb.	• The foot is affected as well as the leg.
• Swelling increases during the day and reduces during the night when the leg is elevated.	• Position does not influence the amount of swelling.
• Swelling does not pit.	• Swelling pits in early lymphoedema but is non-pitting in late disease.
• The skin tends to be thin. Easy bruising and subcutaneous bleeding are common.	• Skin is thickened, fissured and hyperkeratotic.
• Stemmer's sign is absent.	• Stemmer's sign is usually present.

Further reading

Connell F et al. *Ann N Y Acad Sci* 2008; **1131**:140–6.

Kröger K. *Vasa* 2008; **37**:39–51.

Mortimer P. *BMJ* 2000; **320**:1527–9.

Chapter 16

Sun and skin

Contents

Relevant pages in other chapters

See 🕮 Chapter 2, p.17 for the history in suspected photosensitivity and 🕮 Box 4.6, p.71 for the examination findings that suggest photosensitivity. Skin cancer is discussed in 🕮 Chapter 17, p.319.

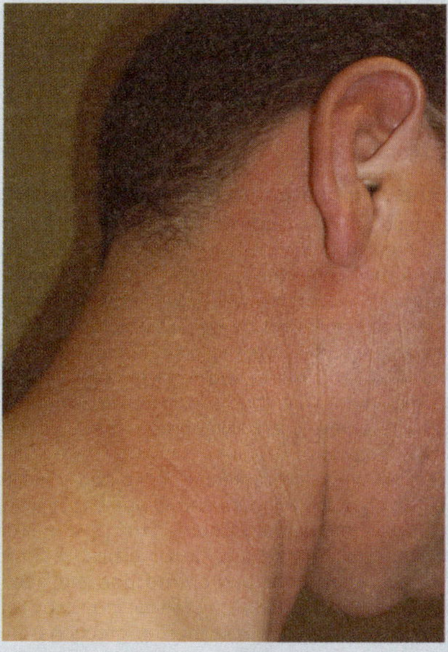

Fig. 16.1 Photosensitive patient with erythema of exposed skin but an abrupt cut-off where skin is covered by clothing.

Introduction

Life on earth depends on the sun's warmth and light. Our spirits rise in the sun and sunny days evoke memories of long holidays (as well as revision for exams). But sun has the potential to harm—there can be 'too much of a good thing'. Sunburn, skin cancer, and most photosensitivity disorders are caused by ultraviolet (UV) radiation.

How does UV radiation affect skin?

The sun emits a broad and continuous spectrum of electromagnetic energy (the solar spectrum)—see Fig. 16.2. UV radiation is divided into short (UVC), medium (UVB), and long (UVA 'black light') wavelength emissions. 98% of the UV radiation that reaches the earth's surface is UVA. All UVC and a little UVB are absorbed in the atmosphere by the ozone layer. UVB is absorbed by nucleic acids and proteins in the epidermis and stimulates the synthesis of vitamin D_3 (cholecalciferol). Some UVA is absorbed in the epidermis, but UVA penetrates into the dermis.

The damage caused by UV radiation depends on the duration of exposure as well as the skin phototype (see Table 16.1).

- UVB causes immediate sunburn with painful erythema and, if severe, blistering. The UVB reaction peaks at 16–24h, then the skin desquamates over 2–3 days, but becomes tanned and may develop solar lentigines (sunburn freckles).
- UV radiation, particularly UVB, damages DNA and cumulative damage causes skin cancer—see 📖 p.324.
- Chronic UV exposure produces many of the signs we associate with ageing (photodamage)—wrinkling, blotchy pigmentation, telangiectasia, a sallow appearance—as well as skin cancer—📖 Box 3.1, p.43.
- UV radiation also causes local and systemic immunosuppression, which not only leads to problems such as recurrent herpes simplex infection, but also contributes to the pathogenesis of skin cancer.

How is the skin protected from sun damage?

Photodamaged DNA is repaired by nucleotide excision repair enzymes, but capacity to repair declines with age (or may be abnormal in some rare photogenodermatoses—see 📖 p.314). Epidermal melanin provides some UV protection by absorbing visible light as well as UV radiation—see 📖 p.12. Melanin also quenches oxygen free radicals.

Darkly pigmented skin has the same number of melanocytes as lightly pigmented skin, but more and slightly differently packaged melanin (melanosomes) within keratinocytes provides greater resistance to solar damage. However, even dark skin burns in the sun if the dose of UV radiation is high enough.

UVA causes immediate darkening of the skin (oxidation of pre-existing melanin) that lasts a few hours and is not photoprotective. UVB is the main stimulus for the delayed tanning detectable 3–5 days after exposure (more melanocytes, synthesis of new melanin, redistribution of melanosomes). This provides some photoprotection and fades slowly.

Sun exposure also induces the injured epidermis to proliferate. Thickening of the horny layer supplies a little more protection from photodamage.

The solar spectrum

The solar spectrum ranges from cosmic rays, gamma rays, and X-rays, through ultraviolet (UV) radiation (100–400nm), visible light (400–800nm), and infrared radiation (800–17 000nm), to radio waves (Fig. 16.2). UVB and UVA contribute to tanning, UVB causes sunburn.

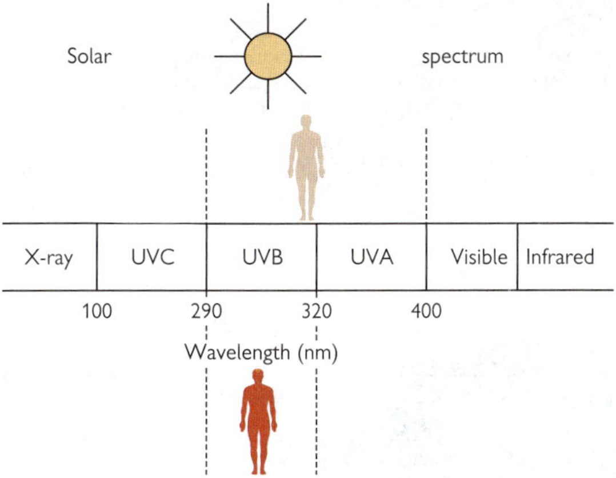

Fig. 16.2 Solar spectrum. UVA and visible light, unlike UVB, penetrate glass.

Skin phototype

Pale skins that burn easily and tan poorly, if at all, are most at risk of chronic photodamage and skin cancer, but it may be difficult to predict the phototype simply from the appearance of the skin. It is better to ask patients how quickly they burn and how easily they tan. The Fitzpatrick classification (Table 16.1) depends on the amount of melanin in the skin.

Table 16.1 Fitzpatrick classification

Skin type	Response of skin to sun	Appearance
I	Always burns, never tans	White or pale skin, many freckles, blond or red hair, blue or green eyes
II	Burns easily, tans poorly	Pale skin, possibly some freckles, blond hair, blue or green eyes
III	May burn, tans lightly	Darker white skin, dark hair, brown eyes
IV	Burns minimally, tans easily	Olive skin, brown or black hair, brown eyes—Mediterranean
V	Rarely burns, always tans	Asian, Latin American, Middle Eastern
VI	Never burns, tans darkly	Black African

Further reading

Hussein MR. *J Cutan Pathol* 2005; **32**:191–205.

Photosensitivity

What is photosensitivity?

- Photosensitivity is defined as an abnormal cutaneous response involving the interaction between photosensitizing substances and sunlight or filtered or artificial light.
- People who are photosensitive burn easily in sunlight and may complain of reddening, swelling, blistering, itching, and/or painful skin after minimal sun exposure—see Box 4.6, p.71.
- ⚠ **Photosensitivity may also lead to early skin cancers**—see p.324.
- Photosensitivity may be primary, but more often is acquired—see Boxes 16.1, 16.3.
- Some skin diseases may be made worse by sunlight (photoaggravated)—see Box 16.2.

Photosensitivity in adults (see Table 16.2 and Box 16.7)

Table 16.2 Common causes of adult photosensitivity

Diagnosis	Clinical features	Action spectra	Frequency
Photoaggravated skin disease e.g. cutaneous LE (Box 16.2)	Features of underlying disease, but more severe on sun-exposed skin	Variable	Common
Drug-induced photosensitivity (Box 16.5, p.305)	Immediate reaction. Signs vary, e.g. sunburn like, eczematous, urticarial, or bullous. Hyperpigmentation common	UVA	Common
Phytophotodermatitis (plant-induced photosensitivity) (Box 16.6, p.305)	Immediate linear erythema followed by blistering. Leaves streaky pigmentation	UVA	Common
Polymorphic light eruption (p.306)	Papular or vesicular rash 1–24h after sun exposure. Lasts 1–3 days or longer	UVA, UVB	Common

Photosensitivity in childhood

- Consider drug-induced photosensitivity, phytophotodermatitis, and polymorphic light eruption before porphyria or a rare genodermatosis.
- Remember that atopic eczema may be photaggravated.

What should I do?—see Box 16.4

Further reading

Yashar SS and Lim HW. *Dermatol Ther* 2003; **16:**1–7.

Box 16.1 Acquired photosensitivity

- Drug-induced photoallergy or phototoxicity—see 📖 p.304.
- Contact photosensitivity:
  - Soaps, tars, perfumes, drugs such as topical NSAIDs.
  - Plants : phytophotodermatitis (plants containing psoralen)—see Box 16.6.
- Porphyria cutanea tarda and pseudoporphyria—see 📖 p.310 and p. 312.

Box 16.2 Skin diseases that may be photoaggravated

- Rosacea.
- Dermatitis—seborrhoeic, atopic.
- Psoriasis (more often helped by sunlight).
- LP, EM.
- LE, especially subacute cutaneous LE.
- Dermatomyositis.
- Darier's disease.
- Autoimmune blistering diseases—pemphigus, bullous pemphigoid.
- Pellagra (niacin deficiency).

Box 16.3 Primary photosensitivity (rare)

- Idiopathic photodermatoses—see Box 16.7.
- Cutaneous porphyrias—see 📖 p.308.
- DNA repair deficiencies (rare)—see 📖 p.314.
  - Xeroderma pigmentosum, trichothiodystrophy, Cockayne's syndrome, Bloom's syndrome.
- Other very rare photogenodermatoses:
  - Kindler–Weary syndrome, Rothmund–Thomson syndrome, Smith–Lemli–Opitz syndrome.

Box 16.4 What should I do?

- Take a full medical history (see 📖 p.28) and examine the patient (see 📖 Box 4.6, p.71).
- Investigation of photosensitivity may include:
  - ANA, ENA (Ro antibodies are linked to photosensitivity).
  - Porphyrins in blood, urine, and stool (ensure the sample is not exposed to light by wrapping the specimen pot in tinfoil).
  - Skin biopsy for histology/fibroblasts for DNA repair disorders.
  - Patch testing and photopatch testing.
  - Phototesting to define the minimal erythema dose (MED) and action spectrum responsible. Skin can be exposed to light that simulates sunlight and also to specific wavebands by using a monochromator to fractionate the light.
  - Metabolic studies (aminoaciduria, hair analysis).
- Advise the patient how to protect the skin from UV light—see 📖 p.316.
- Manage the underlying problem.

Drug-induced photosensitivity

Drugs are the commonest cause of photosensitivity—see Box 16.5. The photosensitivity is caused by phototoxicity more often than photoallergy, but the distinction is not always clear cut. Reactions may also be bullous or lichenoid. Other potential presentations of a drug-induced photosensitivity include pseudoporphyria (see 📖 p.312) and LE (see 📖 p.372).

What is phototoxicity?

Phototoxicity causes an exaggerated sunburn response with pain, erythema, oedema, and sometimes blistering of exposed skin. The action spectrum for phototoxins may be UVB, UVA, or visible solar radiation. The response depends on the amount of UV radiation (the patient may have no problems on a slightly cloudy day) and the dose of the drug, but can occur on first exposure to the drug. The response is usually immediate, but can be delayed. Reactions to amiodarone and chlorpromazine produce pigmentary changes.

Phytophotodermatitis is a phototoxic eruption caused by contact with plant juices containing light-sensitizing furocoumarin chemicals, e.g. psoralens—see Box 16.6.

What is photoallergy?

Photoallergic reactions are idiosyncratic delayed hypersensitivity reactions, similar to an allergic contact dermatitis, that do not develop until the patient has been sensitized by prior exposure to the drug. The action spectrum for most photoallergens is in the UVA range (light coming through window glass causes problems). The response is not dose-dependent and the reaction may spread to affect covered skin. Frequently topical medicaments are implicated. Photopatch testing is positive.

What should I do?

- Withdraw the drug if possible. Phototoxic reactions settle within a week. The signs of photoallergy (erythema) will also disappear within a week but photosensitivity may persist for months after drug withdrawal (sometimes as long as 6 months).
- A potent topical steroid applied ×2/day will help to settle the inflammation. Systemic steroids may be required in severe reactions.
- Sun protection with clothing, a hat, and a high, factor broad, spectrum UVA/UVB sunscreen is essential—see 📖 p.316.
- Photopatch testing may be helpful in suspected photoallergy.

Box 16.5 Drug-induced photosensitivity

- Phototoxicity: amiodarone, doxycycline, thiazides, phenothiazines, NSAIDs, quinolones, quinine, sulphonamides, retinoids, psoralens (in plants), coal tar.
- Photoallergy: topical antimicrobials, fragrances, sunscreens, angiotensin-converting agent inhibitors, non-steroidal anti-inflammatory agents, phenothiazines, sulphonamides, thiazides.
- Pseudoporphyria (a form of phototoxicity with blistering and skin fragility—see 📖 p.312): nalidixic acid, furosemide, ciprofloxacin, bumetanide, NSAIDs.
- Lichenoid reactions resembling LP—see 📖 p.208 (delayed in onset): hydrochlorothiazide, NSAIDs, quinidine-derived drugs.
- Photo-onycholysis (painful): tetracyclines, taxanes.

Box 16.6 What is phytophotodermatitis?

- Phototoxic reactions to light-sensitizing furocoumarin chemicals in plants can occur in anyone and are not an allergy.
- Causes of phytophotodermatitis include members of the Apiaceae family (previously Umbelliferae), e.g. Queen Anne's lace, giant hogweed, parsnip, celery; the Rutaceae family, e.g. garden rue (*Ruta graveolens*), and citrus fruit oils, e.g. lime juice.
- The patient, often a gardener wielding a strimmer, or a child, is outside on a sunny day. Plant juice is deposited in a streaky linear fashion on exposed skin that has brushed against the plant or, with strimmers, the juice is sprayed over the exposed skin.
- The psoralens in the plant juice cause a painful burning (rather than itching) erythema, often with blistering, about 24h after exposure to long-wave UV radiation (UVA).
- The reaction peaks at 48–72h and gradually settles over a few days.
- Linear streaks of hyperpigmentation persist at the site of inflammation and may take months to fade. These may be all you see when the patient presents—see 📖 Fig. 31.11, p.565.
- The diagnosis depends upon the history and the bizarre linear pattern suggesting an external injury. Sometimes child abuse is suspected—see 📖 p.564.

Polymorphic light eruption

Polymorphic light eruption (PMLE, PLE) is the commonest of the idiopathic photodermatoses—see Box 16.7. It is sometimes known as 'sun allergy' or prickly heat. PLE affects about 15% of the young adult female White population in northern Europe, and may present in young adults or childhood. Genetic factors probably play some part in the pathogenesis. The abbreviation is confusing—PLE is not a form of cutaneous lupus erythematosus (LE).

UV radiation (mostly UVA; sometimes UVA and UVB) provokes a T-cell response. The condition may be mediated by a delayed hypersensitivity reaction to an unidentified molecule. Phototesting can be normal.

What should I look for?

- A story of an itching or burning rash that erupts within 2h of exposure to UV radiation, but in some patients may not develop for 24–48h or even longer. (The history is usually diagnostic.)
- A rash that fades within 1–6 days leaving normal skin (no scars).
- Erythematous papules, plaques, vesicles, or, less often, haemorrhagic blisters. The rash is polymorphic in its presentation in populations, but individuals usually have one form of the disease.
- The problem usually presents in spring, but some patients only develop the rash when they go on holiday to a sunny climate. Sunlight reflected from snow may also provoke PLE.
- The rash may be triggered by as little as 10min of direct sunlight.
- Sunlight penetrating window glass (UVA) may cause the rash as can unshielded fluorescent lights and the UVA from sunbeds.
- Chronically exposed skin on face and hands is usually spared.
- The rash usually erupts less frequently as the summer progresses ('hardening') provided exposure to sunlight continues.

What should I do?

- Exclude subacute cutaneous LE (see 📖 p.372) and oral contraceptive (oestrogen)-induced photosensitivity (rare).
- Management options include:
  - Potent topical corticosteroids for acute eruptions.
  - Gradual sunlight exposure to induce tolerance (may be difficult to achieve) and continued sun exposure to maintain tolerance.
  - Protective clothing: broad-brimmed hats, long sleeves—see 📖 p.316.
  - High-factor UVA/UVB sunscreens may prevent PLE. (UVB sunscreens may worsen PLE by allowing UVA through but diminishing the protective immunosuppression produced by UVB).
  - Oral prednisolone 15–20mg a day for 2–3 days may be required to control an acute eruption, e.g. while on holiday.
  - Desensitization using UV radiation (UVB or PUVA) each spring. Treat ×2–3/week for 3–5 weeks. Patients must continue exposure to sunlight to maintain tolerance. Desensitization has to be repeated annually if tolerance is not maintained.
  - Hydroxychloroquine can be helpful in some cases.

Box 16.7 The idiopathic photodermatoses

The pathogenesis of the idiopathic photodermatoses is incompletely understood. All are uncommon, apart from PLE.

Common

- PLE: usually presents under age 30. Onset within hours of sun exposure, not minutes. Symmetrical rash (usually papulonodular or eczematous) that affects skin covered in winter. (Differential diagnosis-subacute cutaneous LE—see 🕮 p.372.)

Uncommon

- Juvenile spring eruption: uncommon. Mainly in boys in spring and summer. Itching, uncomfortable papules and vesicles on exposed helices of the ears. The rest of the skin is usually not affected.
- Solar urticaria: uncommon. May arise at any age. Itchy, urticarial wheals appear within a few minutes of exposure to sunlight and last for <24h. (Differential diagnosis—drug-induced photosensitivity, erythropoietic protoporphyria). Action spectra: UVA, UVB, and visible including fluorescent lights. Antihistamines and desensitization may be helpful.
- Actinic prurigo: rare. Presents in childhood, commonest in Native American tribes. Itching papules evolve into chronic nodules and plaques. Rash is maximal in spring and summer. All exposed skin is affected, but may involve covered sites so the diagnosis is often missed. May simulate atopic eczema. Solar cheilitis of lower lip is common.
- Hydroa vacciniforme: rare. Presents in childhood, usually in boys. Rash appears within minutes of exposure. Tender, itching erythematous papules evolve into haemorrhagic vesicles that crust and heal leaving chickenpox-like scars.
- Chronic actinic dermatitis: uncommon. Usually elderly men (90%) with multiple contact allergies. Compositae (plants) commonest contact allergy. Potent immunosuppressives such as azathioprine may be required.
- Brachioradial pruritus: uncommon. Stinging and burning pain in skin of forearms that is often unexplained. Prevalence unknown. Patients do not have a rash. It may be a form of light-induced chronic neuropathic damage—see 🕮 p.504.

Further reading

Murphy GM. *J Photochem Photobiol B: Biol* 2001; **64:**93–8.

Porphyria

What is porphyria?

The porphyrias are a group of disorders caused by genetic or acquired partial deficiencies in one of the enzymes in the metabolic pathway for haem. Haem precursors accumulate in urine, faeces, plasma, and/or erythrocytes. Disease may be acute neurovisceral, non-acute cutaneous, or mixed—see Table 16.3.

Acute neurovisceral attacks are associated with a rise in 5-aminolaevulinate and porphobilinogen. Blisters and skin fragility are caused by accumulation of water-soluble porphyrins (uroporphyrin and coproporphyrin) in porphyria cutanea tarda (PCT), variegate porphyria, and hereditary coproporphyria, whereas painful photosensitivity is caused by raised protoporphyrin in erythropoietic protoporphyria (EPP).

Although mutations reduce the activity of the enzymes by 50%, most (80%) of those who inherit an autosomal dominant porphyria remain asymptomatic. Other factors that increase the demand for haem and/or decrease enzyme activity are required for the diseases to be expressed.

Acute porphyria: what should I look for?

- Episodic neurovisceral attacks that start between age 15 and 35.
- More common in females (less likely after menopause).
- Severe pain (usually abdominal), nausea, vomiting, constipation.
- Hypertension, tachycardia, low sodium.
- Neurological/psychiatric signs: psychological upset, convulsions, muscle weakness.
- A trigger: e.g. drugs (oestrogens, progesterones, barbiturates, sulphonamides, tetracyclines, etc.), alcohol, infection, calorie restriction.
- Cutaneous involvement (not a feature of acute intermittent porphyria but may be seen in some acute porphyrias, e.g. variegate porphyria) Look for a history of skin fragility, blisters, milia, erosions, and/or scars on exposed sites such as dorsum of hands or face (like PCT—see 🕮 p.310).

Acute porphyria: what should I do?

- Remove precipitating factors (many drugs, including recreational drugs).
- Treat symptomatically: fluids (monitor sodium), analgesia, antiemetics.
- Collect a random fresh sample of urine during attack to measure porphyrins. Protect fresh specimen from light—see 🕮 Box 16.4, p.303. Analyse faecal and plasma porphyrins to determine the type of acute porphyria. Urinary, faecal, and plasma porphyrin concentrations may return to normal during remission in all the autosomal dominant acute porphyrias.
- Consider early administration of intravenous haem arginate to suppress production of haem precursors.
- Screen family members.

Further reading

Badminton MN and Elder GH. *J Inherit Metab. Dis* 2005; **28:**277–86.
European Porphyria Network: http://www.porphyria-europe.org
Poblete-Gutierrez P *et al. Eur J Dermatol* 2006; **16:**230–40.

Table 16.3 Classification of the porphyrias

Porphyria	Enzyme deficiency	Clinical	Comment
Porphyria cutanea tarda (PCT) Sporadic (80%) = type I AD (20%) = type 2	Uropor-phyrinogen decarboxylase	Non-acute. **Cutaneous only.** Blisters, skin fragility, erosions, pigmentation	**Most common type of porphyria** May be acquired or inherited. Increased risk of hepatocellular carcinoma
Erythropoietic protoporphyria (EPP) Inheritance = AD	Ferrochelatase	Non-acute. **Cutaneous only.** Burning, erythema, oedema of light-exposed skin. Subtle scars	**Most common AD type in children.** May develop cholestasis and liver failure
Congenital erythropoietic porphyria (Gunther's disease) Inheritance = AR	Uropor-phyrinogen III	Non-acute. Severe photosensitivity, mutilation, hypertrichosis, red teeth, haemolytic anaemia. Dark urine	Very rare. Presents in infancy. Urine stains napkin purplish red. May have led to folklore of were-wolves emerging at night to avoid sunlight
Acute intermittent porphyria Inheritance = AD	Hydroxy-methylbilane synthase	Acute neurovisceral attacks. **No cutaneous involvement**	**Most common acute porphyria.** Risk of liver cancer and renal failure
Variegate porphyria Inheritance = AD	Protopor-phyrinogen oxidase	Acute neurovisceral attacks (20%) or blisters like PCT (60%) or both (20%)	Common in S. Africa and Chile—founder mutation
Hereditary coproporphyria Inheritance = AD	Copropor-phyrinogen oxidase	Acute neurovisceral attacks. Blisters like PCT (30%)	Very rare
ALA dehydratase deficiency porphyria Inheritance = AR	ALA dehydra-tase	Acute neurovisceral attacks. No cutaneous involvement	Extremely rare! A handful of cases

AD = autosomal dominant; AR = autosomal recessive.

Rare homozygous variants of AD porphyrias are not included.

Porphyria cutanea tarda

Porphyria cutanea tarda (PCT), the commonest porphyria, is the only type that may be either sporadic (80% of cases) or familial (autosomal dominant). Reduced activity of uroporphyrinogen decarboxylase results in overproduction of photoactive porphyrins. Uroporphyrinogen decarboxylase is inactivated by an iron-dependent process that is not fully understood, but a variety of factors can initiate disease (see Box 16.8).

Water-soluble porphyrins cause skin fragility and blistering. Uroporphyrin also stimulates fibroblasts to produce collagen in the skin and this may explain some of the cutaneous features.

What should I look for?

PCT only affects skin and is most common in men. The presentation is subacute and the relationship to sun exposure may be missed.

- Skin fragility: minor knocks produce erosions on dorsum of hands.
- Itching or burning may precede blisters on sun-exposed skin.
- Haemorrhagic vesicles, bullae, and crusted erosions, most often affecting exposed skin on the dorsa of the hands, the face, and upper chest—see Fig. 16.3.
- Superficial scars or milia (firm white pinhead-sized papules—sequelae of subepidermal blisters)—see EBA, 📖 p. 252.
- Dystrophic calcification.
- Hypertrichosis on cheeks and/or forehead.
- Blisters beneath the nail plate; painful discoloration (yellow, blue, or haemorrhagic) of nail; loss of lunula, onycholysis, or dystrophy.
- Diffuse or reticulated hyperpigmentation of sun-exposed skin.
- Waxy yellowish thickening of sun-exposed skin ('sclerodermoid').
- Normal teeth (unlike congenital erythropoietic porphyria).
- Normal mucosa (involved in some autoimmune blistering diseases).

What should I do?

- Confirm the diagnosis and exclude pseudoporphyria (see Box 16.8) by measuring porphyrins in fresh samples of urine and stool—see 📖 p.308. Fresh urine containing excess uroporphyrins is pink and fluoresces bright coral pink under a UVA light (Wood's light).
- Biopsy a fresh blister for histology: subepidermal cell-poor blister, PAS+ve glycoproteins at basement membrane zone (BMZ) and around blood vessels—and for direct immunofluorescence—immunoglobulins deposited at BMZ and around blood vessels.
- Exclude risk factors including hepatitis C—see Box 16.8.
- Withdraw precipitating factors including alcohol and oestrogens.
- Advise strict sun protection—see 📖 p.316.
- Regular venesection (400–500mL every 2 weeks for 3–6 months) depletes iron stores and can be helpful.
- Consider prescribing low-dose hydroxychloroquine (100–125mg × 2/week)—higher doses may cause hepatitis.
- Monitor for development of hepatocellular carcinoma.

Box 16.8 Risk factors for adult PCT

Factors that reduce activity of uroporphyrinogen decarboxylase in the liver can initiate disease in genetically susceptible individuals.

- Alcohol.
- Oral oestrogens: oral contraception and hormone replacement therapy.
- Oral iron.
- Mutations in the hereditary haemochromatosis (*HFE*) gene.
- Hepatitis C virus infection.
- HIV infection.
- Polychlorinated hydrocarbons.
- Chronic haemodialysis (azotaemia reduces activity of uroporphyrinogen decarboxylase; porphyrins are inadequately cleared by hemodialysis). Check plasma and faecal porphyrins as urinary testing is difficult to interpret if patient is on dialysis. If porphyrins are normal consider pseudoporphyria. Venesection is usually contraindicated in renal failure and hydroxychloroquine is ineffective. Human erythropoietin reduces iron stores and may be an effective treatment.

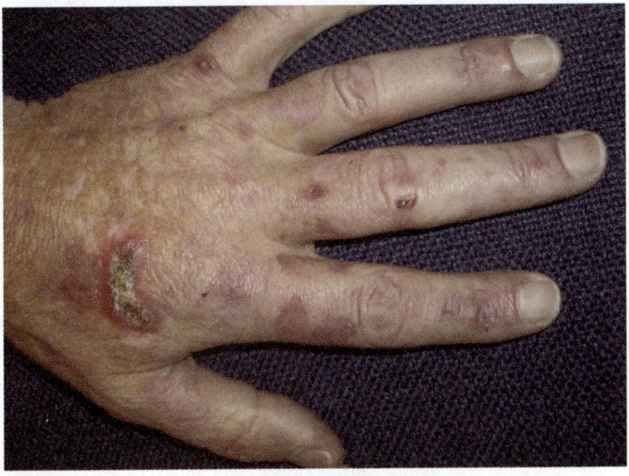

Fig. 16.3 Porphyria cutanea tarda: fragile skin on the back of the hand with crusted erosions and scars.

What is pseudoporphyria?

Pseudoporphyria is an acquired photosensitive blistering disease with clinical and immunohistological features similar to PCT. The pathogenesis is uncertain, but porphyrins are normal.

Patients have PCT-like blistering, erosions, milia, and scars on sun-exposed skin (Fig. 16.3) but, unlike PCT, patients rarely have hyperpigmentation, hypertrichosis, sclerodermoid changes, or dystrophic calcification.

Causes include:

- Chronic renal failure, haemodialysis, peritoneal dialysis (the antioxidant *N*-acetylcysteine may be an effective treatment).
- UVA-tanning beds, PUVA, excess sun exposure (generally women).
- A wide range of drugs including:
  - NSAIDs (most frequent cause): naproxen and others (generally in women).
  - Antibiotics: nalidixic acid, tetracycline, ampicillin-sulbactam, cefepime, fluoroquinolones.
  - Antifungals: voriconazole.
  - Diuretics: furosemide, bumetanide.
  - Antiarrhythmics: amiodarone.
  - Sulphones: dapsone.
  - Vitamins: brewer's yeast, pyridoxine.
  - Retinoids: isotretinoin, etretinate.
  - Muscle relaxants: carisoprodol.
  - Antiandrogens: flutamide.

Further reading

Green JJ and Manders SM. *J Am Acad Dermatol* 2001; **44**:100–8.

⚠ Erythropoietic protoporphyria

Erythropoietic protoporphyria (EPP), caused by reduced activity of ferrochetolase, is a rare form of porphyria presenting in childhood. Intense pain may cause infants to cry bitterly within minutes of sun exposure, but as signs are subtle and skin can look almost normal between episodes, the diagnosis is often missed. In 2% of cases, EPP is complicated by progressive liver failure.

What should I look for?

- Acute episodes of cutaneous photosensitivity that started in infancy. Window glass is not protective (sensitivity to UVA and visible light). Light reflected off snow, sand, or water may cause symptoms.
- Symptoms start in the spring, but reduce in the autumn and winter.
- Burning, tingling, stinging, pain, and/or itching in light-exposed skin occurs within minutes of sun exposure. Children may try to relieve symptoms by plunging hands into cold water.
- Erythema, urticaria, and/or swelling within minutes of sun exposure.
- Occasionally purpuric lesions following sun exposure.
- Waxy skin thickening over knuckles and on the nose.
- Subtle elliptical scars on the nose, cheeks, and/or dorsum of the hands.

What should I do?

- Check porphyrins: protoporphyrin is raised in erythrocytes and stool; urine porphyrins are not increased.
- Check FBC: some patients are anaemic.
- Advise on photoprotection (lifestyle, broad-spectrum sunscreens, clothing, UV blocking films for window glass in home and car)—see 📖 p.316.
- Oral beta-carotene taken from February until October may reduce photosensitivity, but patients may not tolerate the unsightly orange pigmentation.
- UVB phototherapy may improve tolerance to sunlight (probably the most effective treatment).
- Monitor for cholestasis and progressive liver damage.

⚠ Xeroderma pigmentosum

This rare autosomal recessive photodermatosis affects all races and has an equal sex incidence. Patients develop premature photodamage, skin cancers, and ophthalmological abnormalities. 20% of patients have progressive neurological disorders. The disease is devastating and cutaneous malignancies cause early death—see Box 16.9.

Normally, photodamaged DNA is excised and repaired with newly synthesized DNA (excision repair), but xeroderma pigmentosum (XP) cells are unable to repair the damaged DNA—see Box 16.9. The defect affects all cell types. In addition to cutaneous and ocular malignancies, patients have an increased risk of malignancy in other tissues, e.g. oral cavity, breast, lung, liver, gastric, renal, and brain. Gene therapy may hold promise for the future.

Skin is normal at birth, but XP presents within the first few years of life and has a major impact on the lifestyle of the child as well as the family. Clinical features vary, but fair-skinned children are most severely affected.

What should I look for?

- Easy sunburn that usually presents within the first 2 years of life.
- UVB-induced erythema that is delayed in onset and peaks in 2–3 days rather than the usual 24h.
- A history of blistering or burning after very little sun exposure.
- Photophobia in young children.
- Dryness of sun-exposed skin (xeroderma).
- Irregular freckling that appears in the 1st year of life on exposed skin.
- Scarring of exposed skin.
- Signs of premature photodamage—mottled hyperpigmented patches, hypopigmented macules, telangiectasia.
- Hyperkeratotic lower lip (solar cheilitis).
- Eyelid freckling, loss of lashes, ectropion, conjunctival telangiectasia, dry eyes and corneal damage leading to visual impairment.
- Solar keratoses (premalignant change).
- Skin cancers (median age of onset = 8 years)—BCC, SCC, melanoma.
- Parents with a history of skin cancers, but no other signs of XP.

Management

- The diagnosis is confirmed by skin biopsy and demonstration of the DNA repair defect in cultured fibroblasts.
- Care should be provided by a multidisciplinary team that may include paediatricians, dermatologists, ophthalmologists, neurologists, cancer specialist nurses, and plastic surgeons.
- ⚠ ***It is crucial to protect the skin from photodamage*** to slow the onset of life-threatening cutaneous malignancies—see 📖 p.316.
- Carers and/or patients should examine the skin regularly for signs of skin cancer. Cancers are treated surgically.
- Oral retinoids may reduce the incidence of skin cancer.
- Patients should be protected from cigarette smoke.
- Encourage patients to join the XP Patient Support Group—see Box 16.10.

Box 16.9 What is xeroderma pigmentosum (XP)?

- XP is an autosomal recessive disorder caused by defects in one of seven nuclear excision repair (*NER*) genes. Some XP genes are also involved in other processes, e.g. transcription and recombination.
- XP patients are photosensitive and prone to premature skin cancers as well as internal malignancies.
- Patients were separated into different groups when it was found that the defect in excision repair in a cultured cell line from one XP patient could be corrected by fusion with a cell line from a different, unrelated XP patient. Patients whose cell lines failed to complement each other in culture were grouped together.
- 7 complementation groups have been identified (XP-A to XP-G).
- Patients in different complementation groups have different genetic defects. Patients within a complementation group have similar clinical characteristics.
- XP-C is the commonest complementation group worldwide.
- 20% of patients (mostly XP-A and XP-D) have progressive neurological abnormalities, e.g. hyporeflexia, mental retardation, seizures, deafness, ataxia, quadriparesis. Accumulated DNA damage may cause degeneration of neural tissue, which cannot be replaced.
- 30% of XP patients belong to a variant group (XP-V) with a less severe phenotype. XP-V patients have normal NER, but abnormal post-replicational DNA repair caused by defective DNA polymerase.
- Investigation into the genetic basis of XP has provided insights into DNA repair and the pathogenesis of cutaneous malignancy.

Box 16.10 Xeroderma Pigmentosum Support Group

The XP Support Group is a UK charitable trust. The group supports patients and their families, keeps members up to date with the latest research, provides information on XP, and offers practical advice on a wide range of topics including:

- How to deal with schools and education authorities.
- Where to obtain UV protective clothing and UV protective clear window film.
- Grants for UV protective products.
- Annual Owl Patrol night time camps for children and their families.

Further reading

Daya-Grosjean L and Sarasin A. *Mutat Res* 2005; **571**:43–56.

Photoprotection

Patients with photosensitivity disorders must protect their skin from the solar radiation that is responsible—UVA, UVB, visible light, or a combination. Severe photosensitivity may have a catastrophic impact on lifestyle—outdoor activities on sunny days are impossible. Sunglasses, clothing, hats, and shade (indoor activities when sun is strongest between 11.00am and 3.00pm) provide more effective photoprotection than sunscreens.

Clothing, hats, sunglasses, and windows

- Clothing and hats should have a tight weave, sufficiently thick to block transmission of visible light (check transmission of visible light by trying to look through the item held up to the sun).
- Clothing should be loose fitting (photoprotective fabrics are available).
- Patients should wear hats with broad brims (baseball caps do not protect the ears or neck) as well as a flap of cloth to cover the neck, shirts with long sleeves, trousers not shorts, and shoes rather than sandals. Some patients may need gloves for driving.
- UV blocking films can be obtained for window glass, car windscreens, and fluorescent lights if required.
- Sunglasses are needed to protect against UV radiation and blue light.

Sunscreens—see Boxes 16.11 and 16.12

- Sunscreens may be physical or chemical.
- Physical sunscreens (sunblocks) are opaque creams containing particles (titanium dioxide, zinc oxide) that reflect and scatter UV radiation (UVB and UVA) as well as visible light. Physical sunscreens may be less cosmetically acceptable than chemical sunscreens but are probably more effective and may be safer—see Box 16.12, Box 17.3, p.325 and Box 17.4, p.325.
- Chemical sunscreens absorb UV radiation of certain wavelengths, either UVB or UVA. UVB chemical sunscreens protect against UVB-induced sunburn by blocking UVB. They contain cinnamates and other agents. UVA chemical sunscreens provide limited protection and contain chemicals such as oxybenzone. New dual UVB/UVA filters and photon absorbers are being developed.
- Chemical sunscreens may cause contact dermatitis (irritant or allergic).
- Concerns have been raised about the potential chemical sunscreens may have to trigger the development of oestrogen-sensitive cancers and to generate free radicals that could cause skin cancer. Data from long-term studies are needed to address these issues.
- Patients using a UVB absorbing sunscreen that prevents immediate erythema or sunburn should be warned not to stay out longer in the sun, to prevent exposure to excessive UVA.
- Lips should be protected as well as skin.
- The potential of topical or oral antioxidants to reduce photodamage is being investigated.
- Patients avoiding UVB may become vitamin D deficient—see Box 16.13.

Box 16.11 How much UV protection is provided by the sunscreen?

- The sun protection factor (SPF) indicates the UVB photoprotection provided by a sunscreen. An SPF of 10 means that it takes 10 × longer for the skin to go red than unprotected skin exposed to the same amount of UVB. An SPF of 15–20 is adequate for most patients.
- The star rating (maximum 5) indicates the % of UVA absorbed in comparison to UVB. The UVA protection should be at least 1/3 of the labelled SPF.

Box 16.12 Why is the sunscreen ineffective?

- Sunscreen is not blocking the appropriate wavelengths. Broad-spectrum combination sunscreens with an SPF of at least 15 and a high UVA protection are the most effective.
- Sunscreen is not applied sufficiently thickly (at least 6 teaspoons of lotion are needed to cover the body of the average adult). Opaque sunblock creams do not have to be applied very thickly to be effective.
- Sunscreen is not applied evenly to the skin.
- Sunscreen is not applied all exposed skin including lips, sides of neck, ears, and temples.
- Sunscreen is not reapplied every 2–3h.
- Sunscreen is not reapplied straight after swimming or activities causing sweating.
- Patient has become allergic to the sunscreen (refer for photopatch testing).
- But recommend physical barriers—sunglasses, clothing, hats, and shade—rather than encouraging patients to rely on sunscreens.

Box 16.13 Vitamin D synthesis

- UVB stimulates the synthesis of vitamin D_3 (cholecalciferol) in the skin. Adequate levels of vitamin D are maintained if 15% of the body (face, arms, hands) receives about 1/3 of the minimal erythematogenic dose of UVB on most days of week. In the UK, this equates to about 5–10min of sun exposure on arms, legs, and/or face ×2–3/week from May to September (during the rest of the year, sunlight at this latitude is insufficient for vitamin D synthesis).
- Patients who are very photosensitive and cannot tolerate any UVB radiation should take vitamin D supplements.
- Vitamin D supplements may also be needed by individuals living in countries with low levels of UV for much of the year.
- Vitamin D deficiency is common in the elderly, people with darker skin, or those who cover skin when outdoors.

Further reading

González E and González S. *J Am Acad Dermatol* 1996; **35:**871–5.

González S *et al. Clin Dermatol* 2008; **26:**614–26.

Chapter 17

Tumours

Contents

Relevant pages in other chapters

The history and examination in patients with skin tumours are discussed on 📖 p.26 and 📖 p.42. Also see 📖 Chapter 16, Sun and skin, p.300.

Common benign non-melanocytic tumours

Seborrhoeic wart

Also known as seborrhoeic keratosis or basal cell papilloma.

Benign epidermal tumours of unknown cause. Common, particularly in the elderly. They are most common on the trunk, but also affect face and limbs. Patients may have one, several, or hundreds of seborrhoeic warts. Treatment is only required if the seborrhoeic wart is traumatized, when it may become inflamed or bleed, sometimes simulating a malignant melanoma.

What should I look for?

- A well-defined oval pigmented tumour, around 0.5–2cm in diameter that looks as if it has been stuck onto the surface of the skin.
- A rough surface that may feel slightly greasy.
- Dark pits studded over the surface—easier to see with magnification.
- A uniform colour (usually), but may range in colour from a pale pinkish-brown to dark brown or almost black.
- Seborrhoeic warts may be virtually flat or raised by several mm.

Keratoacanthoma

Perhaps best regarded as well-differentiated SCCs. Keratoacanthomas grow rapidly; persist for 2–3 months, and then involute over 4–6 months, leaving a depressed scar. They are usually removed surgically.

What should I look for?

- A history of rapid growth over a few weeks.
- A pinkish symmetrical cup shaped nodule, 1–2cm diameter, on sun-damaged hair-bearing skin, usually the face or neck.
- Smooth rolled edges.
- A central keratin plug.

Chondrodermatitis nodularis helicis chronica

The nodules are caused by prolonged pressure on the skin of the ear, but sun damage or cold may also play a part. The history is usually characteristic and differentiates this nodule from a skin cancer. The affected ear is generally the one on which the patient lies at night and pain prevents the patient from lying on that side. Apparently nuns who wore wimples were affected by chondrodermatitis!

Treatments include relieving pressure, corticosteroids and surgery.

What should I look for?

- A tender nodule on the helix or, less often, the antihelix of the ear.
- A keratotic plug or a small ulcer in the centre of the nodule.

Dermatofibroma

Also known as fibrous histiocytoma or sclerosing haemangioma.

The localized proliferation of fibroblasts is probably triggered by minor trauma such as an insect bite. The tumours are common in young adults, most often women. If you can make a confident diagnosis no treatment is required—excision will merely leave another scar. Multiple dermatofibromas have been reported in conditions such as HIV infection, SLE, and other diseases in which the immune state is altered.

What should I look for?

- A brownish red dermal nodule, 0.5–1cm in diameter, usually on the arm, shoulder, thigh, or leg.
- The overlying epidermis is usually smooth.
- The tumour is firm—this suggests the diagnosis.
- Pinch the skin gently on each side of the tumour and it will sink down into the dermis—the 'buttonhole sign'.

Pyogenic granuloma

Typically this vascular tumour presents at the site of a penetrating injury, e.g. rose thorn, usually on fingers, lips, or face. ⚠ An amelanotic malignant melanoma may look like a pyogenic granuloma—always ask the patient if anything preceded the development of the tumour. Was there a 'mole' at the site or did it arise on normal skin?

What should I look for?

- A history of rapid growth: pyogenic granulomas grow on previously normal skin over a period of weeks to a size of 0.5–4cm.
- A fleshy vascular tumour composed of friable granulation tissue that bleeds readily on contact.
- Exclude any underlying pigmented lesion: inspect any 'pyogenic granuloma' at an atypical site particularly carefully. Melanin can be mistaken for old haemorrhage.

Other common benign tumours or inflammatory nodules

Epidermal

- Viral wart—see 📖 p.152.
- Nodular prurigo (caused by chronic rubbing)—see 📖 Fig. 10.6, p.207.
- Epidermal naevus (warty lesion, present since infancy)—see 📖 p.516.

Dermal

- Epidermoid cyst 'sebaceous' cyst: not sebaceous at all, but arises from the upper part of the hair follicle and has a punctum. Often rupture and become inflamed.
- Pilar cyst: arises from the lower part of the follicle and usually found in scalp—no punctum. Spontaneous rupture uncommon.
- Keloid: dense fibrous scar tissue spreading beyond original wound.
- Spider naevus; Campbell de Morgan spot (cherry angioma).
- Infantile haemangioma (strawberry naevus)—see 📖 p.550.
- Neurofibroma—see 📖 Fig. 27.1, p.511.
- Xanthelasma or xanthoma—see 📖 p.436.

Common benign melanocytic tumours

Melanocytic naevus ('mole' 'naevus')—Fig. 17.1

Melanocytic naevi present at birth, in childhood, or in young adults.

- Acquired melanocytic naevi start as flat evenly pigmented (junctional) naevi in which melanocytes collect in small groups (nests) along the basal layer of the epidermis. As melanocytes migrate down into the dermis, flat moles evolve into raised evenly pigmented dome-shaped papules (compound melanocytic naevi), sometimes hairy. Scalp naevi in children may be an early sign of being 'moley'. Patients with many moles tend to have a 'signature naevus'—i.e all their moles follow a pattern that is characteristic for that patient.
- Finally the epidermal component is lost and moles change into flesh-coloured or pale brown papules (intradermal melanocytic naevi), before disappearing in old age. A pigmented tumour in an elderly patient is much more likely to be a seborrhoeic wart, lentigo (see next section), or melanoma than a melanocytic naevus.
- Congenital melanocytic naevi, usually >1cm diameter (sometimes large and disfiguring = bathing trunk naevus) present at birth or in the early neonatal period. Large congenital melanocytic naevi >20cm have an increased risk of malignant change.
- Halo naevi: a white ring develops around a benign melanocytic naevus which gradually disappears leaving a depigmented macule that usually eventually repigments. Halo naevi are common in adolescence and of no significance. Halo naevi in adults (age 40–50 years) may indicate melanoma elsewhere—check skin, eyes, and mucosal surfaces.

Lentigo (plural = lentigines)

- Simple lentigines are small, round, flat, evenly pigmented lesions that persist in winter, unlike freckles. The basal layer of the epidermis has increased numbers of individual melanocytes. Numerous simple lentigines are found in some genetic disorders, e.g. LEOPARD syndrome, Carney complex, Peutz–Jeghers syndrome—see 📖 p.563.
- Solar (senile) lentigines, 3–12mm diameter, are flat brown marks that present on sun-damaged skin in older patients.

Mongolian spot

- Slate-coloured macular areas of pigmentation are present in newborns—usually on the buttocks or sacrum, where the pigment may simulate a bruise and even be misdiagnosed as a sign of non-accidental injury—see 📖 Fig. 31.10, p.565.
- Mongolian spots are most common in black or Asian infants and gradually disappear with age.
- The melanocytes are deep within the dermis and therefore the pigment appears bluish rather than brown.

Blue naevi

- Benign acquired small slate blue to blue black macules or papules that present most often on the dorsum of the hand or in the scalp.
- Melanocytes are present in the dermis and the tumours appear blue rather than brown.

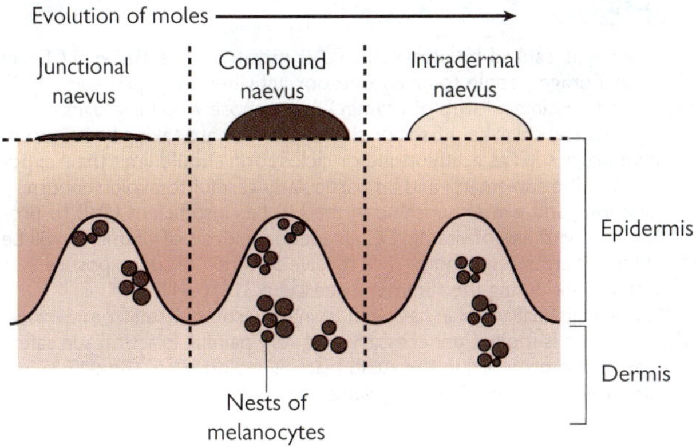

Fig. 17.1 Evolution of melanocytic naevi ('moles').

Avoiding skin cancer

Skin cancer is caused by ultraviolet (UV) radiation (see Boxes 17.1 and 17.2). Encourage people to enjoy outdoor activities (we need some UVB exposure to maintain levels of vitamin D), but those who have signs of sun damage such as solar keratoses or skin cancers or are taking immunosuppressive drugs such as azathioprine or ciclosporin should limit their exposure to sun (be sun-smart) and be particularly careful to avoid sunburn.

The spring and winter sunshine in the UK has insufficient UVB to promote much synthesis of vitamin D, but adequate levels of vitamin D will be maintained if arms, legs, and/or face receive 5–10min of sun exposure 2 or 3 times a week during the summer—see 📖 p.316, p.317.

A tan signals that the skin has been trying to protect itself from damage, while sunburn is foolish, unnecessary, and very painful. Practical sun safety tips have been provided in the Australian 'Slip–Slop–Slap' (Box 17.3) and the UK 'Save our Skin' (Box 17.4) campaigns.

Box 17.1 UV radiation and skin cancer

- UVB is more photocarcinogenic than UVA, but both contribute to the pathogenesis of skin cancer by damaging DNA.
- Photodamaged DNA is usually repaired by nucleotide excision repair enzymes, but repair declines with age and cumulative mutations lead to skin cancer by affecting the function of genes that regulate cell proliferation (oncogenes such as *RAS*, tumour suppressor genes such as *p53*)—see 📖 p.314.
- UV radiation also causes immunosuppression, which may also predispose to skin cancer by interfering with recognition and elimination of abnormal cells.
- Fair skin types I and II (northern European ancestry), with red or blond hair and severe sunburn in childhood or adolescence, increase the risk of developing skin cancer.
- Chronic cumulative UV radiation including PUVA (>200 treatments) and sunbeds also predispose to skin cancer.

For signs of chronic sun damage (photoageing)—see 📖 Box 3.1, p.43.

Box 17.2 Other risk factors for skin cancer

BCC

Previous BCC, X-irradiation, immunosuppression (organ transplant (see 📖 p.464), HIV, lymphatic leukaemia), chronic arsenic exposure, genetic factors (Gorlin's syndrome, albinism, XP).

SCC

Bowen's disease or solar keratosis, previous SCC, pipe smoker (lip), X-irradiation, thermal burns, immunosuppression (organ transplant (see 📖 p.464), HIV, lymphatic leukaemia), HPV infection, chronic wounds (sinuses, scars, or ulcers), tar, chronic arsenic exposure, genetic factors (albinism, XP).

Melanoma

Previous melanoma, >50 melanocytic naevi or many atypical (dysplastic) melanocytic naevi; giant 'bathing-trunk' >20cm diameter congenital melanocytic naevus (melanoma may develop early in childhood in large congenital lesions), immunosuppression, genetic factors: albinism, XP, family history of melanoma (mutations in *CDKN2A* and *CDK4* genes).

See 📖 Chapter 16, p.316 for more about sun and the skin including more detailed information about vitamin D, photoprotection, and sunscreens. See 📖 p.314 for xeroderma pigmentosum (XP).

Box 17.3 Slip–Slop–Slap

- Slip on a shirt: cover exposed skin with loose-fitting cotton clothing that has a tight weave.
- Slop on a sunscreen cream (SPF 15 or more) liberally and frequently to the face and other exposed skin, but creams are no substitute for hats, clothing, and a sensible lifestyle—and they are costly.
- Slap on a hat with a broad brim and tight weave (check how much light comes through the hat by holding it up to the sun). The neck should be protected as well as face and ears. Baseball caps do not provide adequate sun protection.

Box 17.4 SOS: Save Our Skin

- Slip On a Shirt.
- Seek Out the Shade between 11am and 3pm—definitely try to avoid outdoor activities in the midday sun (there is still something to be said for a midday siesta!).
- Step Out of the Sun.
- Slap on Sunscreen—SPF 15 or more.

Further reading

Skin cancer advice and sun safety information including downloadable leaflets and posters. Available at: http://www.bad.org.uk/site/491/default.aspx

Premalignant epidermal tumours

Solar (actinic) keratosis

Solar keratoses are premalignant tumours (the epidermal basal cell layer is dysplastic) that indicate chronic sun damage and are a marker of patients at risk of skin cancer. About 20% regress spontaneously. Progression to SCC is not common (<1 in 1000 per annum)—see Fig. 17.2.

What should I look for?

- Asymptomatic or slightly itchy, brownish-red, discrete flaky or keratotic patches on sun-exposed skin: the bald scalp, face, helix of ear, dorsum of hands, forearms (Fig. 17.3).
- Some may be raised and warty: hypertrophic solar keratosis.
- Induration, inflammation, or ulceration suggesting progression to SCC.
- Other signs of chronic sun damage and skin tumours: BCC, SCC, malignant melanoma.

Treatment is only required if the keratoses are troublesome, but all patients should be advised to monitor their skin for the development of skin cancers and to protect their skin from the sun—see 📖 p.324.

Bowen's disease (intra-epidermal SCC)

Bowen's disease is characterized by full-thickness epidermal dysplasia. Only about 3–5% of plaques progress to SCC—but the risk of metastasis from the SCC is high. Aetiologies include chronic sun exposure, radiation, oncogenic HPV, immunosuppression, and arsenic.

Patients with >1 plaque (10–20% of patients) may have been exposed to arsenic, which is present in Fowler's solution (a tonic once widely available in the UK but finally removed from sale in the 1950s), some traditional remedies in countries such as Pakistan and India; and the water of artesian wells in countries such as Bangladesh or Taiwan.

Plaques are asymptomatic and enlarge slowly over many years. Bowen's disease is often misdiagnosed as 'discoid eczema' or 'ringworm'.

What should I look for?

- A well-defined erythematous scaly or warty plaque (Fig. 17.4).
- A flat edge: stretch the skin gently and inspect the edge closely. A raised thready border suggests superficial BCC rather than Bowen's disease.
- Nodularity or ulceration: this may indicate progression to SCC.

What should I do?

- Take a skin scrape to exclude a fungal infection if indicated.
- Take a skin biopsy to confirm the diagnosis.

Treatment options include surgical removal, topical 5-fluorouracil and topical imiquimod. Patients should protect their skin from the sun—see 📖 p.324.

Further reading

Cox N *et al.* Guidelines for the management of Bowen's disease 2006. Available at: http://www.bad.org.uk/healthcare/guidelines/Bowens_Disease_update_January_2007.pdf

De Berker D *et al.* Guidelines for the management of actinic keratoses 2007. Available at: http://www.bad.org.uk/healthcare/guidelines/Actinic_Keratoses.pdf

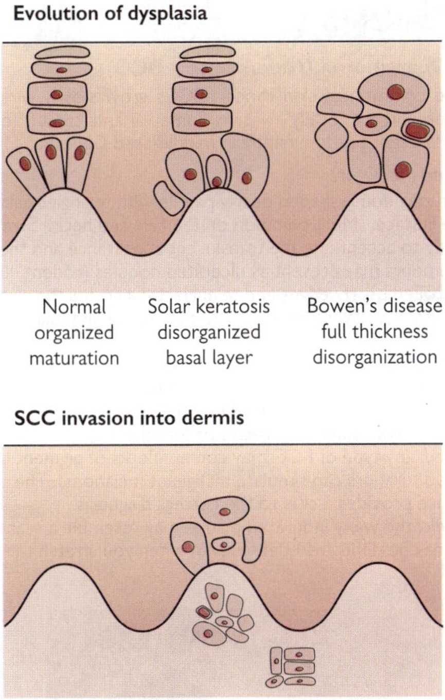

Fig. 17.2 Evolution of dysplasia.

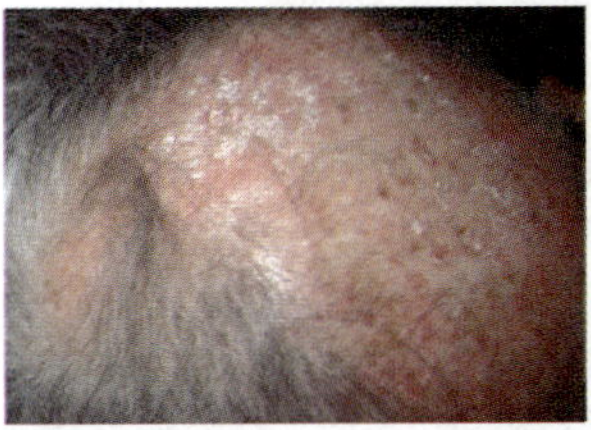

Fig. 17.3 Solar keratoses in sun-damaged skin with solar lentigines (pigmented macules).

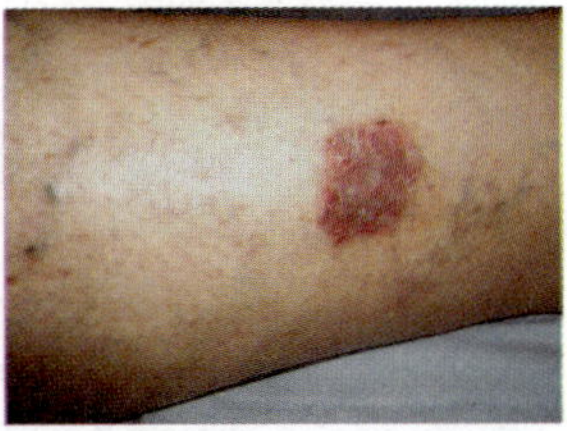

Fig. 17.4 Bowen's disease: an asymptomatic scaly plaque on the leg. The differential includes fungal infection, eczema, and a superficial BCC.

Common skin cancers

Basal cell carcinoma (rodent ulcer, BCC)

BCC is the commonest skin cancer. BCCs grow slowly, virtually never metastasizes, and are locally invasive. Some variants can be very destructive. BCCs present predominantly in middle-aged Caucasians.

What should I look for?

- ***Nodulocystic:*** dome-shaped pearly papule with telangiectasia coursing over the surface. (Most common on the face and neck.) Stretch the skin gently to accentuate the translucent appearance and the borders. Older tumours may present as ulcerated nodules (rodent ulcers) with smooth rolled pearly edges and telangiectasia across the surface—Fig. 17.5. Remove loose crust so you can see the granulating fleshy base.
- ***Superficial:*** 1 or more scaly erythematous plaques (most often on the trunk) with well-defined raised pearly edges. Stretch the skin gently to make the pearly border of superficial BCC more obvious and differentiate from Bowen's disease or fungal infection.
- ***Pigmented:*** any type of BCC may contain flecks of pigment but heavily pigmented tumours can simulate malignant melanoma. The pearly appearance provides a clue to the correct diagnosis.
- ***Morphoeic:*** the waxy indurated plaque may resemble a scar. The border may be difficult to define even when you stretch the skin.

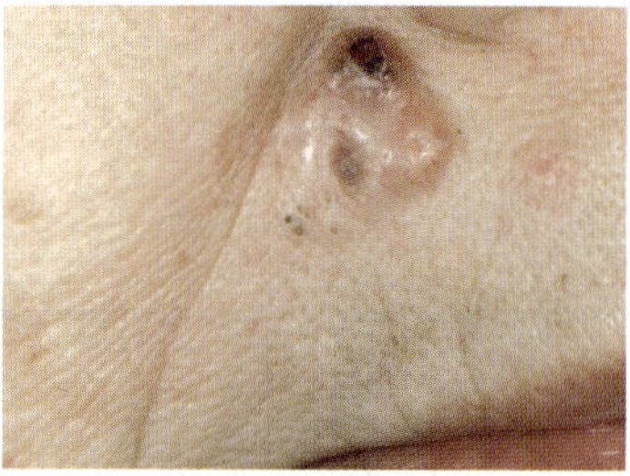

Fig. 17.5 Nodulocystic BCC with a pearly appearance.

Squamous cell carcinoma (SCC)

Cutaneous SCCs are the second most common skin cancer (20% of all non-melanoma cancers). They usually present in elderly patients on sun-exposed sites and are 3× more common in men. The prognosis depends on the potential for metastasis which is influenced by the anatomical site, the tumour (rate of growth, depth, amount of differentiation), and the host response (immunosuppression increases both the incidence of SCC and risk of metastasis).

What should I look for?

- A keratotic nodule or an ulcerated nodule with granulating base and rolled undermined border—Fig. 17.6.
- Induration or ulceration of a solar keratosis or Bowen's disease.
- Regional lymphadenopathy.

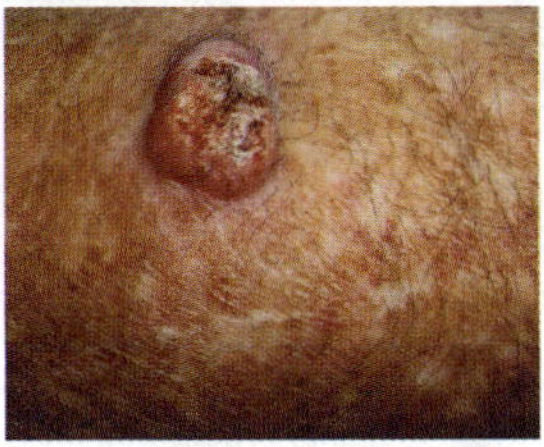

Fig. 17.6 Squamous cell carcinoma arising on severely sun damaged skin with hypo- and hyperpigmentation.

Risk of metastasis

- Very low: SCC on sun-exposed skin (except lip, ear, or Bowen's disease).
- Moderate: SCC of lip or ear (ear higher than lip).
- High: SCC on covered sites, e.g. perineum, sole of foot.
- Very high: SCC in Bowen's disease, areas of X-irradiation, or thermal injury, chronic draining sinuses, or chronic ulcers.

Risk factors for skin cancer—see 📖 p.324 and p.325

Box 17.5 Treatment options for BCC and SCC

Choice of treatment depends on the age of the patient and the history as well as the type and site of the tumour, but options may include:

- Excision (the gold standard); curettage and cautery.
- Mohs micrographic surgery: treatment of choice for locally recurrent skin cancers, cancers in sites where it is important to preserve tissue, e.g. adjacent to eye, or for cancers with ill-defined margins, e.g. morphoeic BCC.
- Topical imiquimod or topical 5-fluorouracil: for superficial BCCs.
- Cryosurgery or photodynamic therapy (PDT) (superficial tumours).
- Radiotherapy.

Further reading

Motley R *et al.* Guidelines for the management of the patient with primary cutaneous squamous cell carcinoma 2009.

Telfer N *et al.* Guidelines for the management of basal cell carcinoma 2008.

These clinical guidelines are available at the BAD website: www.bad.org.uk/site/622/default.aspx

Malignant melanoma

Malignant melanoma is the least common skin cancer, but incidence in the UK has quadrupled since the 1970s (>9500 new cases in 2005). Melanoma is more common in men than in women and almost 1/3 occur in people aged <50 (melanoma is the commonest cancer in young adults). Superficial spreading melanoma is the commonest type in Caucasians (see Box 17.6).

Most melanomas arise de novo, not in pre-existing melanocytic naevi. Risk factors—see 📖 p.324. Melanoma accounts for 75% of deaths associated with skin cancer, but survival rates are improving because tumours are being recognized early.

What should I look for?

- ⚠ Moles that are irregular in colour, outline, or shape (Fig. 17.7).
- Use the ABCDEF criteria to identify suspicious pigmented lesions:
  - *A*symmetry in outline.
  - *B*order irregularity or blurring, sometimes with notching.
  - *C*olour variation with shades of black, brown, and pink.
  - *D*iameter >6mm (cannot be covered by the end of a pencil).
  - *E*volution: a tumour that is changing in size, elevation, and/or colour.
  - *F*unny looking mole (see ugly duckling sign, next).
- Moles that stand out or look different from the others, i.e. 'ugly ducklings'. Better than ABCDE criteria for identifying nodular melanoma.
- New or changing longitudinal pigmented streaks in nails.
- Pigment extending from nailbed onto skin of nailfold (Hutchinson's sign) suggesting melanoma not haematoma.
- Moles that are symptomatic (itching, swollen, tender), but more often than not these turn out to be irritated benign melanocytic naevi rather than malignant melanomas.
- Regional lymphadenopathy.

What should I do?

- Find out more about the history of the tumour from the patient—see 📖 p.26.
- Document any risk factors—see Box 17.1, p.324 and Box 17.2, p.325.
- Record the findings including the site and size of the tumour. Photography is helpful.
- Refer any patient in whom you are concerned about a pigmented lesion for an urgent opinion. Prognosis is determined primarily by the Breslow thickness and mortality is high if the tumour is not removed when it is thin (see Table 📖 p.332).
- Dermoscopy, performed by an expert, may help to confirm the diagnosis of melanoma—see 📖 p.568.
- Excision is the treatment of choice.

Box 17.6 Types of cutaneous malignant melanoma

- Superficial spreading melanoma (80–85%) is the commonest melanoma in Caucasians. Presents as a slowly enlarging, slightly raised, pigmented plaque with irregularity in colour and border. Eventually a nodule appears within the plaque indicating deep invasion. Most often on trunk of men or legs of women—Fig. 17.7.
- Nodular melanoma (10–15%) grows rapidly, invading deeply from the outset. If amelanotic (often some pigment if you look carefully), may be misdiagnosed as a vascular tumour, e.g. pyogenic granuloma.
- Lentigo maligna melanoma (5%) arises within a slow-growing melanoma *in situ* known as lentigo maligna (Hutchinson's freckle). This type of melanoma is associated with chronic sun damage. It usually presents on the head or neck of an elderly patient.
- Acral lentiginous melanoma (2–8%): palms, soles, beneath nail. Most common in Chinese and Japanese.

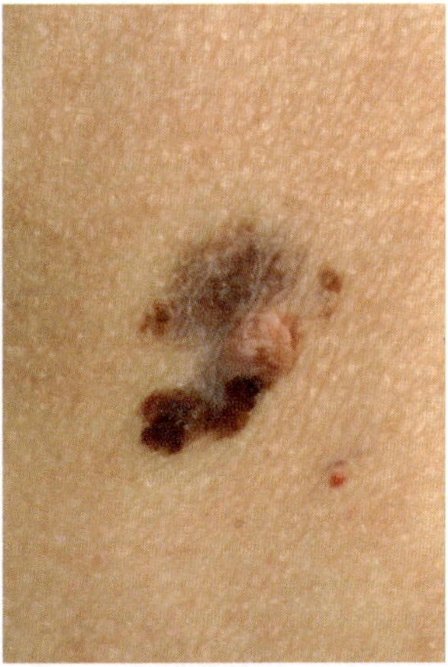

Fig. 17.7 Superficial spreading malignant melanoma with asymmetry in colour and outline. This melanoma did arise in a melanocytic naevus.

Prognosis of malignant melanoma

Breslow thickness	*5-year survival*
Up to 0.75mm	95%
0.76–1.5mm	85%
1.51–4.0mm	65%
>4.0mm	45%
Nodal disease	40%
Metastatic disease	<10%

Further reading

Roberts *et al.* UK guidelines for the management of cutaneous melanoma, 2002. Available at: http://www.bad.org.uk/healthcare/guidelines/Cutaneous_Melanoma.pdf

Cancer research UK: Skin cancer. Available at: http://info.cancerresearchuk.org/cancerstats/types/skin/?a=5441

Other malignancies and skin

Paget's disease

Paget's disease is caused by direct extension of a mammary intraductal adenocarcinoma into skin of the nipple or areola.

What should I look for?

- An erythematous weeping crusted eruption affecting one nipple.
- Is there a past history of atopic eczema? This is common on the nipple and sometimes is unilateral.
- Check the other nipple. Bilateral changes are much more likely to be eczema (atopic or contact) than cancer.
- Check for a breast lump.

What should I do?

- Biopsy any 'eczematous' nipple rash that persists despite potent topical corticosteroid ointments applied ×2/day for 2 weeks.

Metastatic disease

Skin metastasis may be the first sign of an internal malignancy. The skin may be infiltrated by direct invasion of tumour cells or by spread from lymphatics or blood vessels. Tumour may also be implanted into surgical scars. Cancers most often associated with cutaneous metastasis are:

- Breast: skin of chest, scalp, (rarely eyelid).
- Stomach, colon: skin of abdominal wall especially periumbilical.
- Lung: skin of chest, scalp.
- Genitourinary system (uterus, ovary, kidney, bladder): skin of scalp, lower abdomen, external genitalia.

What should I look for?

- Firm intradermal or subcutaneous nodules of varying colour.
- Scalp metastasis may cause a focal scarring alopecia.
- Cutaneous lymphatic invasion initially causes thickening and fibrosis and later firm pink papules or nodules.
- Carcinoma erysipeloides—most often associated with metastatic breast cancer. Lymphatic invasion produces a tender erythematous oedematous plaque, often initially misdiagnosed and treated as infection (erysipelas or cellulitis), but antibiotics are ineffective.
- Extramammary Paget's disease—a slow-growing, itching, erythematous plaque in anogenital skin. Biopsy shows mucin-containing tumour cells within the epidermis. Extramammary Paget's disease is usually associated with an underlying adnexal carcinoma, often of apocrine origin, which may be difficult to localize, but 10–15% of patients have cancer of rectum, prostate, bladder, cervix, or urethra.

Primary cutaneous lymphomas

The primary cutaneous lymphomas are a heterogeneous group of disorders. Most are derived from skin-homing T-cells. Clinical features in combination with histological, immunophenotypic, and molecular studies have helped to delineate subtypes and provide prognostic criteria.

- Mycosis fungoides (MF, Fig. 17.8) and Sézary's syndrome: these cutaneous T-cell lymphomas are discussed on 📖 p.336.

- MF variants: bullous, pigmented, hypopigmented, verrucous, pustular, folliculotrophic. Also Pagetoid reticulosis and granulomatosis slack skin.
- CD30-positive cutaneous T-cell lymphomas: e.g. lymphomatoid papulosis—good prognosis.
- CD30-negative cutaneous T-cell lymphomas: poor prognosis.
- Primary cutaneous B-cell lymphomas (20–25% of cases). Marginal zone and follicle centre: 95% 5-year survival. Diffuse large B-cell lymphoma, leg type: 50% 5-year survival.

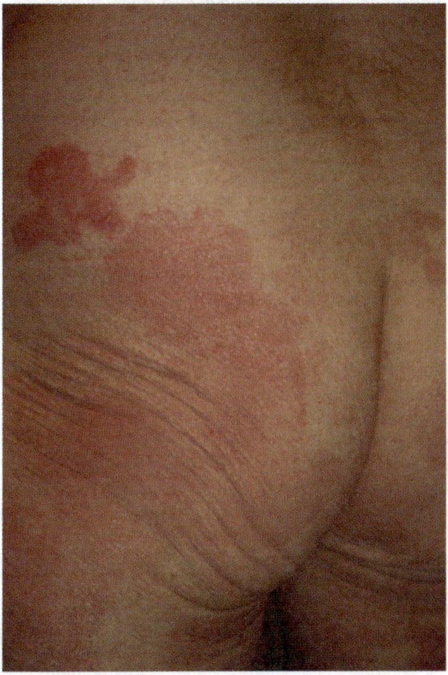

Fig. 17.8 Mycosis fungoides. Finely scaly erythematous patch and a plaque with serpiginous outline.

Adult T-cell leukaemia/lymphoma

CD4-positive lymphoproliferative disorder associated with infection with HTLV-1. Adult T-cell leukaemia/lymphoma is most common in Japan and the Caribbean. Skin signs include patches, plaques, and tumours.

Leukaemia cutis

Leukaemia cutis is rare, but is seen most often with myeloid leukaemias, e.g. acute monocytic or myelomonocytic leukaemias. Cutaneous deposits may precede transformation of myelodysplastic syndrome to leukaemia.

What should I look for?

- Firm purplish plaques or nodules.
- Infiltrates in scars or at injection sites.

Cutaneous T-cell lymphomas

Mycosis fungoides (MF)

MF is the commonest cutaneous T-cell lymphoma. Disease is indolent and diagnosis often delayed (median age 55–60 years). The disease progresses through 3 stages: patches, plaques, and tumours—which may overlap. Aetiology is uncertain, but may involve chronic antigenic stimulation (possibly viral) and mutations in oncogenes or DNA repair genes. Prognosis is worse in patients aged >60 years and in late-stage disease.

Early-stage disease has an excellent prognosis and is managed conservatively. Options include emollients, potent topical corticosteroids, UVB, PUVA, topical nitrogen mustard, and bexarotene, a novel retinoid that activates some retinoid X receptors causing T-cell apoptosis. Radiotherapy is effective for localized thick plaques or tumours. MF is relatively chemoresistant and treatment of advanced disease is still unsatisfactory. Sepsis is a common cause of death.

What should I look for?

- Symptoms: variable itch, ranging from minimal to intense.
- Early MF: 1 or more persistent and/or enlarging well-defined erythematous patches (flat) of variable size and shape with fine scale (compare with thick scale of psoriasis), often on covered sites—buttocks and breasts—see 📖 Fig. 17.8, p.335.
- Atrophy within patches: the skin wrinkles like tissue paper if pinched—not a feature of psoriasis or eczema unless very potent topical steroids have been used for prolonged periods.
- Poikiloderma i.e. mottled pigment and telangiectasia.
- Check extensor surfaces (elbows, knees), scalp and nails: sites usually spared in early MF but often involved in psoriasis.
- Late MF: reddish-brown sharply demarcated infiltrated plaques (elevated) that coalesce into annular or serpiginous shapes see 📖 Fig. 17.8, p.335.
- Hair-bearing skin: follicular plugging and alopecia (hair is retained in psoriasis and eczema).
- Ulcerating mushroom-shaped tumours (late disease).
- Enlargement of lymph nodes, liver and/or spleen (late disease).

What should I do?

- Document % of BSA involved and types of skin lesions.
- Exclude tinea (ringworm) by taking skin scrapes for mycology.
- Take 2 elliptical skin biopsies for histology, immunophenotyping, and molecular studies looking for T-cell receptor gene rearrangement. Repeated biopsies may be required before the diagnosis is established.
- Check FBC, LFT, LDH, renal function.

Further reading

Keehn C *et al. Cancer Control* 2007; **14:**102–11 (MF).

Olsen E *et al. Blood* 2007; **110:**1713–22 (staging of MF).

Senff N *et al. Blood* 2008; **112:**1600–9 (B-cell lymphomas).

Whittaker SJ *et al. Br J Dermatol* 2003; **149:**1095–1107 (management).

Sézary's syndrome

⚠ Sézary's syndrome is a leukaemic form of cutaneous T-cell lymphoma that accounts for about 5% of new cases. The disease is characterized by erythroderma (see 📖 p.102 and Fig. 5.2) lymphadenopathy, and malignant circulating CD4 positive T-cells (Sézary cells) forming >5% total lymphocyte count. The CD4:CD8 ratio may be raised to 10 or more. As disease progresses, the malignant clone of cells expands and the normal CD4 (T helper) and CD8 (T suppressor) populations decrease.

The prognosis is poor (median survival 32 months from diagnosis) and treatment unsatisfactory. PUVA is rarely tolerated. Options include extracorporeal photophoresis, multi-agent chemotherapy, immunotherapy, and oral bexarotene, but prospective clinical trials are needed.

What should I look for?

- Generalized itching, often severe.
- Systemic symptoms such as fever, weight loss, and/or malaise.
- Erythroderma (generalized redness) with or without scale.
- Other cutaneous signs may include:
  - Thickened erythematous skin on face with ectropion.
  - Thickening of skin on palms and soles (keratoderma).
  - Loss of hair and nail dystrophy.
- Widespread lymphadenopathy.

What should I do?

- Carry out a full examination
- Check FBC, film, and count of Sézary cells (T-cells with hyperconvoluted cerebriform nuclei). Some circulating Sézary cells may be found in benign inflammatory skin conditions.
- Take an elliptical skin biopsy for histology.
- Look for T-cell clones in peripheral blood and skin by immunophenotyping and with molecular studies of T-cell receptor gene.
- Check LFT, LDH, renal function.
- Biopsy an enlarged lymph node (removal preferable to needle biopsy).
- If indicated, stage with CXR, CT scan (chest, abdomen, pelvis), and bone marrow biopsy.

Kaposi's sarcoma

Kaposi's sarcoma (KS) is a neoplasm caused by proliferation of lymphatic endothelium and associated with infection of endothelial cells by human herpesvirus-8 (HHV-8). KS may behave as a benign reactive process or pursue an aggressive course that is life-threatening (see Box 17.7).

Secondary skin infections and malignancies (lymphoma) may complicate KS. Pathogenesis is multifactorial. Chronic lymphoedema (see 📖 p.296) may predispose to KS and HIV-I may exacerbate the pathogenicity of HHV-8. Circulating HHV-8 infected endothelial precursor cells localize to sites such as the leg where unregulated spindle cell proliferation is driven by interactions between activated CD8+T-cells, HHV-8 induced intracellular signalling pathways, products of oncogenes (viral and host), and inflammatory cytokines including HHV-8 encoded IL-6 and, in AIDS patients, the product of the HIV-1 *tat* gene.

If immunodeficiency is corrected, e.g. by withdrawing or reducing immunosuppression, KS may regress. KS lesions also shrink in patients treated for HIV infection with highly active antiretroviral therapy (HAART). Localized disease may be controlled with intralesional vinblastine, topical aliretinoin (9-cis-retinoic acid) gel, topical imiquimod, radiotherapy, laser surgery, or cryosurgery. Systemic options for widespread disease include IFNα, multi-agent chemotherapy with anthracyclines (doxorubicin) or paclitaxel (Taxol®). The role of angiogenesis inhibitors, sirolimus, thalidomide, and other drugs is being investigated.

What should I look for? (see Box 17.8)

- KS has a predilection for face, ears, lower limb, including soles of feet, genitalia, and oral mucosa.
- Bruise-like purple or brownish-red macules and patches which may be subtle in early disease. Consider the possibility of KS in any immunosuppressed patient with atypical 'bruises'.
- Blue, purple, red, brown, or brownish-red elliptical vascular papules lying in parallel to the natural lines of cleavage in the skin (Langer's lines). These may involve surgical scars.
- Dark blue or purple vascular nodules or indurated hyperkeratotic plaques that may ulcerate—see 📖 Fig. 17.9, p.340.
- Oral mucosal lesions (vascular patches, papules or plaques) on hard palate or, less often, gums, sometimes with overlying candidiasis. Trauma causes bleeding.
- Lymphadenopathy.
- Lymphoedema affecting face, genitalia, and/or leg caused by vascular obstruction, lymphadenopathy, and local cytokines (more common in AIDS-related KS). Swelling out of proportion to cutaneous signs.

What should I do?

- Take a skin biopsy to confirm the diagnosis.
- Exclude immunosuppression e.g. HIV infection.
- Investigate gastrointestinal tract and/or respiratory tract if indicated.

Box 17.7 Kaposi's sarcoma: clinicopathological subtypes

- Classic: men, aged 40–70, of Mediterranean or central–eastern European (Ashkenazi) Jewish heritage. Affects legs and feet. Indolent and pursues a chronic course. Patients generally die with rather than from KS. Countries bordering the Mediterranean basin have higher rates of HHV-8 infection than the rest of Europe.
- Endemic (African: sub-Saharan Africa): affects younger population than classic KS. Male predominance less marked in childhood. Not linked to AIDS. More aggressive than classic KS. Extensive skin infiltration especially on the lower limbs. High rates of HHV-8 infection in general population in this part of Africa.
- Iatrogenic: particularly in transplant recipients taking calcineurin inhibitors, e.g. ciclosporin, which inhibit T-cell function. Patients either have pre-existing HHV-8 infection or less often acquire HHV-8 when transplanted with an HHV-8 infected organ. KS has also been described in patients taking other immunosuppressive drugs such as prednisolone. KS may regress partially or completely if immunosuppression is withdrawn.
- AIDS-related: predominantly in gay and bisexual men. Trunk, arms, head, and neck involved more frequently than in classic KS. Pursues an aggressive course involving mucosa, lymph nodes and viscera (gastrointestinal tract, respiratory tract). Poor prognosis—death from opportunistic infection, gastrointestinal haemorrhage, cardiac tamponade, or pulmonary obstruction. Treatment of HIV infection with HAART has decreased the incidence of KS. Occasionally the immune reconstitution IRIS seen after treatment with HAART can trigger a flare of KS.

Box 17.8 Kaposi's sarcoma: differential diagnosis

- Melanocytic tumours: melanocytic naevi, melanoma—primary or metastatic—see 🕮 p.330.
- Pyogenic granuloma, haemangiomas, or other vascular tumour.
- Pseudo-KS: vascular nodules seen in venous stasis or in association with arteriovenous malformations. Histology resembles KS.
- Metastatic renal cell carcinoma (also tend to be vascular) or another metastasis.
- Bacillary angiomatosis—see 🕮 p.134. Unlike KS, vascular lesions are uncommon on soles or in the mouth.

Further reading

Schwartz RA *et al. J Am Acad Dermatol* 2008; **59**:179–206.

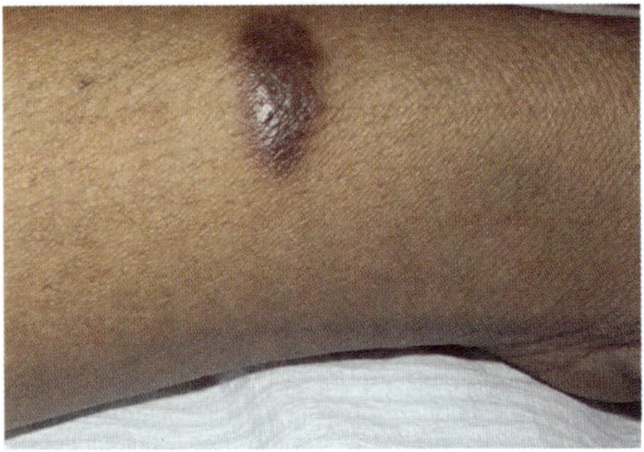

Fig. 17.9 Dark purple vascular nodule in AIDS-related Kaposi's sarcoma.

Cutaneous reactions to drugs

Contents

Relevant pages in other chapters

Adverse effects of topical corticosteroids—see 🕮 p.588

Introduction

Cutaneous adverse drug reactions (see Box 18.1) are common (2–3% of hospitalized patients), the signs extraordinarily diverse, time courses variable, and, worryingly, some are life threatening.

Reactions may be pharmacological or idiosyncratic (see Box 18.2). Predisposition is probably multifactorial, involving genetic and environmental factors—see Box 18.3. In the future, pharmacogenetics may help us to predict which patients are likely to react adversely to certain drugs, as well those likely to have most benefit.

Cutaneous adverse reactions may not be recognized if the reaction simulates a condition such as eczema or if the medication has been taken for months without problems. The exanthem of a viral infection looks like a morbilliform drug reaction, but exanthems are more likely in children than in adults. To compound diagnostic difficulties, reactions may not settle as soon as the drug is withdrawn—some persist for months—and generally there is no definitive test to confirm the diagnosis of 'drug reaction'.

These life-threatening or serious cutaneous adverse drug reactions are discussed in more detail elsewhere:

- Anaphylaxis and angio-oedema—see 🕮 p.98.
- Erythroderma—see 🕮 p.102.
- Stevens–Johnson syndrome (SJS)—see 🕮 p.110.
- Toxic epidermal necrolysis (TEN)—see 🕮 p.110.
- DRESS (drug rash, eosinophilia, systemic symptoms)—see 🕮 p.114.
- Acute generalized exanthematous pustulosis (AGEP)—see 🕮 p.116.
- Anticoagulant induced purpura fulminans and skin necrosis—see 🕮 p.96.
- Vasculitis—see 🕮 p.404.

Box 18.1 What is an adverse drug reaction?

'An appreciably harmful or unpleasant reaction, resulting from an intervention related to the use of a medicinal product, which predicts hazard from future administration and warrants prevention or specific treatment, or alteration of the dosage regimen or withdrawal of the product'.

Edwards IR and Aronson JK. *Lancet* 2000; **356:**1255–9.

Box 18.2 Types of reaction

- Type A (80% of reactions) pharmacological: augmentation of the known pharmacological actions of the drug. Predictable, dose-dependent. Reversed by reducing the dose or withdrawing the drug.
- Type B (20% of reactions) idiosyncratic. Not predictable and may be life threatening. Mechanisms include pharmaceutical variation in drug formulation, receptor abnormalities, abnormalities in drug metabolism, and immune mediated.

Box 18.3 Factors that predispose to drug reactions

- Adults rather than children.
- Female gender.
- Polypharmacy: 50% chance of an adverse interaction if 5 or more drugs are taken concurrently.
- Abnormal drug metabolism: e.g. reduced in renal failure or liver disease; toxic metabolites produced by metabolizing enzymes.
- Genetic polymorphisms: e.g. receptor abnormalities or enzyme deficiencies may cause pharmacological or idiosyncratic reactions.
- Previous hypersensitivity to a related drug.
- Host disease, e.g. SLE, herpesvirus infection, HIV infection. (In HIV infection, the incidence of cutaneous adverse drug reactions, most often morbilliform or urticarial rashes, increases as immune function deteriorates. Trimethoprim-sulphonamides and aminopenicillins cause most reactions.)

Mechanisms of idiosyncratic cutaneous adverse drug reactions

Table 18.1 Mechanisms of idiosyncratic cutaneous adverse drug reactions

Type of reaction	Mechanism	Clinical signs
Type I allergic reaction	IgE-mediated involving release of histamine from mast cells	Urticaria, angio-oedema, anaphylaxis. Minutes to hours after exposure to drug.
Type II allergic reaction	Cytotoxic IgG or IgM antibodies	Blood cell dyscrasia, e.g. allergic thrombocytopenic purpura. Variable time of onset.
Type III allergic reaction	Drug—antibody immune complexes	Vasculitis, serum sickness 1–3 weeks after exposure to drug.
Type IV allergic reaction	T-cell mediated, 'delayed hypersensitivity'	Allergic contact dermatitis 2–7 days after drug is in contact with skin.
Pseudoallergic	Direct mast cell activation with histamine release or inhibition of kinin metabolism	Anaphylactoid reactions with angio-oedema.
Autoimmune	Antinuclear antibodies	E.g. hydralazine-induced LE.
Other	T-cell activation, CD4+ and CD8+	Exanthematic, bullous or pustular rashes. Variable onset.
Other	Cytotoxic T-cells early. Later Fas ligand binding to Fas (death receptors) on keratinocytes may trigger apoptosis	SJS TEN

Further reading

Pichler WJ. *Ann Intern Med* 2003; **139**:683–93.

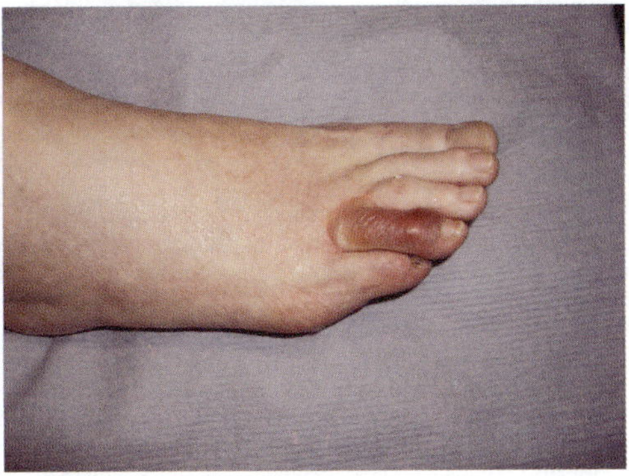

Fig. 18.1 Bullous fixed drug eruption. The blister recurs in the same place each time the patient takes the drug.

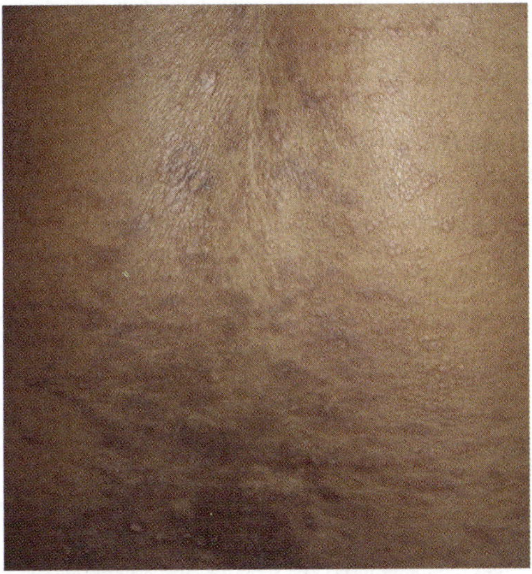

Fig. 18.2 Purplish lichen-planus like eruption caused by ramipril.

Clinical approach

When seeing any patient with a rash, ask yourself if the problem might be a manifestation of an adverse drug reaction and could this be serious. Exclude other causes, such as viral infection, but retain a high index of suspicion.

What should I ask?

- What medicaments is the patient taking or applying to the skin (including herbal or traditional remedies, recreational drugs, long-term medications such as the contraceptive pill, contrast medium, and depot injections)?
- Has the patient been exposed to the medication before?
- When medications were started (dates) and what is the temporal relation to the onset of the rash? You may have to ask the GP to get the answer. The interval between initiation of therapy and the onset of reaction is rarely <1 week, unless the patient has had the drug before, or >1 month.
- Is the reaction less severe if the drug dose is reduced or does it settle if the drug is withdrawn? Pharmacological adverse reactions, unlike idiosyncratic reactions, are usually dose-dependent.
- Are there factors that might predispose to drug reactions? 📖 See Box 18.3, p.343.
- What are the symptoms—malaise, itch, mucosal swelling, cutaneous pain or burning (may indicate TEN), arthralgia, or wheeze?

What should I do?

- Perform a full physical examination, including temperature and blood pressure.
- Document the cutaneous signs—erythema, scale, macules, papules, urticarial wheals (no scale), pustules, vesicles or bullae, purpura—and decide on the predominant pattern of reaction.
- Examine mucosae (mouth, conjunctiva, and genitalia).
- Assess the likelihood of this being a serious reaction—see Box 18.4.
- Consider how the adverse reaction is likely to evolve. Your next steps will be determined by the severity of the reaction—see Box 18.5.
- Document how likely you think it is an adverse drug reaction (certain, likely, possible, or unlikely) and which drug(s) is/are implicated.
- Contact pharmacy if you are not sure about the likelihood of a particular drug causing an adverse reaction.
- Report any possible reaction to the regulatory agency—in the UK return a completed yellow card to the Medicines and Healthcare Products Regulatory Agency (MHRA).
- Ensure that the medical records state that the drug should be avoided in future (it may be possible to continue essential treatment despite a morbilliform reaction) and notify the GP.
- Explain the likely cause to the patient.
- Arrange further investigations once the reaction has resolved—see Box 18.6.

Further reading

Roujeau JC and Stern RS. *N Engl J Med* 1994 **331:**1272–85.

Box 18.4 ⚠ Indications of serious drug reactions (see 📖 p.108)

- General:
  - Fever >40°C, hypotension, lymphadenopathy.
  - Arthralgia, arthritis.
  - Dyspnoea, wheeze.
- Mucocutaneous:
  - Generalized scaly erythema (erythroderma).
  - Swollen face, swelling of tongue, urticaria (anaphylaxis).
  - Skin pain or burning, erosions, shearing stress detaches epidermis from dermis, bullae, mucosal erosions (SJS, TEN)—see 📖 p.110 and Fig. 5.5, p.109.
  - Purpura (vasculitis or anticoagulant-induced).
- Laboratory results:
  - Eosinophilia >1000mm^3, lymphocytosis with abnormal lymphocytes, abnormal LFTs.

Box 18.5 Principles of management

- Withdraw non-essential medications or reduce dose (may be helpful if reaction is pharmacological). Drug withdrawal is not diagnostic immediately. Urticarial reactions settle in a few days, morbilliform rashes in 7–10 days, but other reactions may persist for >8 weeks.
- Start specific management of life-threatening adverse reactions, e.g. anaphylaxis, erythroderma, TEN, vasculitis—see 📖 p.102, p.108, p.112.
- Exclude systemic involvement: FBC (may have eosinophilia or lymphocytosis), renal function, liver function, complement levels.
- Exclude infection with serological tests if indicated e.g. Cytomegalovirus, EBV, Parvovirus B19 in patients with morbilliform rash; hepatitis B and C in urticaria; herpes simplex or mycoplasma in EM.
- Consider a skin biopsy (not helpful in simple morbilliform reactions). The histological findings may not be conclusive.
- Emollients (× 3/day) and soap substitutes will relieve dryness—see 📖 p.584.
- Moderately potent or potent topical corticosteroid ointments × 2/day and sedating antihistamines reduce itch in widespread morbilliform, eczematous, or lichenoid reactions (not helpful in urticaria).
- Non-sedating antihistamines in urticaria (mediated by histamine).

Box 18.6 Further investigation of cutaneous adverse drug reactions

- Once the reaction has resolved, patch testing with standardized dilutions of the suspected drug is helpful in allergic contact dermatitis, and may sometimes be helpful in fixed drug eruptions, AGEP (see 📖 p.116) and hypersensitivity syndrome (DRESS see 📖 p.114).
- Unfortunately skin testing (patch, prick, or intradermal) is rarely helpful in other forms of drug reaction.
- Oral re-challenge is usually inadvisable (except in fixed drug eruption).

Further reading

Barbaud A et al. *Contact Dermatitis* 2001; **45**:321–8.

Generally smooth erythematous drug reactions

Morbilliform (exanthematous)

- The commonest pattern of cutaneous drug reaction.
- Presents within 1–3 weeks of drug exposure.
- A symmetrical morbilliform rash (erythematous macules and papules of 2–10mm in diameter with tendency to confluence) starts on trunk. The rash spreads to arms and legs and may become confluent.
- The rash may be itchy (not painful).
- The patient may have a slight (not high) temperature.
- Mucosae are normal.
- Settles with desquamation within 7–10 days of withdrawing the drug. Thick sheets of scale may detach from palms or soles—do not confuse with the full-thickness loss of epidermis seen in TEN—see 🕮 p.110.
- Erythroderma is a rare complication.
- If the causative drug is essential, it may be possible to treat through a morbilliform reaction, but the patient may become erythrodermic.
- ⚠ Morbilliform reactions may resemble urticaria, but lesions are fixed, or (most often in children) a viral exanthem (take a thorough history).
- Morbilliform reactions may also precede a serious drug reaction such as TEN, hypersensitivity syndrome (DRESS), or serum sickness. Monitor for signs that suggest a serious reaction, e.g. facial swelling, mucosal involvement—see 🕮 Box 18.4, p.347 and p.110.
- Common causes: ampicillin (particularly if the patient has glandular fever), sulphonamides, allopurinol, captopril, barbiturates, thiazides.

Urticaria and/or angio-oedema; anaphylactoid reactions

- Common.
- Ig-E mediated reactions may present within minutes of exposure if previously sensitized. ACE inhibitors are the most common cause of admission with angio-oedema.
- Urticaria: itchy erythematous wheals (no scale) that move around. Wheals fade within 24h to leave normal skin.
- Subcutaneous oedema (angio-oedema) affecting lips, peri-orbital skin, tongue (when patient may have difficulty swallowing or breathing), external genitalia—an emergency—see 🕮 p.98.
- Common causes—penicillins, captopril, cephalosporins, thiazides, phenytoin, NSAIDs, ACE inhibitors (cause angio-oedema without urticaria and may not present until >4 weeks after drug is started), aspirin, radiocontrast agents, opiates, quinine.
- Anaphylactoid reactions (not IgE mediated) may present several weeks after the medication is started. Histamine is released directly from mast cells and basophils. Present as **red man syndrome** with flushing, erythema, and itching of face and upper trunk. Sometimes angio-oedema, hypotension, dyspnoea, and chest pain. Caused by drugs such as vancomycin, ciprofloxacin, amphotericin B, rifampicin, and teicoplanin.

⚠ Drug rash, eosinophilia, systemic symptoms (DRESS) (see 🕮 p.114)

- DRESS is a life-threatening cutaneous drug reaction with systemic symptoms (high fever) that is frequently misdiagnosed as infection.
- The morbilliform rash is associated with facial oedema, simulating angio-oedema.
- Some patients progress to liver failure.
- Causes include allopurinol, anticonvulsants, minocycline, dapsone, sulphonamides, and other antibiotics.

Acute generalized exanthematous pustulosis (see 🕮 p.116)

- Patients suddenly develop an uncomfortable oedematous erythema that burns or itches and then becomes studded with tiny pustules.
- Caused by a wide range of drugs including antibiotics such as penicillins, erythromycin, and tetracyclines.

Serum sickness

- Presents within 1–3 weeks of starting the medication.
- Erythema on sides of fingers, toes, and hands progresses to a widespread morbilliform rash. Some patients also have urticaria.
- Malaise, fever, arthralgia, and arthritis are common.
- Causes include serum preparations and vaccines.

Interstitial granulomatous dermatitis

- Described in association with a range of drugs including calcium channel blockers, betablockers, lipid-lowering agents, ACE inhibitors, antihistamines, anticonvulsants, antidepressants, and TNFα inhibitors. Also seen in association with connective tissue diseases including rheumatoid arthritis, and lymphoproliferative disorders—see 🕮 p.366.
- Presents months to years after initiation of treatment.
- Annular purplish-red (violaceous) plaques on the arms, medial thighs, and flexures. May be mildly itchy.
- Histologically diffuse interstitial granulomatous infiltrate in the mid and deep dermis with lymphocytes, histiocytes, mucin deposition, and variable collagen necrosis.

Erythema nodosum

- Causes: oral contraceptive pill, sulphonamides, gold (but more often triggered by infection (TB) or underlying systemic disease such as sarcoidosis or IBD—see 🕮 p.424).
- Tender erythematous subcutaneous nodules on shins and sometimes forearms.
- Resolves in weeks without loss of fat or scarring.
- NSAIDs relieve discomfort. Gentle compression with stockings that control swelling may speed resolution.

Also consider allergic contact dermatitis and SDRIFE—see 🕮 p.350.

More scaly erythematous drug reactions and pruritus

Allergic contact dermatitis (eczema)

- A localized allergic contact dermatitis is caused by topical preparations to which the patient has been sensitized by previous contact—see 📖 p.200. The reaction appears within 48h of exposure.
- Skin is itchy, oedematous, erythematous, and scaly (may not be scaly if acute). It may blister if the reaction is severe—see 📖 Fig.10.1, p.201.
- Eczema may generalize if contact persists or if the patient takes a cross-reacting oral preparation.
- Consider allergic contact dermatitis in chronic leg ulcers, hand dermatitis, facial dermatitis, otitis externa, or pruritus ani. Causes include topical neomycin, benzocaine, incipients in topical medicaments, topical hydrocortisone.
- Allergy to the constituents of subcutaneous heparin presents with well-demarcated infiltrated eczematous plaques at injection sites.
- Treat eczema with emollients and topical corticosteroid ointments.
- Investigate possible allergic contact dermatitis by patch testing.

SDRIFE: symmetrical drug-related intertriginous and flexural erythema

- A distinctive eczematous flexural reaction that has been described in association with a number of systemic drugs.
- SDRIFE occurs without prior exposure to the drug.
- Itchy bright red (erythematous) papules on buttocks (like a baboon's bottom), groins, and thighs that become confluent. May become bullous. Scale is minimal although pathology is eczematous.
- Similar to 'baboon syndrome' when initial sensitization was by skin contact and subsequently the patient took the agent by mouth.

Drug-induced photosensitivity (see 📖 p.304)

- Drugs are the commonest cause of photosensitivity, more often phototoxicity than photoallergy.
- Look for an eczematous rash on exposed sites sometimes with pigmentation—see 📖 Box 4.6, p.71.
- Drugs may also cause photosensitivity by triggering PCT, pseudoporphyria (see 📖 p.310, p.312), or subacute cutaneous LE (see 📖 p.372).

Lichenoid (lichen planus-like) reaction

- Very itchy flat-topped purplish-red papules that may coalesce into erythematous plaques and become generalized. Often also an eczematous scaly component—see 📖 Fig. 18.2, p.345.
- Examine buccal mucosa for reticulated white areas and erosions—found more often in LP than lichenoid drug reactions—see 📖 p.208.
- Resolution is slow (months) after the drug is stopped.
- The papules fade to leave macular hyperpigmentation that persists for months, particularly in dark skin. Pigmentation tends to be more marked in lichenoid drug reactions than in LP.

- Very potent topical corticosteroid ointments may be required to relieve itch.
- Common causes: gold, antimalarials, penicillamine, beta-blockers, thiazides, non-steroidal anti-inflammatories. Also reported with TNFα antagonists.

⚠ Erythroderma (exfoliative dermatitis)

- Generalized scaly erythema—an emergency—see 📖 p.102.
- Common causes: sulphonamides, gold, carbamazepine, antimalarials, and phenytoin.

Pruritus—see Box 18.7

Box 18.7 Pruritus (itching)

- Itching without any primary rash may be caused by a number of drugs including statins (also dryness of the skin), ACE inhibitors, opiates, barbiturates, antidepressants, and oral retinoids (also dryness of the skin).
- Hydroxyethyl starch (used in many colloid expanders) causes discrete attacks of severe intractable pruritus lasting for minutes up to an hour. Patients may have several episodes a day. Itch may persist for years.
- Signs are those of scratching sometimes superimposed on dry skin.
- Exclude other causes itching including urticaria (the rash is transient) (see 📖 p.212), scabies (see 📖 p.164), and renal, hepatic, thyroid, haematological, or neurological disease including iron deficiency.
- 1% menthol in aqueous cream is a soothing antipruritic. Sedating antihistamines may be helpful (ineffective in hydroxyethyl starch itch).

Also see eczematous reactions 📖 p.362.

Purpuric or pigmented drug reactions

Vasculitis (palpable purpura)

- Usually presents 1–3 weeks after starting the drug, but the interval may be longer.
- Palpable purpura (indicative of small-vessel cutaneous vasculitis) develops initially on legs, but may become widespread. Purpuric papules may evolve into haemorrhagic blisters or purpuric plaques—see 📖 p.404.
- Other signs may include urticaria, ulcers, and nodules.
- Vasculitis may affect kidney, liver, gastrointestinal tract, and/or nervous system.
- Consider other causes of a small-vessel cutaneous vasculitis including infection—see 📖 p.404.
- Common causes: penicillins and other antibiotics, allopurinol, phenytoin, thiazides, and thiouracils.

Macular purpura: may be pigmented

- Aspirin, anticoagulants, calcium channel blockers, ACE inhibitors, analgesics.

Anticoagulant-induced purpura fulminans and skin necrosis

- Rare but life-threatening complication of treatment with warfarin.
- Risk is greatest in obese female patients and in those with hereditary deficiency of protein C, protein S, or antithrombin III.
- Occurs 3–5 days after starting warfarin.
- Painful erythematous indurated plaques develop on fatty areas—breasts, hips, and buttocks. The large irregularly outlined plaques become haemorrhagic, bullous, and eventually necrotic.
- Warfarin causes intravascular thrombosis by reducing protein C levels and other vitamin K dependent coagulation factors.
- ►►Treat by withdrawing warfarin, administering vitamin K, and anticoagulating with heparin.
- Heparin may cause localized necrosis at injection sites, but widespread reactions are much less common. Mechanisms are different from those of warfarin-induced skin necrosis. Deficiencies of protein C or S do not appear to play a part in pathogenesis. Treat with warfarin and antiplatelet drugs to prevent platelet aggregation.

Cutaneous hyperpigmentation

- Mechanisms of hyperpigmentation include increased melanin synthesis and deposition of drug or drug metabolites in the skin.
- Photosensitivity may contribute to the colour change.
- Ask if the colour change was preceded by erythema or itching to differentiate drug induced pigmentation from postinflammatory hyperpigmentation, e.g. after dermatitis, lichenoid rashes or fixed drug eruptions (see 📖 p.354), particularly in individuals with dark skin.
- What is the colour and distribution of the change, e.g. is it predominantly in scars or on light-exposed skin?

- Increased melanin (brown pigmentation) may be caused by drugs such as cytotoxics, hydroxycarbamide (hydroxyurea), pegylated interferon (in chronic hepatitis C infection), ACTH, oral contraceptives (melasma on the face) and some antiretroviral agents (zidovudine and lamivudine).
- Flagellate brown hyperpigmentation is caused by bleomycin—see 📖 p.359.
- Bluish-grey pigmentation is caused by minocycline (often in scars or on the shins (Fig. 18.3)—may be worse on light-exposed skin), phenothiazines, antimalarials, gold, and amiodarone (facial pigmentation with photosensitivity). Vandetanib (inhibitor of epidermal growth factor receptor) is a recently reported cause of photosensitivity and hyperpigmentation.
- Orange pigmentation is caused by the antimalarial mepacrine.
- Pink discoloration is caused by clofazimine.
- Facial hyperpigmentation caused by skin lightening creams containing hydroquinone (acquired onchronosis).
- Resolution of pigmentation may be very slow (months or years) or pigment may persist despite drug withdrawal. Photoprotection is often an important part of management.

Oral mucosal pigmentation

- Changes are often seen along the gingival margins, but may develop on lip, tongue, or palate.
- May be caused by drugs such as oral contraceptives (general darkening) minocycline (grey-blue), antimalarial drugs (grey-blue), and phenothiazines (grey-blue).
- Pigmented macules or patches may develop on the tongue in heroin addicts who inhale smoke.
- A black hairy tongue may be caused by drugs such as oral antibiotics (cephalosporins, chloramphenicol, clarithromycin, penicillins, sulphonamides), as well as corticosteroids and antidepressants.

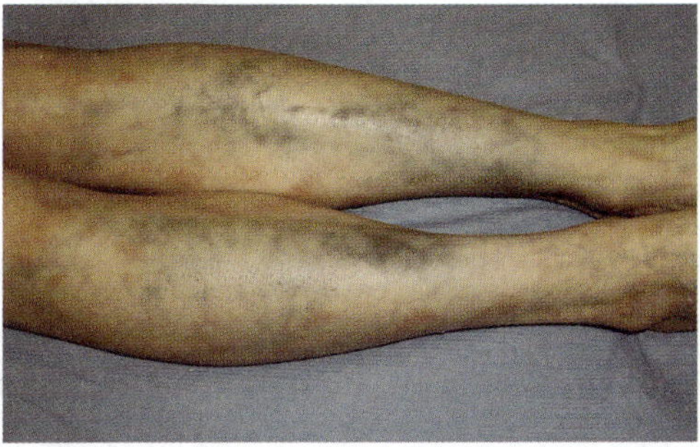

Fig. 18.3 Greyish pigmentation after prolonged treatment with minocycline.

Drug-induced blisters or mucocutaneous ulcers

Blisters may be widespread or localized. Oral manifestations may be erythematous, vesicular, erosive, or ulcerative and can involve the tongue as well as buccal mucosa or gums. Blistering eruptions such as TEN or SJS may cause severe oral ulceration—see 📖 p.110.

⚠ Any persistent oral ulcer should be biopsied to exclude malignancy.

Fixed drug eruption

- 1 or more well-defined circular erythematous plaques that usually blister and then resolve over 7–10 days leaving a hyperpigmented macule. Itching is uncommon (📖 Fig. 18.1, p.345).
- May also affect oral mucosa and in severe cases mucosal lesions may ulcerate.
- Each time the patient is exposed to the drug, the problem recurs within 24h in exactly the same place or places. Recurrent herpes simplex infection is the main differential diagnosis but this does not usually leave macular pigmentation.
- Take a skin biopsy during the reaction to confirm the diagnosis.
- Causes: tetracycline, sulphonamides, allopurinol, aspirin (ask the patient what analgesic is taken for menstrual pain or headaches), phenolphthalein. Also consider herbal medicines and other over-the-counter preparations that are ingested sporadically.
- Oral challenge may help to confirm the diagnosis.

Aphthous ulcers (see 📖 p.262)

- Aphthous ulcers are caused by drugs such as azathioprine, captopril, ciclosporin, fluoxetine, sertraline, and sulphonamides.
- NSAIDs and nicorandil cause oral ulcers that may simulate giant aphthae, but the ulcers do not have the erythematous halo or yellow base of an aphthous ulcer.

Erythema multiforme (EM) (see 📖 p.105)

- EM is an acute, self-limited illness. Infection (most often herpes simplex) is a much more likely trigger than a drug—see 📖 p.144.

⚠ Stevens–Johnson syndrome (SJS) and toxic epidermal necrolysis (TEN) (see 📖 p.110)

Life-threatening cutaneous reactions, with overlapping features, caused by drugs such as sulphonamides, aminopenicillins, antiepileptics, barbiturates, NSAIDs, and allopurinol. Patients may have underlying diseases, particularly AIDS. Course is protracted, lasting at least 3 weeks.

- A tender EM-like rash with severe mucosal involvement (oral, ocular, genital), blistering and erosions that presents 2–3 weeks after the drug is started.
- Epidermal involvement is more severe and widespread in TEN (>30% BSA) than in SJS (<10% BSA).

Coma-induced blisters

- Seen in association with decreased level of consciousness caused by overdose of agents such as barbiturates, benzodiazepines, heroin, methadone, imipramine, and alcohol. (Also reported in some neurological and metabolic causes of reduced levels of consciousness.)
- Blisters, preceded by erythematous plaques, are usually few in number.
- Blisters appear within 24h and resolve in 10–14 days.
- Blisters are predominantly over bony prominences (pressure may cause hypoxic damage) but some may also be found elsewhere.
- Histologically: subepidermal bullae with sweat gland necrosis.

Chemotherapy agents

- Mucosal ulcers are common.

Contact stomatitis

- The patient may notice an oral burning sensation and xerostomia.
- Reactions develop after days or years of exposure.
- Patch testing will confirm the diagnosis.
- Caused by agents such as topical anaesthetics and antiseptic mouthwashes.

Cutaneous ulcers

- Nicorandil causes large deep painful persistent ulcers on perianal skin and other sites. Ulcers may resemble pyoderma gangrenosum.

Other drug-induced blistering reactions

- Pseudoporphyria (see 🕮 p.312).
- Pemphigus foliaceus (see 🕮 Box 13.6, p.249).
- Paraneoplastic pemphigus caused by fludarabine (see 🕮 Box 13.6, p.249).
- Pompholyx caused by IV immunoglobulin. May evolve into a generalized eczematous rash.

Drug-induced abnormalities of hair and nails

Diffuse non-scarring alopecia

- Exclude other causes including iron deficiency, thyroid disease, and telogen effluvium after a severe illness.
- Diffuse alopecia may be caused by drugs such as cytotoxics, anticoagulants (heparin and warfarin), antithyroid drugs, and oral contraceptives.
- Temporary interruption of cell division may cause focal narrowing of hair shafts—Pohl–Pincus marks—and, if severe, hair shafts may fracture (correlates with Beau's lines in nails—see later in this section).

Increased hair growth

- Hirsutes = increased hair growth in females in an androgen-dependent pattern (normal male sexual pattern)—face, lips, chest, arms, thighs. Caused by oral contraceptive pill and other androgenic drugs.
- Hypertrichosis = increased hair growth at all body sites. Caused by drugs including ciclosporin, corticosteroids, acetazolamide, phenytoin, interferon, minoxidil, and cetuximab.

Nail abnormalities

Common causes include tetracyclines, antimalarials, retinoids, antiretroviral agents, and chemotherapy agents. Drug-induced nail changes usually involve many or all of the nails and resolve when the drug is withdrawn. Drugs may cause nail abnormalities by affecting the nail matrix, the nail bed, the periungual tissues, or blood vessels. Several mechanisms may be involved.

- Nail matrix damage:
  - Beau's lines = transverse grooves in nail plate caused by a temporary interruption of cell division in nail matrix (common). If severe, nails may be shed (onychomadesis). (Correlates with Pohl–Pincus marks in hair shafts—see earlier in this section.)
  - Nail fragility.
  - Altered rate of nail growth.
  - Leuconychia.
  - Pigmentation: diffuse or in bands (longitudinal or transverse).
- Nail bed damage:
  - Separation of nail plate from nail bed = onycholysis (common)—Fig. 18.4.
  - Photo-onycholysis (painful, may be pigmented).
  - Splinter haemorrhages.
  - Subungual hyperkeratosis or thickening of nail bed.
- Proximal nail fold damage:
  - Periungual pyogenic granulomas (common).
  - Acute paronychia sometimes with subungual abscess (unusual)—Fig. 18.5.
- Nail blood flow alterations:
  - Ischaemic changes.
  - Subungual haemorrhages (purpura).
  - Nail atrophy.

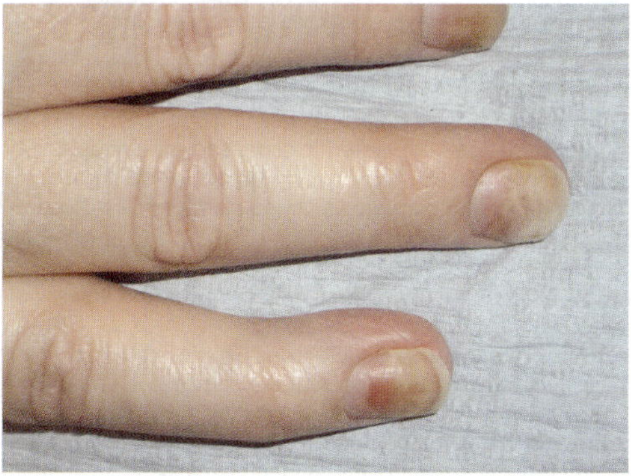

Fig. 18.4 Painful onycholysis caused by chemotherapy.

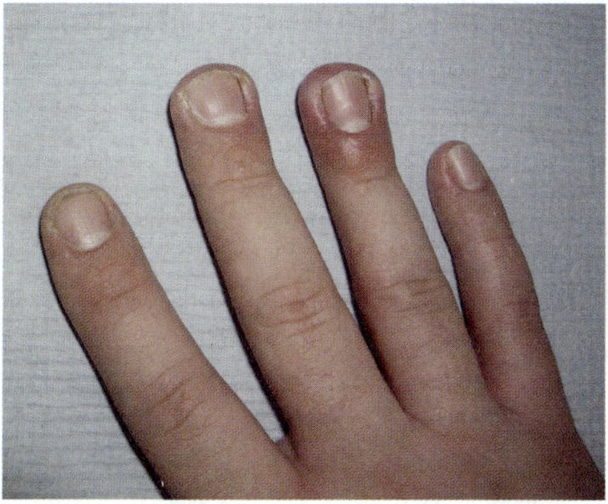

Fig. 18.5 Painful paronychia caused by tretinoin.

Reactions to chemotherapy agents: 1

Chemotherapy-induced hand–foot skin reaction

- Also known as acral erythema or palmar-plantar erythrodysaesthesia.
- Occurs in association with systemic drugs such as cyclophosphamide, cytarabine, capecitabine, doxorubicin hydrochloride, fluorouracil, imatinib, sunitinib, and sorafenib. Eccrine glands are involved in the pathology.
- Before the appearance of signs, patients complain of paraesthesiae, tingling, burning, or pain predominantly of palms and soles. Tolerance to contact with hot objects is reduced.
- Symmetrical erythematous oedematous papules develop on the palms and soles. Skin may fissure, blister, and ulcerate.
- The lateral sides of fingers and periungual skin may be erythematous.
- Sometimes erythema may extend to the dorsum of hands and feet.
- A diffuse keratoderma is a late sign (seen early with sorafenib and tends to be localized to pressure areas or areas of friction over soles and flexures of digits).
- Severity is dose-related. Tenderness and pain may be very distressing, leading to withdrawal of treatment.
- Emollients and topical corticosteroids may be helpful.

Neutrophilic eccrine hidradenitis

- Mainly described in patients receiving chemotherapy for a malignancy, most often haematological such as acute myelogenous leukaemia.
- Delay of about 10 days between start of chemotherapy and onset of rash.
- Rash may be asymptomatic or painful.
- Presents with 1 or more erythematous oedematous papules, nodules, or plaques. Sometimes pustular or purpuric centres to plaques.
- Lesions are either grouped or disseminated widely in an asymmetrical distribution.
- Distribution is mainly proximal, affecting upper trunk, upper limbs, and face, particularly periorbital skin, or distal, involving the extremities.
- Usually spares groins and axillae.
- Mucosae are not affected.
- May show pathergy, i.e. lesions at sites of intravenous injections.
- Fever is common but may be linked to underlying neutropenia rather than the rash.
- Skin biopsy shows neutrophilic infiltrate around degenerative eccrine glands.
- Lesions resolve without scarring in a few days or weeks. Some but not all patients relapse when re-exposed to same drug regimen.
- Topical treatments are ineffective. The role of oral corticosteroids is unproven. NSAIDs may relieve pain and fever.
- Differential diagnosis includes cutaneous infection (culture tissue), leukaemia cutis, EM (symmetrical, target lesions, mucosal ulcers), and Sweet's syndrome—see 📖 p.105, p.480.

Eccrine squamous metaplasia

- Oedematous erythematous plaques or macules that may become confluent. Sometimes vesicles. Typically affects face, axillae, groins, and legs. May also have erythema and oedema on the palms and legs.
- Itchy or painful.
- Possibly a non-specific reaction to damaged eccrine ductal epithelium.
- Triggered by many chemotherapy drugs. Also seen with excessive sweating and in some skin diseases, e.g. infection (herpesvirus, Cytomegalovirus), inflammatory skin diseases, and skin tumours.
- Sometimes considered to be in the spectrum of neutrophilic eccrine hidradenitis.

Flagellate dermatitis

- Mainly seen in association with bleomycin.
- Appears 1 day to several months after administration of the drug.
- Intensely itchy linear erythematous urticated plaques may affect arms, back, and scalp mimicking self-inflicted injury produced by a whip.
- Lesions fade leaving postinflammatory linear (flagellate) pigmentation.
- Treat with sedating antihistamines and potent topical corticosteroids.

Radiation recall dermatitis

- Well-defined cutaneous reaction at a previously irradiated site. Resembles an acute radiation reaction. Mild reactions are characterized by erythema, scale, and pruritus. In more severe reactions oedema and vesiculation may be followed by moist desquamation or haemorrhagic ulceration with necrosis.
- Triggered most often by IV chemotherapy, especially docetaxel, doxorubicin, gemcitabine, and paclitaxel. Cases have been described in association with other drugs including antitubercular drugs, tamoxifen, and simvastatin.
- Recall may be triggered weeks or years after radiotherapy. Reactions tend to be more severe when the recall-triggering drug is given shortly after the end of radiotherapy.
- The reaction settles when the drug is withdrawn. Topical corticosteroids help to control inflammation.
- Response to rechallenge with the drug is unpredictable.

Nail changes are common

See 📖 p.356 and Fig. 18.4, p.357.

Reactions to chemotherapy agents: 2

Epidermal growth factor (EGF) receptor inhibitors

Agents: gefitinib, cetuximab, erlotinib, panitumumab. EGF receptor is expressed by basal keratinocytes and sebocytes as well as the outer root sheath of hair follicles. Cutaneous adverse effects include:

- Initial oedema, redness, and a burning sensation on the face and upper trunk. May be mildly itchy.
- Sterile papulopustular follicular eruption on face and trunk 7–10 days after starting treatment (like acne but no comedones)—see Fig. 18.6. May spare skin previously treated by radiotherapy. The eruption gradually crusts and resolves. Severity is dose-related. The presence of the rash may correlate with more effective treatment and increased survival time.
- Treatment options include topical clindamycin, topical calcineurin inhibitors, oral tetracyclines, and low-dose isotretinoin (20mg daily).
- Painful paronychia, periungual abscess, pyogenic granuloma of nail fold.
- Brittle curly scalp hair, increased facial hair, long eyelashes.

Taxanes

Agents: docetaxel paclitaxel. Cutaneous adverse effects include:

- Hand–foot skin reaction (common)—see 📖 p.358.
- Radiation recall dermatitis see 📖 p.359.
- Alopecia.
- Nail abnormalities:
  - Subungual haemorrhage leading to onycholysis (see Fig. 18.4).
  - Orange-brown discoloration.
  - Beau's lines.
  - Transverse loss of nail plate.
  - Acute paronychia and subungual abscess (see Fig. 18.5).
- Generalized exanthematous pustulosis (AGEP).
- Subacute cutaneous LE, photosensitivity, scleroderma-like changes of legs, and erysipelas-like erythema.

Multikinase inhibitors

Agents: imatinib, dasatinib, nilotinib, sorafenib, and sunitinib. Inhibit a variety of tyrosine kinases such as platelet-derived growth factor receptor and vasoactive endothelial growth factor receptor. Cutaneous adverse effects include:

- Morbilliform rashes.
- Alopecia.
- Hand–foot skin reaction—see 📖 p.358.
- Photosensitivity, pseudoporphyria.
- Dry skin.
- Pigment loss.
- Generalized exanthematous pustulosis (AGEP).

Purine and pyrimidine analogues

Agents: fludarabine, cladribin, capecitabine, tegafur, gemcitabine. Cutaneous adverse effects include:

- Hand–foot skin reaction—see 📖 p.358.
- Acral hyperpigmentation most marked in skin creases.

- Autoimmune phenomena including paraneoplastic pemphigus (linked to fludarabine).
- Inflammation of actinic keratoses (caused by capecitabine which is a prodrug of 5-fluorouracil).

Hydroxycarbamide (hydroxyurea)

Cytostatic agent used in myeloproliferative disorders. Cutaneous adverse effects include:

- Diffuse hyperpigmentation and brown nails.
- Dermatomyositis-like eruption on dorsum of hands (ANA-negative)—see 🕮 Box 19.4, p.381.
- Acral erythema and palmoplantar keratoderma.
- An atrophic poikilodermatous (see 🕮 p.380) appearance on the legs.
- 1 or more persistent painful well-defined shallow leg ulcers, usually over the malleoli, but may affect calf, dorsal foot, or toes. Develop after an average of 5 years of treatment. Surrounding skin may be purpuric and atrophic. Heal when hydroxycarbamide is stopped.
- Oral mucosal ulcers.

Tretinoin

Acid form of vitamin A. Used in acute promyelocytic leukaemia. Cutaneous adverse effects include:

- Pruritus, erythema and dry skin; dry mucosae and cheilitis.
- Alopecia, periungual pyogenic granulomas, acute paronychia—see Fig. 18.5.

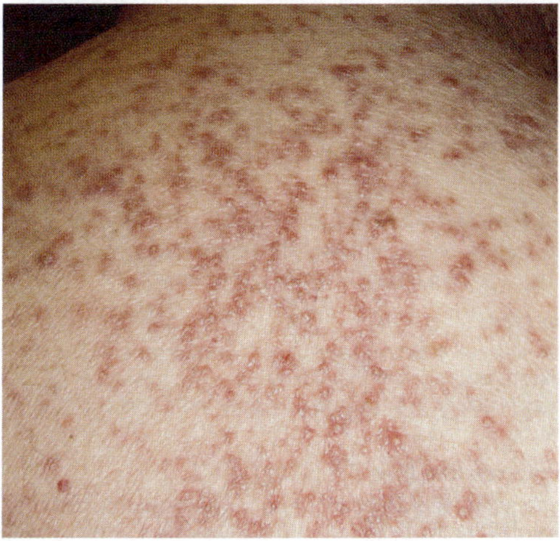

Fig. 18.6 Acne-like eruption caused by erlotinib (EGF receptor inhibitor).

Further reading

Gridelli C *et al. Crit Rev Oncol/Hematol* **66**(2008):155–62.

Heidary N *et al. J Am Acad Dermatol* 2008; **58:**545–70.

Drugs and skin diseases

Psoriasis (see 📖 p.182)

- Lithium: exacerbates existing psoriasis more frequently than inducing new disease.
- Antimalarials may induce or exacerbate psoriasis.
- Systemic corticosteroids: an exacerbation of psoriasis, which may be pustular, can be triggered by withdrawal of systemic corticosteroids prescribed for an unrelated condition.
- Beta-adrenergic receptor blocking agents may exacerbate psoriasis.
- NSAIDs and ACE inhibitors have been reported to exacerbate psoriasis.
- Alcohol: psoriatic patients with a high alcohol intake tend to have more severe disease.
- Anti-TNFα agents have been reported to induce plaque, guttate, and pustular psoriasis, although these drugs are used to treat psoriasis.

Palmoplantar pustulosis (see 📖 p.184)

- TNFα antagonists such as infliximab, etanercept, and adalimumab are used in the treatment of a number of inflammatory diseases including rheumatoid arthritis, IBD, and psoriasis. Cutaneous reactions include palmoplantar pustulosis as well as psoriasis-like eruptions.

Acne or acne-like pustular eruptions (see 📖 p.224)

- Causes include topical and oral corticosteroids—see 📖 p.588, androgens including anabolic steroids, phenytoin, phenobarbital, lithium, bromides, isoniazid, rifampicin, epidermal growth factor receptor inhibitors (see 📖 p.360).
- A papulopustular rash develops within weeks of starting the drug. Comedones are unlikely unless the reaction is caused by exogenous androgens. The rash may take months to resolve, despite treatment for acne.

Rosacea (see 📖 p.234)

- Exacerbated by peripheral vasodilators including glyceryl trinitrate, isosorbide, calcium channel blockers, and alcohol.

Eczema (see 📖 p.198)

- Calcium channel blockers have been linked to generalized chronic eczematous eruptions in the elderly.
- IVIG may precipitate pompholyx (vesicles on palms and soles) and eczema.

Lichen planus-like (see 📖 p.208)

- Widespread lichenoid reactions may appear weeks or months after exposure to the drug—see 📖 p.208 and p.350.
- Discrete papules, resembling LP or plane warts, have been caused by palifermin, a recombinant human keratinocyte growth factor.

Pityriasis rosea-like (see 📖 p.143)

A slightly itchy rash mainly on trunk and proximal upper limbs. Papules and plaques are aligned in a 'Christmas tree' pattern with long axes parallel to the ribs (parallel to Langer's skin lines). Drugs that have been implicated include:

- Gold compounds
- Barbiturates
- Captopril
- Isotretinoin
- Omeprazole
- Imatinib mesylate
- D-penicillamine
- Terbinafine
- Bismuth compounds
- Arsenicals.

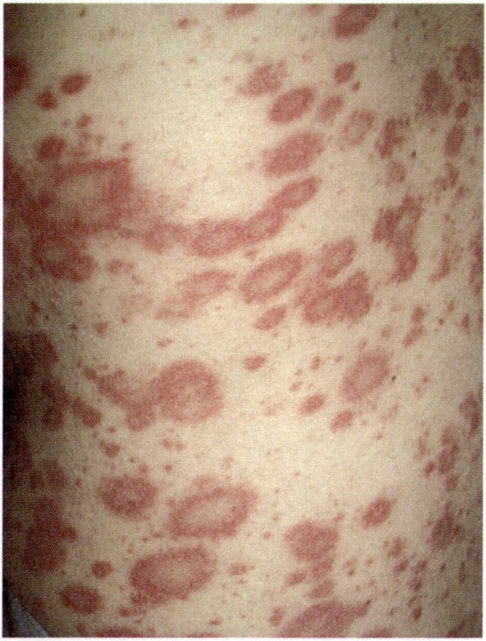

Fig. 18.7 Pityriasis rosea-like drug reaction with annular erythematous lesions.

Subacute cutaneous lupus erythematosus (SCLE) (see 📖 p.372)

SCLE appears weeks to several years after starting the drug and resolves 1–24 weeks after stopping the drug. Anti-Ro antibodies may persist when drug is withdrawn. Consider in older patients presenting with SCLE for the first time. Many drugs have been implicated including:

- Diuretics: hydrochlorothiazide and spironolactone.
- Calcium channel blockers: diltiazem and nifedipine.

- Beta-blockers.
- Antifungals: terbinafine and griseofulvin.
- ACE inhibitors.

Dermatomyositis-like (see 🕮 p.380)

- Most often hydroxycarbamide (hydroxyurea)—see 🕮 p.349.
- Also reported with penicillamine, statins, IFNβ, and others.

Porphyria cutanea tarda (PCT) (see 🕮 p.310)

- In genetically susceptible individuals, some drugs exacerbate PCT including alcohol, oral oestrogens, oral contraception and HRT, oral iron, antimalarials, and griseofulvin.

Pyoderma gangrenosum-like (see 🕮 p.290)

- Nicorandil causes ulcers—see 🕮 p.355.

Chapter 19

Rheumatology

Contents

Relevant pages in other chapters Skin manifestations in spondyloarthropathies such as psoriatic arthritis 🕮 p.192, Reactive arthritis 🕮 p.194, and SAPHO syndrome 🕮 p.228. Vasculitis—see Chapter 20 🕮 p.403, Autoinflammatory diseases 🕮 p.218 and Neutrophilic dermatoses 🕮 p.480, Amyloidosis 🕮 p.460, Alpha-1-antitrypsin deficiency 🕮 p.428, Nephrogenic systemic fibrosis 🕮 p.462, Behçet's disease 🕮 p.264.

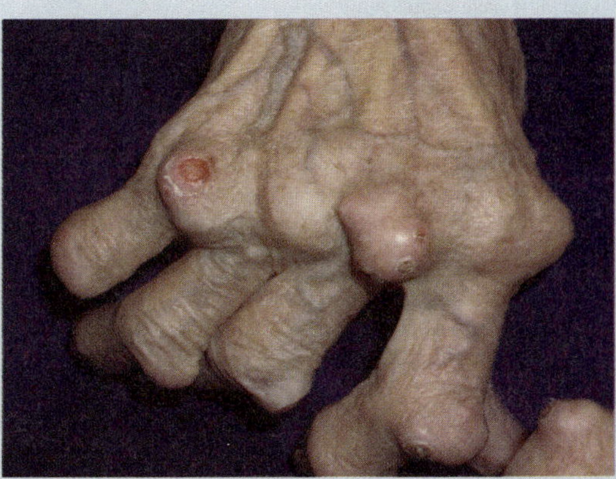

Fig. 19.1 Rheumatoid nodules.

Rheumatoid arthritis

Rheumatoid arthritis (RA) is an autoimmune chronic inflammatory disease of joints and tendon sheaths that may be complicated by a systemic vasculitis with extra-articular manifestations including pericarditis, pleurisy, fibrosing alveolitis, iritis, and neuropathy. Rheumatoid vasculitis is most common in seropositive patients with longstanding nodular disease.

Rheumatoid arthritis: what cutaneous signs should I look for?

- Pale, shiny atrophic skin that is fragile and bruises easily—most obvious on the hands of patients with long-standing disease.
- Palmar erythema.
- Bluish discoloration of finger tips and periungual erythema.
- Nails may be ridged longitudinally and may have red lunulae.
- Firm, skin-coloured, non-tender subcutaneous nodules 5–40mm diameter (20–30% of patients). Rheumatoid nodules are found most often on sites exposed to mild trauma or pressure, e.g. olecranon, knuckles (see Fig. 19.1), knees, and occiput (but may also be found in the lung). Nodules are linked to both seropositivity for rheumatoid factor and severe systemic manifestations. Nodules must be differentiated from tophi in chronic tophaceous gout—see Box 19.2.
- Rarely nodules ulcerate or become infected.
- Signs of small-vessel cutaneous vasculitis: palpable purpura, papulonecrotic lesions, or urticarial vasculitis (see 📖 p.406).
- Vasculitic lesions on the fingers, even in patients without systemic vasculitis, including papules, splinter haemorrhages, linear telangiectasia in the nail fold, petechiae and brownish purpuric lesions of the nail fold or finger pulp (Bywater's lesions) that may infarct and heal leaving small scars. Painless, red-black lesions of nail fold or finger pulp (microinfarcts of superficial dermal vessels) are also seen in SLE.
- Vasculitis involving medium-sized cutaneous vessels presents with livedo reticularis, nodules, and painful punched-out ulcers along the lateral malleoli or pre-tibial region. 20% of patients with severe vasculitis have digital gangrene.
- Leg ulcers (10% of patients with RA) often multifactorial—see Box 19.1.
- Interstitial granulomatous dermatitis: an uncommon condition of unknown cause that may be associated with severe RA as well as other systemic autoimmune diseases. Tender linear indurated bands arise symmetrically on the axilla, trunk, and inner portions of the thighs.
- Rheumatoid neutrophilic dermatitis, a condition of unknown cause associated with severe RA, characterized by papules, plaques, nodules, and urticarial wheals. Biopsy shows a dense dermal infiltrate of neutrophils. Neutrophilic dermatoses have also been described in SLE and dermatomyositis. May resemble Sweet's syndrome—see 📖 p.480.
- Blistering diseases including cicatricial pemphigoid, pemphigus, EBA, and subcorneal pustular dermatosis have been reported in association with RA (see 📖 p.244).

Box 19.1 Leg ulcers in rheumatoid arthritis

- 10% of patients with RA have leg ulcers.
- Pathogenesis is multifactorial and management should address underlying causes, ***but always handle the skin gently***.
- Trauma (beware the footrest of the wheelchair), skin fragility, and immobility with venous stasis are the most common causes of ulcers—see 📖 p.286 for advice on management.
- Systemic corticosteroids delay healing of ulcers and contribute to skin fragility as well as complications such as secondary infection.
- Small-vessel cutaneous vasculitis presents with palpable purpura and if severe may lead to necrotic ulcers with purpuric rims (see 📖 p.406).
- Deeper cutaneous vasculitis may be produced by vasculitis involving medium-sized vessels (see 📖 p.416). Look for livedo reticularis, nodules, and painful punched-out ulcers along the lateral malleoli or in the pre-tibial region.
- Painful, rapidly enlarging ulcers with undermined bluish-red borders may be caused by pyoderma gangrenosum (see 📖 p.290).
- Patients with Felty's syndrome (RA, leucopenia, and splenomegaly) may develop chronic leg ulcers that are refractory to treatment.

Box 19.2 Rheumatoid nodules or tophi?

- Tophi are nodules formed by deposits of urate crystals in cartilage, tendons, and soft tissues.
- Tophi tend to develop in patients with longstanding (>10 years) polyarticular gout and severe hyperuricaemia.
- Tophi are often found along the helix of the ear. Other common sites include the great toe, the fingers, wrist, hand, elbow (olecranon bursa, when tophi may resemble rheumatoid nodules), and Achilles tendon.
- Tophi, unlike rheumatoid nodules, may drain chalky material.
- In gout, uric acid is often raised and rheumatoid factor is usually negative.
- Chronic tophaceous gout causes severe joint destruction if not treated.

Further reading

Jorizzo JL and Daniels, JC *J Am Acad Dermatol* 1983; **8**:439–57.

Sayah A and English JC 3rd *et al.* *J Am Acad Dermatol* 2005; **53**:191–209.

Yamamoto T. *Rheumatol Int* 2009; **29**:979–88.

Lupus erythematosus

Systemic lupus erythematosus (SLE)

- SLE is a chronic multisystem inflammatory disease with autoantibodies.
- The diagnosis of SLE is confirmed once the patient has manifest 4 or more of the American College of Rheumatology diagnostic criteria, either sequentially or simultaneously—see Box 19.3.
- Cutaneous manifestations are the first sign of SLE in around 25% of patients and eventually >90% will develop cutaneous features. 70% of patients are photosensitive.
- Patients with SLE may have cutaneous LE (see next section) as well as non-specific cutaneous signs, such as small-vessel cutaneous vasculitis, that may suggest SLE in the right setting. These non-specific signs are not diagnostic of SLE and many may be seen in other connective tissue diseases—see 🕮 p.406.

Cutaneous lupus erythematosus (LE)

- Cutaneous LE is an inflammatory skin disease that is a specific manifestation of LE. Some but not all patients with cutaneous LE may have SLE. Cutaneous LE is not a vasculitis, but a lichenoid reaction in the skin (Box 19.4). Cutaneous LE is subdivided into:
  - Acute cutaneous LE (only seen in patients with active SLE) (see 🕮 p.372).
  - Subacute cutaneous LE (SCLE)—see 🕮 p.372 and Figs. 19.2, 19.3, and 19.5.
  - Chronic cutaneous LE (including discoid LE)—see 🕮 p.374 and Fig. 19.4.
- Patients may have >1 type of cutaneous LE and all can occur in association with SLE.
- It is confusing because the terms subacute cutaneous LE (SCLE) and discoid LE (DLE) are used in 2 ways, either to describe a type of skin lesion or to refer to subsets of patients who share certain clinical and immunological features, but do not meet the criteria for SLE.

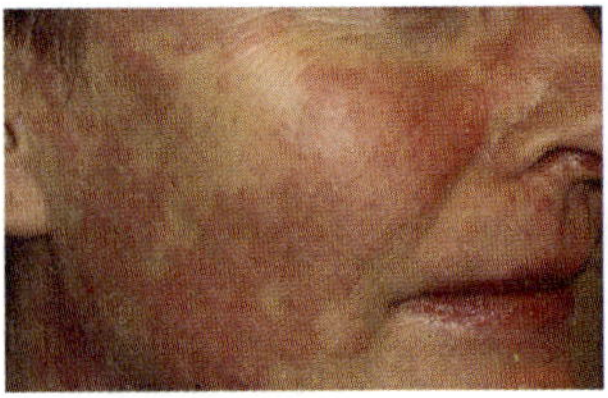

Fig. 19.2 Malar rash in SLE.

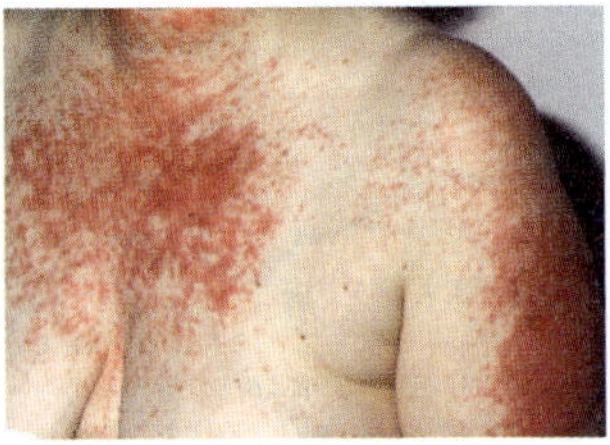

Fig. 19.3 SCLE: scaly papules in a photosensitive distribution.

Box 19.3 The American College of Rheumatology 1982 Revised Criteria for Classification of Systemic Lupus Erythematosus

1. Malar rash (erythematous rash across upper cheeks and bridge of nose—may be asymmetrical)—see Fig 19.2.
2. Discoid rash (scaly plaques that scar if not treated)—see Figs. 19.4 and 19.6, p.374.
3. Photosensitivity.
4. Oral or nasopharyngeal ulcers.
5. Arthritis (non-erosive, involving 2 or more joints).
6. Serositis (pleuritis: pleuritic pain or rub, or pleural effusion, or pericarditis, or pericardial effusion).
7. Renal disorder (persistent proteinuria >0.5g per day or cellular casts).
8. Neurological disorder (seizures or psychosis not caused by a drug or metabolic problem).
9. Haematological disorder (haemolytic anaemia or leucopenia $<4000/mm^3$ on 2 or more checks or lymphopenia $<1500/mm^3$ on 2 or more checks or thrombocytopenia $<100\,000/mm^3$).
10. Immunological disorder. Anti-double stranded (ds) DNA or anti-Smith (Sm) antibody or positive antiphospholipid antibody or false positive serologic test for syphilis (known to be +ve for at least 6 months and confirmed by fluorescent *Treponema pallidum* antibody absorption test). Anti-ds DNA and anti-Sm are virtually specific for SLE.
11. Positive antinuclear antibody (in absence of drugs known to be associated with drug-induced SLE).

For the purpose of identifying patients in clinical studies, a person shall be said to have systemic lupus erythematosus if any 4 or more of the 11 criteria are present, serially or simultaneously, during any interval of observation.

References: Tan EM *et al. Arthritis Rheum* 1982; **25:**1271–7.

Albrecht J. *et al. Lupus* 2004; **13**: 839–49.

Box 19.4 Cutaneous LE: histological findings

- Skin biopsies from cutaneous LE show a lichenoid lymphocytic infiltrate (interface dermatitis), i.e. lymphocytic inflammation at the dermo-epidermal junction with damage to the basal keratinocytes. This involves both the epidermis and hair follicles.
- Inflammation is most marked in chronic lesions.
- There is perivascular inflammation but no vasculitis.

Further reading

Lin JH *et al. Clinic Rev Allerg Immunol* 2007; **33:**85–106.

Sontheimer RD. *Best Pract Res Clin Rheumatol* 2004; **18:**429–62.

Sontheimer RD. *Autoimmun Rev* 2005; **4:**253–63.

Assessment of skin in systemic lupus erythematosus

What should I ask?

- Is the patient sensitive to sun—what happens and how long after exposure? See 🕮 p.28.
- Has the patient any skin problems or mouth ulcers (may be painless)?
- Is the rash leaving scars or pigment change?
- Does the patient notice pustules? (Seen in rosacea or acne but not in cutaneous LE.)
- Is the scalp scaly or the hair changing? (Seborrhoeic dermatitis and psoriasis cause scale and erythema in the scalp, but do not usually cause hair loss.)
- What drugs is the patient taking and what is the relationship of starting drugs to the onset of any rash?

What should I look for?

- Signs suggesting photosensitivity, i.e. the rash is photoaggravated. Does the rash spare skin normally protected from sunlight, such as under the chin, the eyelids (ask the patient to close his/her eyes), beneath hair, or behind ears? See 🕮 p.71 for more information about signs of photosensitivity.
- Signs of cutaneous LE (acute, subacute, or chronic)—see 🕮 p.372 and p.374 for more information.
  - Malar rash: erythematous plaques extending across upper cheeks and bridge of nose. Correlates with photosensitivity.
  - Scalp: perifollicular scale and erythema, hair loss, scarring (follicular orifices lost—may be easier to see with magnification, e.g. dermoscopy). Suggests DLE.
  - Ears (concha and helix): scars, follicular plugs (like 'blackheads'), pigment change. Suggests DLE—see Fig. 19.4.
  - Trunk, arms: erythematous scaly rash, annular scaly lesions, pigment change. Suggests SCLE—see Fig. 19.5, p.373.
  - Mucosal plaques: lips, hard palate, buccal mucosa.
  - Dorsum of hands and fingers: scaly erythematous plaques.
- Non-specific signs suggestive of SLE, including cutaneous vasculitis—see Box 19.5.
  - Look carefully at nail folds for periungual erythema or abnormal capillaries.
  - Check pulps of toes as well as finger pulps and palms for erythema, ulceration, and purpura.
  - Check limbs for livedo reticularis or palpable purpura.

Box 19.5 Non-specific cutaneous features that may be found in patients with SLE

- Urticaria (hives, wheals): itchy smooth, erythematous bumps lasting no more than 48h that fade to leave normal skin.
- Oral ulcers.
- Non-scarring alopecia secondary to:
  - Lupus hairs (hairs break off at the front of the scalp).
  - Telogen effluvium (shedding 8–12 weeks after severe illness).
  - Alopecia areata (autoimmune hair loss).
- Raynaud's phenomenon.
- Vascular involvement: vasculitis or non-inflammatory occlusive vasculopathy—see 📖 p.406 and 418:
  - Periungual erythema.
  - Linear telangiectasia on the posterior nail fold: a sign of a connective tissue disease also found in dermatomyositis, systemic sclerosis, and 5% of cases of RA.
  - Thrombosed nail fold vessels carried forward into a ragged cuticle.
  - Painless, red-black lesions of nail fold or finger pulp (microinfarcts of superficial dermal vessels)—also seen in RA.
  - Papular telangiectasia on the palms or finger tips.
  - Atrophie blanche (streaky telangiectasia interspersed with pale scarred looking skin) on plantar surface of toes or finger pulps.
  - Urticarial vasculitis: tender wheals lasting >48h and resolving to leave bruises; may indicate low complement—see 📖 p.409.
  - Palpable purpura (i.e. non-blanching) at sites of stasis (legs), cooling (ear helix), or pressure (sacrum).
  - Livedo reticularis (discontinuous) that persists if skin is warm or retiform purpura: suggests the antiphospholipid syndrome which is associated with recurrent thromboses and neurological complications—see 📖 p.418 and Box 20.8, 419.
- Neutrophilic Sweet's-like dermatosis: also described in dermatomyositis and RA—see 📖 p.480.

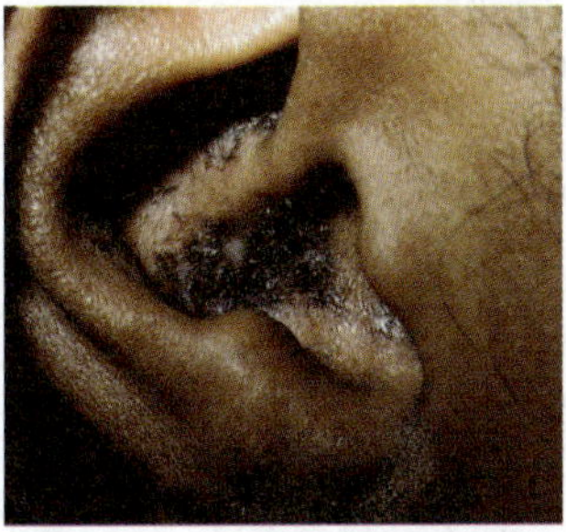

Fig. 19.4 DLE scaly plaques in the ear.

Acute and subacute cutaneous lupus erythematosus

Acute cutaneous LE

Seen in patients with active SLE.

What should I look for?

- Erythematous oedematous rash with minimal scale spreading symmetrically across upper cheeks, i.e. a malar rash suggesting photosensitivity.
- The rash is generally asymptomatic, unlike dermatomyositis which itches, burns, and is painful.
- No scarring and no pustules (pustules suggest rosacea or steroid-induced acne—see 📖 p.224, p.234, p.236).
- Rash disappears quickly once skin is protected from light.
- Erythema may be generalized in very ill patients.
- Rowell's syndrome may occur in acute cutaneous LE or SCLE—see Box 19.6.
- Blisters are uncommon—see 📖 Box 19.9, p.375.

Subacute cutaneous LE (SCLE)

- 50% of patients with SCLE fulfil the criteria for SLE, but only 10–15% will develop severe manifestations of SLE.
- SCLE may be drug-induced: hydrochlorothiazide, calcium channel blockers, NSAIDs, ACE inhibitors, griseofulvin, terbinafine, proton-pump inhibitors, interferons, and statins. The rash commences 4–20 weeks after starting the drug. Drug-induced SCLE does not always reverse, but most eruptions clear within 6–12 weeks after withdrawal of the triggering drug. Rarely SCLE is paraneoplastic.
- In pregnant women, SCLE can affect the neonate—see Box 19.7.

What should I look for?

- Superficial scaly annular lesions involving the V-area of the neck, upper trunk, upper limb, and dorsum of hands (sparing knuckles)—see Fig. 19.5. The rash may be slightly itchy but more often is asymptomatic unlike dermatomyositis—see 📖 p.378. Blisters are unusual—see Box 19.9.
- Scaly red papules resembling psoriasis are less common.
- Non-scarring, but postinflammatory hypopigmentation common.
- Although patients are photosensitive, the face is often spared.
- Differentiate the annular rash from fungal infection (ringworm, 'tinea') by checking the position of the scale. In SCLE, the scale appears after the erythema and on the inner aspect of the ring. In fungal infections, erythema follows the scale which is on the outer edge of the ring.
- Exclude psoriasis by checking for nail pitting, onycholysis, and well-demarcated plaques of psoriasis on knees (sun-protected) or scalp (no hair loss in psoriasis).
- Immunology: anti-Ro antibodies.

What should I do?

See 📖 p.376 for investigation and management.

Box 19.6 What is Rowell's syndrome?

Rowell's syndrome is probably a severe variant of acute or subacute cutaneous LE. The 3 major diagnostic criteria are:

- Diagnosis of LE.
- EM-like erythematous target lesions or erosions simulating TEN, with or without mucosal involvement. Histology shows an interface dermatitis with features of both cutaneous LE and EM.
- Speckled ANA (usually anti-Ro or anti-La antibodies).

Common triggers

- UV radiation.
- Drugs: furosemide, ACE inhibitors, doxycycline, aciclovir, naproxen, hydroxychloroquine, sodium valproate.

Further reading

Zeitouni NC *et al. Br J Dermatol* 2000; **142:**343–6.

⚠ Box 19.7 SCLE in pregnancy

Mothers with SCLE may have infants affected by neonatal LE because anti-Ro antibodies cross the placenta. Rarely these infants develop a connective tissue disease later in life. Affected infants may develop:

- Photosensitive cutaneous lupus (50% of infants) with scaly erythematous papules and plaques that are aggravated by sun exposure. Less often annular patterns. The appearance of the periorbital erythema has been termed 'racoon eyes'. Rash usually resolves over 4–6 months, but may leave atrophy with telangiectasia.
- Congenital heart block which is permanent (10% of infants). At 16–18 weeks' gestation, Ro-positive mothers should be referred for fetal echocardiogram and further monitoring. The risk of congenital heart block is greatest when a previous child has had neonatal lupus or congenital heart block (5–12% recurrence rate in subsequent pregnancies).
- Haemolytic anaemia, thrombocytopenia, leucopenia: all transient.
- Elevated LFTs : transient.

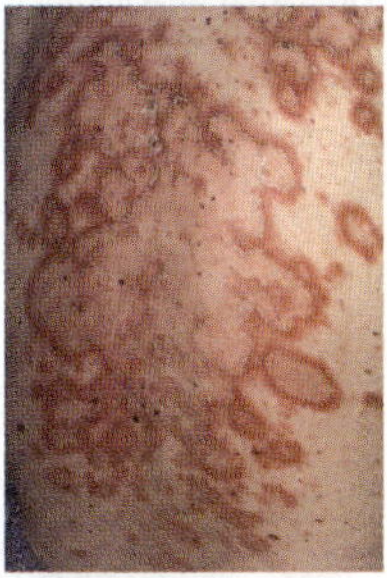

Fig. 19.5 SCLE: annular scaling plaques.

Chronic cutaneous LE

Discoid LE (DLE)

- The commonest form of chronic cutaneous LE (CCLE).
- Most patients with localized DLE (confined to the head and neck) do not develop significant systemic disease and DLE remits eventually in about 50% of patients.
- SLE develops in 5–10% of patients, usually those with widespread DLE. The course of SLE in these patients is benign.

What should I look for?

- Erythematous telangiectatic plaques or hyperkeratotic plaques with adherent keratotic scale most often localized to head and neck. These are usually asymptomatic—see 📖 Fig. 19.4, p.371 and Fig. 19.6.
- Chronic plaques cause scarring and deformity (lupus means wolf, and wolf bites are destructive).
- Plaques on the face tend to spare the nasolabial fold.
- Perifollicular inflammation in scalp causes permanent hair loss (scarring alopecia).
- Acneiform plugged lesions (like blackheads) in the concha of the ears—see 📖 Fig. 19.4, p.371.
- Very hypertrophic lesions may resemble squamous cell skin cancer.
- Plaques may involve the vermillion border of the lips or lower eyelids with loss of lashes and scarring.
- LP-like plaques may involve buccal mucosa or palate—see 📖 p.266.
- Abnormal pigmentation (increased or decreased) is a common outcome in dark skins—see 📖 Fig. 19.4, p.371.
- Blisters are rare—see Box 19.9.
- Immunology: usually antinuclear antibodies are not detected.

What should I do?

- See 📖 p.376 for investigation and management.

The Cutaneous Lupus Disease Area and Severity Index: the CLASI

This tool, which has been validated by both dermatologists and rheumatologists, scores the severity of cutaneous LE. The CLASI takes into account disease activity (erythema, scale, mucous membrane involvement, hair loss or non-scarring alopecia) as well as damage (dyspigmentation and scarring including scarring alopecia).

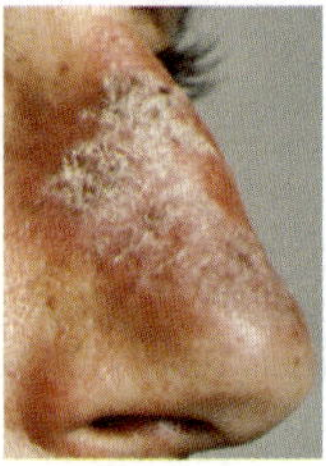

Fig. 19.6 DLE: hyperkeratotic plaque.

Further reading (these references discuss the CLASI)

Albrecht J and Werth V. *Dermatol Ther* 2007; **20:**93–101
Bonilla-Martinez ZL *et al. Arch Dermatol.* 2008; **144:**173–80.

Box 19.8 Less common forms of chronic cutaneous LE

Lupus panniculitis (lupus profundus)
- Subcutaneous nodules on shoulders, upper arm, face, and buttocks.
- Overlying skin may be affected by DLE.
- Fat loss is a disfiguring complication.
- Subcutaneous nodules may calcify and ulcerate.
- Skin biopsies may ulcerate and be slow to heal.
- SLE is unlikely.

Chilblain lupus
- Cold-induced purple plaques on fingers or toes.
- Warty plaques if long-standing.
- May be associated with SLE.

Lupus erythematosus tumidus
- Smooth erythematous 'juicy' nodules on sun-exposed skin without scarring (Jessner's lymphocytic infiltrate is probably the same disease).
- Photosensitive.
- May persist for weeks.
- Biopsy may not be diagnostic.
- SLE is unlikely.

Box 19.9 Vesiculobullous LE

LE-specific vesiculobullous skin disease

Blistering may be a secondary phenomenon in severe cutaneous LE. If the interface dermatitis causes extensive damage to the basal keratinocytes, the epidermis detaches from the dermis. If the epidermal damage is full thickness, the changes may even resemble TEN. Disease has been subdivided into:
- TEN-like acute cutaneous LE.
- TEN-like subacute cutaneous LE.
- TEN in SLE (patients without LE-specific skin lesions in whom no drug-related cause for TEN can be indentified).
- Vesiculobullous annular subacute cutaneous LE.
- Vesiculobullous DLE.

⚠ *LE-non-specific vesiculobullous skin disease*

Blisters may develop in the context of a distinct autoantibody-mediated bullous disease. Histology does not show an interface dermatitis, but the features of the autoimmune blistering disease:
- DH-like vesiculo-bullous LE.
- EBA-like vesiculo-bullous LE.
- BP-like vesiculo-bullous LE.

Further reading

Ting W *et al. Lupus* 2004; **13:**941–50.

Management of cutaneous LE

What should I do?

- Investigate to confirm the diagnosis and exclude systemic disease—see Box 19.11.
- Advise the patient to stop smoking: cutaneous LE is more severe and less responsive to treatment in smokers.
- Advise photoprotection (sun protection) to reduce the need for topical steroids or systemic treatment. Continue even when disease is controlled. See Box 19.12 and 🕮 p.316.
- Very potent topical corticosteroid (clobetasol propionate) ointment applied ×2/day controls most localized cutaneous disease (use topical corticosteroids even if the patient is also taking prednisolone for systemic disease). Apply before application of sunscreen cream. Reduce the strength gradually to less potent preparations such as mometasone furoate (potent—use ×1/day) as soon as inflammation is controlled and lesions have flattened. Gradually reduce frequency of application.
- Scalp: clobetasol propionate scalp application at night.
- Intralesional triamcinolone (10mg/mL) may be effective in resistant plaques of DLE.
- Tacrolimus ointment 0.1% is worth trying if facial DLE is not controlled by very potent topical corticosteroids
- Most patients respond to oral hydroxychloroquine 200mg ×2/day (<6.5mg/kg/day) after 8–12 weeks. Combine with topical corticosteroids and photoprotection.
- If the rash gets worse reconsider the diagnosis—has the patient also got psoriasis, which can be exacerbated by antimalarials? See Box 19.10.
- Check visual acuity if hydroxychloroquine is to be continued. Patients taking hydroxychloroquine should see an optician annually.

Box 19.10 Cutaneous LE is not responding to treatment

If cutaneous LE has not improved after 4 weeks of treatment:

- Ensure that the patient is using photoprotection.
- Ensure that the patient is applying a very potent topical corticosteroid (many patients have steroid phobia). Topical corticosteroids should be used even if the patient is also taking oral prednisolone for systemic disease.
- Is the rash LE? Pustules suggest steroid-induced acne or rosacea not LE; an asymmetrical facial scaling plaque may be caused by a fungal infection; might this be psoriasis triggered by antimalarials?
- Is the patient smoking?
- Is the patient allergic to the sunblock?

Box 19.11 Investigation of cutaneous LE

- SCLE: take a skin scrape from edge of an annular lesion for mycological culture.
- Take a skin biopsy for histology from an active erythematous lesion, not a scar (generally not necessary in acute cutaneous LE).
- Direct immunofluorescence of involved skin for a 'lupus band' is not usually required to diagnose cutaneous LE.
- Detection of a 'lupus band' in a biopsy from sun-protected skin of the forearm has been used to predict the likelihood of renal involvement in SLE, but this test is not in widespread use.
- Does the patient have SLE? Check:
  - Urine RBC, protein, and microscopy—spin down for urinary casts
  - FBC.
  - ESR: raised in both active SLE and in infection.
  - CRP: raised in infection but not in active SLE.
  - Renal function.
  - ANA, anti-double stranded (ds) DNA.
  - ENA (anti-Sm, anti-La, anti-Ro, anti-RNP).
  - Anti-cardiolipin antibody.
  - Complement. C3, C4: may be low in patients with active SLE due to the presence of immune complexes. If C4 is low and patient has cutaneous vasculitis, check for cryoglobulins.

Box 19.12 Photoprotection (see 📖 p.316)

- Discuss lifestyle and importance of limiting sun exposure, particularly between 11am and 2pm.
- Recommend wide-brimmed hats (hold up to sunlight to ensure that weave is sufficient to block transmission of light).
- Recommend dark clothing with long sleeves and a tight weave.
- Prescribe high-factor (>20), broad-spectrum sunscreen creams containing the physical blocker titanium dioxide to block the entire UV and visible light spectrum.
- Patients should apply sunscreen creams liberally in the morning to all exposed sites after application of topical corticosteroids to active cutaneous disease.
- Advise patients to reapply sunscreen creams 4-hourly during the hours of sunlight or after swimming.

Further reading

Callen JP. *Br J Dermatol* 2004; **151:**731–6.

Dermatomyositis

Dermatomyositis is a multi-system autoimmune disease in which inflammatory skin changes are associated with a polymyositis of skeletal muscle. Adults and children of all races are affected but females are affected more often than males.

The prognosis is variable and unpredictable. Interstitial lung disease or underlying malignancy (20–25% of adult-onset patients—see Box 19.13) may be fatal. The disease spectrum encompasses:

- Cutaneous disease without muscle involvement = amyotrophic dermatomyositis. Muscle involvement may not develop until 20 years after the onset of cutaneous dermatomyositis.
- Cutaneous and systemic disease (skin and muscle problems present concurrently in 60% of patients).
- Polymyositis without skin changes (muscle involvement precedes inflammatory cutaneous disease in 10% of patients).

What should I ask?

- Ask about cutaneous symptoms: in dermatomyositis the rash itches, burns, and is painful, unlike the rash of LE. Itch is worse in more severe disease.
- Is the face swollen, particularly around the eyes, and how long does swelling last? Dermatomyositis may simulate angio-oedema, but angio-oedema is transient—see 📖 p.98 and Figs. 19.7 and 19.8.
- Has the skin blistered (sometimes seen with intense oedema)?
- Is the skin sensitive to sun? UV light exacerbates the rash in up to 50% of patients, but many patients are not aware that the skin is sensitive to light.
- Is the scalp erythematous or scaly or the hair thinning? Dermatomyositis, like LE, may cause hair loss and a scarring alopecia.
- Seek evidence of a proximal myopathy: ask about getting out of chairs, going up and down stairs, brushing teeth, or reaching up.
- Check for evidence of interstitial lung disease: dyspnoea, dry cough, and wheeze.
- Probe for symptoms that suggest internal malignancy: weight loss, changes in bowel habit.
- Is the patient taking drugs such as hydroxycarbamide? Some drug-induced rashes may simulate dermatomyositis—see 📖 p.364.

⚠ Box 19.13 Dermatomyositis and internal malignancy

- 20–25% of adult-onset patients develop a malignancy within 2 years of diagnosis.
- History and examination should be directed towards identifying a malignancy.
- Risk is greatest in the 1st year and in women.
- Increased risk may persist for 5 years after diagnosis.
- Cutaneous signs linked to malignancy include:
  - Corticosteroid resistance.
  - Intense erythematous flush on shoulders neck, face, and scalp (malignant suffusion).
  - Ulceration.

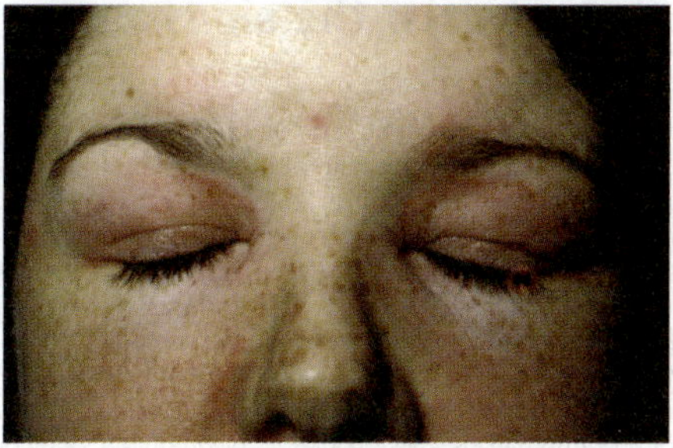

Fig. 19.7 Dermatomyositis with purplish (heliotrope) discoloration of eyelids. Reproduced from Harris A *et al. Br J Dermatol* 1995; **133**:783–5.

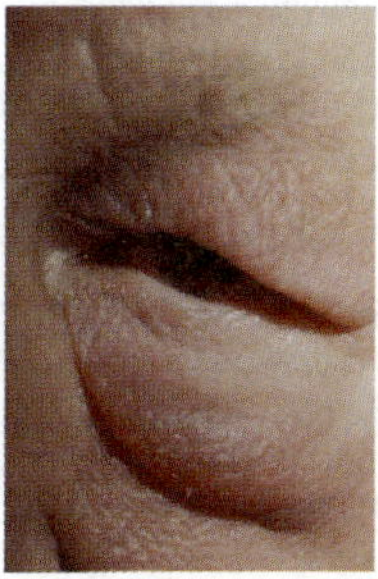

Fig. 19.8 Dermatomyositis: periorbital oedema simulating angio-oedema or an acute contact dermatitis.

Further reading

Santmyire-Rosenberger B and Dugan EM. *Curr Opin Rheumatol* 2003; **15:**714–22.

Sontheimer RD. *Curr Opin Rheumatol* 1999; **11:**475–82.

Dermatomyositis: the signs

What should I look for?

- Diagnostic signs in the hands, fingers, or nail folds—see Box 19.14.
- Assess the blood vessels in the nail fold using an ophthalmoscope or dermatoscope to provide magnification.
- A symmetrical violaceous or heliotrope (violet-red) erythema of eyelids and/or periorbital skin associated with fine scale and periorbital oedema or facial swelling—see Figs. 19.7 and 19.8.
- Perifollicular scale in scalp with erythema sometimes with diffuse hair loss.
- Erythema associated with fine scale affecting upper chest, posterior neck, upper back and shoulders (shawl sign), arms, and/or forearms.
- Symmetrical erythematous scaly papules or plaques over bony prominences of elbows, knees, and/or greater trochanter of hip (holster sign).
- Hypo- and hyperpigmentation, telangiectasia, and atrophy (as a result of chronic inflammation and known as poikiloderma).
- Necrosis and ulceration secondary to vascular damage.
- Calcinosis (more common in children than adults).
- Signs suggesting underlying internal malignancy in adult-onset disease (examine abdomen, lymph nodes, breast and pelvis in women, prostate in men).
- Signs of interstitial lung disease, e.g. fine inspiratory crackles.
- See Box 19.5 for differential diagnosis.

The Dermatomyositis Skin Severity Index: the DSSI

The DSSI is a measure of severity of skin disease in dermatomyositis. The DSSI was developed on the basis of the psoriasis scoring system, the PASI. The score takes into account the extent of disease (body surface area) and the amount of redness, induration and scaling. The total DSSI can range from 0 to 72. However, the score does not take into account muscle disease or the impact of dermatomyositis on quality of life.

Further reading

Carroll CL *et al. Br J Dermatol* 2008; **158:**345–50.

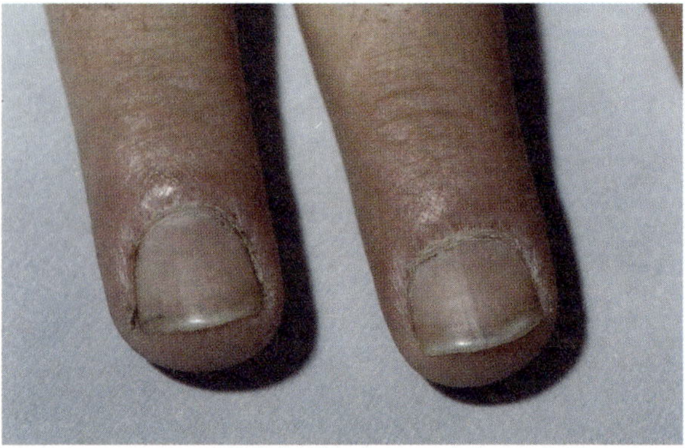

Fig. 19.9 Nail fold telangiectasia in dermatomyositis (also seen in systemic sclerosis and other connective tissue diseases).

Box 19.14 Diagnostic signs in the hands or fingers—see Figs. 19.9 and 19.10

- Periungual erythema.
- Tortuous nail-fold capillaries and capillary drop-out (avascular areas).
- Thickened irregular cuticles with capillary haemorrhage.
- Gottron's papules (flat-topped violaceous scaly papules over dorsal interphalangeal joints) are present in about 1/3 of patients and are pathognomonic of dermatomyositis.
- Gottron's papules evolve into hypopigmented atrophic areas with irregular telangiectasia.
- Linear streaks of erythema over the extensor tendons of fingers.
- 'Mechanic's hands': hyperkeratosis, scaling, and fissuring on the lateral aspects of thumb and fingers simulates contact dermatitis.

Box 19.15 Differential diagnosis

Cutaneous LE
- Intense pruritus is not a feature of cutaneous LE.
- Cutaneous LE tends to spare the skin over the joints on the hands.
- Cutaneous LE is hyperkeratotic not oedematous.

Angio-oedema or urticaria
- Oedema persists for 24–48h in angio-oedema but is long lasting in dermatomyositis.

Seborrhoeic dermatitis
- The greasy ill-defined erythematous papular rash involves the central face but is not oedematous and spares eyelids.
- The scalp may be erythematous and scaly but hair is not usually affected.
- Seborrhoeic dermatitis may also involve central chest, central back, and flexures.

Hand dermatitis: nailfold capillaries are not involved in dermatitis.

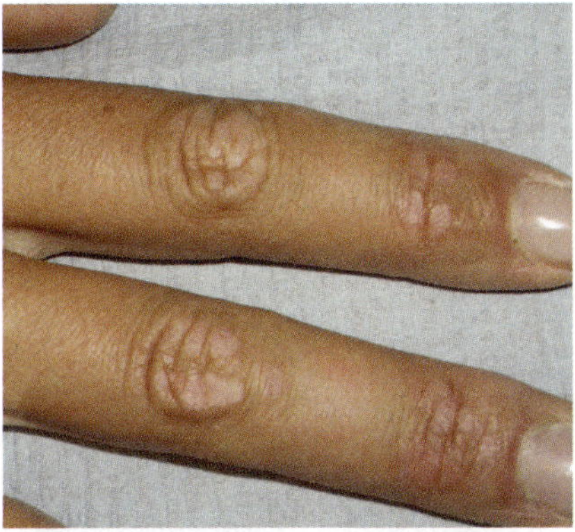

Fig. 19.10 Flat-topped slightly scaly papules over the interphalangeal joints (Gottron's papules).

Dermatomyositis: investigation and management

What should I do?

- Investigation—see Box 19.16.
- Pruritus, skin pain, and burning are difficult to control: try sedating antihistamines such as hydroxyzine 25–50mg × 4/day, cooling baths, aqueous cream with 1% menthol, and moisturizers or soap substitutes.
- Advise on photoprotection using clothing, wide-brimmed hats, and sunscreen creams (see 🕮 p.316).
- Potent or very potent topical corticosteroid ointments or 0.1% tacrolimus ointment applied × 2/day may control limited cutaneous disease.
- A potent steroid (betamethasone) lotion used at night may relieve scalp irritation.
- Hydroxychloroquine (<6.5mg/kg/day) takes 8–12 weeks to have an effect and up to 6 months for maximal benefit, but is less effective in cutaneous dermatomyositis than in cutaneous LE.
- Oral prednisolone (0.5–1mg/kg/day) in reducing doses over 2–3 months may control symptomatic cutaneous disease, while hydroxychloroquine is taking effect.
- Other immunosuppressive drugs have been tried for cutaneous disease with varying success.
- Management of calcinosis is difficult: sometimes painful deposits have to be removed surgically.
- Myositis may prove easier to control with oral prednisolone than cutaneous disease. Other steroid-sparing immunosuppressive drugs that have been recommended include methotrexate, azathioprine, ciclosporin, and mycophenolate mofetil.

Further reading

Sontheimer RD. *Expert Opin Pharmacother* 2004; **5**:1083–99.

Box 19.16 Investigations in dermatomyositis

Skin

- Photography to record extent of disease.
- Biopsy involved skin—see Box 19.17.

Muscles

- Inflammatory markers: ESR, CRP.
- Serum muscle enzymes.
- Myositis-specific antibodies:
  - Jo-1 (a marker for interstitial lung disease), Mi-2, and SRP.
- Myositis-associated antibodies:
  - Ro/SS-A and La/SS-B.
  - PM/Scl (marker of the systemic sclerosis/ dermatomyositis overlap syndrome).
- Electromyography.
- Muscle biopsy or muscle MRI.

Interstitial lung disease

- Chest radiography.
- Lung function tests.
- High-resolution CT scan of lungs.
- ECG and echocardiogram to exclude pulmonary hypertension.

⚠ *Malignancy*

Most cancers present within 2 years of diagnosis.

- FBC, renal function, liver function.
- Chest radiography.
- CT of abdomen and pelvis.
- Mammography.
- Cervical smear.
- CA-125 blood levels.
- Transvaginal ultrasonography.

Box 19.17 Histological findings in the skin

- Skin biopsies show an interface dermatitis (vacuolar degeneration of basal keratinocytes and apoptosis), mild perivascular inflammation, oedema, and dermal mucin.
- These histological features are similar to those of cutaneous LE.

Systemic sclerosis

Systemic sclerosis is a connective tissue disease characterized by collagen accumulation (fibrosis) associated with vascular injury and autoantibodies. Women, particularly black women, are most at risk. Average age of onset is 40–50 years. The disease is divided into 2 major subtypes: diffuse cutaneous systemic sclerosis (10-year survival 21%) and limited cutaneous systemic sclerosis (10-year survival 71%)—see Box 19.19.

Systemic sclerosis is also known as scleroderma, which can lead to confusion with localized scleroderma (morphoea), a self-limited, unrelated condition confined to skin and subcutaneous tissue—see 📖 p.390.

What should I ask?

- Any swelling of hands, feet or face? Develops acutely at onset of diffuse disease.
- Any skin tightness or itching?
- Raynaud's phenomenon? See Box 19.18.
- Joint pain or swelling? (Rheumatoid-like arthritis seen in diffuse disease.)
- Anorexia, fatigue, or weight loss? (More common in diffuse disease.)
- Dyspnoea on exertion or at rest?
- Muscle pain or weakness? (Common in diffuse disease.)
- Dysphagia or dyspepsia?
- Exposure to chemicals or drugs that may induce sclerodermoid changes—see Box 19.20.
- Any features in history suggesting other conditions that may have similar features—see Box 19.20.
- Smoker?
- Assess functional impairment and impact on quality of life.

Box 19.18 Raynaud's phenomenon

- Defined as episodic bilateral, di- or triphasic (pallor, cyanosis, erythema), vascular reactions of the fingers, toes, ears, or nose that are provoked by cold or emotion.
- Occurs in 3–15% of the population.
- May be idiopathic (Raynaud's disease).
- Associated with systemic sclerosis, SLE, and dermatomyositis.
- Also seen with cervical rib, emboli, and vascular trauma including vibration injury.

Further reading

LeRoy C and Medsger TA. *J Rheumatol* 2001; **28:**1573–6.

Box 19.19 Subtypes of systemic sclerosis

Limited cutaneous systemic sclerosis

(Includes CREST: C=calcinosis cutis, R=Raynaud's phenomenon, E=oesophageal distal hypomotility, S=sclerodactyly, T=telangiectasia).

- Occurs in older women more often than diffuse disease.
- Raynaud's phenomenon may precede other features by 10–15 years.
- Skin sclerosis limited to hands, face, feet, and forearms, or absent.
- Cutaneous calcinosis and telangiectatic macules.
- Dilated nailfold capillary loops, usually without capillary dropout.
- Oesophageal distal hypomotility with reflux oesophagitis or dysphagia.
- Late incidence of pulmonary hypertension, with or without interstitial lung disease, biliary cirrhosis, and trigeminal neuralgia.
- Presence of anti-centromere antibodies.

Diffuse cutaneous systemic sclerosis

- Raynaud's phenomenon within 1 year of onset of skin changes.
- Nailfold capillary dilatation and destruction (also seen in dermatomyositis and overlap syndromes).
- Truncal and acral skin involvement.
- Presence of tendon friction rubs.
- Early onset of interstitial lung disease, oliguric renal failure, diffuse gastrointestinal disease, and myocardial involvement.
- Presence of anti-Scl-70 (anti-DNA topoisomerase I) antibodies.
- Absence of anti-centromere antibodies.

Box 19.20 Differential diagnosis

- Morphoea: no Raynaud's phenomenon, normal nail folds (📖 p.390).
- Some features of systemic sclerosis may be present in RA, SLE, dermatomyositis/polymyositis, and Sjögren's syndrome.
- Chemicals (polyvinyl chloride, solvents, pesticides), drugs (bleomycin, pentazocine, ethosuximide, penicillamine), paraffin, aniline-contaminated rapeseed oil, salad oil (toxic oil syndrome), and L-tryptophan may induce a scleroderma-like disease.
- Scleroedema: associated with infection, diabetes, and monoclonal gammopathy. Firm non-pitting oedema of face, neck, upper back (📖 Box 22.2, p.433).
- Scleromyxoedema: associated with paraproteinaemia, myeloma, lymphoma, and leukaemia (📖 Box 26.7, p.499). Waxy, flesh-coloured papules on face, trunk and extremities. Eventually stiffening of the skin causes sclerodactyly and reduced mouth opening. Patients do not have telangiectasia or calcinosis.
- Nephrogenic fibrosing dermopathy—📖 p.462. Seen in patients with renal failure exposed to contrast medium containing gadolinium. Features similar to scleromyxoedema—📖 Box 26.7, p.499.
- Porphyria cutanea tarda: waxy thickening of sun-exposed skin (📖 p.310).
- Chronic GVHD: sclerodermoid form (📖 p.496).

Systemic sclerosis: signs and investigation

Diffuse cutaneous disease: what should I look for?

- Non-pitting oedema of hands, feet, and face.
- Distorted and irregular nailfold capillaries.
- Thickening of the skin proximal to the elbows (diagnostic of diffuse rather than localized disease). Palpate and pinch the skin to assess thickening. Sclerosis spreads to proximal extremities, chest, face, scalp and trunk over 3–12 months or may be present at onset.
- Facial sclerosis giving the face a mask-like stiffness with reduced mouth aperture, radial furrowing around the lips, and pinched nose.
- Neck sign: the skin of the neck skin is ridged and tightened when the head is extended. Positive in >90% of patients.
- Dusky cyanotic fingers and toes—see Fig. 19.11.
- Sclerodactyly and flexion contractures producing a claw-like deformity with painful ulcerations of fingertips and knuckles (rat bite necroses).
- Prayer sign—see next section.
- Pigment change: generalized hyperpigmentation resembling Addison's disease or focal hypo- or hyperpigmentation in areas of sclerosis.
- Tendon friction rubs.
- Swollen painful joints.
- ⚠ Evidence of systemic involvement including hypertension, fine basal inspiratory crackles, right ventricular hypertrophy, heart failure, or pericardial effusion.

Limited cutaneous disease: what should I look for?

- Linear periungual nailfold telangiectasia without any irregularity.
- Atrophy of finger pulps with beaking of fingernails and resorption of bone in the terminal phalanges (also seen in association with Raynaud's phenomenon in diffuse disease).
- Painful ischaemic ulceration of fingertips that heals leaving pitted scarring (also seen in association with Raynaud's phenomenon in diffuse disease—see Fig. 19.11).
- Thickening of skin, but limited to hands, face, feet, and forearms.
- Prayer sign: symmetrical thickening and tightening of the skin distal to the MCP joints (sclerodactyly) restricts opposition of the palms, when wrists are extended. This sign indicates joint or skin pathology or shortening of the finger flexor muscles.
- Well-defined telangiectatic macules on hands, tongue, lips, and face.
- Nodules of cutaneous calcinosis that may become inflamed and ulcerate, discharging chalky material. Cellulitis may complicate ulceration.
- ⚠ Evidence of pulmonary involvement: fine basal inspiratory crackles, right ventricular hypertrophy, heart failure.

What should I do?

See Box 19.21 and 📖 p.388.

Box 19.21 Investigations in systemic sclerosis

- FBC, ESR, renal and liver function tests, creatine kinase.
- Urinalysis and microscopy for casts.
- Immunoglobulins and autoantibodies—see Box 19.22.
- Baseline CXR, lung function tests, ECG, and echocardiogram (repeat annually).
- Further investigations should be guided by clinical findings, but may include pulmonary CT scan, renal ultrasound, gastrointestinal endoscopy, and barium studies.

Box 19.22 Autoantibodies in systemic sclerosis

- 95% of patients have autoantibodies specific for systemic sclerosis or for overlap syndromes with other connective tissue diseases.
- Autoantibodies are usually present at the onset of disease and persist throughout the course of the disease.
- <1% of patients have >1 systemic sclerosis-specific autoantibody.
- It is not clear if autoantibodies have a direct role in the pathogenesis, but autoantibodies predict different subtypes of systemic sclerosis.
- Anti-centromere antibodies: limited cutaneous disease and CREST. High risk for calcinosis, ischaemic digital loss, and pulmonary hypertension, but low risk of pulmonary fibrosis and low mortality.
- Anti-Scl 70 (anti-DNA topoisomerase I): diffuse cutaneous disease, pulmonary fibrosis, high mortality from right ventricular failure secondary to pulmonary disease.
- Antinucleolar system antibodies including:
  - Anti-PM-Scl: polymyositis–scleroderma overlap syndrome (benign and chronic course), limited cutaneous involvement.
  - Antifibrillarin (anti-U3-ribonucleoprotein): diffuse cutaneous systemic sclerosis and, in some populations, myositis, pulmonary hypertension, and renal disease.
  - Anti-Th/To: limited skin involvement, pulmonary hypertension, renal crisis.
  - Anti-RNA-polymerase family: diffuse cutaneous disease, right heart failure (secondary to pulmonary hypertension).

Further reading

Cepeda EJ and Reveille JD. *Curr Opin Rheumatol* 2004; **16**:723–32.

Ho KT and Reveille JD. *Arthritis Res Ther* 2003; **5**:80–93.

Cutaneous systemic sclerosis: management

- Moisturizers, aqueous cream with 1% menthol, soap substitutes, and sedating antihistamines may reduce pruritus.
- Patients should avoid nicotine.
- Keep peripheries warm using thermal underwear to raise core temperatures as well as thermal gloves and/or socks.
- Heat pads (purchased in outdoor activity shops) may be used under gloves or socks.
- Thick-soled padded footwear is essential.
- Warming hands for 5min every 4h in a warm water bath may improve Raynaud's phenomenon. Some patients find it helpful to warm their hands in water before going outdoors.
- Finger tip ulceration: moisturizers (ointments) relieve dryness and cracking of the fingers. Topical antibiotics or antibiotic-steroid combinations may be helpful in superficial ulcers. Hydrocolloid dressings may relieve pain and promote healing.
- GTN patches or calcium antagonists, e.g. nifedipine can reduce vasoconstriction.
- Troublesome fingertip calcinosis may be removed surgically: curettage has been advocated.
- Placebo-controlled trials are needed to evaluate treatments to improve peripheral blood circulation and inhibit fibrosis.

Further reading

Sapadin AN and Fleishmajer R *Arch Dermatol* 2002; **138:**99–105.

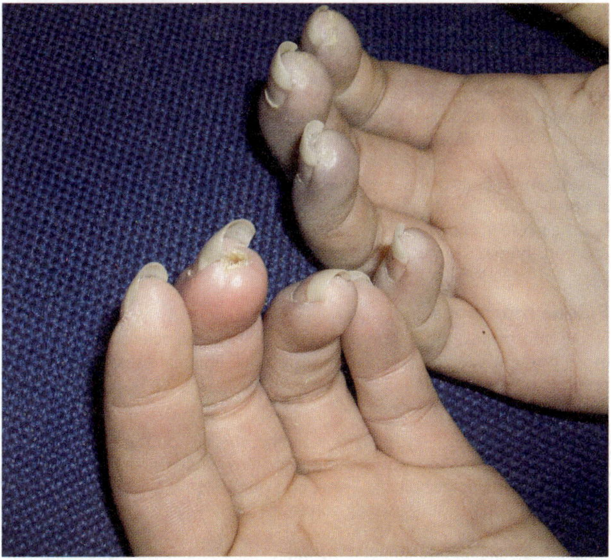

Fig. 19.11 Sclerodactyly with painful ulceration of the fingertips.

Localized scleroderma

Localized scleroderma (morphoea) refers to a group of conditions in which increased collagen deposition causes skin thickening. Internal organs are not involved and localized scleroderma does not progress to systemic sclerosis. Females are affected more often than males. The frequency of the subtypes is different in adults and children. Some patients have >1 type of lesion.

Autoantibodies (antinuclear antibodies, anti-Scl70, anti-centromere antibody, anti-cardiolipin antibody, rheumatoid factor), may be detected, but their role in pathogenesis is unclear. *Borrelia burgdorferi* has been implicated in the pathogenesis of some cases of morphoea, but these findings have not been substantiated.

Plaque morphoea

Plaque morphoea, the commonest type of localized scleroderma, occurs more often in adults than children. It is a self-limiting disease that slowly resolves over 3–5 years.

What should I look for?

- 1 or more smooth erythematous patches, usually on the trunk.
- Patches progress to smooth indurated shiny white or yellowish plaques with violet borders—the 'lilac ring'—see Fig. 19.12.
- Plaques hyperpigment as they soften.

What should I do?

- Consider taking a deep elliptical skin biopsy that extends from normal into abnormal skin, but a biopsy is not always necessary.
- No treatment is required, but a very potent topical corticosteroid ointment may be applied until the inflammatory ring has resolved.

Differential diagnosis

- Granuloma annulare: colour may be similar to morphoea but look for a raised beaded margin in an annular configuration (see 🕮 Box 22.3, p.435).
- Erythema migrans (see 🕮 p.140). Subtle erythema but no thickening.
- Extragenital lichen sclerosus: resembles plaque morphoea, but the surface is slightly hyperkeratotic with follicular plugs. Lichen sclerosus (genital and extragenital) may occur with morphoea—see 🕮 p.268.
- Dermatofibrosarcoma protuberans: a slow-growing fibrosing tumour that may present as a thickened plaque.

⚠ Generalized morphoea

- Much of the skin becomes sclerotic in this very rare variant.
- Involvement of the chest wall may cause disabling restrictive lung defects.
- Treatment is unsatisfactory but phototherapy has been recommended.

Linear scleroderma

This uncommon type of scleroderma is seen more often in children than adults. Once the inflammatory stage has ended, linear scleroderma does not progress.

What should I look for?

- A unilateral sclerotic band, usually extending along a limb, following the lines of Blaschko (see 📖 p.63 and Fig. 19.13).
- In the rare 'en coup de sabre' variant, an atrophic groove gradually extends from the anterior scalp down one side of the face. Involvement of deeper tissues causes disfiguring hemifacial atrophy.
- Neurological complications (seizures, headache, hemiparesis), eye problems, and jaw malalignment in children with facial involvement.
- Hypo- or hyperpigmentation of affected skin (see Fig. 19.13).

What should I do?

- Assess limb length and diameter. Deep atrophy may affect subcutaneous tissues (fat, muscle, bone) so that the limb is short and wasted.
- ⚠ Complications such as limb length discrepancy, joint contractures, or jaw malocclusion should be managed by a multidisciplinary team.
- ⚠ If affecting the face, arrange ophthalmological assessment and consider MRI to detect CNS involvement.
- Placebo-controlled trials are needed to evaluate the impact of treatments such as phototherapy, oral prednisolone, intralesional triamcinolone, IV methylprednisolone, and/or methotrexate.
- Reconstructive surgery may reduce deformity, once disease is inactive.
- Cosmetic camouflage may be helpful.

Eosinophilic fasciitis (Shulman's syndrome)

Vigorous exercise may trigger this variant of scleroderma which involves deep fascia and initially may simulate cellulitis.

What should I look for?

- Symmetrical non-tender reddish-brown oedematous plaques, usually on the limbs, that develop into indurated brawny plaques.
- Sclerosis extending into subcutaneous tissues restricts movement of tendons in affected limb, e.g. patients are unable to extend wrist and fingers simultaneously if flexor muscles of forearm are involved.

What should I do?

- FBC looking for a peripheral eosinophilia.
- Arrange a deep biopsy of fascia and muscle.
- Oral corticosteroids, methotrexate, and azathioprine have been advocated for treatment, but controlled trials are lacking and disease remits spontaneously in about 1/3 patients.

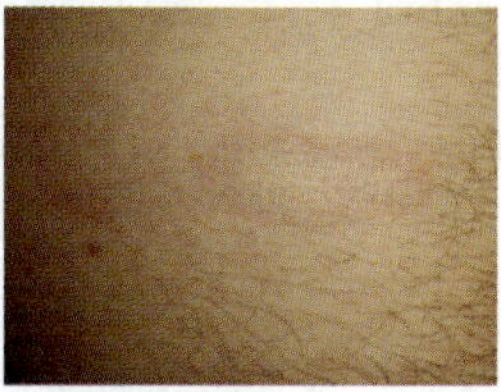

Fig. 19.12 Morphoea: smooth shiny white plaque with a violet border.

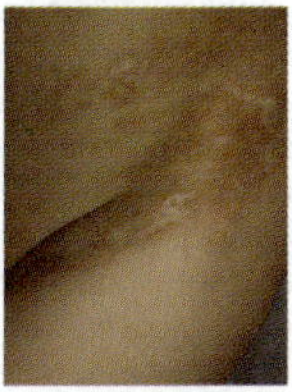

Fig. 19.13 Linear scleroderma with a mix of hypo- and hyperpigmentation.

Relapsing polychondritis

This rare disorder is characterized by episodes of inflammation of cartilage leading to destruction with deformity. Relapsing polychondritis affects cartilage in ear, nose, larynx, trachea, bronchi, and joints as well as proteoglycan-rich tissues such as the skin, eyes, aorta, and heart. Antibodies to type II collagen have been found in cartilage. Onset is usually between the ages of 20–60 years. Relapsing polychondritis may be mild or rapidly progressive—about 25% of patients die of their disease after 5–7 years. Causes of death include pulmonary infection, systemic vasculitis, airway collapse, and renal failure.

What should I look for? (see Box 19.23)

- Fever, anorexia, weight loss and/or myalgia.
- Erythema, tenderness, warmth, and swelling of the cartilaginous portion of the ear—usually both ears and the non-cartilaginous ear lobe is always spared, unlike cellulitis—see Fig. 19.14. (85% of patients—diagnostic sign). Episodes last from days to weeks. Repeated episodes may lead to a droopy pinna or cauliflower ear (destruction of cartilage).
- Asymmetric, usually migratory non-erosive oligoarthritis or polyarthritis (50–75% of patients): most often MCP and PIP joints and knees (may have RA).
- Episodic acute painful inflammation of nasal cartilage with rhinorrhoea, epistaxis, and, eventually, deformity (saddle nose) (54% of patients).
- Painful red eye: commonly episcleritis, scleritis, or keratitis (60% of patients).
- Laryngotracheobronchial disease (50% of patients): cough, hoarseness, dyspnoea, wheezing, choking. Tenderness over the thyroid cartilage and trachea. Airway obstruction or collapse. Secondary chest infections.
- Narrowing of external auditory meatus with hearing loss. Vestibular dysfunction causes dizziness, ataxia, and nausea.
- Large-vessel vasculitis leads to aortic aneurysms.
- Aortic or mitral valve disease (5–10% of patients).
- Skin problems (50% of patients) including small-vessel cutaneous vasculitis (p.406), livedo reticularis (p.418), urticaria or angio-oedema (p.98) erythema nodosum (p.424), and Sweet's syndrome (p.480).
- Migratory superficial thrombophlebitis.
- Neurological problems secondary to vasculitis.
- Renal disease (10% of patients)—may be fatal.
- Associated disease (25–35% of patients):
  - Connective tissue disease, e.g. RA, SLE.
  - Systemic vasculitides, e.g. Wegener's granulomatosis.
  - Haematological disease, e.g. myelodysplastic syndrome, IgA myeloma, lymphoma.
  - Gastrointestinal disease, e.g. Crohn's disease, ulcerative colitis.
  - Skin disease, e.g. vitiligo, psoriasis, lichen planus.
  - Endocrine disease, e.g. autoimmune thyroid disease, diabetes, thymoma.
- See Box 19.24 for differential diagnoses.

What should I do?

- The diagnosis is based on clinical criteria—see Box 19.23.
- Biopsy of inflamed cartilage may be required to exclude other pathology.
- FBC (anaemia, leucocytosis, thrombocytosis).
- ESR (raised).
- Urinalysis and creatinine.
- ANA, RF (may be detected, but not helpful diagnostically).
- Further investigation should be guided by the clinical findings but may include CXR, pulmonary function tests, high-resolution laryngotracheal CT scans, ENT assessment, and ophthalmological review.
- Recommended treatments include oral corticosteroids, NSAIDs, dapsone, and colchicine. Other steroid-sparing immunosuppressive agents that have been tried include methotrexate, hydroxychloroquine, cyclophosphamide, ciclosporin, and anti-TNF agents (infliximab).

Box 19.23 Relapsing polychondritis: diagnostic criteria

3 of these criteria should be present to make the diagnosis:
- Bilateral auricular chondritis—see Fig. 19.14.
- Non-erosive seronegative inflammatory polyarthritis.
- Nasal chondritis.
- Ocular inflammation including keratitis, scleritis, episcleritis.
- Respiratory tract chondritis involving laryngeal and tracheal cartilages.
- Cochlear or vestibular damage manifested by neurosensory hearing loss, tinnitus, and vertigo.

Box 19.24 Relapsing polychondritis: differential diagnosis

- Ear: cellulitis or dermatitis. Sparing of ear lobe rules out these diagnoses. Most cases of cellulitis are unilateral. Relapsing polychondritis is usually bilateral.
- Wegener's granulomatosis and PAN do not cause chondritis of ear or respiratory tract.
- Saddle nose: consider infection including congenital syphilis, Wegener's granulomatosis.

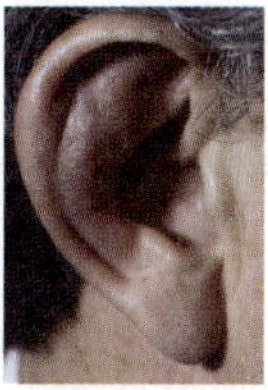

Fig. 19.14 Erythema and swelling in relapsing polychondritis do not affect the ear lobe.

Further reading

Letko E *et al. Semin Arthritis Rheum* 2002; **31:**384–95.

Rapini RP and Warner NB. *Clin Dermatol* 2006; **24:**482–5.

⚠ Multicentric reticulohistiocytosis

If you recognize the cutaneous manifestations of this very rare disease, you will make the diagnosis. Patients, most often middle-aged women, present with systemic complaints, a destructive arthropathy, and, at some stage, a characteristic rash. 2/3 of patients present with arthritis (skin signs appear within months or a few years) and about 1/5 with skin signs (arthritis appears at any time). Multicentric reticulohistiocytosis may be a paraneoplastic disorder.

What should I look for?

- Systemic symptoms: weight loss, weakness, and fever.
- A rapidly progressive, disabling, symmetrical arthritis involving DIP joints in 75% of patients (may be confused with Heberden's nodes), sometimes with involvement of PIP joints (producing an 'opera glass' deformity) and MCP joints, knees, shoulders, wrists, hips, ankles, feet, elbows and vertebrae—see 🕮 Box 19.25.
- Smooth reddish brown papules and nodules ranging in size from a few mm to 2cm diameter on ears, nose, dorsum, and lateral aspect of fingers, neck and, sometimes, trunk. Nodules over PIP, MCP and DIP joints may resemble Gottron's papules seen in dermatomyositis (see 🕮 p.381), but are not scaly or hyperkeratotic—see 🕮 Fig. 19.5, p.373.
- Periungual nodules and papules with a 'coral bead' appearance—see Fig. 19.5.
- Papules and nodules on the lips, buccal mucosa, tongue, gingival, and nasal septum.
- Associated diseases:
  - Hyperlipidemia (30–58% of cases).
  - ⚠ Malignancy (25% of cases) most commonly breast or stomach, but also cervix, colon, lung, ovary, lymphoma, leukaemia, sarcoma, and melanoma.

What should I do?

- Skin biopsy shows characteristic lipid-laden multinucleated giant cells of a foreign-body type with 'ground glass' cytoplasm. Similar histiocytes also invade the synovium.
- Radiographs demonstrate a circumscribed erosive arthritis. Erosions advance from joint margins to involve the entire joint surface. The joint space is widened with loss of cartilage and resorption of subchondral bone, but without osteopenia or periosteal new bone formation.
- Very potent topical corticosteroids may speed resolution of the cutaneous papules. Cutaneous signs resolve before the arthritis.
- Arthritis is difficult to control. Corticosteroids provide symptomatic relief without inducing remission. Drugs such as methotrexate, cyclophosphamide, alendronate, and anti-TNF agents have been recommended, but controlled trials are lacking.

Box 19.25 Multicentric reticulohistiocytosis: differential diagnosis

The cutaneous signs are diagnostic but may not develop until some months or years after the arthritis. Consider:

- RA
- Psoriatic arthritis
- Reiter's disease
- Erosive osteoarthritis
- Crystal-induced arthropathies.

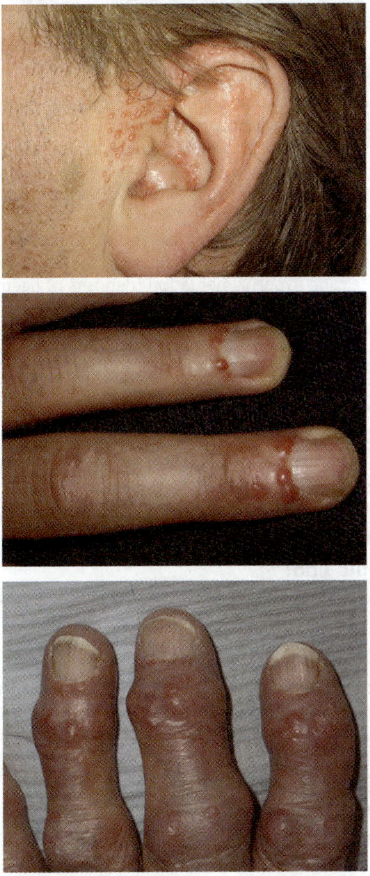

(a) (b) (c)

Fig. 19.15 (a, b, and c) Smooth reddish-brown papules and nodules on an ear (a) and fingers (b,c) in multicentric reticulohistiocytosis.

Ehlers–Danlos syndrome (EDS)

EDS is a heterogeneous spectrum of inherited disorders with overlapping clinical features that may include hyperextensible skin, hypermobile joints, and generalized tissue fragility. ⚠ Vascular EDS carries a high risk of life-threatening uterine or vascular rupture. EDS is caused by mutations in genes that modify collagen proteins—see Table 19.1.

What should I ask?

- Skin: easy bruising or stretchy skin (apparent in early childhood).
- Joint hypermobility: pain, sprains, or dislocation.
- Surgical complications: delayed wound healing, postoperative hernia.
- Family history of similar problems or, in vascular EDS, sudden death.

What should I look for?

- Soft, doughy, velvety skin.
- Hyperextensible skin that once released quickly snaps back to its original state (skin returns slowly to its former position in cutis laxa). Test at a site that is not subjected to mechanical forces or scarring, e.g. flexor surface of the forearm.
- Thin transparent skin with easily visible vessels (chest, abdomen, limbs): seen in vascular EDS.
- Subcutaneous nodules on forearms and shins. Nodules may calcify.
- Spontaneous bruising: bruises reappear in the same areas, often shins or knees, leaving hyperpigmentation (deposits of haemosiderin).
- Wide atrophic 'cigarette-paper' scars over pressure points (knee, elbow, forehead, chin).
- Molluscoid pseudotumours (small spongy tumours over scars and pressure points).
- Elastosis perforans serpiginosa—see 📖 Box 19.27 and Fig. 19.16, p.399 (a rare association).
- Joint hypermobility: influenced by age, sex, ethnicity, and family background. Do little fingers dorsiflex passively to >90°; do elbows or knees hyperextend beyond 10°; is it possible to flex the thumb down onto the flexor surface of the forearm? Benign joint hypermobility syndrome may be misdiagnosed as EDS.

What should I do?

- Confirm diagnosis with skin biopsy, biochemical analysis of collagen, and/or genetic testing.
- Refer to medical geneticist for counselling if diagnosis is confirmed.
- Patients should be managed in a specialist centre by a multidisciplinary team.
- Echocardiography (mitral valve/tricuspid valve prolapse).
- Advise patients with easy bruising to avoid contact sports.
- Surgeons should take steps to minimize the risk of the risk of poor wound healing—avoid wound tension, use plentiful deep sutures, leave skin sutures in place for longer than usual, apply steristrips to reduce stretching of scars.

Further reading

Beighton P *et al. Am J Med Genet* 1998; **77:**31–7.

Callewaert B *et al. Best Pract Res Clin Rheumatol* 2008; **22:**165–89.

Table 19.1 Some subtypes of Ehlers–Danlos syndrome. Many variants cannot be classified into one of the known subtypes

Subtype and inheritance	Major clinical features	Protein defect
Hypermobility Autosomal dominant (most common subtype)	Marked joint hypermobility Joint pain Mild skin hyperextensibility	Unclear but may involve type V collagen or tenascin-X (regulates deposition of collagen by fibroblasts)
Classic Autosomal dominant	Skin hyperextensibility Widened atrophic scarring Smooth and velvety skin Joint hypermobility Surgical complications	Genetic heterogeneity Type V collagen (50%) or unknown
Vascular Autosomal dominant	Easy bruising Thin, translucent skin (not hyperextensible) Arterial/intestinal/uterine rupture—sudden death Characteristic facial appearance—acrogeria Hypermobility, tendon rupture Pneumothorax	Type III collagen
Kyphoscoliosis Autosomal recessive	Hypermobility Hypotonia at birth Kyphoscoliosis at birth Ocular fragility, rupture of globe	Lysyl hydroxylase-1 (responsible for cross-linking of collagen fibres to give tensile strength) or unknown
Arthrochalasia Autosomal dominant	Severe generalized joint hypermobility Congenital hip dislocation Skin hyperextensibility Wide atrophic scars	Type 1 collagen (loss of a procollagen-N-proteinase cleavage site)
Dermatosparaxis Autosomal recessive	Skin fragility; sagging, redundant skin; excessive bruising. Characteristic facies (oedema of eyelids, downslanting palpebral fissures, epicanthic folds, blue sclerae, gingival hyperplasia, micrognathia) Umbilical hernia	Procollagen-N-proteinase

Marfan's syndrome

Marfan's syndrome is an autosomal dominant condition linked to mutations in the *FBNI* gene that encodes the extracellular matrix protein, fibrillin-1. Fibrillin-1 deficiency may affect the development of tissues by dysregulating TGFβ signalling pathways. Several hundred mutations have been described. Diagnostic criteria are shown in Box 19.26. ⚠ Aortic root dissection or ruptured aortic aneurysms may be fatal.

What should I look for?

- Skin: striae not associated with weight change, usually seen on the shoulders, back, or thighs (low specificity).
- Recurrent inguinal or incisional hernias.
- Musculoskeletal: limbs disproportionately long for the trunk, scoliosis, pectus excavatum or carinatum, arachnodactyly (fully flexed thumb extends beyond the ulnar border of the palm; distal phalanges of the thumb and 5th finger overlap fully when grasping the contralateral wrist), muscle hypoplasia and myalgia.
- Facies: downslanting palpebral fissures, enophthalmia, and retrognathia.
- High arched palate with tooth crowding.
- Cardiovascular: mitral valve prolapse, dilatation of the ascending aorta with risk of fatal rupture or dissection, aortic regurgitation.
- Ocular: lens dislocation, myopia, retinal detachment, cataract, or glaucoma. May cause visual impairment or blindness. Slit lamp examination is required to diagnose ectopia lentis.
- Pneumothorax and pulmonary emphysema (rare).
- Family history of marfanoid features or sudden death.
- Elastosis perforans serpiginosa—rare association (see Box 19.27).

What should I do?

- Diagnosis is clinical—see Box 19.26.
- Patients should be managed in a specialist centre by a multidisciplinary team.
- Refer for genetic counselling.
- Recommend that patients avoid competitive sport, straining, or isometric exercise that might raise the blood pressure.
- Avoid contact sports that might precipitate aortic dissection.
- Beta-adrenergic blockade is recommended to control blood pressure and slow the rate of aortic growth.
- Annual echocardiography is required to monitor the aortic root.
- Annual review by an ophthalmologist is recommended.
- Pregnancy carries high risk of aortic complications.

Further reading

Callewaert B *et al. Best Pract Res Clin Rheumatol* 2008; **22**:165–89.

De Paepe A *et al. Am J Med Genet* 1996; **62**:417–26.

Box 19.26 Ghent nosology of Marfan's syndrome

Major criteria

Skeletal system (4 or more skeletal features)

- Pectus carinatum, pectus excavatum requiring surgery.
- Arm span to height ratio >1.05, wrist and thumb signs (see 📖 p.398).
- Scoliosis >20° or spondylolisthesis.
- Elbow extension <170°, pes planus.
- Protrusio acetabuli (on radiography).

Dura: lumbosacral dural ectasia on CT or MRI.

Ocular system: ectopia lentis.

Cardiovascular system

- Dilatation of ascending aorta, maximal at sinuses of Valsalva.
- Dissection of ascending aorta.

Family/genetic history

- First-degree relative with Marfan's syndrome.
- Presence of *FBN1* mutation.

Diagnosis

For index case diagnosis requires major criteria in at least 2 different organ systems and involvement of a 3rd organ system.

For a relative of an index case diagnosis requires major criterion in 1 organ system and involvement of a 2nd organ system.

Box 19.27 Elastosis perforans serpiginosa (EPS)

- A rare disorder of elastic fibres.
- May be sporadic.
- Reported in association with disorders of connective tissue including Marfan's syndrome, EDS, PXE, and systemic sclerosis.
- Also seen in Down's syndrome and in patients taking penicillamine.
- Most often affects face, neck, and upper limbs.
- Abnormal dermal elastic fibres are eliminated through channels in the epidermis (transepidermal elimination) producing skin-coloured or erythematous keratotic papules with central plugs.
- Papules may erupt in annular or serpiginous patterns.

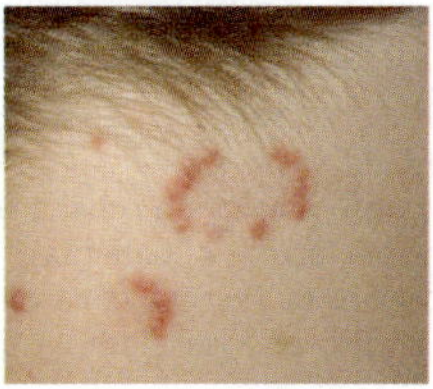

Fig. 19.16 EPS: papules with central keratotic plugs.

Pseudoxanthoma elasticum

Pseudoxanthoma elasticum (PXE) is a rare inherited disorder in which elastic fibres become fragmented and calcified. PXE is caused by mutations in an ABC-transporter gene encoding a transmembrane protein mainly found in the liver and kidney (multidrug resistance associated protein 6, MRP6). PXE may be a systemic metabolic disorder with secondary mineralization of connective tissues.

The inheritance pattern is usually autosomal recessive and PXE is more common in women. Clinical features, including age of onset, vary within and between families, but skin changes are not usually apparent until puberty (average age of onset = 13 years). Diagnostic criteria—see Box 19.28.

(⚠Consider screening fundoscopies in young patients presenting with gastrointestinal haemorrhage, macular degeneration or unexplained claudication.)

What should I ask?

- Skin changes (mainly a cosmetic problem).
- Visual impairment (reduced visual acuity is a late problem).
- Cardiovascular disease: intermittent claudication (30% of patients), angina, and myocardial infarction (commence in 3rd– 5th decades—caused by calcification of the internal elastic lamina of medium-sized arteries).
- Bleeding: gastrointestinal (most common). Other sites include subarachnoid, retinal, renal, uterine, bladder, nasal, and and/or joints (spontaneous bleeding is seen in 10% of patients).
- Family history.

What should I look for?

- Asymptomatic yellowish, grouped 'cobblestone' papules giving the appearance of 'plucked chicken' skin. Examine the sides of the neck, axillae, antecubital fossae, popliteal fossae, groins, and periumbilical skin. Yellowish plaques form when papules coalesce.
- Redundant skin folds or lax yellowish skin. The sagging skin gives a prematurely aged appearance (advanced disease).
- Yellowish papules on the mucosal surface of the lower lip (common).
- Calcium extruded from the skin in perforating PXE (advanced disease).
- Less common cutaneous manifestations include acneiform lesions, brown macules in a reticulate pattern, and EPS—see Box 19.27.
- Yellowish mottling 'peau d'orange' of the retina (may be the first ocular sign).
- Angioid streaks: present in >85% of patients. Breaks in the elastic lamina of the Bruch membrane produce single or multiple, dark red, brown or grey bands usually radiating from the optic disc. Onset is between ages of 15–25 years, usually after the cutaneous signs.
- Reduced peripheral pulses.
- Hypertension (obstruction of calcified renal arteries causes renovascular hypertension in 25% of patients).
- Signs of mitral valve disease or restrictive cardiomyopathy caused by calcification of valves and/or endocardium.

Box 19.28 Diagnostic criteria for PXE

Patients with 3 criteria definitely have PXE:

- Characteristic skin signs (yellow papules in flexural areas).
- Characteristic ophthalmologic features (angioid streaks, mottled 'peau d'orange' retinal pigmentation, maculopathy).
- Characteristic histological features in lesional skin: fragmentation, clumping, and calcification of dermal elastic fibres.

Box 19.29 What should I do?

- Take a skin biopsy from involved skin to confirm the diagnosis (wound healing may be slow). Consider biopsying a scar or flexural skin if no cutaneous signs.
- Eyes: refer for an ophthalmological assessment. Patients should be reviewed every 6–12 months: subretinal neovascularization and haemorrhages may result in loss of central vision.
- Refer for genetic counselling and screen first-degree relatives by examining skin and fundi.
- Arrange echocardiography to exclude mitral valve prolapse, mitral valve stenosis, and/or restrictive cardiomyopathy.
- Monitor blood pressure, peripheral pulses, and cardiac function.
- Minimize cardiovascular risk factors: control weight, advise patients to avoid nicotine, lower cholesterol, encourage regular exercise.
- Advise patients to avoid heavy straining, such as weightlifting, and contact sports with a risk of head trauma, e.g. football, wrestling.
- Avoid drugs such as warfarin, aspirin, and NSAIDs that may increase the risk of bleeding.

Box 19.30 Differential diagnosis

- Sun damage produces a waxy yellowish appearance (solar elastosis) on chronically exposed skin (neck, face) associated with deep furrows—see 📖 Box 3.1, p.43.
- Thalassaaemia and sickle cell syndromes: a PXE-like syndrome occurs with skin, ocular (angioid streaks), and vascular manifestations.
- PXE-like skin lesions may develop in chronic end-stage renal disease, L-tryptophan-induced eosinophilia myalgia syndrome, amyloid elastosis, and patients taking penicillamine.
- PXE-like papules occur in papillary dermal elastolysis (an acquired condition of older women).
- Angioid streaks may be seen in EDS, Marfan's syndrome, Paget's disease of the bone, and lead poisoning.

Further reading

Jiang Q *et al. J Invest Dermatol* 2009; **129:**348–54.

Laube S and Moss C. *Arch Dis Child* 2005; **90**:754–6.

Le Saux *et al. J Invest Dermatol* 2006; **126:**1497–505.

Chapter 20
Vasculitis

Contents

Relevant pages in other chapters

Kawasaki's disease—see 🕮 p.142
Behçet's disease—see 🕮 p.264
Connective tissue diseases—see 🕮 p.365
Alpha-1-antitrypsin deficiency—see 🕮 p.428

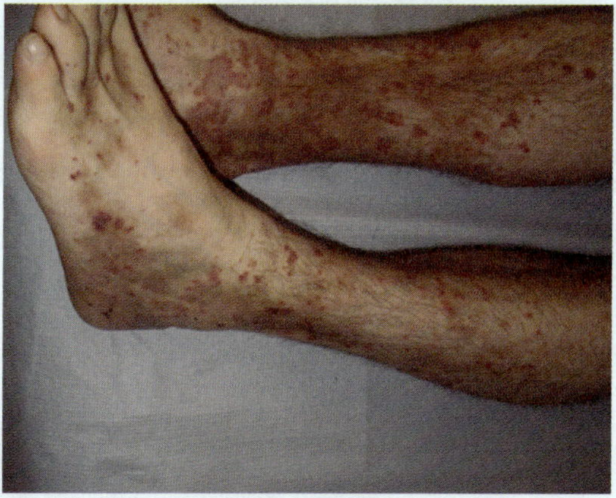

Fig. 20.1 Small-vessel cutaneous vasculitis with a symmetrical palpable purpuric rash and haemosiderin deposition.

Introduction

What is cutaneous vasculitis?

Vasculitis (angiitis) is a necrotizing inflammation of the blood vessels caused by various mechanisms (Box 20.1). Necrosis of blood-vessel walls leads to extravasation of RBCs (purpura), vascular obstruction, and tissue ischaemia or infarction. Vasculitis may affect vessels of different sizes in the skin, kidneys, gut, respiratory tract, peripheral nerves, and/or skeletal muscle.

The histological findings in vasculitis may include:

- Perivascular neutrophilic inflammation extending into vessel walls.
- Swelling and injury of endothelial cells.
- Necrosis of vessel walls.
- Fibrinoid deposition around vessels (fibrinoid necrosis).
- Extravasation of RBCs (clinically evident as purpura in the skin).
- Nuclear dust indicative of leucocytoclasis (fragmentation of the nuclei of neutrophils).

Symptoms and signs vary, but palpable purpura is the hallmark of a small-vessel cutaneous vasculitis (see Box 20.1 and Figs. 20.1 and 20.2).

Clinical findings should be integrated with the results of serological, pathological, and imaging studies to reach a diagnosis.

What is occlusive vasculopathy?

Vasculitis in the skin must be differentiated from an occlusive vasculopathy. Skin biopsy shows that the vessels are occluded without significant vascular inflammation—see 📖 p.418, p.294.

Purpura: differential diagnosis (see 📖 p.69)

Further reading

Fiorentino DF. *J Am Acad Dermatol* 2003 **48:**311–40.

Ghersetich I *et al. Clin Dermatol* 1999 **17:**499–503.

Box 20.1 Vasculitic reaction patterns (patterns overlap)

- Allergic vasculitis (type I reaction) causing urticarial vasculitis—see Fig. 20.3.
- Antibody-associated vasculitis (type II reaction) e.g. anti-neutrophil cytoplasmic antibody (ANCA)-mediated vasculitis in Wegener's granulomatosis and microscopic polyangiitis; antibodies binding to endothelial cell antigens generating a thrombogenic vasculopathy in SLE, rheumatoid arthritis, or systemic sclerosis.
- Immune complex vasculitis (type III reaction) e.g. small-vessel cutaneous vasculitis such as Henoch–Schönlein purpura (HSP) with complement activation, deposition of immunoglobulin in vessel walls, and release of Th2-type cytokines (IL-10, IL-6)—see Fig. 20.2.
- T-cell-mediated hypersensitivity (type IV reaction), e.g. granulomatous large-vessel vasculitides such as temporal arteritis. Lymphocytes and monocytes invade blood vessel walls and CD4+ Th1-type cells produce IFN-gamma.

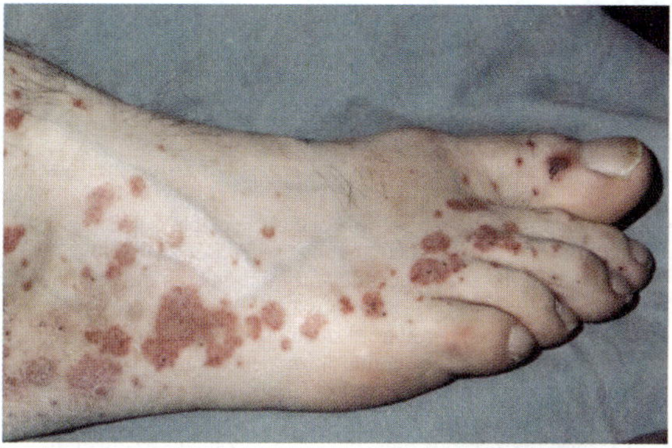

Fig. 20.2 Palpable purpura.

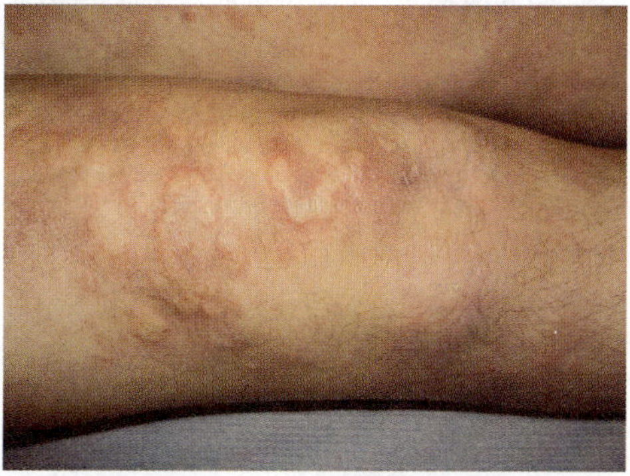

Fig. 20.3 Urticarial vasculitis and livedo reticularis.

Small-vessel cutaneous vasculitis

Synonyms: leucocytoclastic angiitis/vasculitis, cutaneous small-vessel necrotizing vasculitis, allergic vasculitis, hypersensitivity angiitis.

This is the most common vasculitis affecting the skin. The vasculitic lesions in idiopathic small-vessel cutaneous vasculitis are identical to those in a small-vessel cutaneous vasculitis occurring as part of a systemic disease associated with circulating immune complexes (Box 20.2).

Idiopathic small-vessel cutaneous vasculitis confined to the skin usually resolves within a few weeks or months. 10% have recurrent disease lasting months or years.

What should I ask?

- Explore the distribution and evolution of the rash.
- Search for an underlying cause (Box 20.2).
- Enquire about symptoms such as orogenital ulcers, dry eyes, dry mouth, gastrointestinal symptoms, myalgia, arthralgia, or joint swelling.

What should I look for?

- Distribution:
  - Vasculitis involves dependent areas such as the leg, sites of trauma, pressure sites (elbows, sacrum, waist band), or cool skin (tip of nose, ears, fingers)—see Fig. 20.1.
- Morphology:
  - Is the rash purpuric? Purpura, unlike erythema, does not blanch with light pressure—see Fig. 20.2.
  - Are the spots flat or raised (palpable)? Palpable purpura is the hallmark of small-vessel cutaneous vasculitis. Flat (macular) purpuric lesions are associated with non-inflammatory pathology (see 🕮 p.69).
  - How does the rash evolve? In small-vessel cutaneous vasculitis, small round or oval erythematous macules rapidly become raised and purpuric. Papules may coalesce into larger polycyclic or annular lesions.
  - Are there blisters, pustules, or ulcers secondary to inflammation?
  - What is left? Vasculitis fades gradually over 3 or 4 weeks leaving macular pigmentation (haemosiderin) or atrophic scars.
- Note the position of leg ulcers and check for signs of stasis or arterial disease, see 🕮 Box 15.5, p.279. Is there purpura around the edge of the ulcer (a feature of some vasculitic ulcers)?
- Look for livedo reticularis, retiform purpura, or ulcerated nodules indicating a necrotizing vasculitis affecting deeper vessels or an occlusive vasculopathy e.g. cholesterol emboli (see 🕮 p.418).
- Is there evidence of a systemic disease (Box 20.2)?

What should I do? See Box 20.3.

Further reading

Lotti T *et al. J Am Acad Dermatol* 1998; **39**:667–87.

Box 20.2 Causes of small-vessel cutaneous vasculitis

- Uncertain 'idiopathic': 50%.
- Infections: 15–20%. Remember hepatitis B or C in adults, HSP in children—see 📖 p.408.
- Drugs: 10–15%. 7–21 days after commencing the drug.
- Connective tissue diseases: 15–20%. Rheumatoid vasculitis is most common in seropositive patients with long-standing nodular disease.
- Malignancies: 5%. Most often lymphoproliferative disorders: e.g. Hodgkin's disease, mycosis fungoides, lymphosarcoma, adult T-cell leukaemia, multiple myeloma.
- Inflammatory bowel disease.
- Other: e.g. prolonged exercise such as long distance walks—marathons may trigger a cutaneous vasculitis on the leg 'exercise-induced purpura'. This fades within days.

Box 20.3 What should I do?

Investigations

- Guiac testing of stool (in children with HSP).
- Urinalysis: including microscopy to check for cellular casts.
- FBC.
- Inflammatory markers (ESR, CRP).
- Renal function tests, LFTs, HBV/HCV serologies.
- Complement levels (C3, C4), cryoglobulins if C4 is low.
- Immunoglobulins, RF, and ANA.
- ANCA if evidence of systemic disease.
- CXR if concern about interstitial lung disease.
- Skin biopsy: cutaneous vasculitis can be diagnosed using standard histological techniques, but the histology is unlikely to reveal the cause, exclude systemic disease, or distinguish one form of systemic vasculitis from another. Take a biopsy from a purpuric papule about 12–24h old.
- Direct IMF of frozen tissue may be requested to look for deposits of immunoglobulin in vessel walls, e.g. IgA in HSP, but it is not necessary to demonstrate immune complexes to diagnose vasculitis. Immune complexes are not found in older lesions so take a punch biopsy from the edge of a fresh lesion and immediately freeze the specimen.

Management

- Eliminate precipitating agents (drugs or infections), but it may take several weeks for vasculitis to settle.
- Minimize local triggers by avoiding cooling or trauma and reducing stasis (elevate legs, provide support stockings, encourage exercise).
- Most patients with small-vessel vasculitis limited to the skin do not require systemic corticosteroids or immunosuppressive agents.
- If cutaneous vasculitis is symptomatic, dapsone (50–200mg/day) may be helpful. Alternatives include colchicine (0.5mg $\times$2/day) or low-dose methotrexate (10–25mg/week).

Henoch–Schönlein purpura

Henoch-Schönlein purpura (HSP) is the most common small-vessel systemic vasculitis in children, but HSP may also affect adults. HSP is triggered by infection, often in the upper respiratory tract. IgA immune complexes are present in the circulation and vessel walls.

Clinical features

- Palpable purpura (indicating a small-vessel cutaneous vasculitis) is present on extensor surfaces of the limbs, buttocks, and back. The distribution probably reflects stasis and pressure.
- In children, the purpura may be oedematous; early lesions may be urticarial (wheal-like); and scalp, ears, hands, feet, and scrotum may be oedematous.
- Infantile acute haemorrhagic oedema of the skin is possibly a variant of HSP in which the oedematous component is particularly marked.

Features of systemic involvement in children include:

- Migratory arthralgia or arthritis, usually of knees and ankles (60–90%).
- Colicky abdominal pain (50–70%) sometimes with blood in the stool or melaena.
- Haematuria, microscopic or gross, caused by glomerulonephritis (60%), but proteinuria, hypertension, and decreased renal function are less common.

What should I do?

- Direct the history, examination, and investigations towards confirming the diagnosis and determining the extent of systemic involvement—see 🕮 p.406.
- Treat with:
  - Antibiotics if indicated for underlying infection.
  - Paracetamol for pain control.
  - Fluids, bowel rest, and nutrition.
- The value of oral corticosteroids is controversial.

Prognosis

HSP is self-limiting but mild recurrences are common for a few months. Rapidly progressive renal failure is rare and the prognosis is excellent.

Further reading

Roberts PF *et al. South Med J* 2007; **100:**821–4.

Urticarial vasculitis

Patients with urticarial vasculitis have signs that indicate a mix of dermal oedema (urticarial wheals) and small-vessel cutaneous vasculitis (palpable purpura). The smooth erythematous papules (wheals) are uncomfortable (tender or burn) but may also itch; individual wheals last up to 72h; and wheals resolve leaving bruising. Some patients have angio-oedema-like lesions. Simple urticaria is itchy, individual wheals last around 24h and wheals fade to leave normal skin (see 📖 p.212).

Associations

- Connective tissue diseases: some patients with low complement levels have anti-C1q antibodies and overlapping features with SLE including pleuritis, glomerulonephritis, eye symptoms, and positive ANAs.
- Serum sickness (10 days after the administration of drugs or vaccines).
- Infections including HCV.
- Haematological malignancies; IgM or IgG gammopathy.

What should I ask?

- Document the evolution of individual lesions. If the duration is uncertain, ask the patient to draw around fresh lesions and note how long they last.
- Does the wheal blanch or is it purpuric? Patients may have a mix of urticarial and purpuric lesions as well as angio-oedema-like swellings. Is there residual bruising when lesions resolve?
- Ask about musculoskeletal symptoms (common: 50–75% of patients) or gastrointestinal symptoms (less common).

What should I do?

- Search for an underlying cause and check FBC (anaemia is common), ESR (often raised), complement (low complement, detected in 18% of patients, suggests underlying systemic disease), and autoantibodies including anti-C1q antibodies.
- Exclude systemic vasculitis (see Box 20.3, p.407).
- Take a skin biopsy from a purpuric lesion to confirm the presence of a leukocytoclastic vasculitis.

Treatment options include:

- Antihistamines.
- Dapsone, colchicine, or hydroxychloroquine.
- NSAIDs.
- Severe disease: prednisolone or steroid sparing agents (azathioprine, cyclophosphamide, ciclosporin, mycophenolate mofetil).

Further reading

Kallenberg CG. *Autoimmun Rev* 2008; **7:**612–15.

Venzor J *et al. Clin Rev Allergy Immunol* 2002; **23:**201–16.

Cryoglobulinaemic vasculitis and obstructive vasculopathy

Cryoglobulins are immunoglobulins that precipitate at low temperatures.

Type I cryoglobulinaemia

- Type 1: monoclonal IgG or IgM immunoglobulins (25% of cases).
- The cryoglobulins obstruct vessels (obstructive vasculopathy) causing RBC extravasation without inflammation (no vasculitis).
- ***Associations:*** chronic lymphatic leukaemia, multiple myeloma, Waldenström's macroglobulinemia.

What should I look for?

- Patients are sensitive to cold and complain of Raynaud's phenomenon.
- Mottling of the skin or blotchy cyanosis of the helices of the ears as well as fingers and toes.
- Initially cold-induced lesions may be urticarial (see 🕮 p.214), but then become purpuric and blister or ulcerate.

Type II and type III mixed cryoglobulinaemia

- Type II: monoclonal and polyclonal immunoglobulins (25% of cases).
- Type III: polyclonal immunoglobulins (50% of cases).
- Immune complexes precipitated in vessel walls induce a small-vessel vasculitis that can affect many organs.
- ***Associations:*** connective tissue diseases, e.g. rheumatoid arthritis or SLE; infections especially hepatitis C virus (HCV) infection in type II mixed cryoglobulinaemia. HCV infection triggers B-cell clonal expansions that may be associated with monoclonal gammopathy or, rarely, non-Hodgkin B-cell lymphoma.

What should I look for?

- Palpable purpura: the first sign in most patients.
- Arthralgia (70%).
- Sensorimotor neuropathy (60%).
- Raynaud's phenomenon (30%).
- Renal involvement (20–30%).
- Chronic leg ulcers (15%), usually above the malleoli, surrounded by purpura, but without signs of venous stasis.

What should I do?

See Boxes 20.4–20.6 for investigation and management.

Box 20.4 Investigation of cryoglobulinaemia

- Type II or III mixed cryoglobulinaemia: measure complement C4, which is low in mixed cryoglobulinaemia and is easier to measure than cryoglobulins as the blood does not have to be kept warm. If C4 is low, measure cryoglobulins—see Box 20.5.
- Type 1 cryoglobulinaemia: measure cryoglobulins and RF.
- Take a skin biopsy from a purpuric lesion or the edge of an ulcer.

Dermal blood vessels are plugged by homogeneous eosinophilic material in monoclonal cryoglobulinaemia. You will see a vasculitis in mixed cryoglobulinaemia.

Box 20.5 Measuring cryoglobins

- The clotted blood specimen must be kept warm (37°C).
- Place the container in a Thermos flask for transportation to the laboratory.
- It may be easier to send the patient to the laboratory for venesection.

Box 20.6 Management of cryoglobulinaemia

- Treat underlying disease.
- Warmth:
  - Keep the trunk warm with thermal underwear.
  - Recommend thermal gloves and thermal socks.
  - Footwear should have thick soles.
- Control venous stasis with compression bandaging to promote healing of leg ulcers. Badly applied ridged bandages with uneven skin pressure may exacerbate cutaneous vasculitis—see 📖 p.286.
- Consider corticosteroids in combination with cytotoxic agents, but response is variable.
- Plasmapheresis has been used to treat progressive vasculitis.

Further reading

Sansonno D and Dammacco F. *Lancet Infect Dis* 2005; **5**:227–36.

ANCA-associated vasculitis

ANCA-associated vasculitis is rare, but is the commonest primary systemic vasculitis affecting adults. The vasculitis involves both small and medium-sized vessels.

Cutaneous findings are not specific. The diagnosis is based on the evidence of systemic vasculitis, which may be life threatening, not the cutaneous findings.

Subtypes

The 3 major subtypes have overlapping features:

- Wegener's granulomatosis: granulomatous inflammation of the upper and lower airways, necrotizing small-vessel vasculitis and necrotizing glomerulonephritis. Patients may have non-specific symptoms such as nasal stuffiness, nose bleeds, sinus pain, ear pain, or red eye.
- Microscopic polyangiitis: necrotizing glomerulonephritis, pulmonary capillaritis without asthma, necrotizing small-vessel vasculitis.
- Churg–Strauss syndrome: allergic rhinitis and asthma, eosinophilia, necrotizing small-vessel vasculitis, and eosinophil-rich and granulomatous inflammation involving the respiratory tract.

What should I look for?

- Evidence of systemic disease: take a thorough history and perform a full physical examination including fundoscopy and a neurological examination.
- Systemic symptoms such as fever, malaise, arthralgia, and myalgia.
- A palpable purpuric rash on legs secondary to small-vessel cutaneous vasculitis is common in all types of ANCA-associated vasculitis.
- Livedo reticularis, ulcers, or subcutaneous nodules indicate involvement of larger cutaneous vessels (see 📖 p.418).
- Progressive painful ulceration of the face, neck or perianal skin, resembling pyoderma gangrenosum (see 📖 p.290) is associated with Wegener's granulomatosis.
- Ulcerated papules on the limbs, particularly the elbows (like rheumatoid nodules), but also on the face and scalp may occur in Wegener's granulomatosis and Churg–Strauss syndrome.
- An underlying cause: e.g. infection including HIV, autoimmune disease, drugs, malignancy.

What should I do?

- Baseline investigations to assess disease activity and organ involvement—see 📖 Box 20.7.
- Further investigation will be guided by the findings, e.g. patients with nodules on the chest radiograph may need high-resolution CT.
- Biopsy of internal organs is usually required to confirm the diagnosis.
- Biopsy of cutaneous lesions may show a vasculitis, but will not distinguish between different forms of ANCA-associated vasculitis.
- ANCA-associated vasculitides are managed using immunosuppressive drugs such as prednisolone, azathioprine, and cyclophosphamide. There may be a role for drugs such as rituximab, which depletes B-cells.

Box 20.7 Baseline investigations in systemic vasculitis

- Urine dipstick: if proteinuria is detected, quantify protein loss with a 24-h urine or protein-creatinine ratio.
- Urine microscopy to look for cellular casts.
- FBC.
- ESR, CRP.
- Renal function.
- Complement levels.
- ANA, RF, ANCA.
- Antiphospholipid antibodies and lupus anticoagulant when indicated e.g. in patients with SLE who have recurrent venous/arterial thrombosis, cerebral thrombosis, recurrent fetal loss, pulmonary hypertension, and/or livedo reticularis.
- CXR.
- Cutaneous nodules: take a deep incisional biopsy extending down to fat to detect pathology in arterioles or small arteries. The pathology will not distinguish between different forms of ANCA-associated vasculitis.

Further reading

Chen KO and Carlson JA. *Am J Clin Dermatol* 2008; **9**:71–92.

Septic cutaneous vasculitis

Vascular damage may occur in infective endocarditis, meningococcaemia, chronic gonococcaemia, Gram-negative septicaemia, and rickettsial infections. Septic vasculitis can also follow any intravascular procedure.

The vasculitis tends to involve both small and medium-sized vessels. Organisms damage blood vessels by direct invasion, release of endotoxins that provoke thrombosis (disseminated intravascular coagulation (DIC)), and immune complex-mediated vasculitis.

⚠ Infective endocarditis

Signs include splinter haemorrhages in nails, mucosal petechiae, Osler's nodes (tender erythematous spots on the pulps of fingertips and toes), and Janeway's lesions (non-tender red or haemorrhagic macules or nodules on palms and soles).

►► Acute meningococcaemia

A life-threatening illness that must be treated immediately with IV antibiotics, e.g. cefotaxime 2g. Purpuric lesions develop on limbs or trunk within 12–36h of the onset of infection. These may be small and few in number. Purpura fulminans with DIC is a devastating complication—see 📖 p.96.

Fibrin thrombi occlude capillaries, venules, and vessels in the deeper dermis and subcutis leading to ischaemia and infarction. Persistent cyanosis of the extremities is an early warning sign. Large irregular indurated ecchymoses become necrotic, blister, and may progress to extensive gangrene.

⚠ Gram-negative septicaemia (*Escherichia coli*, *Pseudomonas*, or *Klebsiella*)

Septic emboli produce erythematous wheals and papules that become irregularly purpuric and necrotic.

Chronic meningococcaemia and chronic disseminated gonococcaemia

Rare immune-complex mediated illnesses associated with fever, arthralgia, arthritis, and a cutaneous vasculitis. Look for scattered purpuric papules and vesicopustules on trunk and extremities (meningococcaemia) or palms, fingers, and toes (gonococcaemia). These may be few in number.

⚠ Rocky Mountain spotted fever

Rickettsia rickettsii invades the walls of small cutaneous vessels inducing a focal lymphocytic vasculitis. Look for an erythematous maculopapular rash that becomes petechial and purpuric within 24–48h.

⚠ Septic vasculitis after percutaneous arterial puncture

Signs suggest unilateral cutaneous emboli: local infarction, livedo, and/or retiform purpura.

Cutaneous involvement in medium-sized and large-vessel vasculitis

Polyarteritis nodosa

Polyarteritis nodosa (PAN) is a life-threatening systemic necrotizing segmental vasculitis that involves vessels ranging in size from arterioles to medium-sized arteries.

Cutaneous manifestations are infrequent but may include palpable purpura (small-vessel cutaneous vasculitis) or, less often, livedo reticularis, cutaneous nodules, ulcers, and peripheral gangrene (medium to large vessel vasculitis).

Cutaneous polyarteritis nodosa

A necrotizing vasculitis affects small and medium-sized muscular wall arteries in the deep dermis and subcutis. Major organs are not involved, but the disease is chronic and recurrent.

What should I look for?

- Painful cutaneous nodules, palpable purpura, ulceration, and livedo reticularis on the legs.
- Fever, malaise, arthralgia, and myalgia.
- Peripheral neuropathy.

What should I do?

- Screen for systemic vasculitis. Laboratory findings are unremarkable, except for leucocytosis and an elevated ESR.
- Ensure patient is not hypertensive.
- Take a deep incisional biopsy to demonstrate vascular pathology in arterioles or small arteries.
- Control pain with NSAIDs, paracetamol, morphine, or amitriptyline.
- Try compression bandaging (may not be tolerated).
- Consider pentoxifylline or low-dose methotrexate (evidence lacking for efficacy).

Nodular vasculitis

See 📖 p.426.

⚠ Giant cell arteritis (temporal arteritis)

This granulomatous panarteritis of the large and medium-sized arteries, particularly those of the head and neck, generally affects patients >60 years of age. Some patients also have polymyalgia rheumatica. Both conditions are more common in women.

Complications include retinal artery inflammation with sudden irreversible blindness or, less often, stroke.

What should I look for?

- A history of recent severe headache, scalp tenderness (noticed when combing hair or lying on a pillow), jaw claudication, and/or visual disturbance (transient loss, diplopia, ptosis).
- Systemic symptoms such as fever, malaise, or weight loss.

- Rarely, a tender non-pulsatile temporal artery or a tender scalp nodule that may resemble a BCC, particularly if ulcerated.
- Pallor of the optic disc, retinal haemorrhages and exudates, optic atrophy (late finding).

What should I do?
- Measure ESR and CRP: usually very high.
- Arrange a biopsy of the temporal artery, but disease is patchy and the artery may look normal.
- ►► Prescribe high-dose oral corticosteroids, prednisolone 30mg/day for headaches, and, if visual symptoms, >40mg/day immediately to prevent blindness without waiting for the diagnosis to be confirmed.

Thrombo-occlusive vasculopathies

These conditions are characterized by vascular occlusion without frank vasculitis. Also see 📖 p.414 and p.96.

⚠ Livedo reticularis (livedo racemosa)

Livedo reticularis is seen most often on the legs. The mottled reddish-purple reticulated discoloration reflects sluggish vascular flow in the superficial dermis. A continuous livedo network is likely to be physiological and will disappear when the skin is warmed.

A broken (discontinuous) persistent livedo reticularis is seen with:

- Hyperviscosity states: polycythaemia rubra vera, antiphospholipid syndrome—see Box 20.8, type 1 cryoglobulinaemia (see 📖 p.410).
- Medium- or large-vessel vasculitis: connective tissue diseases, PAN, Wegener's granulomatosis (see 📖 p.412).
- Cholesterol emboli and other emboli; calciphylaxis (see 📖 p.292).

What should I look for? (Fig. 20.4)

- A mottled reddish-purple reticulated discoloration, usually on limbs.
- Retiform purpura (purpura in a reticulate or net-like distribution).
- Is the skin cold? Does the discoloration disappear when the skin is warmed, indicating a physiological change of no significance?
- Is the discoloration a continuous network or discontinuous?
- Signs of a vasculitis affecting medium or large cutaneous vessels, e.g. subcutaneous nodules or ulcers.

Differential diagnosis

- Erythema ab igne, a reticulated brown staining that can develop if skin is exposed chronically to heat from a radiator, open fire, or hot water bottle (Fig. 20.5).

What should I do?

- If the livedo is physiological, no investigation or treatment is required.
- If the livedo is discontinuous and persistent:
  - Screen for underlying disease—see earlier in this section.
  - Take deep biopsies that extend into fat to demonstrate diagnostic pathology in arterioles or small arteries such as cholesterol emboli or hyaline thrombi.

Livedoid vasculopathy with ulceration

Synonyms: segmental hyalinizing vasculitis, livedo reticularis with summer/winter ulceration, livedoid vasculitis.

This thrombo-occlusive vasculopathy affects young to middle-aged women. Hyaline thrombi occlude small vessels in the upper and mid-dermis leading to painful ulceration that is chronic and recurrent—see 📖 p.294.

Further reading

Jorizzo JL. *Arch Dermatol* 1998; **134:**491–3.

Box 20.8 ⚠ What is the antiphospholipid syndrome?

This thrombo-occlusive vasculopathy presents most often in females. Anticardiolipin antibodies, lupus anticoagulant antibodies, and/or anti-β2 glycoprotein 1 antibodies cause microvascular occlusion. Many patients have SLE. Anticoagulants or antiplatelet agents are the mainstay of treatment. Cutaneous features include:

- Livedo reticularis and retiform purpura; livedoid vasculopathy—see 📖 p.294.
- Purpuric lesions simulating vasculitis.
- Atrophie blanche-like scars—see 📖 Fig. 12.3, p.227.
- Raynaud's phenomenon and digital gangrene.
- Nail fold ulcers, splinter haemorrhages.
- Superficial thrombophlebitis migrans, leg ulcers.
- Cutaneous necrosis which may be limited or, rarely, widespread.

Extracutaneous features include:

- Complications in pregnancy such as unexplained fetal deaths, premature births, or unexplained spontaneous abortions.
- Sneddon's syndrome: CVAs with livedo reticularis and labile hypertension.
- Pulmonary embolus, DVT.

Further reading

George D and Erkan D. *Prog Cardiovasc Dis* 2009; **52**:115–25.

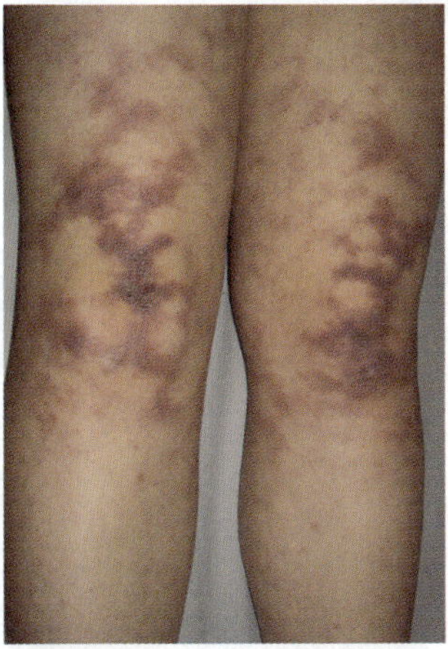

Fig. 20.4 Livedo reticularis in a discontinuous network.

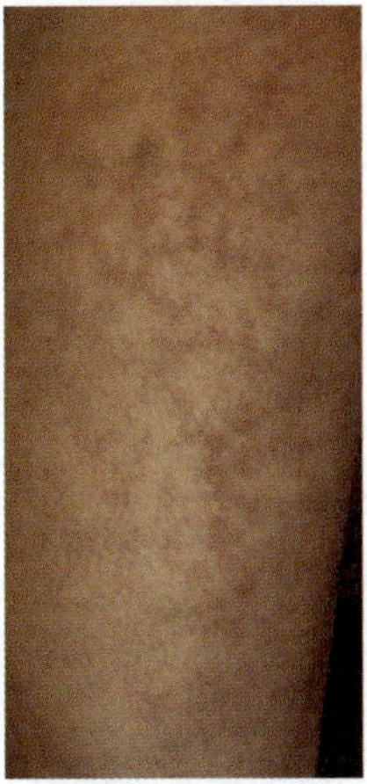

Fig. 20.5 Erythema ab igne—reticulate brownish pigmentation on the thigh of a patient who was snuggling up to a hot water bottle.

Chapter 21

Panniculitis

Contents

Introduction

Inflammation of subcutaneous fat is known as panniculitis. Panniculitis is characterized by erythematous nodules. Depending on the cause of panniculitis, nodules may resolve without loss of fat and change in contour, or cause fat necrosis (that may discharge) and leave a depression.

The inflammation may commence in the fat or spread into the fat from the adjacent dermis. The panniculitides are classified histologically into predominantly septal or predominantly lobular patterns of inflammation and some types are associated with vasculitis—see Box 21.1.

Some types of panniculitis, such as erythema nodosum, may indicate an underlying systemic disease.

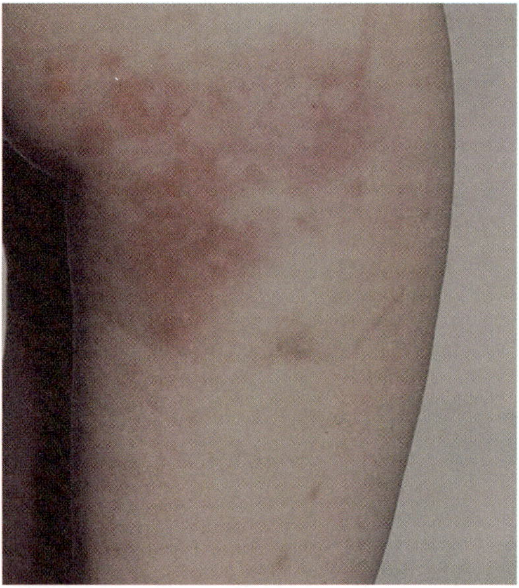

Fig. 21.1 Cold panniculitis in a young female horse-rider.

Further reading

Requena L *et al. J Am Acad Dermatol* 2001; **45:**163–83.
Requena L *et al. J Am Acad Dermatol* 2001; **45:**325–61.

Box 21.1 Types of panniculitis

Septal panniculitis

With large vessel vasculitis:

- Superficial thrombophlebitis.
- Cutaneous polyarteritis nodosa—see 📖 p.416.

No vasculitis:

- Erythema nodosum—see 📖 p.424.
- Rheumatoid nodule—see 📖 p.365, 366.
- Necrobiosis lipoidica—see 📖 p.434.
- Scleroderma and eosinophilic fasciitis—see 📖 p.390.

Lobular panniculitis

With large vessel vasculitis:

- Nodular vasculitis—see 📖 p.426.

No vasculitis:

- α1-Antitrypsin deficiency—see 📖 p.428.
- Cold panniculitis: seen most often in the winter in plump, young female horse-riders wearing tight jodhpurs that provide insufficient insulation and restrict the blood supply to the subcutaneous fat. Mottled bluish-red chilblain-like plaques appear on thighs 'Chiltern chaps' and buttocks 'Berkshire buttocks'—📖 Fig. 21.1, p.422. The plaques resolve without scarring. Riders should wear loose-fitting warm clothing.
- Sclerosing panniculitis (also known as lipodermatosclerosis)—seen on the lower leg in association with venous insufficiency (see 📖 p.288).
- Calcific uraemic arteriolopathy (calciphylaxis)—see 📖 p.292.
- Lupus panniculitis (lupus profundus)—see 📖 Box 19.8, p.375.
- Pancreatic panniculitis—see 📖 p.428.
- Infective panniculitis (infections of subcutaneous fat in immunosuppressed patients).
- Traumatic or factitious panniculitis—see 📖 p.524.
- Cytophagic histiocytic panniculitis and subcutaneous T-cell lymphoma.

Weber–Christian disease

Weber-Christian disease is no longer considered to be a distinct entity. This term was used to describe a nodular, relapsing panniculitis with fever and lipoatrophy. Subsequently most cases considered to be examples of Weber–Christian disease have been given more specific diagnoses.

Reference: White JW *et al. J Am Acad Dermatol* 1998; **39**:56–62. (Discusses Weber–Christian panniculitis.)

Erythema nodosum

What is erythema nodosum (EN)?

EN is the most common type of panniculitis. It is a septal panniculitis. Vasculitis is not a feature of typical erythema nodosum.

EN may be a hypersensitivity response to an infection or to an underlying inflammatory disease (see Box 21.2) but no cause is identified in about 1/3 of cases.

Most cases appear between the 2nd and 4th decades, with a peak incidence between the ages of 20–30. EN is more common in women. Cases usually occur in the first half of the year, possibly because of an increase in streptococcal infections. The prognosis depends on the underlying disease. Idiopathic EN is a self-limiting condition with an excellent prognosis. Relapses are uncommon.

What should I look for?

- Underlying triggers—see Box 21.2.
- Tender, erythematous (no purpura), warm nodules, measuring 1–5cm or more in diameter (Fig. 21.2).
- A symmetrical distribution on the shins, ankles, and knees—see Box 21.3 and 📖 Table 21.1, p.427, for differential diagnosis.
- Less often nodules appear on the arms or trunk.
- EN does not ulcerate.
- Fever, malaise, arthralgia, and headache.
- Sometimes gastrointestinal problems such as abdominal pain, vomiting, or diarrhoea.
- Nodules fade over 2–6 weeks (more quickly in children) leaving a purplish bruise-like appearance that slowly resolves.
- Absence of scarring (nodules do not leave a depression—contour goes back to normal).
- A chronic migratory variant (subacute nodular migratory panniculitis, erythema nodosum migrans) is much less common. The tender indurated erythematous plaque may be asymmetrical.

What should I do?

- Check FBC, ESR, urinalysis, and chest radiography.
- Further investigations should be guided by the history, examination, and local prevalence of aetiological factors such as bacterial, viral, fungal, or protozoal infections.
- If required, take a deep elliptical biopsy that includes fat (biopsy is usually unnecessary).
- Manage any underlying problem such as infection.
- Provide pain relief with NSAIDs.
- Elevation may relieve pain in acute disease.
- Support stockings control swelling and may speed resolution.
- Potassium iodide 200–600mg/day has been recommended in persistent disease.
- Rarely oral corticosteroids are required, but exclude infection before prescribing.

Box 21.2 Causes of erythema nodosum

No cause is identified in about 1/3 of cases:

- Infection: bacterial (often streptococcal in children), viral, protozoal, and fungal.
- Drugs.
- Sarcoidosis (EN and bilateral hilar adenopathy)—see 📖 p.486.
- Inflammatory bowel disease.
- Pregnancy.
- Miscellaneous conditions.

Box 21.3 Differential diagnosis of erythema nodosum

1 or more erythematous nodules in an asymmetrical distribution consider:

- Trauma.
- Cellulitis.
- Insect bite.
- Superficial thrombophlebitis—cord-like nodules usually on the side of one leg.

Symmetrical nodules consider:

- Nodular vasculitis (erythema induratum of Bazin). The nodules, which tend to be on calves rather than shins, ulcerate and heal with scarring (loss of fat)—see 📖 p.426 and Table 21.1, p.427.

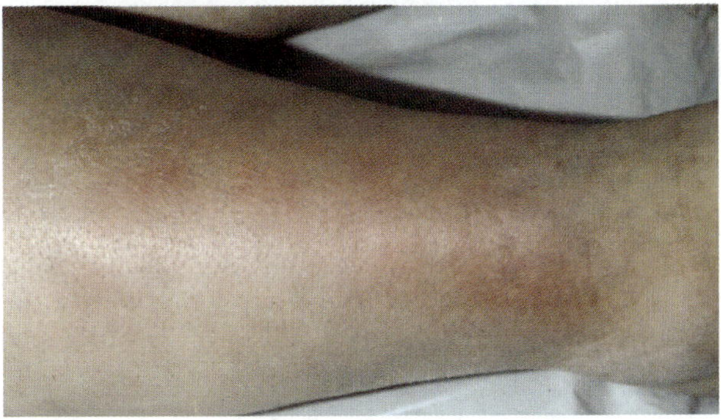

Fig. 21.2 Erythema nodosum with smooth tender erythematous nodules on both shins.

Nodular vasculitis (erythema induratum of Bazin)

What is nodular vasculitis?

Nodular vasculitis is the most common form of lobular panniculitis with vasculitis. It is considered to be a 'reactive disorder'. Bazin described this form of vasculitis in 1861 and a link with TB was recognized in the early 1900s. *Mycobacterium tuberculosis* DNA has been demonstrated in cutaneous biopsy specimens.

In many patients no underlying trigger is identified. Nodular vasculitis is common in obese middle-aged women in whom venous stasis and cooling may play some part in the localization to the leg. The condition runs a protracted course over many years.

What should I look for?

- History of recurrent nodules that form slowly and equally slowly resolve.
- Tender erythematous indurated nodules and plaques on the calves (rather than the shins) of fat legs where skin is cyanotic and cold.
- Ulceration of nodules (unlike EN—see Table 21.1).
- Atrophic scars (depressions) where ulcerated nodules have healed.
- Venous insufficiency of the lower legs (a frequent association).
- Any indications in history and examination of an underlying disease such as TB.

What should I do?

- Take a deep incisional biopsy to demonstrate the pathology.
- Exclude TB by chest radiography and Mantoux test. Treat TB if identified.
- Control venous stasis by weight loss, compression bandages, elevation, and exercise.
- Relieve pain with NSAIDs.
- Corticosteroids are not indicated.

Table 21.1 Differential diagnosis

	Erythema nodosum	Nodular vasculitis
Presentation	Acute	Indolent
Distribution	Shins	Calves
Signs	Tender warm erythematous nodules	Tender erythematous nodules and plaques that may ulcerate
Resolution	Resolves in a few weeks leaving a bruise-like mark that slowly fades	Heals slowly over months leaving an atrophic scar
Prognosis	Relapses uncommon	Relapse common. Course is protracted lasting many years

Uncommon causes of panniculitis

⚠ Alpha-1-antitrypsin (AAT) deficiency panniculitis

AAT is a circulating serine protease inhibitor (serpin). AAT inhibits enzymes (e.g. trypsin, collagenase, elastase) involved in the proteolytic degradation of tissues, has effects on the immune system, and inhibits activation of complement.

Mutations in the AAT gene may cause enzyme deficiency or abnormal enzyme function. Patients may develop emphysema, pancreatitis, chronic liver disease with cirrhosis, glomerulonephritis, rheumatoid arthritis, vasculitis, and/or angio-oedema. Rarely AAT deficiency is associated with an acute lobular panniculitis accompanied by fat necrosis (seen in adults more often than children). Patients with a partial deficiency of AAT may have panniculitis without systemic disease.

Approximately 70 000–100 000 individuals in the USA and Europe have AAT deficiency. Enzyme function may be significantly impaired despite normal serum levels of AAT, but most cases associated with panniculitis have the ZZ phenotype with AAT levels below normal.

What should I look for?

- Recurrent erythematous plaques and nodules in a proximal distribution on hips, thighs, and buttocks.
- Panniculitis that is induced or exacerbated by trauma.
- Characteristically nodules suppurate with the release of oily material (uncommon in other forms of panniculitis).
- Associated diseases including emphysema, hepatitis and/or cirrhosis, vasculitis, and angio-oedema.

What should I do?

- Take a deep biopsy from a fresh nodule to reveal the suppurative lobular panniculitis.
- Only check the serum level of AAT and the AAT phenotype if the clinical and histological findings are compatible with panniculitis associated with AAT deficiency.
- Dapsone may be effective in mild cases (inhibits neutrophil migration and function).
- Oral tetracyclines (doxycycline 200mg ×2/day) may have a direct effect on serine proteases released from neutrophils and can help some patients.
- NSAIDs and hydroxychloroquine have been recommended.
- Replacement therapy using IV infusions of AAT controls panniculitis effectively.

Pancreatic panniculitis

A characteristic form of panniculitis has been described (rarely) in association with a number of pancreatic diseases including:

- Acute or chronic pancreatitis
- Pancreatic islet cell tumours
- Ductal adenocarcinoma
- Acinar-cell carcinoma

- Post-traumatic pancreatitis
- Pancreatic pseudocysts.

Circulating lipase and/or amylase may be responsible for destruction of fat. The cutaneous signs may present some months before the manifestations of pancreatic disease. Disseminated fat necrosis is associated with a high mortality.

What should I look for?

- Subcutaneous erythematous or reddish-brown nodules, usually on the legs, but sometimes on thighs, arms, buttock, and/or trunk—see Fig. 21.3.
- Nodules may soften in the centre.
- Nodules may be painful or painless.
- In mild cases, nodules heal with atrophic scarring.
- In severe cases, nodules may ulcerate and discharge sterile brown oily material (necrotic fat).
- May be associated with arthritis (necrosis of periarticular fat) and plural effusions.

What should I do?

- Search for evidence of pancreatic disease including measurement of serum amylase.
- Biopsy a nodule. The histology of pancreatic panniculitis is characteristic with fat necrosis, basophilic granular material (fatty acids combine with calcium to form calcium soap), and 'ghost-like' cells (adipocytes with thick shadowy walls- the cell membrane resists lipase).
- Treat underlying condition.

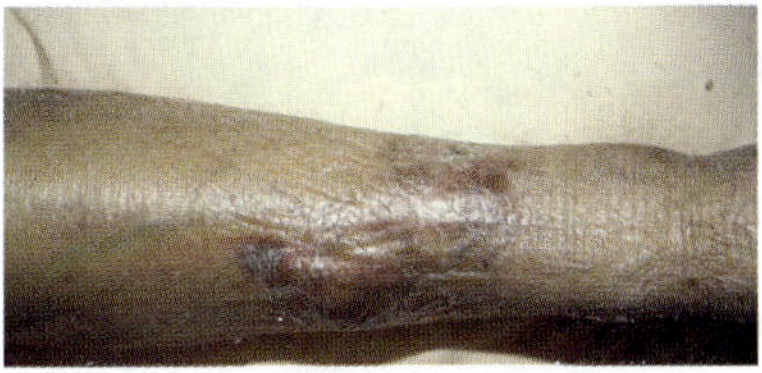

Fig. 21.3 Reddish-brown nodules that discharged oily fluid in a patient with pancreatic cancer.

Chapter 22

Diabetes and endocrinology

Contents

Relevant pages in other chapters

Flushing 📖 p.70, 482.
Erythrasma 📖 p.124.
Bacterial folliculitis 📖 p.126.
Cellulitis 📖 p.130.
Candida 📖 p.158.
Ulcers 📖 p.274.
Calcific uraemic arteriolopathy 📖 p.292.
Neuropathies 📖 p.504, 506.
Melasma 📖 Box 30.1, p.539.

Diabetes mellitus and the skin

Chronic diabetes affects microcirculation as well as skin collagen and cutaneous problems are common. These include specific manifestations of diabetes, complications such as neuropathy (see 📖 p.504, 506), skin infections (Box 22.1), and cutaneous adverse effects related to treatment. Type 1 diabetes (autoimmune) is less common than type 2 diabetes (defective insulin action or secretion).

Diabetes: what should I look for?

- Linear periungual telangiectasia without loss of capillary loops—compare with systemic sclerosis in which capillaries are lost.
- Periungual erythema, ragged cuticles, and tender fingertips.
- Diabetic hand syndrome: scleroderma-like thickening on dorsum of hands with knuckle pads and papules on periungual skin and sides of fingers; and sclerosing tenosynovitis of palmar flexor tendons with stiffness of metacarpophalangeal and proximal interphalangeal joints. Mild flexion contractures may limit ability to press hand flat on a table or to oppose palmar surfaces of fingers. May also have Dupuytren's contractures and carpal tunnel syndrome.
- Diabetic dermopathy or shin spots (round or oval erythematous papules or pigmented scars on shins). Associated with microvascular complications.
- Neuropathic ulcers on feet (check shoes), onychomycosis, or tinea pedis.
- Necrobiosis lipoidica diabeticorum on shins. May ulcerate—see 📖 p.434.
- Diabetic bullae: asymptomatic bullae on non-inflamed skin. Seen most often on legs and feet. Cause is unknown but the differential includes bullous impetigo, porphyria cutanea tarda, and autoimmune blistering diseases. Bullae resolve without scarring in 2–3 weeks.
- Vitiligo: well-demarcated, depigmented macules and patches with a smooth surface. Check for other autoimmune diseases—see 📖 p.452.
- Lipohypertrophy (like a lipoma) at sites of insulin injections. Lipoatrophy is uncommon since the introduction of recombinant human insulin.
- Lipodystrophy, acquired or inherited, is a very rare cause of insulin resistance with diabetes and hypertriglyceridaemia—see 📖 Box 22.4, p.437.
- Neuropathic itch—see 📖 p.504.
- Eruptive xanthoma (itchy yellow papules on extensor surfaces and buttocks) seen in association with elevated triglycerides—see 📖 p.436.
- Skin tags and (pseudo) acanthosis nigricans: velvety thickening in skin folds. Seen in obese patients with insulin resistance and high levels of circulating insulin. Insulin has a growth-hormone-like action on skin. Encourage patients to lose weight. Acanthosis nigricans may respond to a topical retinoid such as 0.05% tazarotene gel. Also see HAIR-AN syndrome—see 📖 p.442
- Scleroedema diabeticorum (see Box 22.2).
- Calcific uraemic arteriolopathy (see 📖 p.292), acquired perforating dermatosis in diabetes with renal failure—see 📖 Fig. 23.1, p.457 and p.458.

Box 22.1 Cutaneous infections in diabetes mellitus

Candidal infections

- Look for scaly flexural erythema with satellite pustules. Chronic paronychia (inflammation of nail fold) may also be caused by *Candida*.
- *Candida* causing angular cheilitis, vulvitis, or balanitis may be a presenting sign of diabetes. Pruritus vulvae or ani is often caused by *Candida* infection.

Dermatophyte infections

- Look for a well-demarcated scaly rash, most often in an asymmetrical distribution, involving palms or soles. May also have onychomycosis.
- Ulceration produced by a thickened toenail digging into the adjacent toe, or fissuring of the dry scaly skin, may provide a portal of entry for bacterial infection.

Bacterial infections

- Impetigo, folliculitis, and erysipelas may be severe and widespread in patients with diabetes.
- Erythrasma presents with a glazed erythema or hyperpigmentation in flexures. Look for coral fluorescence when examined with a Wood's lamp—see 🕮 p. 568.
- Life-threatening cutaneous infections may be caused by organisms such as *Pseudomonas aeruginosa* and *Clostridium* species, particularly when diabetes is not well controlled.

Box 22.2 What is scleroedema diabeticorum?

This slowly progressive and persistent cutaneous mucinosis occurs in longstanding poorly controlled diabetes. (Compare with scleroedema of Buschke in which dermal thickening of skin on face, arms and hands develops suddenly after infection and resolves in months or years.) Phototherapy with UV-A1 may reduce induration and improve mobility, but long-term controlled studies of therapy are needed. Look for:

- Thickening of the skin of the posterior neck and upper back limiting mobility of the neck and shoulders. Occasionally changes extend to the deltoid and lumbar regions.
- Non-pitting induration with a peau d'orange appearance.
- Sometimes reduced sensitivity to pain and touch.
- Normal FBC, unlike eosinophilic fasciitis (eosinophilia)—see 🕮 p.391.
- No paraprotein, unlike scleromyxoedema (paraproteinaemia)—see 🕮 Box 26.7, p.499.
- Histopathologically: swollen dermal collagen bundles separated by mucin, but skin biopsy is not usually required to make the diagnosis.

Further reading

Van Hattem S *et al.* *Cleveland Clin J Med* 2008 **75:**774–86.

Yosipovitch G *et al.* *Diabetes Care* 1998 **21:**506–9.

Necrobiosis lipoidica

Necrobiosis lipoidica occurs most often in women. It usually presents on the shins but may affect other areas. The reddish-yellow plaques enlarge slowly and are generally asymptomatic unless they ulcerate. The pathogenesis of the granulomatous inflammation (see 📖 Box 32.5, p.579) is uncertain, but many cases are associated with diabetes (necrobiosis lipoidica diabeticorum). Necrobiosis lipoidica shares some features with granuloma annulare, another granulomatous condition, but one which is associated with diabetes only rarely—see Box 22.3.

What should I look for?

- Oval, well-demarcated papules or plaques, usually on the shin (may be bilateral) that expand slowly and may coalesce (Fig. 22.1).
- Reddish-brown plaques that are smooth, shiny, and telangiectatic.
- The border is erythematous and may be scalloped in outline.
- In older plaques, the reddish centre is more yellow and may be atrophic, revealing deeper subcutaneous vessels (Fig. 22.1).
- Plaques may ulcerate, but the surrounding intact skin generally has some features of necrobiosis lipoidica.
- Some patients also have granuloma annulare—see Box 22.3 and Fig. 22.2.

What should I do?

- If necessary take a deep elliptical biopsy to confirm the diagnosis but the wound may not heal. The histological features, which overlap with those of granuloma annulare, include extensive dermal necrobiosis (alteration of collagen bundles) outlined by histiocytes and giant cells.
- Treatment options include topical and intra-lesional corticosteroids, and topical 0.1% tacrolimus, but response is variable.
- Topical corticosteroids, pentoxifylline, and nicotinamide with minocycline have been advocated for ulcerated necrobiosis lipoidica.

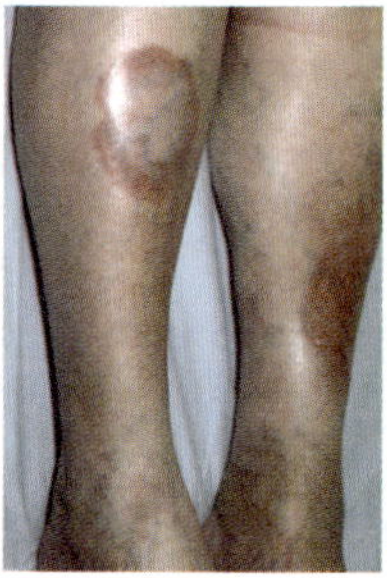

Fig. 22.1 Necrobiosis lipoidica.

Box 22.3 What is granuloma annulare?

- Granuloma annulare is a chronic non-infectious inflammatory condition. The cause is unknown, but rarely extensive disease is linked to diabetes. Sometimes patients also have necrobiosis lipoidica.
- Any age group can be affected, but granuloma annulare is most common in children.
- 1 or more asymptomatic skin-coloured or erythematous ring-like marks appear on the skin, most often on limbs.
- Most people only have 1 or 2 annular lesions, but granuloma annulare may be widespread (disseminated) (Fig. 22.2).
- In children granuloma annulare tends to affect the backs of the hands or the dorsum of the feet.
- Stretch the skin and you will see that the raised border is composed of coalescing papules that may be umbilicated.
- The surface is smooth (unlike tinea which is scaly).
- Rings slowly expand and develop a purplish-red colour.
- The lesions may persist for several years but eventually fade to leave normal skin.
- Subcutaneous granuloma annulare presents as nodules, sometimes on the fingers when they may simulate rheumatoid nodules.
- The histological features (granulomatous inflammation with necrobiosis) overlap with those of necrobiosis lipoidica.
- Treatment is unsatisfactory, but generally is not required. Topical corticosteroids, intralesional corticosteroids, oral retinoids, tetracyclines, and phototherapy have been used with variable success.

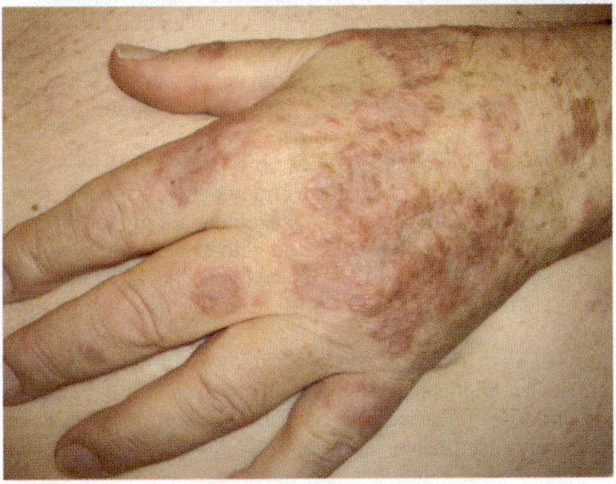

Fig. 22.2 Granuloma annulare with disseminated smooth purplish papules and annular plaques.

Hyperlipoproteinaemias

The hyperlipoproteinaemias are classified according to which of the 4 classes of lipoproteins (chylomicrons, very low-density lipoprotein = VLDL, low-density lipoprotein = LDL or beta-VLDL) are elevated (Table 22.1). Hyperlipoproteinaemia may be primary or secondary to an underlying problem such as obesity, diabetes mellitus, renal disease, cholestatic liver disease, alcohol abuse, hypothyroidism, hyperuricaemia, or drugs.

Lipodystrophy is a rare cause of diabetes with hypertriglyceridaemia—see Box 22.4.

Identification is important because of the risk of coronary artery disease. Cutaneous xanthomas (lipid deposits in the skin) are a marker of hyperlipoproteinaemia. The type of xanthoma correlates with the underlying cause—see Table 22.1.

What should I look for?

- Eruptive xanthomas: clusters of yellowish papules with erythematous halos on the extensor surfaces of arms and legs, shoulders, and buttocks. Itch is common as they regress (primary and secondary hypertriglyceridaemia).
- Tendon xanthomas: firm subcutaneous nodules on Achilles tendon and over other extensor tendons including the dorsum of interphalangeal joints (knuckles), patellae, and elbows. May become inflamed. Skin is a normal colour and is not yellow (primary and secondary hypercholesterolaemia)
- Tuberous xanthomas: firm yellow papules and nodules found over large joints (knees, elbows), the heels, or the dorsum of interphalangeal joints (primary and secondary hyperlipidaemia).
- Plane xanthomas: yellow macules with a predilection for face, upper trunk, and scars. Orange-yellow plane xanthomas may also be found in palmar creases (striate palmar xanthomas, 'bread and butter' palms). (type III and secondary hypercholesterolemia). Generalized plane xanthoma may be found in myeloma.
- Xanthelasma: soft yellowish papules on eyelids or below eyes. Common in the normal population and not a very specific sign, but may be associated with hypercholesterolaemia if present in young patients. Xanthelasmas are associated with cholestatic liver disease.
- Corneal arcus may be linked to familial hypercholesterolaemia but is more likely to be significant if present in adolescence or early adulthood.
- Lipaemia retinalis (pallor of the optic fundus with white retinal veins and arteries) seen in severe hypertriglyceridaemia.
- Signs of underlying disease such as diabetes, hypothyroidism, nephrotic syndrome, cholestatic liver disease, or, very rarely, lipodystrophy.

Table 22.1 Primary hyperlipidaemias and xanthomas

Frederickson classification	Biochemistry	Signs
Type I familial hyperchylomicronaemia	Severe hypertriglyceridaemia (raised chylomicrons)	Eruptive xanthomas, lipaemia retinalis hepatosplenomegaly
Type IIa familial hypercholesterolaemia or familial defective apoB	Hypercholesterolaemia (raised LDL)	Tendon xanthomas Tuberous xanthomas
Type IIb familial combined hyperlipidaemia	Hypercholesterolaemia with hypertriglyceridaemia (raised LDL and VLDL)	Usually no xanthomas
Type III familial dysbetalipoproteinaemia (Broad beta disease)	Hypercholesterolaemia with hypertriglyceridaemia (raised beta-VLDL)	Plane xanthomas on palms Tuberous xanthomas
Type IV familial hypertriglyceridaemia (may be secondary to diabetes or excess alcohol)	Moderate hypertriglyceridaemia (raised VLDL)	Usually no xanthomas
Type V familial hypertriglyceridaemia	Severe hypertriglyceridaemia (raised chylomicrons and VLDL)	Eruptive xanthomas lipaemia retinalis hepatosplenomegaly

Box 22.4 Lipodystrophies

Acquired lipodystrophies

- Localized secondary to pressure, injected drugs (corticosteroids), panniculitis or unknown causes.
- HIV infection treated with protease inhibitors—subcutaneous fat lost from face and limbs. Subcutaneous fat deposited on trunk.
- Low serum C3 and glomerulonephritis with autoantibodies (C3 nephritic factor) to an alternative complement pathway enzyme—loss of fat from face, neck, arms, and trunk. Excess fat on lower limbs.
- Generalized panniculitis may be followed by fat loss with tender nodules.

⚠ ***Inherited:*** all rare and caused by different genetic mutations. Lipodystrophy may be complete or partial.

Complications of lipodystrophies may include insulin resistance with diabetes, hypertriglyceridaemia, acute pancreatitis, and hepatic cirrhosis. Psychological distress is common.

Thyroid disorders and the skin

Hyperthyroidism: what cutaneous signs should I look for?

- Warm moist skin.
- Palmar erythema.
- Onycholysis.
- Fine hair sometimes with diffuse alopecia (may be predominantly parietal hair loss).
- Thyroid-associated ophthalmopathy—upper lid retraction, periorbital oedema, scleral injection, conjunctival oedema, and proptosis (50% of patients with Graves' disease).
- Pretibial myxoedema (<5% of patients with Graves' disease)—see Box 22.5, Figs. 22.3 and 22.4.
- Autoimmune hyperthyroidism may be associated with vitiligo and/or alopecia areata—see 🕮 p.452 and p.454.
- Thyroid acropachy (<1% of patients with Graves' disease)—see Box 22.6.
- Evidence of scratching (generalized pruritus is not common).
- Chronic urticaria.

Hypothyroidism: what cutaneous signs should I look for?

- Pale skin with a yellow tinge.
- Puffy face especially skin below the eyes.
- Puffy hands and feet (non-pitting).
- Cool peripheral extremities.
- Coarse rough dry skin particularly on extensor surfaces of limbs, e.g. shins. In severe cases, the changes may simulate ichthyosis.
- Reduced sweating.
- Coarse dry brittle hair.
- Diffuse alopecia (may be predominantly frontal hair loss).
- Thinning of outer third of eyebrows.
- Autoimmune hypothyroidism may also be associated with vitiligo and alopecia areata—see 🕮 p.452 and p.454.
- Eruptive and tuberous xanthomas (unusual—see 🕮 p.436).

Box 22.5 What is pretibial myxoedema

Synonyms: localized myxoedema, thyroid dermopathy

- Pretibial myxoedema is an autoimmune manifestation of Graves' disease. Less often it is seen in association with Hashimoto's thyroiditis.
- All patients have high serum concentrations of antibodies to thyroid-stimulating hormone receptor. Humoral and cellular immune mechanisms may stimulate dermal fibroblasts with the production of large amounts of glycosaminoglycans.
- Pretibial myxoedema is preceded by ophthalmopathy and may be associated with thyroid acropachy (usually without bone changes).
- Look for:
  - Non-pitting erythematous or flesh-coloured indurated nodules or plaques on both shins. Nodules may also develop on dorsum of feet as well as other sites (Fig. 22.3).
  - The surface has a waxy appearance.
  - The skin is not warm or tender (unlike cellulitis).

Box 22.5 (Cont.)

- Rarely, extensive infiltration by mucin causes gross non-pitting thickening of skin on the legs and foot. The thickened skin has a waxy papular surface. Indurated folds may overhang the ankles simulating the changes secondary to lymphoedema (Fig. 22.4).
- Mild disease may be a cosmetic problem but does not require treatment.
- Potent topical or intralesional corticosteroids may be helpful in symptomatic disease.
- Lymphoedematous pretibial myxoedema may benefit from compression stockings.

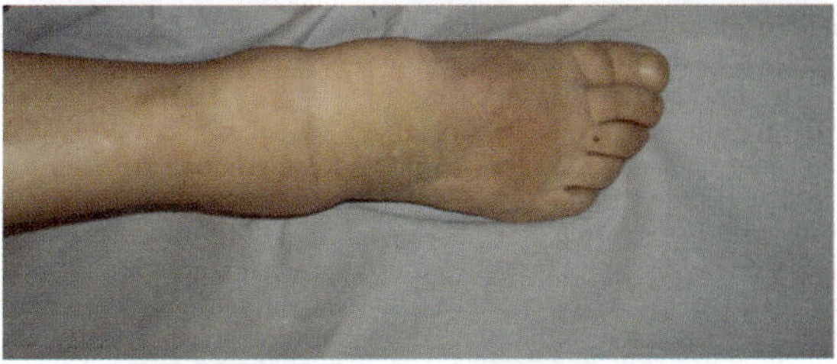

Fig. 22.3 Pretibial myxoedema—firm nodules and mild erythema.

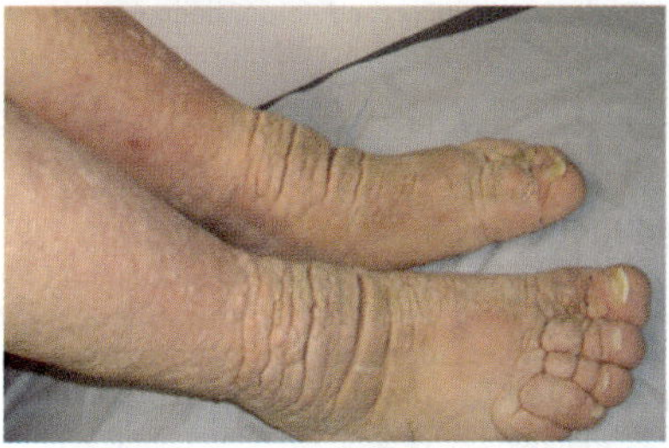

Fig. 22.4 Extensive pretibial myxoedema simulating lymphoedema (see 🕮 p.296).

Box 22.6 What is thyroid acropachy?

- Thyroid acropachy is the triad of nail clubbing, swollen fingers, and a periosteal reaction.
- Typically the periosteal reaction affects the metacarpal bones of the thumb, index, and little fingers and their proximal and middle phalanges as well as the first metatarsals.
- The periosteum of the long bones of the forearms and leg is involved less often.
- The periosteal reaction is usually asymptomatic, but occasionally causes bone or joint pain.
- Acropachy is strongly associated with Graves' disease, thyroid-associated ophthalmopathy, and pretibial myxoedema (thyroid dermopathy).

Hirsutes and hypertrichosis

Hirsutes is defined as excess terminal (coarse, pigmented) hair that appears in a male pattern in a woman. It affects about 10% of Caucasian women (more Mediterranean and African women) and usually results from subtle increases in androgens—see p.356, but rarely may presage a serious underlying condition—see Box 22.7.

In contrast, hypertrichosis is independent of androgens. The increased hair growth may be localized or generalized and affect any part of the body. Hypertrichosis may be racial, hereditary, or caused by drugs—see p.356 and some diseases—see p.88 and Box 22.7.

What should I ask?

- Enquire about onset, sites involved, and progression. Sudden onset and rapid progression may indicate a virilizing tumour (rare).
- What is the psychological impact?
- What treatments have been tried?
- Any other problems suggesting hyperandrogenism or polycystic ovary syndrome (PCOS), e.g. acne, androgenetic alopecia, menstrual irregularities or infertility? See p.442.
- Symptoms suggesting hyperprolactinaemia (galactorrhoea), adrenal pathology (see p.448), or pituitary tumour (visual disturbance, headache).
- Symptoms suggesting late onset congenital adrenal hyperplasia (hirsutes pre-puberty, premature pubarche, menstrual irregularity, primary amenorrhea).
- Symptoms of virilization (increased libido, deep voice).
- Drug history including oral contraceptives—see Box 22.7 and p.356.
- Family history of hirsutism, PCOS, androgenetic alopecia, or congenital adrenal hyperplasia.

What should I look for?

- Exclude hypertrichosis by ensuring excess hair is limited to androgen-dependent areas and score using the Ferriman-Gallwey scale—Box 22.8.
- Other cutaneous manifestations of excess androgens:
  - Female pattern hair loss: frontal hair-line is preserved in women (unlike men) but hair on the vertex of the scalp thins diffusely—see p.446.
  - Acne and seborrhoea (oily skin on the central face).
- Signs of PCOS (the commonest cause) or another underlying cause—see Box 22.7
- ⚠ Signs of virilization: deep voice, cliteromegaly, breast atrophy, muscularity. If present examine for an ovarian or adrenal mass.
- Signs of a visual field defect if you suspect a pituitary adenoma.

What should I do?

- Investigation is recommended in moderate or severe hirsutism; hirsutism of any severity if it is sudden in onset or progressing rapidly; and hirsutism associated with menstrual irregularity or infertility, central obesity, acanthosis nigricans, or cliteromegaly—see Box 22.9.
- Management of hirsutes—see p.444.
- Treat underlying cause.

Box 22.7 Causes of hirsutes

- Idiopathic (normal menstrual cycle, normal androgens, but may have a subclinical abnormality in androgens or response to androgens).
- Polycystic ovary syndrome (PCOS), the commonest hormonal cause, ovarian hyperandrogenism, or ovarian tumours—see 📖 p.442.
- HAIR-AN syndrome—see 📖 p.442.
- Adrenal hyperandrogenism including non-classical congenital adrenal hyperplasia (21-hydroxylase deficiency) and rarely virilizing tumours.
- Other endocrine disorders: Cushing's syndrome or disease, acromegaly, or hyperprolactinaemia.
- Pregnancy-related hyperandrogenism.
- Drugs including oral contraceptives with androgenic progestins (levonorgestrel, norgestrel, norethindrone), anabolic and androgenic steroids. (Non-androgenic drugs that cause hypertrichosis rather than hirsutes include ciclosporin, phenytoin, diazoxide, minocycline, and high-dose corticosteroids.)

Box 22.8 What is the Ferriman–Gallwey score?

- Hair growth is rated from 0 (no growth of terminal hair) to 4 (complete and heavy cover) in 9 locations—upper lip, chin, chest, upper back, lower back, upper abdomen, lower abdomen, the upper arms, and the thighs.
- It is difficult to score accurately as most women will have removed some of the excess hair.
- Score does not correlate closely with androgen level probably because the response of the pilosebaceous unit to androgen is variable.
- Caucasian women: 8–15 = mild hirsutes.

Box 22.9 Investigation of hirsutes

Investigation should be guided by the clinical findings but consider:

- Pregnancy test, in patients with amenorrhea.
- Total testosterone, ideally in early morning. Discuss with your laboratory—some have reliable assays that compute free testosterone by also measuring sex hormone-binding globulin (SHBG).
- Transvaginal ultrasound for polycystic ovaries or ovarian neoplasm.
- Prolactin level to exclude hyperprolactinemia.
- Early morning 17-hydroxyprogesterone (17-OHP) to exclude adrenal hyperandrogenism in high-risk populations (positive family history or ethnic groups at high risk: Ashkenazi Jews, Hispanics, and Slavs).
- Screen for Cushing's syndrome/disease, thyroid disease, or acromegaly if clinically indicated.
- Obese hirsute women: assess for type II diabetes and hyperlipidaemia (metabolic syndrome) as well as thyroid disease.

Further reading

Martin KA *et al. J Clin Endocrinol Metab* 2008, **93:**1105–20.

Polycystic ovary syndrome

Polycystic ovary (ovarian) syndrome (PCOS) is common (affects 5–10% of Caucasian women of reproductive age), and is the most common hormonal cause of hirsutes, which may be the presenting complaint. Diagnostic criteria for PCOS are shown in Box 22.10.

PCOS is caused by a combination of genetic and non-hereditable factors but the pathogenesis is incompletely understood—see Box 22.11.

Many patients also have the metabolic syndrome (central obesity, glucose or insulin abnormalities, dyslipidaemias, elevated blood pressure) and are at risk of cardiovascular disease (stroke, coronary artery disease, congestive heart failure). Lipodystrophy is a rare association—see Box 22.4.

What should I ask?

- Menstrual history/history of infertility?
- Family or personal history of diabetes, hyperlipidaemia, acne, or hirsutism?

What should I look for?

- Cutaneous manifestations of excess androgens:
  - Hirsutes: which may be mild (or altered by treatment).
  - Female pattern hair loss: frontal hair-line is preserved in women (unlike men) but hair on the vertex of the scalp thins diffusely.
  - Acne.
  - Seborrhoea: oily skin on central face (nose and forehead).
- Acanthosis nigricans usually secondary to obesity with insulin resistance.
- HAIR-AN syndrome: hyperandrogenism (acne), insulin resistance, and acanthosis nigricans. May also have hirsutes.
- Central obesity (record waist–hip ratio or waist circumference).
- Evidence of metabolic syndrome including hypertension. Record height and weight and calculate BMI.
- Rarely lipodystrophy—Box 22.4.

What should I do?

- Pregnancy test, in patients with amenorrhea.
- Measure plasma testosterone ideally in early morning (normal or increased).
- Transvaginal ultrasound to detect polycystic ovaries.
- LH/FSH ratio >2 suggests PCOS, but as the ratio is raised in fewer than 50% of cases, it is not a useful test for confirming PCOS.
- Fasting glucose and lipids (metabolic syndrome is common).
- PCOS is the commonest cause of hirsutes but consider excluding other causes of hirsutism if clinically relevant—see Box 22.7.

Box 22.10 Diagnostic criteria for PCOS

Diagnosis of PCOS requires 2 of the following 3 criteria:
- Polycystic ovaries (not pathognomonic).
- Oligo or anovulation (menstrual irregularity, infertility).
- Biochemical or clinical signs of hyperandrogenism such as hirsutes, acne, or androgenetic alopecia.

Reference: Setji TL and Brown AJ. *Am J Med* 2007; **120:**128–32.

Box 22.11 Factors involved in the pathogenesis of PCOS

The pathogenesis is still incompletely understood but is multifactorial:
- Intrinsic dysfunction of ovaries and adrenal glands probably contributes to hyperandrogenaemia.
- Central obesity (40% of patients with PCOS):
  - Adipocytes containing excess triglycerides are insulin resistant and this triggers compensatory hyperinsulinaemia. Hyperinsulinaemia stimulates production of ovarian androgens.
  - Increased conversion of androgen to oestrogen by adipocytes stimulates release of LH and reduces FSH.
- LH also stimulates production of ovarian androgens (testosterone, androstenedione, and dehydroepiandrosterone).
- Hyperinsulinaemia and elevated androgen inhibit production of sex hormone-binding globulin (SHBG).
- Reduced SHBG leads to an increase in the proportion of plasma testosterone that is free (unbound) and therefore is available for conversion to dihydrotestosterone in the pilosebaceous unit (by the enzyme 5 alpha-reductase).
- Dihydrotestosterone binds more strongly to the androgen receptor in follicles than testosterone and is the primary mediator of androgenetic effects on the pilosebaceous unit (acne, hirsutes, androgenetic alopecia). Hyperinsulinaemia may increase the responsiveness of the pilosebaceous unit to androgen.

Management of hirsutes

Women with hirsutes may be too embarrassed to discuss the condition or what they have been doing to remove the excess hair. Hirsutes can have a major impact on quality of life and many women will be anxious, have a low self-esteem, or have concerns about sexual self-worth.

Although there is no single easy answer, treatments can make a difference and most women will value the opportunity to talk to a sensitive physician about what can be done. Any underlying cause of androgen excess should be controlled and drugs contributing to hirsutes withdrawn. The choice of treatment for reducing or removing hair will depend on the patient's preference, the distribution and severity of hirsutes, and the cost of treatment (most are not provided through the NHS).

Topical treatments

- Bleaching with hydrogen peroxide preparations may make dark facial hair less obvious, but can be irritant.
- Depilatory creams or foams containing thioglycolates that dissolve hair are widely available, but smell unpleasant, are irritant, and are not very effective for coarse hair.
- Eflornithine cream (inhibitor of ornithine decarboxylase) applied twice daily reduces the rate of growth of hair after 6–8 weeks. Once treatment is discontinued the hair growth returns to pre-treatment levels. Eflornithine is helpful in combination with mechanical treatments.

Mechanical treatments

- Shaving. Re-growing hairs have a blunt tip which may make them look thicker than before. Although women are prepared to shave their legs or axillae, most do not find it acceptable to shave the face. Shaving may cause a folliculitis, particularly on thighs.
- Epilation: plucking, waxing, threading, or sugaring to extract hairs. Contrary to popular opinion, epilation does not make hairs grow back more thickly. Epilation is uncomfortable. Irritation and folliculitis are common. Postinflammatory hyperpigmentation may be a problem in dark skins.
- Electrolysis can permanently destroy some hair follicles (about 60%), but the outcome depends on the skill of the operator. Complications include scarring and infection.
- Laser hair removal (photoepilation) is most effective for dark hairs on fair skin (laser energy is absorbed by melanin in the hair follicle and not the surrounding epidermis). Treatment interrupts hair growth temporarily, but regrowing hairs may be finer and lighter. Some permanent hair loss may be achieved after repeated treatments. Laser treatment is considerably more expensive than electrolysis but is also more effective and faster.

Oral therapy See Box 22.12.

Box 22.12 Oral therapy for hirsutes

- Combined oral contraceptive containing the progestin, cyproterone acetate (2mg). Cyproterone acetate blocks the androgen receptor in the pilosebaceous unit and, to a lesser extent, the activity of 5-alpha reductase. First-line therapy for premenopausal women. Treat for at least 6 months. Adverse effects: liver toxicity, weight gain, fatigue, loss of libido, mastodynia, nausea, headaches, and depression. Monitor liver function.
- Spironolactone (androgen receptor antagonist) 100mg/day: monitor for hyperkalaemia. Treat for at least 6 months. Causes breast soreness and menstrual irregularities
- Finasteride (inhibits 5-alpha reductase) 5mg/day. Treat for at least 6 months.
- Ensure that premenopausal women taking antiandrogens always use effective contraception to avoid the potential risk of feminization of a male fetus.
- Insulin-sensitizing drugs e.g. metformin lower insulin levels in hyperinsulinaemia by increasing sensitivity to insulin. Metformin also attenuates both hyperinsulinaemia and hyperandrogenaemia and may reduce hirsutes in patients with PCOS, but is less effective than spironolactone.

Further reading

Blume-Peytavi U and Hahn S. *Dermatol Ther* 2008; **21:**329–39.

Martin KA *et al. J Clin Endocrinol Metab* 2008; **93:**1105–120.

Somani N *et al. Dermatol Ther* 2008; **21:**376–91.

Wanitphakdeedecha R and Alster TS. *Dermatol Ther* 2008; **21:**392–401.

Male and female pattern hair loss

Synonyms: male pattern baldness, androgenetic alopecia

Hair loss (alopecia) is common as people age, but the pattern of loss is different in men and women. Androgens play a pivotal role in male pattern hair loss but their role in female pattern hair loss is less certain and other mechanisms may be involved. Genetically determined susceptibility is important (prevalence varies in different populations).

Male pattern hair loss—what should I look for?

- About 25% of men begin to lose hair by age 30.
- Androgens cause follicular miniaturization with progressive decrease in the width of the hair shaft.
- A receding frontal hairline is common, particularly on the temples (may commence in the mid-teens).
- Gradual thinning of the hair on the vertex is eventually followed by complete loss of hair over the vertex (loss may be preceded by curling and coarsening of hair—acquired progressive kinking).
- A rim of hair is retained around the back and sides of the scalp (occipital follicles are not dependent on androgens and are a source of follicles for hair transplants).

Female pattern hair loss—what should I look for?

- Female pattern loss occurs any time after the onset of puberty. Prevalence increases to 29–42% in women aged >70.
- Some patients notice increased shedding; others just complain of gradual diffuse thinning over the crown, parietal, and/or frontal scalp.
- Women may say 'I can see my scalp' or complain that the central parting gets sunburnt.
- The density of hair on top of the scalp is reduced either in a diffuse central pattern or with accentuated loss frontally, but the frontal hair line is preserved. A hair pull (see 📖 Box 3.3, p.45) may be positive in early loss, but is usually negative in longstanding loss.
- Some temporal thinning is common, but unlike men, women do not progress to complete balding on the vertex. Even in advanced female pattern hair loss, when the hair may be very sparse over the top of the scalp, a rim of hair is still retained along the frontal margin.
- Rapidly progressive hair loss in a male pattern suggests virilization—look for other symptoms or signs such as oligomenorrhoea or amenorrhoea, hirsutes, severe acne, or cliteromegaly—see 📖 p.440. Some hyperandrogenic women show a female pattern of hair loss.
- Exclude other causes of diffuse non-scarring alopecia—see Boxes 22.13 and 22.14. In particular ask about menstrual history, dieting, recent illnesses, and drugs.

What should I do?

See Box 22.15.

Further reading

Olsen EA *et al. J Am Acad Dermatol* 2005; **52**:301–11.

Box 22.13 Differential diagnosis in diffuse non-scarring alopecia

- Female pattern hair loss.
- Telogen effluvium: seek a trigger in previous 2–5 months including pregnancy. If acute, hair falls out in handfuls. Remits in 12 months. If chronic (lasts months–years) can be difficult to distinguish from female pattern hair loss.
- Diffuse alopecia areata: positive hair pull, may have lost hair at other site—see 🕮 p.454. Dermoscopic features include cadaverized hairs, exclamation mark hairs, broken hairs, and yellow dots. Look for nail pitting, autoimmune thyroid disease.
- Traction alopecia: is the patient pulling back the hair tightly into a ponytail?
- Systemic disease or drugs—see Box 22.14.

Box 22.14 Systemic causes of diffuse non-scarring alopecia

- Iron deficiency (often associated with heavy menses).
- Hypothyroidism (often frontal hair loss) or hyperthyroidism (often parietal hair loss) but may resemble female pattern hair loss.
- Hypoparathyroidism, hypopituitarism.
- SLE (frontal alopecia is most common).
- Protein malnutrition, crash dieting, or anorexia nervosa.
- Severe chronic disease including malignancy.
- Cytotoxic drugs, vitamin A, and oral retinoids.

Box 22.15 Management of male and female pattern hair loss

- If the woman has no symptoms or signs suggesting hyperandrogenaemia, investigation of androgen status is not indicated.
- Investigate and treat coexisting problems such as iron deficiency or thyroid disease.
- Explain to women that they are unlikely to go bald, that shorter layered hair styles make hair look fuller, and that boosting the volume of the hair with rollers, mousses, or a gentle permanent wave is not going to increase hair loss—this reassurance may be all that is required by many women with mild thinning.
- Explain that treatment will only have a modest impact (stabilize loss, thicken residual hair shafts) but will not reverse hair loss.
- Topical 2% or 5% minoxidil lotion ×2/day may produce some regrowth in men and women. Treat for 12 months and if helpful continue treatment.
- Women—antiandrogens: the combined oral contraceptive containing the progestin cyproterone acetate, or spironolactone 100mg/day. Treat for at least 6 months (see management of hirsutes—see 🕮 Box 22.12, p.445)
- Monitor with photographs or hair counts (if shedding).
- Wigs are an option for some patients.

Other endocrinopathies

Panhypopituitarism

Cutaneous signs include:
- Smooth facial skin with fine wrinkles, loss of facial hair and decreased body hair.
- Decreased ability to tan and pale yellowish skin (deficiency of ACTH, which has a role in regulating melanin pigmentation).

Addison's disease

Primary adrenal failure is caused most often by autoimmune adrenalitis or by infection (TB, fungal, cytomegalovirus, AIDs). High levels of circulating pituitary peptides, such as proopiomelanocortin, ACTH β-lipotropin, and melanocyte stimulating hormone, induce melanocyte activity. Look for:
- Hyperpigmentation of sun-exposed skin.
- Hyperpigmentation in palmar creases, axillae, nipples, old scars, and sites of pressure or friction such as knuckles and waist line.
- Pigmented mucous membranes (lips, gums, buccal, vaginal, vulval, anal).
- Darkening of melanocytic naevi and hair.
- If caused by autoimmune adrenalitis, you may find vitiligo.

Note that hyperpigmentation does not occur if adrenal failure is secondary to ACTH deficiency, e.g. after withdrawing oral glucocorticoids.

Cushing's syndrome

Cushing's syndrome is associated with inappropriately elevated levels of free plasma glucocorticoid. Causes—see Box 22.16. Cutaneous signs include:
- Central obesity with thin arms and legs.
- Dorsal neck and supraclavicular fat pads.
- Plethoric telangiectatic round 'moon' face.
- Hirsutism with fine hair on cheeks.
- Atrophic skin with purple striae on trunk, upper thighs, and arms.
- Easy bruising.
- Cutaneous fungal infections: pityriasis versicolor, widespread *Trichophyton rubrum* (nails, trunk, buttocks), nail candidiasis.
- Acne: pustules and perifollicular papules, but no comedones.
- Signs of virilism if an adrenal tumour is producing androgens—see 📖 p.440.
- Hyperpigmentation if associated with high levels of ACTH, e.g. in ectopic ACTH syndrome—see 📖 Addison's disease and 📖 Nelson's syndrome (see Box 22.17).
- ⚠ Signs of Carney's syndrome or McCune–Albright syndrome—see Box 22.16.

Acromegaly

Excess secretion of growth hormone by pituitary tumours. Look for:
- Thick greasy, coarse, furrowed skin on face and neck.
- Frontal bossing, thick lips, and broad nose; doughy hands.
- Cutis verticis gyrate (thick ridges and furrows on the scalp).
- Hyperhidrosis (common). Hyperpigmentation: 40% of patients. Hirsutism: 50% of patients.

Multiple endocrine neoplasia (MEN)—see Box 22.18

Box 22.16 Causes of Cushing's syndrome

- Cushing's disease: pituitary-dependent bilateral adrenocortical hyperplasia, usually secondary to a pituitary adenoma. The commonest cause of Cushing's syndrome (50–70% of patients).
- Adrenal adenomas or carcinomas (20–30% of patients)
- Iatrogenic
- Ectopic ACTH: ACTH released by non-pituitary tumours, e.g. small-cell carcinoma of the bronchus (16% of patients).
- Carney's syndrome: cutaneous and mucosal freckling, mesenchymal tumours (atrial myxoma), peripheral nerve tumours, endocrine tumours.
- McCune–Albright syndrome: fibrous dysplasia and cutaneous pigmentation (large café au lait patches with an irregular outline), may be associated with pituitary, thyroid, adrenal, and gonadal hyperfunction.

Box 22.17 ⚠ What is Nelson's syndrome?

- This rare syndrome presents in patients with Cushing's disease who have been treated by bilateral adrenalectomy.
- The pituitary adenoma, no longer inhibited by cortisol released from the adrenals, continues to enlarge and release ACTH.
- High levels of ACTH produce Addisonian hyperpigmentation.

Box 22.18 ⚠ Multiple endocrine neoplasia (MEN)

Multiple endocrine neoplasia type 1

- Inherited as an autosomal dominant.
- Predisposition to tumours of the parathyroid glands, anterior pituitary, pancreatic islets cells (gastrinoma, insulinoma).
- Cutaneous signs: multiple cutaneous angiofibromas (flesh-coloured papules), collagenoma (thickened yellow plaque), café au lait spots.

Multiple endocrine neoplasia type 2A

- Inherited as an autosomal dominant.
- Predisposition to medullary thyroid cancer, phaeochromocytoma, and primary parathyroid hyperplasia.
- Cutaneous signs: cutaneous lichen amyloidosis—see 📖 Box 23.3 p.461.

Multiple endocrine neoplasia type 2B

- Inherited as an autosomal dominant.
- Predisposition to medullary thyroid cancer and phaeochromocytoma.
- Intestine ganglioneuromas.
- Cutaneous signs: mucosal neuromas on lips, tongue buccal mucosa, gingiva, and palate. Café au lait spots. Marfanoid appearance (📖 p.398).

Autoimmune polyendocrine syndromes

Synonym: autoimmune polyendocrinopathy–candidiasis–ectodermal dystrophy (APECED).

Interactions between genetic and environmental factors influence susceptibility. Vitiligo is common in all types (Fig. 22.5).

⚠ Polyglandular autoimmune syndrome type 1

Very rare: mutations of autoimmune regulator gene on chromosome 21.

- At least 2 of the following: chronic mucocutaneous candidiasis (includes nails) often apparent in first few months of life, usually apparent before age 5; chronic hypoparathyroidism (paraesthesiae, muscle twitching, or spasms, may have dry skin, brittle hair and nails) usually apparent before age 15; and/or Addison's disease.
- Defect in T lymphocytes demonstrated by skin anergy to *Candida* and tuberculin antigens.
- Associated conditions may include alopecia (totalis or areata) (Fig. 22.6), vitiligo, hypergonadotropic hypogonadism, autoimmune thyroid disease, pernicious anaemia, chronic active hepatitis, and/or steatorrhoea (malabsorption), type 1 diabetes mellitus (rare).
- Malignant neoplasias, e.g. oral SCC, adenocarcinoma stomach.

⚠ Polyglandular autoimmune syndrome type 2

Rare, associated with HLA DR3/DR4 = Schmidt's syndrome.

- Addison's disease (always present) and autoimmune thyroid disease and/or type 1 diabetes mellitus.
- Associated conditions including alopecia (totalis or areata) (Fig. 22.6), vitiligo, primary hypogonadism, autoimmune hepatitis, pernicious anaemia.

⚠ Polyglandular autoimmune syndrome type 3

(Has been subdivided into types A, B , C, and D.)

- Autoimmune thyroid disease (Hashimoto's thyroiditis, idiopathic myxoedema, asymptomatic thyroiditis, Graves' disease, endocrine ophthalmopathy, pretibial myxoedema) associated with another autoimmune disease (excluding Addison's disease, and/or hypoparathyroidism).
- Examples of other diseases include vitiligo (common), type 1 diabetes mellitus, alopecia areata, pernicious anaemia, coeliac disease, myasthenia gravis, rheumatoid arthritis, or Sjögrens's syndrome.

⚠ Polyglandular autoimmune syndrome type 4

- Combination of organ-specific autoimmune diseases not included in other groups, e.g. vitiligo and alopecia, type 1 diabetes mellitus, and vitiligo.

Further reading

Amerio A et *al. Clin Expt Dermatol* 2006; **31**:746–749.

Betterle C and Zanchetta R. *Acta Biomed* 2003; **74**:9–33.

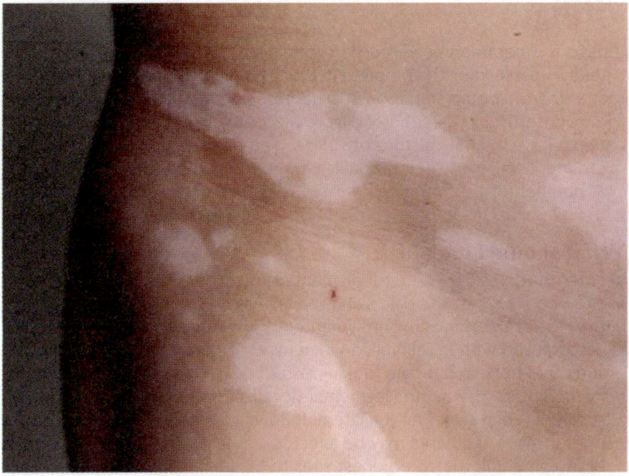

Fig. 22.5 Vitiligo: smooth depigmented patches.

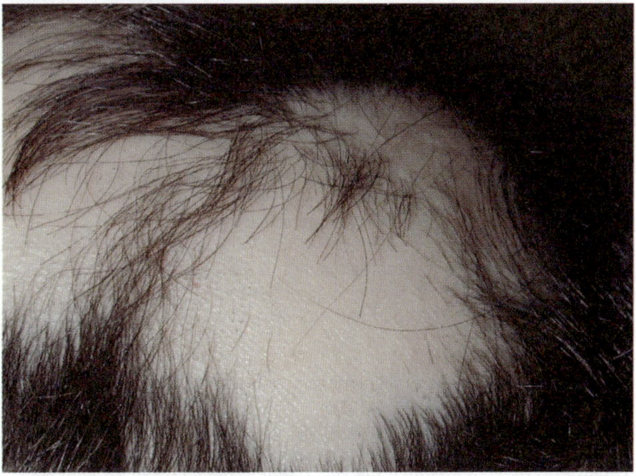

Fig. 22.6 Alopecia areata: well circumscribed patches of non-scarring alopecia. The skin is not scaly or inflamed.

Vitiligo

Vitiligo is a common acquired skin condition in which epidermal melanocytes are lost leading to complete loss of pigmentation, i.e. depigmentation rather than hypopigmentation (partial pigment loss) (Fig. 22.5). Average age of onset is 20 years, but vitiligo may commence in childhood. 18% of patients have a family history of vitiligo. The psychological impact may be profound, particularly in individuals who have darkly pigmented skin.

A number of autoimmune diseases have been reported in association with vitiligo, particularly thyroid disease—see 📖 Box 22.19, p.450.

What should I look for?

- Smooth (no scale) white (depigmented) macules and/or patches.
- Are you sure that the pale skin is abnormal? Might it be possible that the rest of the skin is hyperpigmented? For example, melasma may be confused with facial vitiligo when hyperpigmented facial lesions surround normal but pale looking skin.
- Pigment loss may be nonsegmental (localized, generalized, or acrofacial) or segmental (unilateral following a dermatomal distribution; one or more segments may be affected)—see Table 22.2.
- Nonsegmental: the commonest sites to be affected are fingers, wrists, axillae, groins, perioral and periorbital skin, and genitalia. Look for vitiligo at sites sensitive to pressure, friction or trauma (Köbner's phenomenon)—e.g. belt-line, beneath watch strap.
- A rim of depigmented skin around melanocytic naevi. These halo naevi are 10 × more common in vitiligo. The melanocytic naevi regress leaving depigmented macules.
- Vitiligo or lichen sclerosus (see 📖 p.268) affecting genitalia—the patient may be too embarrassed to report the vitiligo. Lichen sclerosus may coexist with vitiligo.
- White hairs in eyelashes and scalp as well as white body hair within areas of vitiligo.
- A 'trichrome' appearance with a white depigmented centre, a surrounding light brown zone of varying width, and dark brown normal skin. Seen rarely in developing patches in dark skin.
- Inflammation at the advancing edge of a macule—uncommon.
- Mucosae may be affected in patients with dark skin.

What should I do?

- Exclude other causes of pigment loss: differential diagnosis—see 📖 p.84.
- Assess psychological impact of vitiligo using DLQI—see 📖 p.32.
- Check thyroid function.
- You may wish to examine the skin under a Wood's light to confirm the diagnosis (the depigmented skin appears bright white) and determine the extent of disease, particularly in pale skins.
- Record extent of vitiligo with photographs.
- Management is difficult but sun protection is important—see Box 22.20.

Box 22.19 Autoimmune diseases associated with vitiligo

- Thyroid disease, type 1 diabetes mellitus and adrenal insufficiency.
- Autoimmune polyendocrinopathy syndromes—see 📖 p.450.
- Lupus erythematosus, rheumatoid arthritis, sarcoidosis, myasthenia gravis, pernicious anaemia, autoimmune hepatitis.
- Alopecia areata, psoriasis, lichen planus, lichen sclerosus.

Table 22.2 Types of vitiligo

Non-segmental vitiligo	Segmental vitiligo
Late onset is more common	Often begins in childhood when it may be difficult to distinguish from naevus depigmentosus
Is progressive, with flare-ups	Has rapid onset but stabilizes
Involves hair compartment late	Involves hair compartment early
Often associated with personal or family history of autoimmunity	Usually not accompanied by other autoimmune diseases

Box 22.20 Management of vitiligo

- Advise about sun protection (pale skinned individuals can also use sunblocks to prevent normal skin from tanning so that vitiligo is less obvious), cosmetic camouflage (fake tanning products) and the Vitiligo Society.
- Minimize trauma to the skin.
- Very potent (clobetasol propionate) topical corticosteroid cream or 0.1% tacrolimus ointment may induce some repigmentation in vitiligo of recent onset.
- UVB phototherapy or PUVA may be indicated in adults with widespread disease that has not responded to conservative treatment, but prolonged courses are required and the response is variable. Partial follicular repigmentation may be even more disfiguring and the normal skin darkens making vitiligo more obvious.
- Skin grafts or epidermal suspension transplants have been advocated, particularly for segmental vitiligo.

Further reading

Gawkrodger DJ *et al.* *Br J Dermatol* 2008; **159:**1051–76.

Taieb A and Picardo M. *N Engl J Med* 2009; **360:**160–9.

Alopecia areata

Alopecia areata is a common (1–2% of the population), T-cell mediated cause of non-scarring alopecia. It presents at any age, but is seen most often in children and young adults, when it may cause considerable psychological distress, particularly if hair loss is widespread. Genetic and environmental factors are involved in pathogenesis and alopecia areata is associated with autoimmune diseases such as vitiligo and autoimmune thyroiditis, as well as with atopy.

T-cells clustering around the lower part of growing (anagen) hair follicles like a 'swarm of bees' disturb the normal cycle of hair growth. Hair follicles in the growing part of the cycle are pushed prematurely into the resting (telogen) phase. Affected follicles still have the potential for regrowth as there is no scarring. Patients have circulating IgG antibodies to anagen hair follicles, but it is not clear if these are pathogenic.

Disease is both dynamic and unpredictable. Stress may trigger onset. Severity ranges from transient loss in a few patches to persistent loss of all scalp and body hair. Alopecia areata is chronic in 7–10% of patients.

Poor prognostic factors include:

- Young age of onset.
- Family history of alopecia areata (20% of patients).
- History of autoimmune diseases or atopy.
- Nail involvement.
- Extensive hair loss or ophiasic pattern of loss (see below).
- Recurrent episodes of hair loss or longstanding loss.

What should I look for?

- One or more well-circumscribed, smooth, round, or oval patches of non-scarring alopecia on the scalp (the commonest pattern). The skin is not inflamed and the patches are asymptomatic—see Box 22.21 for differential diagnosis.
- Often sparing of grey or white hair. Regrowing hairs white at first.
- Exclamation mark hairs (short and tapering to a point) at the edge of patches of complete loss are pathognomonic of alopecia areata, but not found often. They are easier to see using a dermatoscope, which may also reveal cadaverized hairs (black dots), broken hairs, yellow dots, and clustered short vellus hairs.
- In active disease, a hair pull may be positive at the edge of the patch. >6 hairs are pulled out by the root when a small clump is tugged gently but firmly—see 🕮 p.45.
- Patches of hair loss in beard area, loss of eyebrows or eyelashes.
- Nail pitting (10–60% of cases).
- Other patterns of loss include:
    - A band of loss around the periphery of the scalp (ophiasic pattern).
    - Diffuse thinning that resembles female pattern hair loss (see 🕮 p.446).
    - Complete loss of scalp hair (alopecia totalis). Sudden onset of alopecia totalis can make a patient's hair appear to 'go white overnight' because white hairs are retained.
    - Complete loss of scalp hair and body hair (alopecia universalis).

What should I do?

See Boxes 22.22 and 22.23.

Box 22.21 Alopecia areata: differential diagnosis

The characteristic dermoscopic findings of alopecia areata will help to exclude other diagnoses such as:

- Telogen effluvium: hair loss is generalized and not patchy.
- Tinea capitis: the scalp is erythematous and scaly, but signs may be subtle particularly in infections caused by *T. tonsurans*.
- Trichotillomania (deliberate pulling hair): broken hairs or regrowing hairs are still firmly anchored to the scalp.
- Drug-induced anagen effluvium may mimic diffuse alopecia areata.
- Female pattern hair loss (see 🕮 p.446) may mimic diffuse alopecia areata.
- SLE (usually frontal alopecia).
- Secondary syphilis (patchy moth-eaten appearance).
- Early scarring alopecia—see 🕮 Box 3.2, p.45.

Box 22.22 Investigations in alopecia areata

- Usually none required.
- Although autoimmune diseases are increased in frequency, current UK guidelines do not recommend routine screening.
- If the diagnosis is in doubt consider:
  - Fungal culture of plucked hairs.
  - Skin biopsy: rarely necessary.
  - Serology for SLE and syphilis.

Box 22.23 Management of alopecia areata

- Alopecia areata is difficult to treat as nothing has been shown to affect the course of disease or the long-term outcome.
- Remember that most patients (80%) will have spontaneous regrowth of hair in any individual patch within 3 months of onset.
- Topical corticosteroids are safe and used widely, although there is little evidence that they are effective.
- Intralesional corticosteroids temporarily stimulate tufts of hair growth, but repeated injections cause atrophy. Intralesional steroids near the eye may cause cataract or raised intraocular pressure.
- Other treatments that have been tried include short courses of oral prednisolone, contact immunotherapy, and phototherapy, but there is no evidence that any hair that regrows will persist.
- Patients with extensive loss or recurrent episodes may benefit from psychological support or contact with the alopecia areata website http://www.alopeciaareata.com
- For some, a wig or hairpiece may be the best option.

Further reading

Delamere *et al. Cochrane Database Syst Rev.* Interventions for alopecia areata. 2008. http://www.cochrane.org/reviews/en/ab004413.html.

Chapter 23

Skin and renal disease

Contents

Relevant pages in other chapters

Calcific uraemic arteriolopathy (calciphylaxis) 🕮 p.292
Porphyria 🕮 p.310 and pseudoporphyria 🕮 p.312
Vasculitis 🕮 p.404
Alpha-1-antitrypsin deficiency 🕮 p.428
Lipodystrophy 🕮 p.437
Cancer syndromes 🕮 p.500

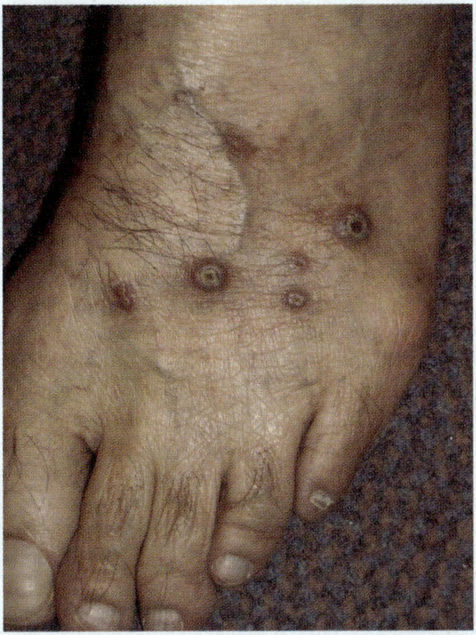

Fig. 23.1 Itchy dome-shaped nodules with a central hyperkeratotic plug in acquired perforating dermatosis.

Skin in renal failure

General examination

- Dry skin; pale skin secondary to chronic anaemia.
- Yellowish tinge to skin (accumulation of carotenoids, urochromes, and lipoochromes) or diffuse hyperpigmentation (increased melanin).
- Macular purpura: increased vessel fragility, heparin during dialysis.
- Sparse body hair, diffuse alopecia, and/or dry hair; nail changes—see Box 23.1.
- Pseudo-Kaposi's sarcoma adjacent to arteriovenous fistula: purplish papules that may evolve into scaly, crusted, violaceous plaques (manifestation of venous hypertension).

Uraemic pruritus—see Box 23.2 for management

- Itching is a common and distressing problem both in chronic renal failure and in patients receiving dialysis (60–90% of patients).
- Itch, whether intermittent or persistent, generalized or localized, may have a major impact on quality of life, e.g. insomnia, depression.
- Pathogenesis is unclear, but accumulation of metabolic toxins and immunological mechanisms may be involved. Dryness and impairment of the integrity of the stratum corneum may also play some part.
- Signs include excoriations, skin thickening (lichen simplex) caused by chronic rubbing and nodules (nodular prurigo—see 🕮 p.206).
- Always consider other causes of itching including scabies: is anyone else in the family itchy? Check for burrows between fingers and on genitalia—see 🕮 p.164 and Box 23.2.

Acquired perforating dermatosis

Synonym: reactive perforating collagenosis.

- Most often seen in diabetic patients with chronic renal failure.
- Itchy dome-shaped nodules erupt on trunk and extensor surfaces of limbs. Each nodule has a central depression filled with crust (Fig. 23.1).
- Skin biopsy shows collagen with other dermal components being eliminated through transepidermal channels ('perforations').
- Scratching may play some part in the pathogenesis.
- Often resolves spontaneously.
- Topical steroids, occlusion, UVB, or retinoids may be helpful.

Other cutaneous problems

- Cutaneous vasculitis related to underlying problems such as SLE—see 🕮 p.404.
- Porphyria cutanea tarda and pseudoporphyria present with skin fragility, erosions, and blisters on exposed skin, usually the dorsum of the hands—see 🕮 p.310 and p.312. Take a detailed drug history as a wide range of drugs may be implicated in the pathogenesis of pseudoporphyria.
- Calcific uraemic arteriolopathy (calciphylaxis): a life-threatening condition, seen most often in patients on dialysis. Presents acutely with a painful mottled erythema that becomes necrotic—see 🕮 p.292.
- Nephrogenic systemic fibrosis (see 🕮 p.462); drug reactions (see 🕮 p.342).

Box 23.1 Nail changes

- Transverse white bands (Mees' lines): acute renal failure.
- Paired narrow transverse white lines on several nails (Muehrcke's lines): hypoalbuminaemia in nephrotic syndrome. Bands fade if the nail plate is compressed, unlike Mees' lines.
- 'Half-and-half' nails (proximal white, distal brownish-pink = Lindsay's nails): uraemia.
- Less frequent changes seen in chronic renal failure:
  - Absence of lunula.
  - Splinter haemorrhages.
  - Brittle nails.
  - Koilonychia.

Box 23.2 Management of uraemic pruritus

Exclude other causes of itch including drugs, scabies, iron deficiency, and thyroid disease—see 📖 p.60. Optimize dialysis and control hyperparathyroidism and/or hyperphosphataemia. High permeability haemodialysis has been advocated to clear medium and large sized molecules acting as toxins.

Strategies worth trying include:

- Trim nails short to prevent damage to skin from scratching.
- Reduce body temperature by using cool cotton clothing.
- Keeping the room cool, particularly at night (avoid too many bedclothes).
- Avoid soap or excessive bathing (water temperature should not be too hot).
- Copious emollients as well as soap substitutes to relieve dryness.
- Aqueous cream with 1% menthol.
- Occlusion with paste bandages such as Zipzoc®.
- 0.025% capsaicin cream (initially causes a burning discomfort).
- 0.03% or 0.1% tacrolimus ointment (potentially carcinogenic and not suitable for long-term treatment).
- Topical gamma-linolenic acid.
- Sedating antihistamines (non-sedating antihistamines are ineffective). Oral doxepin is a powerful antipruritic—start with a low dose. Doxepin is metabolized via the liver cytochrome P450 3A pathway. Avoid if also prescribing macrolide antibiotics or imidazole antifungals.
- Phototherapy with UVB.
- Systemic treatments that have been used with variable success include colestyramine (inconsistent results, risk of acidosis), thalidomide, naltrexone, ondansetron, gabapentin, and sodium cromoglicate.

Further reading

Chen ZJ *et al. Clin Exp Dermatol* 2009; **34:**679–83.

Kurban MS *et al. Clinics Dermatol* 2008; **26:**255–64.

Mettang T *et al. Nephrol Dial Transplant* 2002; **17:**1558–63.

Yosipovitch G *et al. Nephrol Dial Transplant* 2007; **22:**3268–72.

Amyloidosis

What is amyloid?

The amyloidoses are disorders of protein folding. At least 20 different proteins can form the extracellular deposits of non-functional beta-pleated sheets that typify amyloid fibrils. The fibrils stain with Congo red dye and produce apple-green birefringence under polarized light.

Amyloid protein may be deposited in virtually any tissue including kidney, gastrointestinal tract, heart, skin, muscle, brain, and/or blood vessels. Accumulation of protein eventually causes organ failure (often renal).

Reactive systemic amyloidosis (AA) develops in association with chronic inflammation including chronic infections, e.g. leprosy, TB, or osteomyelitis, and chronic inflammatory diseases, e.g. rheumatoid arthritis and ankylosing spondylitis. Amyloidosis is also a frequent complication in patients with renal failure on maintenance haemodialysis. Rarely systemic amyloidosis may be hereditary e.g. in association with FMF (see 📖 p.218).

Monoclonal immunoglobulin light-chain amyloidosis (AL), which has similar clinical features to AA, is seen in association with diseases involving B-lymphocytes such as multiple myeloma, B-cell lymphomas, and macroglobulinemia.

The most common forms of primary localized cutaneous amyloidosis (macular and lichenoid) are caused by deposition of keratin filaments in the skin and are not associated with systemic amyloidosis—see Box 23.3.

Systemic amyloidosis: what should I look for?

- Smooth yellowish or rather waxy, translucent looking, but firm papules, nodules, or plaques on the face (eyelids, nasolabial folds, perioral), neck or trunk (chest, flexures, periumbilical). Some may be purpuric or become purpuric if rubbed.
- Petechiae and/or purpura arising spontaneously.
- Pinch purpura: pinching or rubbing the skin causes purpura.
- Purpura of face or neck induced by coughing or vomiting.
- Periorbital purpura including 'post-proctoscopy palpebral purpura' (Fig. 23.2) (purpura on the eyelids of patients who have been positioned head down for investigation by proctoscopy).
- Mucosal infiltration:
    - Smooth, pale, enlarged indurated tongue (rare but virtually pathognomonic). The teeth may produce scalloped indentations on the sides of the tongue.
    - Thickened gingiva that bleed easily.
    - Pale red or yellow papules on buccal, conjunctival, nasal, vaginal, or anal mucosa.
- Hepatosplenomegaly.
- Evidence of systemic involvement such as nephrotic syndrome, renal failure, sensory or autonomic neuropathy, heart failure, arrhythmias, malabsorption, or gastrointestinal haemorrhage.

Box 23.3 Primary localized cutaneous amyloidosis

Lichen amyloidosis

Intensely itchy shiny or hyperkeratotic hyperpigmented papules, often on the shins. Most common in South East Asia and South American countries.

Macular amyloidosis

Itchy oval greyish-brown poorly defined patches with rather rippled or whorled patterns of hyperpigmentation. Often on the upper back.

Macular and lichen amyloid are secondary to chronic rubbing or friction, sometimes with rough towels or brushes. Small globular deposits of amyloid, formed from keratin filaments, are found in the papillary dermis just beneath the basement membrane zone.

Macular and lichen amyloid may coexist. These forms of cutaneous amyloid are never associated with systemic amyloidosis.

⚠ ***Familial primary localized cutaneous amyloidosis*** is a rare variant caused by missense mutations in the *OSMR* gene, encoding oncostatin M-specific receptor beta, a cytokine receptor complex. The molecular studies have provided new insights into the pathogenesis of itch.

Nodular localized primary cutaneous amyloidosis

A very rare variant, usually presenting in the 6th or 7th decades, with 1 or more waxy translucent nodules or plaques that may become purpuric if traumatized. Nodules are formed by deposits of immunoglobulin light chains (amyloid L protein, AL). AL infiltrates dermis, subcutis, and blood vessel walls.

Such patients must be screened for underlying systemic disease and should be monitored if no systemic disease is identified, but few (<10%) will develop systemic amyloidosis.

Further reading

Woollons A and Black MM. *Br J Dermatol* 2001; **145:**105–9.

Tanaka A *et al.* *Br J Dermatol* 2009; **161:**127–24.

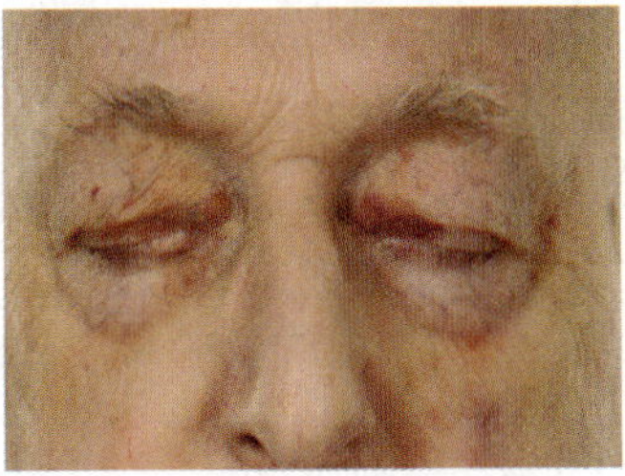

Fig. 23.2 Systemic amyloidosis: periorbital purpura. Reproduced with permission from Warrell D *et al.* (eds) *Oxford Textbook of Medicine*, 5th edn, 2010. Oxford: Oxford University Press.

Nephrogenic systemic fibrosis

⚠ What is nephrogenic systemic fibrosis (NSF)?

NSF is a rare, but devastating, cutaneous fibrosing dermopathy seen in patients with end-stage renal disease who have been exposed to the gadolinium-based contrast agents used in MRI. NSF may affect lungs, heart, liver, and muscles as well as skin and subcutaneous tissues. Complications such as cardiomyopathy, pulmonary fibrosis, pulmonary hypertension, and/or diaphragmatic paralysis may be fatal (mortality rate 30%).

Gadolinium is deposited in affected tissues. Circulating fibrocytes may be involved in the pathogenesis of fibrosis and certain cofactors may increase the risk of developing NSF—see Box 23.4.

What should I ask?

- Symptoms: progressive painful tightening of skin leading to disabling joint contractures. Bone pain is common.
- Has the patient been investigated by a contrast-enhanced MRI in previous weeks or months?
- Explore other causes of skin thickening: see Box 23.5. For example, symptoms such as itch, Raynaud's phenomenon, or difficulty swallowing suggest systemic sclerosis rather than NSF.

What should I look for?

- Symmetrical erythematous oedematous hyperpigmented patches or plaques most often on lower limbs, but may affect trunk and upper limbs. Face and neck are spared.
- Papules, nodules, and/or well-demarcated indurated plaques with an irregular outline.
- Woody thickening of skin and fascia gives a cobblestone or 'peau d'orange' appearance.
- Yellow scleral plaques.
- Normal nail folds (unlike systemic sclerosis).
- Flexion contractures of joints in association with skin thickening.

What should I do?

- Take a deep elliptical skin biopsy looking for fibrosis, dermal fibroblast-like cells (CD34 positive), thickening of collagen, and increased elastic and mucin.
- Consider a muscle biopsy.
- Exclude other causes of skin thickening—see Box 23.5:
    - FBC (no eosinophilia), anti-Scl 70 and anti-centromere antibodies (absent). ANA may be positive in NSF and is not a helpful discriminator, paraproteins (absent), thyroid antibodies (absent).
- Echocardiogram, CXR, lung function to exclude systemic disease.
- Treatment—see Box 23.6. May improve if renal function improves.

Box 23.4 Cofactors that may increase risk of NSF

NSF develops in patients with severe renal insufficiency (GFR <30mL/min/1.73m^2) who are exposed to gadolinium-based contrast agents. Cofactors that possibly increase risk of NSF may include:

- Erythropoiesis stimulating agents.
- Acidosis.
- Recent surgery.
- Hepatic disease.
- Proinflammatory events such as infection.

Box 23.5 Differential diagnosis of NSF

- Systemic sclerosis: localized cutaneous or diffuse cutaneous. Look for Raynaud's phenomenon, hand signs, involvement of face, and presence of specific antibodies (Scl-70, anti-centromere)—see 🕮 Box 19.18, p.384.
- Plaque morphoea (scleroderma): 1 lesion. Asymmetrical—see 🕮 p.390.
- Eosinophilic fasciitis (= subcutaneous morphoea): eosinophilia—see 🕮 p.391.
- Scleromyxoedema: associated with a monoclonal paraprotein. Face is involved—see 🕮 Box 26.7, p.499.
- Chronic GVHD—see 🕮 p.496.
- Pre-tibial myxoedema: positive thyroid antibodies—see 🕮 Box 22.5, p.438.
- Porphyria cutanea tarda—see 🕮 p.310.
- Other rare causes of skin thickening include Spanish toxic oil syndrome, vinyl chloride exposure, and eosinophilia–myalgia syndrome.

Box 23.6 Treatment of NSF

Generally disease progresses relentlessly. Thickening and hardening of the skin has a major impact on quality of life.

These therapies have been tried:

- Topical corticosteroids, calcipotriol ointment.
- Oral corticosteroids, cyclophosphamide, ciclosporin.
- Phototherapy, extracorporeal photophoresis.
- High-dose IV immunoglobulin.
- Plasmapheresis.
- Tyrosine kinase inhibitors (imatinib mesylate).

Further reading

Bangsgaard N *et al. Arch Dermatol* 2009; **145:** 183–7.
Nainani N and Panesar M. *Am J Nephrol* 2009; **29:**1–9.
Prchal D *et al. Kidney Int* 2008; **73:**1335–7.

Skin cancer in renal transplant recipients

⚠ Skin cancer, lymphoma/lymphoproliferative malignancies, and solid-organ tumours are common in renal transplant recipients and a leading cause of death. By 5 years after transplantation, the risk of developing a SCC is approximately 100 × greater than in an immunocompetent patient. Most patients have multiple cancers.

Pathogenesis of skin cancer is multifactorial—see Box 23.7. The risk relates to the level as well as the chronicity of immunosuppression, e.g. patients who receive ciclosporin, prednisolone, and azathioprine have a 3 × higher risk of SCC than those taking prednisolone and azathioprine alone. The introduction of immunosuppressant drugs such as mycophenolate mofetil and sirolimus may reduce the risk of cancer in the future.

What should I look for?

- Photodamage: telangiectasia, solar elastosis, erythema, pigmentation. Common in fair skins most at risk of skin cancer (see 🕮 Box 3.1, p.43).
- Persistent HPV-induced warts and pre-cancers e.g. Bowen's disease, solar keratoses on sun-exposed skin. Large numbers of seborrhoeic warts are linked to increased risk of skin cancer.
- New warty papules or tender keratotic nodules on sun-exposed skin: SCCs are the most common skin cancer (65–250-fold increase in risk) and may resemble viral warts. SCCs are much more common in immunosuppressed patients than BCCs, a reversal of the usual ratio of 3BCCs:1SCC.
- Other skin cancers include BCC (10–16-fold increase), malignant melanoma (3–8 fold increase), Kaposi's sarcoma (84-fold increase, HHV-8 related), and Merkel cell cancer (polyomavirus-related).
- Non-melanoma skin cancers are more common in pale skinned individuals living in tropical or subtropical countries.
- Post-transplant lymphoproliferative disorders (mostly B-cell and EBV-related) rarely present in the skin with erythematous patches or nodules.

What should I do?

- Clinical accuracy of diagnosis is poor: cancers may appear banal but conversely warts or hypertrophic solar keratoses may simulate SCC. Have a high index of suspicion and biopsy or excise changing lesions for histological examination, particularly new tender nodules on sun-exposed skin. Cancer on lip and ear may be particularly subtle.
- Ensure the patient understands the importance of rigorous sun protection and reinforce the message regularly—see 🕮 p.316.
- Ensure that patients with chronic renal failure, who may eventually need a renal transplant, are also educated about the importance of sun protection and regular self-examination.
- Examine all the skin of transplant recipients regularly.
- Oral acitretin 20–25mg/day may reduce the incidence of skin cancers.

Box 23.7 Pathogenesis of skin cancer in renal transplant recipients

- Chronic exposure to ultraviolet radiation—see 📖 p.324.
- Impaired immunosurveillance—relates to level of immunosuppression as well as length of time patient has been immunosuppressed.
- Genetic factors including skin type.
- Human papilloma virus (HPV) may play some part in the pathogenesis of skin cancer. Transplant patients have great quantities of low- and medium-risk HPV types in skin.
- Other viruses, e.g. HHV-8 (Kaposi's sarcoma) and polyomavirus (Merckle cell cancer).

Further reading

Bordea C *et al. Transplantation* 2004; **77:**574–9.
Buell JF *et al. Transplantation* 2005; **80:**S254–S264.
Ho WL and Murphy GM. *Br J Dermatol* 2008; **158:**217–24.
Lally A *et al. J Eur Acad Dermatol Venereol* 2009; epublication.
Le Mire L *et al. Br J Dermatol* 2006; **154:**472–7.

Fabry's disease

Synonyms: Anderson–Fabry disease; angiokeratoma corporis diffusum.

⚠ Cutaneous signs may be an early manifestation of this rare X-linked lysosomal storage disease caused by a deficiency in alpha-galactosidase A. Globotriaosylceramide accumulates in endothelial cells, vascular smooth muscle, cutaneous fibroblasts and erector pilori muscles, myocardium, corneal epithelial cells, and organs such as the kidney, heart, lungs, bowel, and eye.

Complications include renal failure, angina, myocardial infarction, transient ischaemic attacks, and stroke. Severe neuropathic pain causes depression or even suicide. Males with Fabry's disease die around age 40–50 and life expectancy is also shortened in heterozygous females. Patients who have cutaneous angiokeratomas and telangiectases are more likely to have major organ involvement.

Prevalence may be higher than previously realized, for example, 2–5% patients with cryptogenic stroke may have milder forms of Fabry's disease. Enzyme replacement therapy may improve quality of life by relieving symptoms such as pain and slowing progression of disease, but is not curative.

What should I ask?

- Patients complain of excruciating neuropathic pain (lancinating, burning) in the extremities (onset in childhood). Exercise, heat, and alcohol make pain worse.
- Asymptomatic telangiectasias and dark red papules (angiokeratomas) may appear in childhood and become more numerous with age.
- Reduced sweating (50% of males, 28% of females) or anhidrosis (25% of males, 4% of females) causes heat intolerance. Patients may collapse after exercise. Rarely patients may have hyperhidrosis.
- Other problems may include hearing loss, visual loss, nausea and abdominal pain, episodic diarrhoea/constipation, but presentation is variable.

What should I look for?

- Facial features: males have prominent supraorbital ridges, frontal bossing, and thickening of the lips.
- Angiokeratomas (slightly keratotic vascular papules, like Campbell de Morgan spots) on the thighs, hips, buttocks, genitalia, and lower back and abdomen, i.e. between the knees and the umbilicus in a 'bathing trunk' distribution (66% of males, 36% of females).
- Telangiectases, vascular macules and/or papules distributed sparsely other areas, e.g. palms and soles, fingers and toes, nail folds, vermillion border of lips, and labial mucosa.
- Reversible oedema/lymphoedema of lower extremities (16–25% of males, 6–17% of females).

What should I do? See Box 23.8.

Box 23.8 Confirming diagnosis of Fabry's disease

- Refer to ophthalmology for a slit-lamp examination to detect changes such as cornea verticillata (vortex opacities located in the superficial corneal layers), tortuous conjunctival, and retinal vessels or Fabry cataract (posterior lens opacities with a radiating appearance).
- Assess renal, cardiac, respiratory, and nervous systems.
- Males: measure alpha-galactosidase in plasma or white cells.
- Genotype females.

Further reading

Hughes DA *et al.* Guidelines for diagnosis and management of Anderson-Fabry disease, 2005. Available at: http://www.dh.gov.uk/en/Publicationsandstatistics/Publications/PublicationsPolicyAndGuidance/DH_4118404

Orteu CH *et al. Br J Dermatol* 2007; **157:**331–7.

Chapter 24

Skin and gastroenterology

Contents

Relevant pages in other chapters

These conditions that may be associated with manifestations in the gastrointestinal tract are discussed in more detail elsewhere:

Aphthous ulcers 🕮 p.262
Pyoderma gangrenosum 🕮 p.290
Porphyria cutanea tarda 🕮 p.310
Kaposi's sarcoma 🕮 p.338
Henoch–Schönlein purpura 🕮 p.408
Erythema nodosum 🕮 p.424
Alpha-1-antitrypsin deficiency 🕮 p.428
Pancreatic panniculitis 🕮 p.428
Systemic amyloidosis 🕮 p.460

Cirrhosis

Cutaneous signs will depend on the cause of cirrhosis.

Mucocutaneous signs in cirrhosis

- Colour change:
  - Dry yellow skin and yellow sclerae.
  - Hyperpigmentation of exposed skin.
  - Generalized hyperpigmentation with sparing of the interscapular and scapular skin has been described in primary biliary cirrhosis.
  - Generalized slate-grey pigmentation (melanin) or bronzed pigmentation of legs (iron and melanin deposition) 'bronze diabetes' in haemochromatosis.
  - Greyish skin and bluish lunulae in Wilson's disease (also Kayser–Fleischer rings—copper in the limbus of the cornea).
- Excoriations. Itch may be very distressing, particularly in primary biliary cirrhosis. Precise cause is unknown but presumably relates to impaired biliary excretion of an irritating substance or substances. Bile acids injected into skin cause itch, but the intensity of pruritus is not related to the levels of bile acids. Biliary obstruction leads to increased intrahepatic synthesis of opioid peptides which are released into the circulation and may contribute to itch—see Box 24.1.
- Spider telangiectasia in the distribution of the superior vena cava.
- Bruising and purpura, gingival bleeding.
- Males: loss of body hair (axillary, pubic) and gynaecomastia.
- White nails (Terry's nails) or parallel white bands (Muehrcke's lines).
- Nail clubbing.
- Palmar erythema, erythematous tips to fingers.
- Peripheral oedema and ascites.
- Dilated superficial veins on the abdomen and chest if portal hypertension.
- Xanthomas in primary biliary cirrhosis and hyperlipidemia—see 📖 p.436.
- Limited cutaneous systemic sclerosis may be associated with primary biliary cirrhosis—see 📖 p.386.
- Signs of porphyria cutanea tarda (photosensitivity, skin fragility, blisters) associated with iron overload (haemochromatosis), alcoholic cirrhosis, and hepatitis C infection—see 📖 p.310.
- Panniculitis in alpha-1-antitrypsin deficiency—see 📖 p.428.

Box 24.1 Management of itch in primary biliary cirrhosis

- Exclude other causes of itching including drugs, scabies, iron deficiency, and thyroid disease— see 📖 p.60.
- Trim nails short to prevent damage to skin from scratching.
- Reduce body temperature by using cool cotton clothing and keeping the room cool, particularly at night (avoid too many bedclothes).
- Avoid soap or excessive bathing (water should not be too hot).
- Copious emollients as well as soap substitutes will relieve dryness.
- Aqueous cream with 1% menthol may be helpful.
- Ursodeoxycholic acid (UDCA), 13–15mg/kg/day, delays progression of hepatic fibrosis in primary biliary cirrhosis but may not relieve itch.
- Colestyramine 4–12g/day (binds bile acids and other biliary molecules). Take before and after breakfast (when gallbladder empties). At least 4h should elapse between the administration of colestyramine and other medications.
- Rifampicin 150mg ×2/day or ×3/day (max. dose 600mg/day), may help, but may cause hepatitis.
- Other options include:
  - UVB.
  - Sertraline (75–100mg/day), a serotonin reuptake inhibitor.
  - Naloxone (opioid antagonist). Start with a low dose and increase very gradually. May cause symptoms of narcotic withdrawal.
  - Plasmapheresis.

Kumagi T and Heathcote EJ. *Orphanet J Rare Dis* 2008; **3:**1–17.

Inflammatory bowel disease (IBD)

Cutaneous signs are common in both Crohn's disease and ulcerative colitis and may precede the diagnosis by several years. Abdominal stomas also cause skin problems—see Box 24.2.

What should I look for?

- Nail clubbing and palmar erythema.
- Erythema nodosum—see p.424.
- Aphthous ulcers and glossitis—see p.262.
- Thrombophlebitis.
- Perianal fissures, fistulae, and abscesses—more severe in Crohn's disease than ulcerative colitis—see Box 24.3.
- Genital or orofacial Crohn's disease—see Box 24.3 (biopsy shows non-caseating, sarcoidal granulomas with multinucleated giant cells in dermis and subcutaneous tissue).
- Peri-stomal dermatitis or folliculitis—see Box 24.2.
- Cutaneous adverse drug reactions including reactions to sulphasalazine (patients may be photosensitive).
- Manifestations of nutritional deficiency including an acrodermatitis enteropathica-like syndrome (acquired zinc deficiency)—see p.474.
- Psoriasis (increased prevalence in Crohn's disease).
- Chronic palmoplantar pustulosis sometimes linked to SAPHO syndrome—see p.228.
- Neutrophilic dermatoses such as pyoderma gangrenosum including peri-stomal pyoderma (see Box 24.2 and see p.290), Sweet's syndrome (see p.480), and bowel-associated dermatosis-arthritis syndrome (see p.481).
- ⚠ Pyostomatitis vegetans: a rare pustular disorder that is a marker of IBD and usually precedes the onset. Friable grey-yellow pustules may involve oral, vaginal, nasal, and, rarely, periocular mucosa. Ruptured pustules leave vegetating erosions or ulcers. Symptoms are mild. Differentiate from pemphigus by histology and immunofluorescence—see p.248. Skin involvement has been reported (pyodermatitis vegetans).
- Cutaneous granulomatous vasculitis (in Crohn's disease).
- Vitiligo.
- Autoimmune bullous diseases: bullous pemphigoid, linear IgA disease and EBA—see p.250–52.
- Skin manifestations of systemic amyloidosis—see p.460.

Extra-intestinal non-cutaneous signs

- Inflammatory arthropathies with sacroilietis, peripheral arthritis with or without enthesitis, tenosynovitis, and dactylitis. Some patients develop SAPHO syndrome—see p.228.
- Episcleritis, scleritis, and uveitis.

Box 24.2 Skin and abdominal stomas

Hydrocolloids are widely used both for securing stoma devices and for protecting the skin, but skin disorders are reported in >70% of patients with an abdominal stoma. These include:

- Irritant dermatitis: common and may be secondarily infected. Chronic irritation leads to over-granulation or erosions at the mucocutaneous junction. Treat with topical corticosteroids. Sucralfate powder prevents further irritation and may promote healing of erosions.
- Allergic contact dermatitis is uncommon but consider patch testing to reassure patient and stoma nurse.
- Bacterial folliculitis occurs when shaving is used to help the bag to adhere to the skin. Swab, treat with antibiotics, and triclosan wash.
- Peri-stomal psoriasis: treat with topical corticosteroids.
- Peri-stomal pyoderma gangrenosum: treat with a very potent topical corticosteroid or 0.1% tacrolimus (in carmellose sodium paste). May need systemic treatment, e.g. oral ciclosporin.

Topical corticosteroids

Creams, gels, or oils will impair adhesion of the bag. Apply betamethasone valerate (0.1%) lotion to the adhesive surface of the stoma appliance. Let alcohol evaporate before placing appliance on skin. Alternatively, spray on steroid powder from an aerosol inhaler.

Further reading

Lyon CC et al. *Br J Dermatol* 2000; **143:**1248–60.

Box 24.3 Cutaneous Crohn's disease

Perianal

- Perianal: polypoid tags, moist plaques, erythema, swelling, induration, fissures, fistulas, scarring, abscesses, and sinus tracts.
- Aphthous ulcers in the anal canal, ulcers of anal sphincter.

Orofacial

- Granulomatous infiltration of oral mucosa with oedema, aphthous ulcers, and a 'cobblestone' papular hyperplasia.
- Angular cheilitis with fissuring.
- Gingival erythema and oedematous gingival nodules.
- Persistent swelling of lips and/or cheeks.

'Metastatic' i.e. separated from the gastrointestinal tract by normal tissue:

- Swelling or induration of genitalia sometimes with erythema (more common in children).
- Genital papules, plaques, fissures, and ulcers
- Erythematous papules, plaques, nodules or ulcers exuding pus, mainly in the lower extremities and flexures.

Signs may suggest lymphoedema, hereditary angio-oedema, cellulitis, chronic HSV infection, sarcoid, hidradenitis suppuritiva (see 📖 p.230) or a sexually transmitted infection such as syphilis.

Treatment options include potent topical corticosteroids, 0.1% tacrolimus ointment, and oral metronidazole.

Nutritional deficiencies

Starvation is the most common cause of nutritional deficiency in the developing world. In Africa, 1 of every 3 children is underweight. Malnutrition contributes to more than 1/2 of the nearly 12 million under-5 deaths in developing countries each year.

In the developed world, patients who are seriously ill, unable to care for themselves, or have problems such as malabsorption, chronic alcoholism, chronic diarrhoea, or bowel fistulae may also be malnourished. Some patients choose to restrict their diets, perhaps because of religious beliefs, concerns about food allergy, or eating disorders. Parents of children with atopic eczema may omit essential nutrients such as milk from the child's diet in the well-intentioned but mistaken belief that this may cure the eczema. Bariatric surgery, used to restrict the stomach's capacity in obesity, may cause nutritional deficiency. Rarely, genetic or metabolic defects cause nutritional deficiency. (Cystic fibrosis—see 📖 Box 24.6 p.479.)

Cutaneous signs depend on the deficiency—protein, carbohydrate, vitamins, minerals, and/or essential trace elements. Some patients have a number of deficiencies.

Cutaneous signs in malabsorption

Increased faecal excretion of fat is associated with variable deficiency in proteins, minerals, trace elements, fat-soluble vitamins, and carbohydrates as well as water. Signs include combinations of:

- Itching, dry skin which may be very scaly (ichthyotic).
- Hyperpigmentation (chloasma-like facial, generalized Addisonian, or pellagra-like—see 📖 p.475).
- Pallor (iron deficiency and anaemia).
- Brittle nails and hair loss.
- Follicular hyperkeratosis also known as phrynoderma. Mainly affects extensor surfaces of extremities (vitamin A deficiency).
- Bruising, petechiae, oral bleeding (lack of vitamin K).
- Angular stomatitis, cheilitis, glossitis (smooth sore red tongue), mucosal erosions (lack of vitamin B complex or folic acid).
- Seborrhoeic dermatitis-like rash (lack of vitamin B complex).

Cutaneous signs in kwashiorkor

This common childhood disorder, seen in developing countries, is caused by protein malnutrition in the presence of reasonable calories. Kwashiorkor develops after the child is weaned (age 1–4), when diet is mainly starchy vegetables. Signs include:

- Erythematous or purplish hyperkeratotic plaques with fissuring like 'flaky paint' or 'crazy paving'.
- Hypopigmented dry skin. Fine desquamation is common.
- Sparse dry, brittle hair.
- Normal dark brown hair becomes orangish red. The flag sign—alternating bands of pale and dark hair—with intermittent protein intake.
- Cheilitis, angular stomatitis, oral erosions, vulvovaginitis.
- Swollen abdomen.
- Pitting oedema of lower extremities and muscle wasting.

Cutaneous signs in pellagra: niacin (vitamin B3) deficiency

Pellagra is characterized by dermatitis (the only sign in 3% of patients), diarrhoea, and dementia. Pellagra may complicate chronic alcoholism. Look for:

- Erythema and superficial scaling on sun-exposed skin that fades to leave reddish-brown pigmentation.
  - 'Butterfly rash' (malar) on face.
  - Well-demarcated erythema on anterior neck (Casal's necklace).
- Erythema and scaling of skin exposed to heat, friction or pressure.

Cutaneous signs in scurvy: vitamin C deficiency

- Follicular keratoses on upper arms, back, buttocks and lower extremities containing 'corkscrew' coiled hairs.
- Petechiae, perifollicular haemorrhage, and bruising.
- Gingival hypertrophy and bleeding gums.
- Delayed wound healing.

Cutaneous signs in acrodermatitis enteropathica: zinc deficiency

Acrodermatitis enteropathica is an autosomal recessive disorder in which intestinal absorption of zinc is inadequate. Disease usually presents 4–6 weeks after weaning but may develop earlier if the infant is not given breast milk, which enhances zinc absorption. Zinc deficiency has also been described following total parenteral nutrition without zinc and in association with alcoholism, Crohn's disease, and chronic pancreatitis.

Zinc deficiency causes acral dermatitis, alopecia, and diarrhoea as well as (in infants) failure to thrive with apathy and irritability. Look for:

- Vesiculobullous or pustular dermatitis on hands and feet.
- Pustular paronychia.
- Periorificial (perioral, periorbital, and perianal) crusted papules and plaques which may be pustular.
- Photophobia with blepharitis and conjunctivitis.
- Slow hair growth, generalized alopecia, and a nail dystrophy with Beau's lines in chronic zinc deficiency.
- Delayed healing of ulcers; secondary bacterial and fungal infections.

Cutaneous signs in essential fatty acid deficiency

- Dry leathery skin and follicular keratoses.
- Dry hair and brittle nails.
- Periorificial plaques resembling acrodermatitis enteropathica have been described, but patients may also be zinc deficient.

Cutaneous signs in iron deficiency

In addition to the pallor of anaemia, iron deficiency may lead to

- Hair loss.
- Itching.

Further reading

Oumeish OY and Oumeish I. *Clin Dermatol* 2003; **21**:260–3.

Coeliac disease (coeliac sprue)

Coeliac disease is a gluten-sensitive enteropathy primarily found in Caucasians that is associated with IgA anti-gliadin, anti-endomysial, and anti-transglutaminase 2 antibodies. Genes for specific class II human leukocyte antigens (HLA) DQ2 and DQ8 confer susceptibility to coeliac disease. Presentation varies but may include failure to thrive (children), delayed puberty, chronic diarrhoea, and abdominal distension or pain. Malabsorption leads to nutrient and mineral deficiencies with problems such as anaemia (folate and iron deficiency), osteomalacia, or osteoporosis. Symptoms are controlled by a gluten-free diet.

Coeliac disease is associated with an increased prevalence of other disorders including splenic atrophy, autoimmune endocrine disorders (hypothyroidism, diabetes, and Addison's disease), primary biliary cirrhosis, neurological disorders, and IgA deficiency (5% of patients). Patients have an increased risk of intestinal lymphoma and, rarely, other gastrointestinal cancers. The risk is reduced by a strict gluten-free diet. Dermatitis herpetiformis occurs in 10–20% of patients but is rare in children.

What is dermatitis herpetiformis (DH)?

DH is a rare IgA-mediated bullous disease that is associated with sensitivity to gluten. All patients have coeliac disease which is never severe and is usually subclinical. Serum IgA autoantibodies to epidermal transglutaminase probably play some part in the pathogenesis—see 📖 p.477. DH may be associated with other autoimmune diseases—see Box 24.4.

For more information see 📖 p.254.

Pathogenesis of coeliac disease and dermatitis herpetiformis

- An inflammatory response to certain proteins in wheat (gliadin, the alcohol-soluble component of gluten), and related proteins in rye and barley, damages the mucosa of the small intestine leading to malabsorption. Oats do not cause problems provided they have not been contaminated with wheat proteins when ground in the mill.
- Gluten peptides cross the intestinal epithelial barrier.
- Tissue transglutaminase (transglutaminase 2) in small bowel binds to and deaminates gliadins producing immunogenetic peptides that activate a T-cell response. Antigen-presenting cells expressing the HLA-DQ2 and HLA-DQ8 molecules have an increased affinity for these peptides.
- Activated gluten-specific T-cells stimulate B-cell production of IgA anti-gliadin and anti-transglutaminase 2 antibodies. (The antigen recognized by antiendomysial antibody is tissue transglutaminase.)
- Inflammation causes intestinal mucosal damage, crypt cell hyperproliferation, and villous atrophy.
- IgA antibodies to tissue transglutaminase cross-react with epidermal transglutaminase but patients with DH also produce specific IgA antibodies to epidermal transglutaminase (TG3).
- Anti-epidermal transglutaminase antibodies in immune complexes play a role in the pathogenesis of DH.

Box 24.4 Diseases associated with DH

- Vitiligo and alopecia areata.
- Autoimmune thyroid disease (common), diabetes mellitus, Addison's disease.
- SLE, Sjögren's syndrome, rheumatoid arthritis.
- ⚠ Intestinal lymphoma.

Further reading

Briani C *et al. Autoimmun Rev* 2008; **7:**644–50.

Kárpáti S. *J Dermatol Sci* 2004; **34:**83–90.

Rose C *et al. J Am Acad Dermatol* 2009; **61:**39–43.

Pancreas

See Box 24.5 for cutaneous signs of pancreatic disease.

⚠ Necrolytic migratory erythema

This very rare, but striking, skin condition should prompt an urgent search for a glucagon-producing tumour in the pancreatic alpha cells. Unfortunately many patients already have metastases at the time of diagnosis. The full syndrome includes necrolytic migratory erythema, diabetes mellitus (mild), stomatitis, cheilitis, weight loss, diarrhoea, venous thrombosis, and neuropsychiatric symptoms.

'Pseudoglucagonoma syndromes'—necrolytic migratory erythema has been described in association with other conditions including pancreatic cancers, chronic pancreatitis, coeliac disease, jejunal adenocarcinoma, and hepatic cirrhosis.

What should I look for?

- Recurrent outbreaks of itchy, uncomfortable erythematous papules or plaques most marked on face, flexures, and sites of friction, but may be widespread.
- Superficial flaccid vesicles and bullae within erythematous patches. These rupture rapidly leaving crusted erosions.
- The crusted edges of patches extend outward in serpiginous patterns.
- After 1–2 weeks, patches heal centrally often leaving hyperpigmentation.
- Perioral erythematous crusted patches with peripheral scale.
- Genital or perianal skin may be involved and some features may resemble acrodermatitis enteropathica—see 📖 p.475.
- Patients may have glossitis.

What should I do?

- Check serum glucagon levels, which are markedly raised.
- Check serum zinc levels, which are normal.
- Take a skin biopsy from the edge of an early lesion. Histological features (which may be non-specific) include parakeratosis, subcorneal neutrophils, intracellular oedema in the upper layers of the epidermis and degeneration (necrolysis) of superficial keratinocytes.
- Investigate for a pancreatic tumour initially by abdominal CT scan.

Cystic fibrosis

See Box 24.6 for cutaneous features.

Box 24.5 Pancreatic disease and the skin

- Acute pancreatitis may be associated with purpura in the left flank (Grey Turner's sign) or periumbilical purpura (Cullen's sign).
- Pancreatic panniculitis occurs in association with acute or chronic pancreatitis, pancreatic islet cell tumours, ductal adenocarcinoma, and acinar-cell carcinoma. The reddish-brown subcutaneous nodules are found most often on the legs. Nodules may ulcerate and discharge necrotic fat—see 📖 p.428.
- Necrolytic migratory erythema—glucagon-producing tumour in the pancreatic alpha cells—see 📖 p.478.
- Manifestations of nutritional deficiency in cystic fibrosis—see Box 24.6.

Box 24.6 Cystic fibrosis (CF)

CF is inherited in an autosomal recessive pattern and is characterized by chronic bacterial infection of airways and sinuses, fat malabsorption, male infertility, and elevated concentrations of chloride in sweat. Mutations in the cystic fibrosis transmembrane conductance regulator (*CFTR*) gene cause abnormalities in ion transport.

Cutaneous features include:

- Aquagenic skin wrinkling. Itchy or tingling oedematous white papules and plaques appear on palms and soles within 2min of exposure to water. Remits within a few hours. Mechanism uncertain—elevated sweat chloride may increase keratin binding to water, or regulation of water membrane channels may be abnormal or eccrine ducts may be dysfunctional.
- Nutrient deficiency dermatitis (age 2 weeks to 6 months). Features overlap with those of acrodermatitis enteropathica, essential fatty acid deficiency and kwashiorkor (see 📖 p.474). Erythematous papules (may be annular) present in napkin area, periorbital and perioral skin but may spread to the extremities and progress to extensive desquamating plaques.
- Cutaneous adverse drug reactions (30% of patients), e.g. morbilliform, urticaria, angioedema, SJS, and leucocytoclastic vasculitis.
- Atopic eczema (increased prevalence).
- Cutaneous vasculitis.

Further reading

Bernstein ML *et al Paed Dermatol* 2008; **25**: 150–157.

Neutrophilic dermatoses

The neutrophilic dermatoses associated with bowel disease include pyoderma gangrenosum (see 📖 p.290), Sweet's syndrome, and bowel associated dermatosis-arthritis syndrome.

Sweet's syndrome (acute febrile neutrophilic dermatosis)

This syndrome is characterized by intense neutrophilic infiltration of the skin. It is more common in women.

Associations

- Infection: 70% of patients. Most often 1–3 weeks after infection of upper respiratory tract.
- Chronic inflammation: 15% of patients, e.g. inflammatory bowel disease, connective tissue diseases such as polychondritis, sarcoidosis.
- ⚠ Malignancy: 10–20% of patients—particularly haematological malignancies, e.g. acute myelogenous leukaemia, myeloproliferative disease or myelodysplastic syndromes, lymphoma, and paraproteinaemias.
- Drugs: e.g. oral contraceptive, minocycline, diazepam, granulocyte colony-stimulating factor (G-CSF), and bortezomib (a proteasome inhibitor).
- Immunodeficiency: primary or secondary.
- Pregnancy.

What should I look for?

- Fever and neutrophilia with a raised ESR often suggesting sepsis.
- Tender well-demarcated oedematous erythematous papules and large plaques, most often on face and upper trunk (may be misdiagnosed as cellulitis or herpes infection, particularly if a solitary lesion) (Fig. 24.1).
- The surface of plaques may appear to be vesicular (pseudo-vesicles) reflecting the intense dermal oedema, but it is rare to find discrete vesicles or bullae that can be ruptured. Occasionally plaques become pustular.
- Panniculitis: nodules rupture releasing necrotic fat (uncommon).
- Iritis, episcleritis, and/or conjunctivitis.
- Arthralgia, polyarthritis, and myalgia.
- Oral mucosal ulcers (mimic aphthae) (uncommon).
- Patients may also have pyoderma gangrenosum—see 📖 p.290.

What should I do?

- Exclude infection by taking blood for culture and swabs from pustular skin lesions. Cultures are sterile in Sweet's syndrome.
- Check FBC and ESR, and exclude an underlying disease.
- Take a skin biopsy from a well-developed plaque. In Sweet's syndrome you will find a dense dermal neutrophilic infiltrate with leucocytoclasis but without vasculitis. Gram stain is negative.
- Treat with systemic corticosteroids (initially prednisolone 30mg/day) and very potent topical corticosteroids ×2/day.
- Recurrences are common. Steroid-sparing agents that may be helpful include dapsone, colchicine, and ciclosporin.

Bowel-associated dermatosis-arthritis syndrome

The overgrowth of bacteria in a blind loop with the deposition of immune complexes is thought to trigger disease. The histopathological changes resemble those of Sweet's syndrome.

Associations

- Bowel bypass surgery to treat morbid obesity.
- Extensive resection of small bowel.
- Patients with an abnormal segment of bowel in diseases such as diverticulosis or IBD.

What should I look for?

- A history of gastrointestinal disease or gastrointestinal surgery.
- Crops of erythematous macules, purpuric papules, and small vesicopustules on upper trunk and extremities.
- Migratory polyarthralgia or a non-erosive polyarthritis.
- Malaise and fever.

What should I do?

- Confirm diagnosis by skin biopsy which shows a neutrophilic dermatosis like Sweet's syndrome.
- Correct the underlying cause.

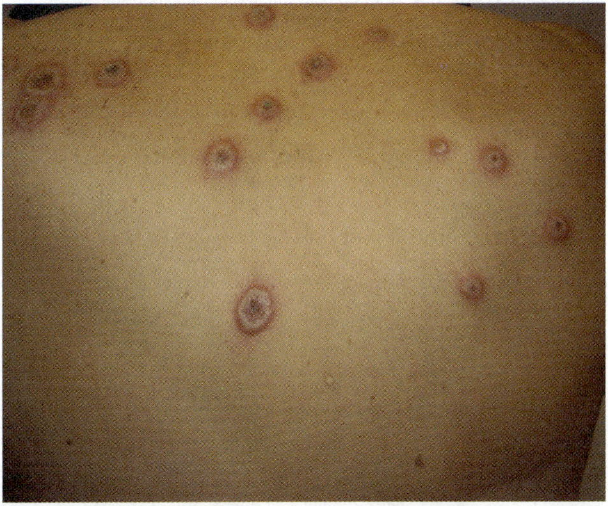

Fig. 24.1 Sweet's syndrome: well-demarcated oedematous plaques.

Rare syndromes

⚠ Carcinoid syndrome

Carcinoid tumours are found most often in the gastrointestinal tract (55%) and bronchopulmonary system (30%). Carcinoids arise from enterochromaffin cells of the gastrointestinal tract and the tumours release a variety of polypeptides, pyogenic amines, and prostaglandins, which are responsible for the carcinoid syndrome. Tumours are rare and the syndrome even rarer, occurring in <10% of patients with a tumour.

What should I look for?

Features of carcinoid syndrome comprise:

- Episodic cutaneous flushing (85% of patients) lasting 20–30s.
- Flushes may be spontaneous or triggered by eating, alcohol, defecation, changes in temperature, emotional stress, or palpation of the liver.
- Flushing starts suddenly on the face, neck, and upper chest.
- A mild burning sensation is common or skin may be intensely itchy.
- Severe flushes may be accompanied by hypotension and tachycardia.
- Diarrhoea may be explosive and disabling.
- Wheezing and dyspnoea are common, particularly during episodes of flushing.
- Flushes may last from hours to days in bronchial carcinoid.
- Chronic disease leads to persistent facial oedema and facial venous telangiectasia that may simulate rosacea, but patients do not have pustules or papules.
- Persistent brawny facial oedema.
- Scleroderma-like fibrosis probably caused by impaired tryptophan metabolism.
- Pellagra (dietary tryptophan is diverted for synthesis of serotonin)—rough scaly skin, glossitis, angular stomatitis, and confusion.

What should I do?

- Exclude more common causes of a red face—see Box 24.7 and 📖 p.70.
- If clinically indicated, measure 24-h urinary excretion of 5-hydroxyindoleacetic acid (HIAA) which is increased in carcinoid syndrome.
- Localize the tumour e.g. abdominal CT.

Box 24.7 Flushing: what should I do?

- Flushing of face, chest and neck is common in individuals with a fair complexion, particularly Celts and northern Europeans.
- Easy flushing may precede the development of rosacea—look for papules, pustules, swelling, and telangiectasia—see 📖 p.234.
- Exclude seborrhoeic dermatitis, psoriasis, or contact dermatitis as a cause of facial redness.
- Exclude photosensitivity (drugs) or a photoaggravated dermatosis (cutaneous LE, atopic eczema)—see 📖 p.302.

Box 24.7 (Cont.)

- Carcinoid syndrome is very rare and investigation is only indicated if flushing is accompanied by systemic symptoms such as abdominal pain, diarrhoea, dyspnoea, or hypotension.
- Treatment options for idiopathic flushing are limited:
  - Reduce anxiety levels.
  - Beta-blockers (propranolol 10–40mg ×2–3/day).
  - Clonidine has been recommended.

See Box 24.8 for cutaneous signs in other rare conditions.

Box 24.8 Cutaneous signs in other rare conditions

Hereditary haemorrhagic telangiectasia (Osler–Weber–Rendu disease): telangiectasias on skin and mucous membranes (stretch the lip to see the branching vessels); nail clubbing if patient has pulmonary arterio-venous fistulae. Look for telangiectasias and a history of nasal bleeds in any patient with anaemia or melaena. 80% of cases have a positive family history (inheritance is autosomal dominant). Patients may also have von Willebrand's disease.

Blue rubber-bleb naevus syndrome: cavernous hemangiomas in skin and gastrointestinal tract with gastrointestinal bleeding.

Pseudoxanthoma elasticum: gastrointestinal bleeds are a major complication—see 📖 p.400.

Gardner's syndrome: premalignant colonic and rectal polyps; many sebaceous cysts on face, other cutaneous tumours, osteomas—see 📖 p.501.

Peutz–Jeghers syndrome: intestinal polyps; pigmented macules (lentigines) on vermillion borders of lips, oral mucosa, perioral, perianal, and periorbital skin, over joints, and on palms and soles—see 📖 p.501.

Cronkhite–Canada syndrome: nail dystrophy, alopecia, and hyperpigmentation; intestinal polyps cause diarrhoea, malabsorption, and weight loss; rapidly fatal in 1/3 of patients.

Muir–Torre syndrome: sebaceous neoplasms with gastrointestinal and genitourinary cancers—see 📖 p.501.

Degos' disease: crops of erythematous papules evolve into porcelain-white macules with an erythematous rim. An occlusive vasculopathy produces wedge-shaped infarcts in the skin. Similar pathology in gastro-intestinal tract or cerebral vessels may be fatal.

Familial Mediterranean fever: abdominal pain, tender erythematous, patches (like erysipelas) and arthritis—see 📖 p.218.

Further reading

Braverman IM. *Gastroenterology* 2003; **124:**1595–614.

Chapter 25

Skin and chest diseases

Contents

Relevant pages in other chapters

Superior vena cava obstruction 📖 p.70
Cutaneous tuberculosis 📖 p.136
Atopic eczema 📖 p.202
Erythema nodosum 📖 p.424
Alpha-1-antitrypsin deficiency 📖 p.428
Cystic fibrosis 📖 Box 24.6, p.479
Carcinoid syndrome 📖 p.482
Cancer syndromes 📖 p.500
Familial cancer syndrome 📖 p.500
Paraneoplastic skin changes 📖 p.502

Sarcoidosis

Sarcoidosis is an idiopathic granulomatous disease of unknown cause (see Box 25.1) that predominantly affects the lung, but may involve virtually any organ. Skin is affected in 25% of patients. Sarcoidosis has been described in association with other diseases—see Box 25.2.

What should I look for?

Specific cutaneous lesions

The skin is easier to biopsy to confirm the diagnosis than internal organs, so look hard for cutaneous involvement. Cutaneous sarcoidosis is a great imitator. Specific cutaneous lesions have a granulomatous histology (see 📖 Box 32.5, p.579) and may include:

- Asymptomatic translucent yellowish-brown firm papules (often periorbital), nodules or plaques (round, oval, or annular) (Fig. 25.1) on an erythematous background. Smooth or scaly. Use diascopy to reveal the yellow-brown colour—see Box 25.3. Usually resolve spontaneously.
- Changing scars: infiltration gives skin a purplish-red colour (see Fig. 25.2). May be tender. Sarcoid may also involve tattoos.
- Firm subcutaneous nodules (Darier–Roussy sarcoid) most often on forearms. Often associated with systemic disease.
- Lupus pernio: indolent reddish-purple destructive plaques and nodules on nose, cheeks, lips, and ears (sites where skin is cool). Most common in women. Lesions may ulcerate and heal with telangiectatic scars (see Fig. 25.3). Poor prognosis. Associated with more severe pulmonary disease.
- Alopecia: scarring or non-scarring.
- Ulcers, most often on legs: seen most often in African Americans.
- Ichthyosis-like scaling on legs.
- Psoriasiform erythematous or reddish-brown scaly plaques.
- Hyopigmented macules or patches or hypopigmentation over papules.

Non-specific cutaneous lesions

- Erythema nodosum is a 'reactive' panniculitis, that tends to be associated with an acute form of sarcoid, which resolves without treatment. Löfgren's syndrome (erythema nodosum with bilateral hilar adenopathy, fever and acute ankle arthritis) is diagnostic of sarcoid.

Involvement of other organs

- Lungs: asymptomatic in 60%. May have cough, dyspnoea, or pleuritic chest pain. 10–30% develop chronic pulmonary disease. Pulmonary fibrosis causes respiratory failure.
- Eyes: blurring or loss of vision, painful red eye, or photophobia. Signs include macular oedema and papilloedema.
- Lacrimal or salivary gland swelling (with dry eye/dry mouth).
- Peripheral lymphadenopathy.
- Heart: arrhythmias, left ventricular dysfunction.
- CNS: palsy of VIIth cranial nerve, mono- or polyneuropathies.
- Liver: abnormal LFTs.
- Renal failure secondary to hypercalciuria or hypercalcaemia.

What should I do?

See 📖 p.488.

Box 25.1 Pathogenesis of sarcoidosis

- Genetic susceptibility: more severe in African Americans (black Americans) than white Americans.
- Chronic cell-mediated immune response to unknown antigen:
  - Activated macrophages and CD4+ T-lymphocytes release cytokines that trigger formation of granulomas.
  - Elevated interferon-gamma, interleukin-2 and interleukin-12.
  - Overproduction of TNF-α at the sites of disease.
- Relative anergy *in vivo* possibly secondary to regulatory T-cells inhibiting IL-2 and T-cell proliferation.

Box 25.2 Associations between sarcoidosis and other diseases

Sarcoidosis may be associated with other conditions including:

- Scleroderma, Sjögren's syndrome, and ankylosing spondylitis.
- Primary biliary cirrhosis.
- Autoimmune thyroid disease.
- Crohn's disease.
- Lymphoproliferative and solid malignancies.

Box 25.3 How to perform diascopy

- Gently press a glass slide onto a sarcoidal papule or plaque.
- The pressure enhances the yellow-brown 'apple jelly' colour by removing the background erythema.
- Cutaneous tuberculosis has a similar appearance.

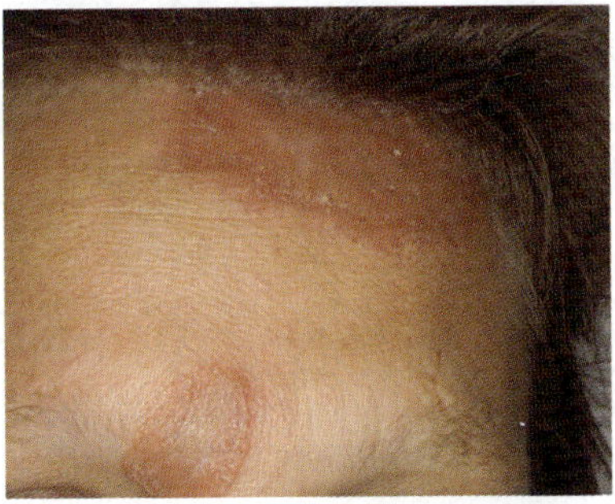

Fig. 25.1 Reddish-brown slightly scaly, plaques with raised border.

Further reading

Marchell RM and Judson MA. *Clin Dermatol* 2007; **25:**295–302.

Iannuzzi MC *et al. N Engl J Med* 2007; **357:**2153–65.

Judson MA. *Am J Med Sci* 2008; **335:**26–33.

Management of cutaneous sarcoid

⚠ The diagnosis is one of exclusion. Always search hard for another explanation for the granulomatous histology, particularly mycobacterial or fungal diseases—see Box 25.4.

What should I do?

- Take a biopsy from a specific cutaneous lesion (much easier than taking a biopsy from an internal organ).
- If the histology is granulomatous, exclude mycobacterial and fungal infection by culture of involved skin.
- Tuberculin skin test (may be anergic in sarcoid).
- FBC, renal function, and liver function.
- Serum and urinary calcium (risk of hypercalcaemia and hypercalciuria). 1-alpha hydroxylase is activated by macrophages in granulomas and converts 25-hydroxyvitamin D_3 to 1,25-dihydroxyvitamin D_3, the active form of the vitamin. Absorption of calcium from the gut increases, as does renal excretion.
- Although serum ACE may be elevated in active sarcoidosis, this test is insufficiently sensitive or specific to be of diagnostic help.
- Serum protein electrophoresis: 50% have a polyclonal hypergammaglobulinemia. ⚠ If hypogammaglobulinemia, check for variable common immunodeficiency or lymphoma.
- Chest radiograph and pulmonary function tests.
- Electrocardiogram (ECG).
- Refer for an ophthalmological assessment.

Treatment of cutaneous sarcoid

- No treatment required if not symptomatic. Skin manifestations may resolve spontaneously.
- Very potent topical corticosteroids: may be used under a hydrocolloid occlusive dressing (see 📖 p.590). Haelan® tape is an alternative.
- Intralesional triamcinolone (3–20mg/mL): repeated injections required.
- Topical 0.1% tacrolimus ointment.
- Systemic agents that have been recommended for cutaneous disease (few controlled trials) include:
  - Hydroxychloroquine 200–400mg/day (no more than 6.5mg/kg/day). Should see optician annually.
  - Methotrexate 10–20mg/week.
  - Oral tetracyclines.
  - Oral prednisolone 20–40mg/day is indicated in recalcitrant extensive or destructive skin disease. May be combined with hydroxychloroquine or methotrexate.
  - Other drugs that have been advocated include isotretinoin, fumaric acid esters, leflunomide, mycophenolate mofetil, thalidomide, and infliximab.

Box 25.4 Cutaneous sarcoid: histological differential diagnosis

- Cutaneous tuberculosis and atypical mycobacterial infections.
- Deep fungal infection.
- Foreign body reaction: zirconium, beryllium, tattoo, paraffin, etc.
- Rheumatoid nodule.
- Leishmaniasis.
- Melkersson–Rosenthal syndrome: recurrent or persistent orofacial swellings (especially the lower lip and around the eyes), a fissured tongue, and intermittent paralysis of peripheral facial nerve.

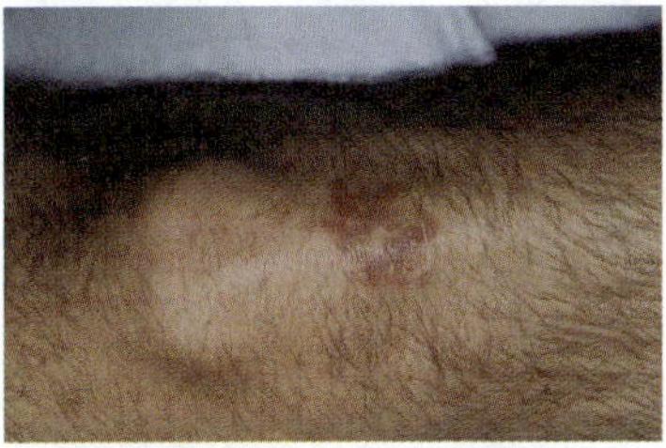

Fig. 25.2 Purplish red discoloration of an old scar secondary to sarcoidal infiltration.

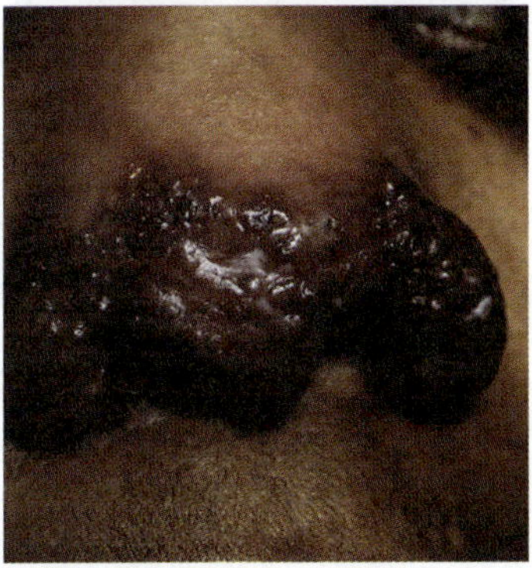

Fig. 25.3 Lupus pernio with destruction of the nose.

Further reading

Baughman RP and Lower EE. *Clin Dermatol* 2007; **25:**334–40.

Doherty CB and Rosen T. *Drugs* 2008; **68:**1361–83.

Kalajian AH *et al. Arch Dermatol* 2009; **145:**905–9.

Chapter 26

Skin and haematology/ oncology

Contents

Relevant pages in other chapters

Reactions to chemotherapy 🕮 p.358, Radiation recall dermatitis 🕮 p.359, Neutrophilic dermatoses including Sweet's syndrome 🕮 p.480, Neutrophilic eccrine hidradenitis 🕮 p.358, and Pyoderma gangrenosum 🕮 p.290, Cryoglobulinaemia 🕮 p.410, Kaposis's sarcoma 🕮 p.338, Cutaneous T-cell lymphoma 🕮 p.336, Infections 🕮 Chapters 6, p.121 and 7, p.141, Demodicosis in immunocompromised 🕮 p.168, Amyloidosis 🕮 p.460, Immunodeficiency syndromes 🕮 p.562.

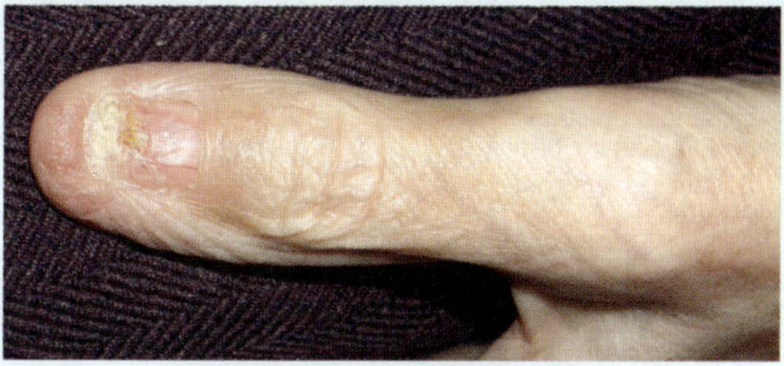

Fig. 26.1 Destruction of nails in lichenoid chronic GVHD.

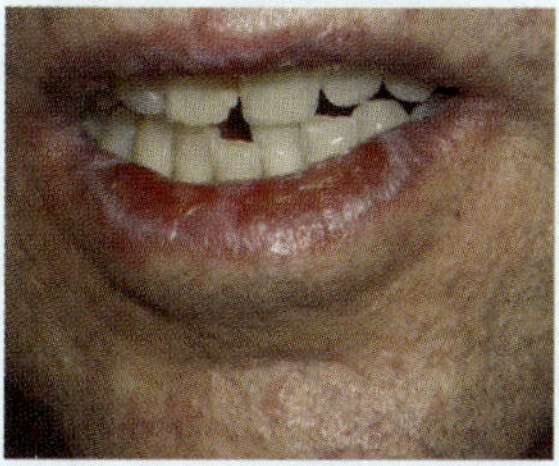

Fig. 26.2 Erosions and whitish discoloration of the lips simulate lichen planus in lichenoid GVHD.

Radiotherapy

Early reactions in radiation field

Acute side effects resolve in around 4–6 weeks, usually without treatment, but moisturizers and soap substitutes may be helpful.

Reactions include:

- Erythematous dry skin and mild oedema (like sunburn).
- Oedema, marked erythema, and moist desquamation.
- Blisters, ulcers, and haemorrhagic crusting (infrequent because doses of radiotherapy are controlled more precisely than in the past).
- Hyperpigmentation (more common in dark skin).
- Hair loss.

Late reactions in radiation field

Late reactions in the radiation field may appear years after radiotherapy and changes gradually progress. Reactions include:

- Telangiectasia, hypo- and hyperpigmentation.
- Epidermal atrophy and fragility.
- Necrosis leading to ulceration (may simulate cutaneous malignancy).
- Dermal and subcutaneous fibrosis (within first 3 months).

Generalized skin diseases induced by radiation

- Herpes zoster.
- Erythema multiforme (EM).
- Auto-immune blistering diseases (bullous pemphigoid, pemphigus).

Skin diseases induced by radiation but localized to the radiation field

- Acneiform lesions with comedones.
- Lichenoid reactions:
  - EM, GVHD, LP.
- Bullous pemphigoid.
- Fibrosing reactions:
  - Morphoea: abrupt onset with erythema and induration 1 month to 3 years after radiotherapy. Usually affects the breast. Treatment is not very effective but topical, intralesional, and oral corticosteroids have been recommended.
  - Lichen sclerosus.
  - Post-irradiation pseudosclerodermatous panniculitis 1–8 months after megavoltage (deeply penetrating) radiotherapy. Usually affects the breast. May resemble metastatic disease. Can improve spontaneously.
- Vasculopathy with fibrosis, atherosclerosis, and rupture of vessels.
- Malignancy.

Further reading

Carrasco L *et al. Am J Dermatopathol* 2001; **23:**283–7.

Reddy SM *et al. Semin Arthritis Rheum* 2005; **34:**728–34.

Acute cutaneous graft-versus-host disease

What is graft-versus-host disease (GVHD)?

Haemopoietic stem cell transplants (HSCTs) are used to treat conditions such as leukaemia, myeloma, lymphoma, aplastic anaemia, and immunodeficiency. GVHD complicates >50% of allogeneic HSCTs and is caused by the donor immunocompetent T-cells reacting against the immunocompromised host tissues. New, less aggressive approaches (reduced-intensity conditioning and umbilical-cord blood transplantation) have expanded the indications for HSCTs and the number of patients with GVHD is rising. Some GVHD may be desired for the graft-versus-malignancy effect, but chronic GVHD is a major cause of morbidity and mortality. Risk factors—see Box 26.1.

The boundary between acute and chronic GVHD is blurred and diagnosis depends on clinical features not on timing in relation to transplant. Although the prevalence of acute GVHD is directly related to the amount of mismatch between HLA proteins in donor and recipient, acute GVHD has been reported after autologous HSCT possibly because regulatory T-cells are depleted allowing the autologous graft to recognize self-antigens.

What should I look for?

- Sudden onset of a burning or itching morbilliform rash which is often perifollicular initially.
- Macular blotchy erythema of palms, soles, and face is a common early sign.
- Commonly involves pinnae, cheeks, lateral neck, and upper back. Scalp is usually spared. Patient may become erythrodermic.
- Mucosal involvement is frequent, especially conjunctivae.
- Generalized erythema, blistering, and erosions simulate TEN in severe acute GVHD—see 🕮 p.110.
- Other features:
  - Fever.
  - Abdominal pain, nausea, vomiting, and watery or bloody diarrhoea.
  - Abnormal liver function—raised bilirubin and alkaline phosphatase.

What should I do?

- Consider alternative diagnoses—see Box 26.2.
- Exclude infection with cultures of blood, urine, sputum, and stool.
- If the diagnosis is uncertain take a skin biopsy from a well-established perifollicular lesion, but the histology may not distinguish between a severe drug reaction and acute cutaneous GVHD.
- Potent topical corticosteroids may control mild acute cutaneous GVHD, but severe cases require high-dose systemic corticosteroids.

Box 26.1 Risk factors for GVHD

- Older age.
- Previous acute GVHD increases risk of chronic GVHD.
- HLA disparity.
- Intense preparative regimen.
- Haemopoietic cells from peripheral blood not bone marrow (more T-cells).
- Less aggressive immunosuppression after transplantation.
- Donor T-lymphocyte infusions (given to incite a graft-versus-malignancy effect).

Box 26.2 Morbilliform rash after HSCT: differential diagnosis

- Drug eruption (including early TEN): chemotherapeutic agents, antibiotics, etc.
- Viral exanthema.
- EM secondary to herpes simplex infection.
- Acute GVHD.
- Eruption of lymphocyte recovery (ELR):
  - Occurs 1–4 weeks after chemotherapy when immunocompetent lymphocytes return to peripheral circulation and skin.
  - Mild fever.
  - No mucosal involvement. No systemic involvement.
  - Rash fades spontaneously with desquamation within 1–3 weeks.
- Engraftment syndrome (ES, capillary leak syndrome):
  - Occurs within 96h of engraftment. Neutrophil recovery is associated with release of cytokines and neutrophil degranulation.
  - Described most often after autologous HSCT (may be confused with early acute GVHD in allogeneic HSCT).
  - Fever >38.3°C without infection.
  - Non-cardiogenic pulmonary oedema or haemorrhage with diffuse pulmonary infiltrates.
  - Generalized oedema with weight gain.
  - Multiorgan failure and increased mortality.
- Stem cell transplantation erythema (SCTE, only recently defined):
  - Occurs 3–15 days after HSCT.
  - Itchy widespread symmetrical erythematous eruption. Discrete circular macules that may become confluent. Marked at acral sites. May develop tender plaques, occasionally surrounded by microvesicles or pustules. No purpura or bullae. Lesions darken then desquamate.

Further reading

Burnett JW *et al. Arch Dermatol* 2008; **144:**902–7.

Ferrara JL *et al. Lancet* 2009; **373:**1550–6.

Häusermann P *et al. Dermatology* 2008; **216:**287–304.

Lee SJ and Flowers ME. *Hematology Am Soc Hematol Educ Program* 2008; **2008:**134–41.

Schaffer JV. *Semin Cutan Med Surg* 2006; **25:**190–200.

Chronic cutaneous graft-versus-host disease

Chronic GVHD has an insidious onset. The disease is multisystem, but skin, mouth, and eyes are major targets. Donor-derived, alloreactive CD4- and CD8-positive T-cells are thought to play a part in the pathogenesis. Some aspects of chronic GVHD share features with other autoimmune diseases such as primary biliary cirrhosis, bronchiolitis obliterans, and Sjögren's syndrome.

Patients should be cared for by a multidisciplinary team that includes ophthalmologists and dermatologists as well as haematologists. 50% have limited cutaneous disease and a good prognosis, but the outcome in widespread chronic cutaneous GVHD is poor.

What should I look for?

- Manifestations vary and patients often have overlapping patterns of disease with combinations of lichenoid and sclerodermoid features.
- Check hair and nails as well as skin—see Box 26.3.
- Examine mucosae including genitalia—see Box 26.4.
- Assess joint mobility and impact of disease.
- ⚠ These patients have been exposed to chemotherapy and prolonged immunosuppression so are also at risk of cutaneous malignancies as well as unusual cutaneous infections (fungal, atypical mycobacterial).
- Chronic GVHD may also involve
  - Gastrointestinal tract causing abdominal symptoms and weight loss.
  - Liver with abnormal LFTs; lungs causing shortness of breath.

What should I do?

- Biopsy atypical cutaneous lesions to exclude malignancy or infection.
- Emollients and soap substitutes with antiseptics, e.g. Dermol® lotion may reduce itch, improve the skin barrier, and reduce risk of infection.
- Artificial saliva, topical local anaesthetic gels, and topical corticosteroids are indicated for painful oral disease (see 📖 Box 14.4, p.263).
- Prescribe artificial tears for dry eyes.
- Lichenoid disease: potent corticosteroid ointments or 0.1% tacrolimus ointment ×2/day may reduce inflammation.
- Sclerodermoid disease: UVB, PUVA, or UVA1 may be helpful in early disease. Extracorporeal photophoresis (ECP) may have a role in widespread disease—see Box 26.5. ECP may induce antigen-specific regulatory T-cells that suppress GVHD, but the mechanisms of action are not clear.
- The combination of systemic corticosteroids and immunosuppressive agents is generally used as first-line treatment. Complications such as infection increase mortality. More trials are needed.

Further reading

Ferrara J *et al. Lancet* 2009; **373:**1550–6.
White JM *et al. Br J Dermatol* 2007; **156:**1032–8.

Box 26.3 Signs of chronic cutaneous GVHD

- Lichenoid (like lichen planus):
  - Flat-topped violaceous papules that may be perifollicular and involve scars (sites of central lines, scars of herpes zoster).
  - Hands, forearm, trunk, nails, and mucosa are often involved.
  - May be photosensitive.
- Sclerodermoid GVHD:
  - Also tends to involve scars (köbnerization).
  - Lichen sclerosus-like. Hypopigmented with wrinkling and follicular plugging. Involves neck, upper trunk, and vulva. Progresses to more morphoeaform or sclerodermoid (generalized) pattern.
  - Morphoeaform. Single or many plaques that may progress to generalized tight, thickened skin with contractures (see 📖 p.390).
  - Disfiguring hypo- and hyperpigmentation is common.
  - Atrophy with fragility, blistering, and ulceration.
  - Eosinophilic fasciitis-like disease with deep sclerosis and contractures. Acute onset of pain and oedema in extremities sparing hands and feet. Sometimes preceded by vigorous exercise. Peripheral eosinophilia in 60% (see 📖 p.391).
- Appendageal involvement:
  - Brittle hair, premature greying, scarring alopecia, loss of body hair.
  - Dystrophic nails with longitudinal ridging, thinning, fragility, scarring (pterygium) and loss of nails (like lichen planus)—Fig. 26.1.
  - Loss of sweat glands causes heat sensitivity.
- Other features that have been described:
  - Asteatotic eczema or ichthyosis.
  - Intensely itchy diffuse erythema with fine scaling and palmoplantar hyperkeratosis. Frequent impetiginization ('eczematoid' GVHD).
  - Keratosis pilaris-like rash.
  - Cutaneous focal mucinosis.
  - Eruptive angiomas, nodular fibromas.

Box 26.4 Mucosal involvement in chronic GVHD—Fig. 26.2

- Mouth with LP-like lacy white buccal involvement (early sign), ulceration, and fibrosis (late). Sicca syndrome causes pain, dryness, sensitivity, and dental caries. Viral or fungal infections are common.
- Eyes with burning, irritation, dryness, and photophobia.
- Vaginal dryness, pain, erythema, LP-like changes, lichen sclerosus-like changes, and strictures.

Box 26.5 What is ECP?

- The patient's blood is collected and WBCs are separated.
- The RBC and plasma are returned to the patient.
- The WBCs are photosensitized by mixing with a psoralen and then exposed to UVA which induces apoptosis.
- The treated cells are returned to the patient.

Haematological diseases and skin

Polycythaemia rubra vera

- Itching or paraesthesiae, typically after a hot shower or bath.
- Erythromelalgia. Attacks of burning pain in the legs often worse in bed, when the patient is unable to tolerate the heat under the bed clothes. He/she may resort to sitting with the legs in a bucket of cold water to relieve pain. Skin is erythematous but cool and the legs may be slightly swollen. Platelets are raised. Aspirin is helpful. Resolves when polycythaemia is controlled—see 📖 p.504.

Essential throbocythaemia

- Livedo reticularis and/or retiform purpura with painful leg ulcers secondary to vasculopathy—see 📖 p.294.
- Erythromelalgia—see above and 📖 p.504.

Leukaemias and lymphomas

- Neutrophilic dermatoses: Sweet's syndrome (see 📖 p.480) and pyoderma gangrenosum (see 📖 p.290).
- Interstitial granulomatous dermatitis (see 📖 p.349).
- Cutaneous lymphoma, Sézary's syndrome and leukaemia cutis (see 📖 p.336).
- Adverse reactions in skin and nails secondary to chemotherapy (see 📖 p.358, 360).
- ⚠ Paraneoplastic pemphigus—see 📖 p.248. Seen most often in non-Hodgkin's lymphoma, Castleman's disease (a rare lymphoproliferative disorder), and chronic lymphocytic lymphoma, but occurs in other cancers.

Hyperglobulinaemic purpura

Hyperglobulinaemia occurs in association with many chronic inflammatory diseases including LE, rheumatoid arthritis, Sjögren's syndrome, sarcoidosis, chronic hepatitis, inflammatory bowel disease, and chronic infections. Asymptomatic diffuse petechiae and purpuric macules develop at sites of pressure, minor trauma, or stasis. Purpura may be precipitated by exercise. Occasionally paraesthesiae precede the rash.

Multiple myeloma

Skin lesions are uncommon and occur late in the course of disease.

- Plasma cell tumours: erythematous or purplish nodules—direct extension into the skin from underlying bone disease or metastatic disease.
- Amyloidosis may have cutaneous manifestations (see 📖 p.460).
- Type1 cryoglobulinaemia: cold sensitivity, mottling, cyanosis, purpura, blisters, ulcers (obstructive vasculopathy—see 📖 p.410).
- POEMS syndrome—rare (see Box 26.6).
- Follicular spicules particularly on nose. Also scalp and neck.
- Papular mucinosis (lichen myxoedema, scleromyxoedema) (see Box 26.7).

Waldenström's macroglobulinaemia

- Epistaxis and oral mucosal bleeding.
- Cutaneous macroglobulinosis—flesh-coloured papules on extensor surfaces.
- Evidence of type1 cryoglobulinaemia as in myeloma—see 🕮 p.410.

Box 26.6 ⚠ POEMS syndrome

A rare syndrome associated with plasma cell disorders. The syndrome comprises:

- **P**olyneuropathy: motor and sensory. Starts distally and spreads proximally.
- **O**rganomegaly: liver, spleen, lymph nodes.
- **E**ndocrinopathy: impotence, gynaecomastia, amenorrhoea (secondary to raised oestrogen), diabetes, hypothyroidism, hyperprolactinaemia, hypoparathyroidism.
- **M**onoclonal gammopathy.
- **S**kin changes: hyperpigmentation, skin thickening, sclerodermoid changes, hypertrichosis, nail changes (clubbing, white nails), oedema, and hyperhidrosis.

15% of patients have evidence of Castleman's disease (giant angiofollicular hyperplasia, multicentric plasma cell variant).

Box 26.7 ⚠ Papular mucinosis

These uncommon mucinoses are associated with a serum monoclonal IgG paraprotein. A minority of patients develop myeloma. Mucin is deposited in the dermis.

- Lichen myxoedema: 2–3mm waxy flat-topped papules on hands, elbows, forearms, upper trunk, face, and neck. May be linear.
- Scleromyxoedema: papules coalesce. The waxy indurated skin may resemble scleroderma. Involvement of the forehead produces furrowing and may mimic acromegaly. Thickening of the skin limits movement of limbs and mouth opening. Patients may have systemic involvement with mucin in vocal cords, kidneys, pulmonary and coronary vessels, and other organs.

Compare with scleroedema—see 🕮 Box 22.2, p.433.

Familial cancer syndromes

Gorlin's syndrome (basal cell naevus syndrome)

- Autosomal dominant inheritance. Mutation in *PTCH1* tumour suppressor gene on 9q22.3–q31.
- Medulloblastoma (frequent and early onset; avoid radiotherapy which may induce numerous BCCs within the field). Intracranial ectopic calcification.
- Multiple BCCs resembling pigmented or non-pigmented 'moles', milia, dermal and epidermoid cysts, pits on palms and soles.
- Skeletal abnormalities including macrocephaly with frontal bossing, bifid ribs, short 4th metacarpal, and scoliosis.
- Odontogenic keratocysts of the jaws, cleft lip, and/or palate.
- May have abnormalities of ocular, genitourinary, auditory, cardiac and/or respiratory systems.

Melanoma/pancreatic cancer syndrome (familial atypical multiple mole melanoma-pancreatic cancer syndrome)

- Mutation of gene encoding cyclin-dependent kinase inhibitor-2A (*CDKN2A*) on chromosome 9p21.
- Malignant melanoma and pancreatic cancer. Possibly breast cancer.
- Many large melanocytic naevi with irregular pigmentation and outlines.

Birt–Hogg–Dubé syndrome

- Autosomal dominant inheritance. Mutation in the 17p11.2 gene encoding folliculin.
- Lung cysts and spontaneous pneumothorax.
- Renal carcinoma.
- Skin tags and benign hair follicle tumours (fibrofolliculomas and trichodiscomas) present as skin-coloured papules.

Cowden's syndrome (multiple hamartoma syndrome)

- Autosomal dominant inheritance. Mutations in *PTEN/MMAC1* tumour suppressor gene on chromosome 10q22–23.
- Fibrocystic breast disease and breast cancer, thyroid tumours, endometrial cancer, lung cancer, gastrointestinal polyps, and colon cancer.
- Flesh-coloured papules on head and neck (trichilemmomas).
- Smooth papules (cobblestone-like) on oral mucosal surfaces: labial, palatal, and gingival (benign fibromas). Furrowed tongue.
- Flat wart-like papules on dorsum of hands and feet.
- Keratoses on palms, soles and sides of feet.
- Lipomas and haemangiomas; café au lait spots.

Howell–Evans syndrome

- Autosomal dominant inheritance. Gene unknown.
- Oesophageal cancer.
- Keratoderma (thickened hyperkeratotic skin on palms and soles).

Hereditary leiomyomatosis/renal cell cancer syndrome

- Autosomal dominant inheritance. Mutation of gene encoding fumarate hydratase at locus 1q42.3–43.
- Papillary renal cell cancer.
- Leiomyomas of skin: firm reddish-brown painful tumours of smooth muscle (benign) that may be in a band-like distribution or diffuse.
- Leiomyomas of the uterus. Also increased risk of uterine fibroids at a young age.

Peutz–Jeghers syndrome

- Autosomal dominant inheritance. Mutations in the *STK11/LKB1* tumour suppressor gene on chromosome 19p13.3.
- Hamartomatous polyps throughout the gastrointestinal tract, particularly in the jejunum. Intussusception causes bleeding and pain.
- Increased risk of gastrointestinal cancer especially stomach and duodenum.
- Other cancers: pancreas, gallbladder, lung, breast, uterus, and ovary.
- Pigmented macules (lentigines) on perioral skin, lips, buccal mucosa, palms and soles.

Gardener's syndrome

- A variant of familial adenomatous polyposis coli.
- Autosomal dominant inheritance-mutation in adenomatosis polyposis coli gene (*APC*) at locus 5q21–22. APC protein is involved in regulation of cell division.
- Adenomatous polyps throughout the colon with high risk of colorectal cancer.
- Other cancers (thyroid, osteosarcoma, chondrosarcoma, liposarcoma, hepatoblastoma).
- Multiple epidermoid ('sebaceous') cysts on face, scalp, and extremities-most common skin finding.
- Also fibromas, desmoid tumours, lipomas, and leiomyomas.
- Dental abnormalities (unerupted teeth, supernumerary teeth).
- Hypertrophy of retinal pigment epithelium.
- Osteomas of mandible, skull and, less often, long bones.

Muir–Torre syndrome

- Autosomal dominant inheritance. A subset of the non-polyposis colon cancer syndrome. Mutations in DNA mismatch repair genes.
- Gastrointestinal cancers. Also breast cancer, genitourinary cancer, and haematological malignancies.
- Many sebaceous gland tumours (hyperplasia, adenomas, carcinomas), keratoacanthomas with sebaceous differentiation.

Also see 📖 p.508; 📖 Box 22.8, p.441.

Paraneoplastic skin changes

Most of these paraneoplastic phenomena are uncommon. Look for a more banal explanation for the skin changes.

- Nail clubbing with hypertrophic osteoarthropathy (phalanges) seen in lung cancer.
- Ichthyosis (dry scaly skin). May be seen in lymphoma and other lymphoproliferative diseases.
- Dermatomyositis—see 📖 p.378. 10–30% of adult patients have an associated malignancy.
- Subacute cutaneous LE may be triggered by an underlying malignancy (rare)—see 📖 p.372.
- Neutrophilic dermatoses (Sweet's syndrome, pyoderma gangrenosum)—see 📖 p.290 and p.480.
- Acanthosis nigricans: more often seen in insulin resistance and obesity (see 📖 p.432) than in malignancy (generally adenocarcinoma of stomach). Flexural skin is hyperpigmented and thickened with a velvety texture. Skin tags are common. May be associated with a wrinkled ridged appearance on the palms (tripe palms).
- Diffuse pigmentation may be caused by an ACTH-secreting tumour (ectopic ACTH). Malignancies include small-cell carcinoma of lung, carcinoid tumours, and pancreatic islet cell tumours.
- Carcinoid syndrome (rare). Episodic flushing eventually leads to persistent facial oedema and telangiectasia—see 📖 p.482.
- Necrolytic migratory erythema (rare) seen in association with alpha cell tumours of the pancreas—see 📖 p.478.
- Eruptive seborrhoeic warts (sign of Leser–Trelat). The sudden appearance of large numbers of seborrhoeic warts is seen rarely in association with cancer of gastrointestinal tract, genitourinary cancers, and lymphoproliferative disease. Seborrhoeic warts are very common in the elderly and in most patients are of no significance. Eruptive seborrhoeic warts may also be triggered by widespread inflammatory skin diseases such as eczema.
- Bazex's syndrome (acrokeratosis paraneoplastica). Psoriasiform rash on ears, nose, cheeks, hands, feet, and knees with a nail dystrophy. Rare and associated with carcinomas of larynx, pharynx, trachea, bronchus, or upper oesophagus.
- Acquired hypertrichosis lanuginosa. Long silky non-pigmented hair (lanugo hair) on face and trunk. Most often associated with adenocarcinoma of gastrointestinal tract (rare). Consider other causes of hypertrichosis (increased hair growth on any part of the body, independent of androgens) including drugs and porphyria cutanea tarda—see 📖 p.88.
- Paraneoplastic pemphigus (rare). Associated with B-cell lymphoma, thymoma, and Castleman's tumour—see 📖 Box 13.6, p.249.
- Erythema gyratum repens—see 📖 p.220. Urticated wavy erythematous bands like the grain of wood that advance outward by about 1cm a day. Most often seen in association with carcinoma of the lung (rare).

Further reading

Thiers BH *et al. CA Cancer J Clin* 2009; **59:**73–98.

Chapter 27

Skin and neurology

Contents

Relevant pages in other chapters

Seborrhoeic dermatitis (common in Parkinson's disease) 📖 p.202
Neuropathic ulcers 📖 p.274
Porphyria 📖 p.308
Xeroderma pigmentosum 📖 p.314
Pompholyx induced by IVIg 📖 p.362
Rheumatology 📖 Chapter 19, p.365
Vasculitis 📖 Chapter 20, p.403
Amyloidosis 📖 p.460
Fabry's disease 📖 p.466
Sarcoidosis 📖 p.486
Congenital cutaneous lesions 📖 p.548
Ataxia telangiectasia 📖 p.562
Immunodeficiency syndromes 📖 p.562

Sensory symptoms and the skin

Neuropathic itch

Patients with localized itching or paraesthesiae usually attribute their puzzling symptoms to the skin. But sensory neuropathy may cause itch or contribute to itch in conditions such as chronic renal failure.

What should I look for?

- Ask about burning, tingling, stinging, hypoaesthesia, or hyperalgesia.
- Is the distribution distal symmetrical (polyneuropathy), individual nerve territories (mononeuritis multiplex, e.g. vasculitis), dermatomal (radiculopathy), or 1 side of body (central)?
- The skin may show evidence of rubbing (lichen simplex) or scratching.
- Examine for sensory signs—check light touch, vibration, proprioception, pain, and temperature (use a cold tuning fork).
- Examine for weakness and autonomic dysfunction in the same distribution as sensory disturbance.

Causes of generalized neuropathic itch

- Small-fibre neuropathy (Aδ and C-fibres) seen in diabetes and HIV infection may cause itch as well as pain.
- Centrally driven neuropathic itch has been described in association with brain tumours, strokes, spinal tumours, and multiple sclerosis.

Causes of localized neuropathic itch

- Peripheral nerve or root impingement may underlie puzzling conditions such as notalgia paraesthetica (see Box 27.1) and brachioradial pruritus (severe irritation of dorsolateral aspect of the arms, possibly aggravated by sun exposure, that may be relieved by ice-packs, capsaicin cream, or oral gabapentine).
- Herpes zoster may cause itch as well as pain—see 🕮 Box 7.7, p.149.
- Trigeminal trophic syndrome—see Box 27.2.
- Keloids may be associated with neuropathic itch, but the cause is uncertain. Pain fibres may be trapped in proliferating collagen.

⚠ Erythermalgia and erythromelalgia

Primary erythermalgia is a rare autosomal dominant channelopathy caused by gain-of-function mutations in *SCN9A*, the gene encoding a voltage-gated sodium channel, Na(v)1.7. Hyperexcitable autonomic and nociceptive neurons cause incapacitating pain, refractory to analgesia.

Acquired erythromelalgia has a similar presentation, but is most often secondary to a myeloproliferative disorder associated with raised platelets (less often to an autoimmune disease). Aspirin relieves pain—see 🕮 p.498.

What should I look for?

- Attacks of severe burning pain, warmth, and redness of legs, feet, and, occasionally, hands. Symptoms are provoked by warmth, e.g. by bedding at night and by exercise and may last for minutes or hours.
- Patients may soak feet or legs in icy water to relieve pain.
- Oedema and erythema (skin may appear normal between attacks).

Box 27.1 What is notalgia paraesthetica?

- Notalgia paraesthetica is thought to be caused by impingement of the posterior rami of T2–T6 nerve roots because it is associated with degenerative changes in the thoracic spine.
- Patients present with a localized area of itch and paraesthesiae over the lower border of the scapula. Other symptoms may include tingling, burning, formication, and hyperalgesia.
- The skin may be normal, lichenified, or pigmented. Notalgia paraesthetica has also been labelled a 'puzzling posterior pigmented pruritic patch'. Sensory examination may be normal or the involved skin may be hypoaesthesic to pin-prick or hyperaesthetic.
- Amyloid may be deposited within the affected skin (macular amyloid), probably secondary to chronic rubbing—see 📖 Box 23.3, p.461.
- Capsaicin, which depletes neuropeptides from C-type sensory nerve fibres may be helpful. Other options include topical local anaesthetic cream (e.g. lidocaine 2.5% with prilocaine 2.5%) or oral gabapentin.

Box 27.2 What is trigeminal trophic syndrome?

- Trigeminal trophic syndrome is an uncommon complication of damage to the trigeminal nerve. The syndrome most often follows trigeminal ablation by rhizotomy or alcohol injection into the Gasserian ganglion, but may be triggered by other causes of damage to the trigeminal nerve or its central connections such as CVA, acoustic neuromas, syringobulbia, herpes zoster, or trauma.
- Irritating paraesthesiae or dysaesthesiae in the affected dermatome or a sensation of nasal congestion provoke compulsive self-mutilation. Picking and rubbing lead to ulceration.
- Patients may not be aware of their actions.
- Typically ulcers involve the ala nasi, sometimes spreading to the adjacent lip and cheek. Scalp, forehead, ear, palate, or jaw may be affected.
- The tip of the nose (anterior ethmoidal nerve) and angle of jaw (greater auricular nerve) are spared.
- Differential diagnosis includes infection (herpes simplex and zoster, deep fungal, syphilis, yaws, TB, leprosy), malignancy (BCC, SCC, lymphoma), vasculitis (Wegener's granulomatosis), and pyoderma gangrenosum.
- Biopsy shows non-specific inflammation.
- Management is difficult and requires a multidisciplinary approach. Educate the patient and protect the skin with occlusive dressings. Carbamazepine, diazepam, and amitriptyline are of limited help. Surgical repair with a skin flap has been recommended.

Further reading

Drenth JP *et al.* *Arch Dermatol* 2008; **144:**320–4.

Lauria G *et al.* *Histopathology* 2009; **54:**273–85 (Discusses role of skin biopsy for small fibre neuropathy.)

Yosipovitch G and Samuel LS. *Dermatol Ther* 2008; **21:**32–41.

Autonomic and motor dysfunction

Autonomic dysfunction and the skin

Autonomic dysfunction occurs in disease of peripheral small fibres (e.g. diabetes, vasculitis, HIV), disease affecting autonomic ganglia, and CNS disease (e.g. Parkinson's disease, multiple system atrophy). Manifestations may be cardiac (e.g. postural hypotension, tachycardia, exercise intolerance), gastrointestinal (e.g. dysphagia, abdominal pain, nausea, vomiting, malabsorption, diarrhoea, and constipation), genitourinary (e.g. erectile dysfunction), and metabolic (e.g. hypoglycaemia). Diabetes is one of the commonest causes of autonomic neuropathy, when it is usually accompanied by a sensory neuropathy.

Complex regional pain syndrome (reflex sympathetic dystrophy), a painful disabling condition that most often affects the hand, is associated with dysfunction of autonomic nerves.

What should I look for?

- Alterations in microvascular skin circulation affect skin colour (erythema, cyanosis, oedema, delayed capillary refill, livedo reticularis) and may impair skin nutrition contributing to dryness and cracking.
- Alterations in sweating.
- Dryness of the feet which predisposes to cracking and provides a portal of entry for infection. Diabetic patients with sudomotor dysfunction are more likely to develop foot ulcers—see 🕮 Box 15.1, p.275 and Fig, 15.4, p.277.
- Gustatory sweating (hyperhidrosis associated with eating).
- Compensatory hyperhidrosis in normal skin if patients have focal loss of sweating.
- Harlequin syndrome: one half of the face fails to flush during thermal or emotional stress as a result of damage to vasodilator sympathetic fibres. May be associated with Adie's tonic pupil and impaired sweating on the same side (Ross's syndrome).

The motor system and the skin

Muscle weakness with abnormalities in gait or musculoskeletal deformity may be associated with the development of callosities. Immobility may lead to pressure sores. Use tone, power, coordination, and reflexes to determine whether pathology is central, peripheral, or both.

POEMS syndrome in patients with plasma cell disorders is a rare cause of motor and sensory neuropathy that starts distally and spreads proximally—see 🕮 Box 26.6, p.499.

Neurofibromatosis type 1

Synonym: von Recklinghausen's disease.

Neurofibromatosis type 1 (NF1) is one of the commonest autosomal dominantly inherited conditions (1 in 3000 births). NF1 is caused by mutations in a large tumour suppressor gene at locus 17q11.2 that encodes a 2818 amino acid protein, neurofibromin, involved in regulating cell growth and differentiation. Pathogenesis is complex. NFI is associated with other conditions—see Box 27.3.

The diagnosis is clinical. See Box 27.4 for some of the causes of café au lait spots. Lipomas and the tumours of proteus syndrome (see Box 27.9, 📖 p.517) may simulate the neurofibromas of NF1.

Diagnostic criteria: what should I look for?

To make the diagnosis, an individual must have ***2 or more*** of the following criteria:

- 6 or more café au lait spots (macules or patches). These increase in number and size with age. Spots in prepubertal individuals should be >5mm in diameter, but postpuberty >15mm. Spots usually have smooth outlines, but larger ones may be irregular. Intensity of colour varies, but most are pale brown.
- Axillary or inguinal freckles, 1–3mm diameter, develop later than café au lait spots. Freckling may also appear around the neck and in other skin folds (see 📖 p.563 for other causes of freckling).
- 2 or more neurofibromas of any type or 1 plexiform neurofibroma. Dermal neurofibromas also appear later than café au lait spots. Large numbers only develop in adulthood. They may occur at any skin site, but usually spare exposed skin (e.g. face) except in severe cases (Fig. 27.1). Apply gentle pressure to small neurofibromas and they sink down into the skin, 'buttonholing'—a virtually pathognomonic sign. Neurofibromas are soft and may become pedunculated. Patients may develop thousands of disfiguring neurofibromas. Large soft subcutaneous neurofibromas (plexiform) are associated with local hypertrophy of bone and soft tissues (including skin) and overlying skin may be hyperpigmented with increased hair growth (hypertrichosis). Nodular neurofibromas (5% of patients) may involve major peripheral nerves or nerve roots.
- Optic glioma.
- 2 or more Lisch nodules (iris hamartomas). Look for yellowish-brown nodules within the iris. These appear before neurofibromas and will confirm the diagnosis, but they are easier to see with a slit-lamp than with the naked eye.
- Sphenoid wing dysplasia or thinning of the long bone cortex with or without pseudarthrosis.
- First-degree relative with 2 or more of the preceding criteria.

Box 27.3 Other features associated with NF1

- Epilepsy and learning difficulties (often mild).
- Neurofibromas in bone or gastrointestinal tract (may bleed), spinal neurofibromas, CNS tumours, peripheral nerve sarcoma—greatest risk in nodular plexiform neurofibromas. (Dermal neurofibromas do not undergo sarcomatous change.)
- Phaeochromocytoma (5–20% of patients).
- Renal artery stenosis, cerebrovascular disease.
- Skeletal deformity, e.g. scoliosis, bowing of legs, short stature, macrocephaly, hypertelorism.
- Other tumours: pelvic rhabdomyosarcoma, childhood leukaemia.

Box 27.4 Café au lait spots

Use an ultraviolet (Wood's) light to accentuate epidermal pigmentation in individuals with pale skin so that café au lait spots are easier to see—📖 p.568.

Light brown, evenly pigmented, well defined, flat café au lait spots occur in a variety of situations and rare syndromes:

- 10% of normal people have 1 or 2 café au lait spots.
- NF1: 6 or more café au lait spots.
- NF2: rarely >5 café au lait spots—see 📖 p.510.
- Segmental NF1: café au lait spots localized to 1 segment of body (mosaicism for mutation—see 📖 p.510).
- Juvenile xanthogranulomas: rarely associated with myelomonocytic leukaemia and with NF.
- Tuberous sclerosis: <6 café au lait spots—see 📖 p.512.
- McCune–Albright syndrome. <6 café au lait spots. Darker brown with a more irregular outline (like a map) and larger than in NF1. Usually unilateral (do not cross midline) and most often trunk or proximal limbs. No axillary freckling. Also precocious puberty, endocrine abnormalities. Mutations in a gene encoding a protein that stimulates activity of adenylate cyclase are present in affected tissue. Individuals are mosaics—see 📖 p.514. It is presumed that the mutation would be lethal if it involved all cells.
- Cowden's syndrome—see 📖 p.500; Carney complex—see 📖 p.563.
- LEOPARD syndrome: multiple lentigines, sometimes café au lait spots—see 📖 p.563.
- Multiple endocrine neoplasia type 1 and type 2B—see 📖 Box 22.18, p.449.
- Autosomal mismatch repair gene mutations, ring chromosome syndromes, and DNA repair syndromes such as ataxia telangiectasia—see 📖 p.562.
- Proteus syndrome—see 📖 Box 27.9, p.517.

Further reading

Boyd KP *et al. J Am Acad Dermatol* 2009; **61:**1–14.

Jentarra G *et al. Semin Pediatr Neurol* 2006; **13:** 43–7.

Other neurofibromatoses

Neurofibromatosis type 2 (NF2)

NF2 is a rare condition inherited as an autosomal dominant disorder (prevalence about 1 in 40 000). The *NF2* gene encodes a protein (Merlin) that appears to play a role in mediating communication between the cytoskeleton and the extracellular environment. The diagnosis is confirmed if the individual has bilateral vestibular schwannomas or a family history of NF2 in a first-degree relative plus a unilateral vestibular schwannoma diagnosed by age 30 or any 2 of: meningioma, glioma, schwannoma, juvenile posterior subcapsular lenticular opacities/juvenile cataracts.

Cutaneous signs include:

- Café au lait spots: rarely >5 so do not meet criteria for NF1.
- Peripheral nerve tumours: less frequent than in NF1. Most often small (<2cm) discrete plaques with a rough surface (may be pigmented or hypertrichotic) or subcutaneous schwannomas. Dermal neurofibroma-like tumours are uncommon and few in numbers.

Segmental neurofibromatosis 1

Patients with a somatic mosaicism for a mutation in the *NF1* gene present with 1 or more features of NF1 limited to 1 segment of the body. The clinical features are determined by the timing of the mutation during the development of the embryo. Involvement follows Blaschko's lines—Fig. 27.1 and 🕮 Fig. 27.2, p.515, and inside back cover.

Such patients have no risk of developing generalized NF1, but should be advised about the low risk of having a child with generalized NF1.

Children may present with unilateral lentigines in axilla or groin.

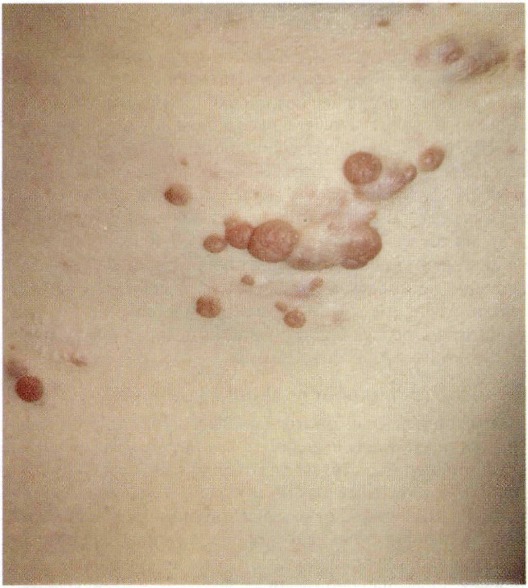

Fig. 27.1 Soft neurofibromas in a linear band in a patient with segmental NF.

Tuberous sclerosis

Synonyms: Bourneville's disease, Pringle's disease, epiloia.

A dominantly inherited condition (prevalence around 1 in 10 000) associated with learning difficulties (50% of individuals) and epilepsy (35% of individuals) as well as involvement of almost any organ including skin—see Box 27.5. Many cases are new mutations.

1 of 2 tumour suppressor genes (*TSC1* or *TSC2*) is involved in the pathogenesis of the hamartomas that are the hallmark of the disease. *TSC1* encodes a protein called hamartin, while tuberin is the product of *TSC2*. Hamartin and tuberin combine to produce a functional protein. A mutation in either gene results in the same phenotype.

Cutaneous signs, especially hypopigmented macules, may be of considerable help in making the diagnosis particularly in children presenting with learning disorders, behavioural problems, or epilepsy. 10% of children with infantile spasms have tuberous sclerosis.

What mucocutaneous signs should I look for?

- Hypopigmented macules on trunk and limbs. May be present at birth. Few or scattered widely in a confetti-like pattern. Hair within macules is hypopigmented (look for white streak in scalp hair). Ash leaf patch is a misnomer as macules may be any shape. Cutaneous hypopigmentation is accentuated by examination of the skin under a Wood's light. But remember other causes of hypopigmentation, particularly post-inflammatory hypopigmentation—see Box 27.6.
- Forehead plaques may be present at birth. Develop on scalp, face, or neck. Initially resemble a capillary haemangioma, but evolve into firm, red or yellowish brown plaques with histology of angiofibroma.
- Facial angiofibromas ('adenoma sebaceum') on nasolabial folds and cheeks. The erythematous papules and/or nodules appear in 85% of individuals after age 5 and slowly increase in number. Associated with telangiectasia. Often misdiagnosed as acne or rosacea—but no pustules, see 🕮 p.234.
- Shagreen patch (connective tissue naevus with increased collagen). Rare in infancy, but usually appear in adolescence. The orange-red patches develop most often on lower back or thigh varying in size from a few mm to 15cm. Dermal thickening may give the skin the feel of soft rubber. The surface may be dimpled like orange peel or slightly rough. The appearance is said to resemble untanned leather or pig-skin. Small 'gooseflesh' bumps may surround a larger central patch.
- Periungual fibromas (garlic clove tumours). Check toes as well as fingers. The small smooth fleshy tumours arise from beneath the nail fold and may press down on the nail plate to produce a longitudinal groove. A single fibroma may occur in a normal individual.
- Skin tags around the neck: molluscum fibrosum pendulum.
- Subcutaneous occipital angiofibromas.
- Oral angiofibromas on lips, gingiva, dorsum of tongue, palate.
- Café au lait spots (<6) occasionally.

Box 27.5 Organ involvement in tuberous sclerosis

- Skin: see 🕮 p.512.
- CNS: cortical 'tubers' (giant cell astrocytoma) are associated with epilepsy (infantile spasms, partial seizures, absence seizures, and tonic–clonic seizures); and behavioural problems, e.g. autism, hyperactivity, and/or learning disorders (both associated with seizures). Patients may have focal neurological deficits, e.g. mild hemiparesis. Growth of giant cell astrocytoma may cause life-threatening raised intracranial pressure.
- Retinal astrocytomas (25% of patients): often asymptomatic.
- Cardiac rhabdomyomas (60% of patients at birth). Detect by echocardiography. May be multiple. Often asymptomatic but may cause heart failure (e.g. by outflow obstruction), arrhythmia including Wolff–Parkinson–White syndrome, thromboembolism, or sudden cardiac death.
- Renal angiomyolipomas may cause haematuria. Renal cancer is rare.
- Renal cysts may cause hypertension and renal failure. *TSC2* is localized very close to the gene for autosomal dominant polycystic kidney disease, and some patients have both conditions, but renal cysts also occur in tuberous sclerosis.
- Pulmonary lymphangioleiomyomatosis causes pneumothorax, haemoptysis, and respiratory insufficiency.
- Bone cysts and periosteal new bone formation—asymptomatic.

Box 27.6 Pale macules and patches

Hypopigmented macules or patches

Loss of pigment is partial. Skin is creamy rather than bright white. A few hypopigmented macules may occur in normal individuals. Large numbers are more likely to be associated with an underlying condition—see 🕮 p.85. You should decide:

- Was pigment loss preceded by inflammation? Postinflammatory hypopigmentation is common in dark coloured skins—see Box 4.9, 🕮 p.87.
- Is skin scaly? Consider pityriasis versicolor in young adults—see 🕮 p.160.
- Is texture normal? Localized scleroderma causes hypopigmentation, but skin is thickened—see 🕮 p.390.
- 1–5% of normal individuals have a congenital naevus depigmentosus (despite the name, pigment loss is partial).

Depigmented macules or patches

The skin has a bright white tone and is a brighter white than hypopigmented skin when examined under Wood's light.

- Vitiligo is the commonest cause of acquired smooth depigmented macules or patches—see 🕮 p.452.

Further reading

Inoki K and Guan K-L. *Hum Mol Genet* 2009; **18:**R94–R100.

Cutaneous mosaicism

What is mosaicism?

A mutation during development that is propagated in only a limited number of the adult cells causes mosaicism. Germline mosaicism affects gonadal cells and somatic mosaicism affects other cells. In X-linked disorders, mosaicism is caused by random X-inactivation (Lyonization).

Skin and nerves are both derived from ectoderm and therefore cutaneous mosaicism is often associated with abnormalities in the nervous system. Mutations arising early in development are associated with widespread changes and abnormalities in other organs. Involvement of germline cells (hypothesized to be more likely in individuals with extensive skin involvement) could cause a widespread skin disorder in the offspring.

What are Blaschko's lines? (📖 see inside back cover for diagram)

Alfred Blaschko was a dermatologist from Berlin who observed that epidermal naevi and some acquired skin diseases followed similar patterns: linear on limbs, arcs on the chest, S-shapes on the abdomen, or V-shapes near the midline of the back. The patterns were not related to dermatomes (segments of skin defined by sensory innervations) or any known cause of linear skin markings such as Langer's lines of cleavage, axial lines separating cranial and caudal dermatomes, lymphatic drainage, vascular flow, embryonic clefts, or pigmentary demarcation lines—see 📖 p.62. The lines probably reflect keratinocyte mosaicism and correspond to the pathways followed by keratinocytes migrating from the neural crest during embryogenesis.

How do I recognize cutaneous mosaicism?

5 patterns have been described—see Fig. 27.2. The pattern is influenced by the pathway of migration of the affected cell as well as other factors such as the timing of the mutation:

- Keratinocyte: Blaschko-linear pattern. Each clone of keratinocytes forms a continuous line as the cells migrate outwards by directional proliferation following surface forces.
- Melanoblast: block or phylloid but may be Blaschko-linear patterns. Melanoblasts migrate as single cells and proliferate locally in the skin.
- Nerve cells: dermatomal. Nerve cells migrate along future dermatomes.
- Mesodermal tissues (blood vessels, fibroblasts): segmental or dermatomal. Cells migrate within segments or dermatomes.

Further reading

Bolognia JL *et al. J Am Acad Dermatol* 1994; **31:**157–90.

Happle R. *Acta Pædiatrica* 2006; Suppl **451:**16–23.

Paller AS. *J Clin Invest* 2004; **114:**1407–9.

Torrelo A *et al. Eur J Dermatol* 2005; **15:**439–50.

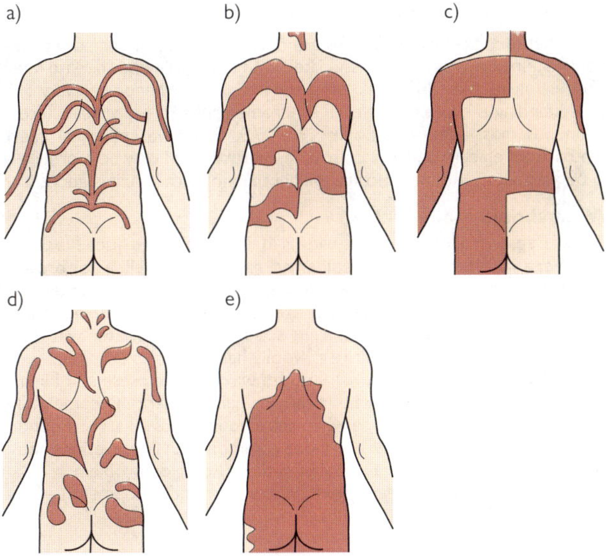

Fig. 27.2 Patterns of cutaneous mosaicism. a) Lines of Blascko, narrow bands. b) Lines of Blaschko, broad bands. c) Checkerboard pattern. d) Phylloid pattern e) Patchy pattern without midline separation. Adapted with permission from Happle R. *Arch Dermatol* 1993; **129**: 1460–70.

Epidermal naevus syndromes

These neurocutaneous syndromes are defined as the presence of epidermal and adnexal hamartomas associated with extracutaneous disease most often involving the CNS, eyes, or skeletal systems. Phenotypes vary and understanding is evolving, but each syndrome probably reflects a different cutaneous mosaicism—see Boxes 27.7–27.9. Extensive epidermal naevi, centro-facial epidermal naevi, or scalp epidermal naevi may be more likely to be associated with neurological or ophthalmological manifestations.

What should I look for?

- Linear epidermal or sebaceous naevus in Blaschko's lines—see 🕮 p.514:
  - Verrucous (keratinocyte) epidermal naevus: pink, yellow, or brown linear array of papules usually present at birth. Becomes darker, more raised, and wart-like with age. Less common on the head and neck than trunk or limbs. If in the scalp may be associated with alopecia or abnormal hair (e.g. woolly hair naevus).
  - Sebaceous naevus: yellowish smooth waxy plaque present at birth. Most often on face or scalp (overlying hair is absent). Become more prominent in adolescence when sebaceous glands enlarge. (Round or oval sebaceous naevi are more common than linear lesions and much less likely to be associated with neurological problems, probably because linear lesions arise earlier in development.)—See 🕮 Fig. 31.2, p.549.
- Other skin signs:
  - Hypo- or hyperpigmentation or café au lait macules.
  - Scalp aplasia cutis—see 🕮 p.548 and Fig. 31.1, p.549.
- CNS abnormalities including:
  - Seizures, infantile spasms, or hemiparesis.
  - Mental retardation or developmental delay.
- Eye problems including:
  - Strabismus, lipodermoids, choristomas (congenital overgrowth of ectopic tissue) and colobomas (congenital defect when part of the eye does not form—may affect choroid, iris, lens, optic nerve, or retina).
- Skeletal abnormalities including:
  - Bony hypoplasia, bone cysts, abnormal skull shape, limb hypertrophy, kyphoscoliosis.
  - Spontaneous fractures, hypophosphataemic vitamin D-resistant rickets (described in association with both keratinocyte and sebaceous epidermal naevi).

Further reading

Happle R. *J Am Acad Dermatol* 1991; **25:**550–6.

Sugarman JL. *Semin Cutan Med Surg* 2007; **26:**221–30.

Box 27.7 Sebaceous naevus syndrome (uncommon)

Linear or extensive sebaceous naevus of the head (often centrofacial), associated with neurological and/or ocular abnormalities that may include:
- Mental retardation.
- Seizures, especially infantile spasms, hemiparesis.
- Choristomas, colobomas.
- Skull asymmetry on the same side as the naevus.

All children with large sebaceous naevi should be assessed for neurological or ophthalmological problems.

Secondary tumours derived from adnexal structures may develop within sebaceous naevi. These are usually benign.

Box 27.8 Phacomatosis pigmentokeratotica (rare)

The condition is characterized by the combination of a linear sebaceous naevus that follows the lines of Blaschko and a speckled-lentiginous melanocytic naevus in a checkerboard pattern (the pigmented patches do not cross the midline).

Associated problems may include:
- Mild mental retardation and seizures.
- Segmental sensory abnormalities and segmental hyperhidrosis on the same side as the speckled lentiginous melanocytic naevus.
- Deafness.
- Ptosis and strabismus.
- Hemiatrophy with muscle weakness.

Box 27.9 ⚠ Proteus syndrome (very rare)

This syndrome is named after the Greek demigod Proteus, who could change his appearance. The condition is characterized by asymmetrical overgrowth (macrosomia) in a variety of tissues. Individual digits, limbs, or 1/2 of the body may be grossly enlarged. Before the features were delineated, patients were often considered to have NF1. The elephant man, Joseph Merrick, probably had severe proteus syndrome rather than neurofibromatosis. Intelligence is usually normal. Clinical features vary but may include:
- Hemifacial macrosomia or macroglossia.
- Skeletal anomalies including hemihypertrophy, limb gigantism, and asymmetrical macrodactyly.
- Linear verrucous epidermal naevi following lines of Blaschko.
- Vascular malformations especially port wine stains.
- Connective tissue naevi causing localized 'ceribriform' thickening of palmar or plantar soft tissues—may be misdiagnosed as plexiform neurofibroma, lipomas, or lipoatrophy.
- Visceral hamartomas.
- Choristoma of the eye.
- Café au lait macules have been reported.

Pigmented skin conditions with neurological features

⚠ Incontinentia pigmenti (IP)

Synonym: Bloch–Sulzberger incontinentia pigmenti.

IP is a rare X-linked dominant cutaneous disorder that is lethal in males. IP is caused by mutations in the NF-κB essential modulator gene (*NEMO*). The NEMO protein activates NF-κB, which protects against apoptosis. 80% of affected children have other problems, e.g. strabismus, visual loss, epilepsy, spastic paralysis, developmental delay, hypotonia, microcephaly, and scoliosis. Skin signs follow Blaschko's lines—see 📖 p.516.

What should I look for?

The classic presentation evolves through 4 stages but sometimes these stages overlap or the 1st and/or 2nd stage (s) may not be manifest at all. Stages typically comprise:

1. *A linear erythematous or vesiculobullous eruption* on limbs or trunk, following the lines of Blaschko, appears within 6 weeks of birth, but may be present at birth. Blisters usually clear in 6 months. The recurring crops of blisters may be associated with a circulating eosinophilia. A smear taken from a blister will also show eosinophils. Differential diagnosis includes erythema toxicum and infection (herpes simplex, herpes zoster, or varicella), but the child is well (see 📖 p.144, p.148).
2. *A verrucous stage* with a linear hyperkeratotic or pustular rash, mostly acral (fingers, ankles), which commences around age 2 months and may persist for up to 3 years.
3. *Linear streaks or swirls of macular hyperpigmentation* following Blaschko's lines are usually apparent by age 6 months, fade during adolescence and disappear by around 16 years. Differentiate from pigmentary mosaicism—see Box 27.10.
4. *An atrophic stage* with pale hairless patches or streaks most often on arms and legs is seen in adult females and rarely in children.

Other ectodermal signs may include:

- A self-limiting nail dystrophy in 40% of children with ridging, pitting, and/or onychomycosis-like thickening.
- Linear absence of sweat glands.
- Delayed dentition or missing or conical teeth.
- Asymmetrical breast development or supernumerary nipples.

What should I do?

- Take a full medical history from the mother and specifically enquire about miscarriages (male infants) or dental problems. Examine mother for subtle pigment change on limbs.
- Take a skin biopsy from involved skin in the infant. The inflammatory stage shows eosinophilic spongiosis and dyskeratotic keratinocytes.
- Refer for genetic counselling and neurological, ophthalmological, and dental assessment.

Box 27.10 Pigmentary mosaicism

Synonyms: chromosomal mosaicism, hypomelanosis of Ito, incontinentia pigmenti achromians, linear and whorled naevoid hypermelanosis.

Males and females are affected in this heterogeneous condition that reflects genetic mosaicism. Skin may be hypo- or hyperpigmented.

What should I look for?

- Linear or whorled hypo- or hyperpigmentation present from birth and following Blaschko's lines—see 🕮 p.516. Pigment change is easier to see under UV (Wood's) light.
- No inflammatory or verrucous stages (in contrast to incontinentia pigmenti).
- Areas of hypopigmentation may be hypohidrotic or anhidrotic in some patients (demonstrated using a starch iodine test).
- Hair abnormalities in some patients, e.g. colour or textural variation or alopecia.
- Involvement of other systems including nervous system (epilepsy, autistic behaviour, learning disability), musculoskeletal system (joint contractures, kyphoscoliosis, digital abnormalities), eyes (micropthalmia, iris coloboma, heterochromia of iris), or teeth (hypodontia, absent teeth).

Box 27.11 ⚠ Focal dermal hypoplasia of Goltz

This rare X-linked dominantly inherited condition is lethal in males. Random inactivation of the X chromosome accounts for mosaicism with the distribution of skin lesions in Blaschko's lines—see 🕮 p.516.

What should I look for?

- Congenital linear hypo- or hyperpigmented lesions following the lines of Blaschko (no inflammation or blisters, unlike incontinentia pigmenti).
- Streaky atrophy of affected skin with telangiectasia and herniation of fat.
- Hyperkeratosis, aplasia cutis (see 🕮 Box 31.6, p.549), and scarring within lesions.
- Skeletal abnormalities including limb reduction, cleft hand or foot deformities, syndactyly, short stature, asymmetrical growth.
- Ocular abnormalities including strabismus, and microphthalmia.
- Malformed teeth.
- Less often renal anomalies or congenital heart defects.

Further reading

Berlin AL *et al. J Am Acad Dermatol* 2002; **47:**169–87.

Capillary malformations

Slow-flow capillary malformations in the skin present at birth as port wine stains (PWSs). Rarely PWSs develop later in life. These vascular malformations never regress and may be associated with overgrowth of underlying tissues and ocular or neurological problems. In adults, PWSs darken to deep purple and, on the face, may become hypertrophic. Laser surgery may be an effective cosmetic treatment if carried out in infancy.

What should I look for?

- A red patch, present at birth, that enlarges with the growth of the child. Facial PWSs follow the distribution of the sensory trigeminal nerve: V1 = forehead and upper eyelid; V2 = maxillary; V3 = mandibular—see Fig. 27.3 and 📖 Fig. 31.4, p.553.
- ⚠ Neurological and ocular abnormalities in patients with facial PWSs involving the forehead and upper eyelid (Sturge–Weber syndrome)—see Box 27.12. More common if PWS is bilateral.
- Naevus anaemicus with a well-defined serpiginous outline. A naevus anaemicus does not go red if skin is rubbed, but stands out more clearly from surrounding erythematous skin. Diascopy can also be used to confirm the diagnosis—see 📖 p.569. Found in phakomatosis pigmentovascularis—see Box 27.13. May be sporadic.
- Naevus spilus or dermal melanocytosis (Mongolian spot) see 📖 Fig. 31.10, p.565 suggesting phakomatosis pigmentovascularis—see Box 27.13.
- Overgrowth of an affected limb: Klippel–Trenaunay (venous) or Parkes–Weber (arteriovenous) syndromes.
- ⚠ Evidence of occult spinal dysraphism in patients with a midline lumbosacral PWS. Look for other signs such as a midline pit or dimple above gluteal cleft, sinus, fibroma, or tuft of hair (faun's tail). Confirm with MRI. Also see 📖 p.548.

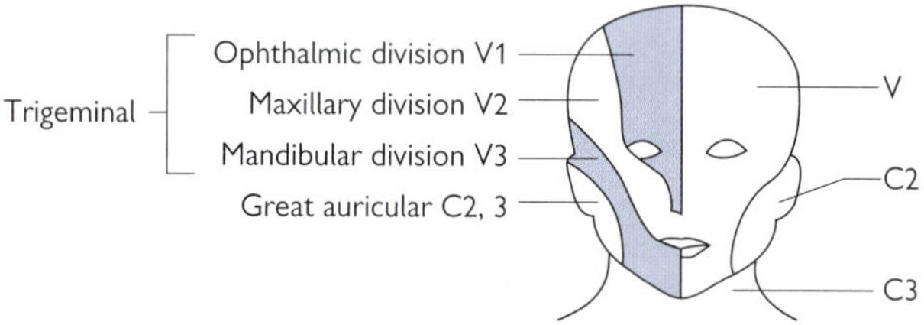

Fig. 27.3 Facial branches of trigeminal nerve. Reproduced with permission from Giele H and Cassell O. *Plastic and Reconstructive Surgery*, 2008. Oxford: Oxford University Press.

Box 27.12 Sturge–Weber syndrome—see 🕮 Fig. 31.4, p.553

Neurological and ocular abnormalities occur in 10–15% of patients with a facial PWS in V1 distribution (forehead and upper eyelid). The PWS is often extensive and may be bilateral.

- ⚠ Ocular involvement is secondary to choroidal vascular malformation and includes:
  - Buphthalmos (congenital glaucoma).
  - Glaucoma: may develop slowly or present acutely with a cloudy cornea. This is a medical emergency. Need annual checks of pressures.
- Neurological symptoms caused by a capillary-venous malformation in the pia mater on the same side as the PWS may include:
  - Seizures on opposite side of body or generalized.
  - Contralateral hemiparesis or hemiplegia.
  - Developmental delay.
  - Emotional or behavioural problems, attention deficit.
  - Migraine.

Refer infants for ocular and neurological assessment.

Box 27.13 What is phacomatosis pigmentovascularis?

Definition: association of a widespread vascular nevus with an extensive pigmentary nevus. Associated with extracutaneous defects. A number of types have been described including:

- Mongolian spots, dermal melanocytosis and one or more PWSs. Patients may also have naevus anaemicus and hypoplastic nails. Associations include CNS defects, ocular anomalies, asymmetrical length of limbs, and dysplastic veins or lymph vessels.
- Nevus spilus (speckled lentiginous nevus) and a pale pink telangiectatic nevus. May be associated with unilateral lymphoedema, hemiparesis, seizures, or asymmetrical length of legs.
- Nevus cesius (blue spot, aberrant Mongolian spot) and cutis marmorata telangiectatica congenita (reticulated vascular skin markings present since birth). Reported in association with asymmetry of hemispheres and ventricles, limb hyperplasia.

Chapter 28

Skin and psychiatry

Contents

Relevant pages in other chapters

Porphyria 📖 p.308

Self-induced dermatoses

Synonym: dermatitis artefacta.

Self-mutilation

Lip-licking, hair-pulling (trichotillomania), and nail-biting are common childhood habits with a good prognosis that are not usually linked to an emotional disorder, but self-mutilation is used by some adults, usually young women, to relieve emotional stress. Tensions involving family or work may precede onset. Self-mutilation may also be associated with learning difficulties and psychiatric conditions such as personality disorders, eating disorders, or mood disorders. Although patients may know what they are doing, they cannot easily stop the damaging behaviour. Serious self-harm associated with suicidal intent is a different problem.

- Cutting the skin is probably the commonest form of episodic self-mutilation. The cuts are made in privacy to relieve tension and are usually kept hidden.
- Patients with obsessive–compulsive disorder who wash their hands repeatedly may develop irritant contact hand dermatitis—see p.200.
- Some patients cannot resist the impulse to endlessly pick, scratch, or gouge previously normal skin (neurotic excoriations, psychogenic pruritus). Management is challenging—see Box 28.1 and Box 10.4, p.207.
- Acne excoriée (picking and squeezing acne pustules and papules—see p.224) is a form of psychogenic pruritus that may be associated with obsessive–compulsive disorder or other body image disorders such as anorexia nervosa. Self-inflicted scarring reinforces a negative self-image.

Factitious disorders (Münchausen's syndrome)

Deliberate and highly visible self-induced damage may be used by patients who want to adopt the sick role to attract attention from other people, particularly doctors. This form of dermatitis artefacta presents most often in women, often working in healthcare-related professions, and may be associated with psychiatric problems such as eating disorders.

- Self-inflicted skin lesions present on normal looking, exposed, and highly visible skin that is accessible to the patient, e.g. the face.
- The pattern is asymmetrical.
- The morphology depends on how the lesions are induced, but well defined, irregular, jagged, rather geometric outlines are common and quite unlike the smooth outlines of an endogenous skin disease. Signs may include crusted erosions, erythematous patches, and blisters sometimes with a linear streak suggesting contact with a caustic liquid that has dripped, purpura (produced by suction), ulcers, and oedema.
- Alternative diagnoses should always be considered—see Box 28.2.
- Patients deny damaging their skin, appear to lack insight into the problem, and are often reluctant to accept psychiatric help. Confrontation, with the offer of support, may precipitate a different pattern of destructive behaviour or, very rarely, suicide.

Box 28.1 Management of psychogenic pruritus

- Assess thoughts and emotions before, during, and after the excoriation episode; enquire about sleep patterns, history of depression, suicidal ideations, and self-mutilating behaviours; and record previous use of psychiatric medications as well as their effect on itch.
- What drugs is the patient taking? Any history of substance abuse?
- Do not accept the diagnosis of psychogenic itch without excluding other contributory factors, especially scabies (see 🕮 p.164), no matter how long the history of itch.
- Exclude systemic causes of itching—iron deficiency, thyroid disease, renal failure, chronic liver disease, malignancies, HIV—see 🕮 p.60.
- Look for excoriations, nodules, or ulcers on skin that can be reached by the patient—the centre of the back is spared.
- Refer to a psychologist or psychiatrist for management of underlying psychological or psychiatric problem.
- Remember that patients with an organic basis for their itch may also have a psychogenic component and might benefit from psychological support.
- Trim nails.
- Prescribe soap substitutes and emollients if skin is dry—see 🕮 p.584.
- Occlusion, e.g. with Zipzoc®, will protect the skin from further damage—see 🕮 p.590.
- Systemic options include antidepressants such as selective serotonin reuptake inhibitors or low-dose tricyclic antidepressants (amitriptyline, doxepin) which act as 'neuromodulators'. These drugs are often poorly tolerated so start with a very low dose, e.g. amitriptyline 10mg at night.
- Topical corticosteroids are not helpful unless the skin is inflamed.

Box 28.2 Dermatitis artefacta: differential diagnosis

- Contact dermatitis: allergic or irritant.
- Phytophotodermatitis.
- Infection: bacterial, viral, fungal.
- Fixed drug eruption.
- Pyoderma gangrenosum.

Further reading

Gupta MA. *Int Rev Psychiatry* 2006; **18**:41–7.

Lee CS *et al. Dermatol Therapy* 2008; **21:**69–82.

Yosipovitch G and Samuel LS. *Dermatol Ther* 2008; **21:**32–41.

Localized dysaesthesias

Some patients complain of localized itching, pain, or burning without any objective physical findings. These dysaesthesias are frequently associated with underlying psychological factors and are exacerbated by stress. Women are affected more often than men. Some patients have fears of cancer or they may have an associated body dysmorphic disorder—see 📖 p.528.

Patients seek relief by trying a wide range of topical medicaments and the conditions may be complicated by iatrogenic problems such as corticosteroid-induced skin atrophy or contact dermatitis (irritant or allergic).

The most frequent presentations are:

- Tingling, itching, or burning in the scalp.
- Burning scrotum.
- Burning vulva (vulvodynia).
- Burning mouth syndrome (often associated with an unpleasant taste) or glossodynia (usually affecting the anterior portion of the tongue).

What should I do?

- Exclude a physical cause for the symptoms such as irritant contact dermatitis.
- Refer for patch testing to exclude allergy.
- Check FBC, iron studies, and thyroid function.
- Set aside enough time to listen to the patient's concerns (this consultation is likely to be lengthy).
- Reassure the patient that you understand the problem and that the condition is well-described—sometimes patients have been dismissed by other professionals and despair of getting help.
- Explain that the skin/mucosa looks entirely normal and that the sensations may be a result of very sensitive nerve endings (whether this is true or not it can be a helpful way of looking at things).
- Reassure the patient that the symptoms are not a sign of cancer or another serious disease.
- Prescribe soothing topical treatments such as emollients and soap substitutes—see 📖 p.584.
- Avoid potent topical corticosteroids.
- A low dose of amitriptyline can be very helpful, but may be poorly tolerated so start with a very low dose (amitriptyline 10mg at night). Doxepin is an alternative. These drugs are prescribed for their action as 'neuromodulators' rather than antidepressants.
- Psychological support: a support group or cognitive behavioural therapy may be helpful.

Further reading

Lee CS *et al.* *Dermatol Therapy* 2008; **21**:69–82.

Delusions

What is a delusion?

See Box 28.3

Body dysmorphic disorder

Synonyms: dysmorphophobia; dermatologic non-disease.

Patients with a normal appearance become preoccupied by imaginary problems such as too much or too little hair, scars, vascular marks, acne, facial redness, or facial asymmetry. Patients attribute their personal failings at work or social difficulties to the 'defect' and may be tempted to spend large sums of money in an attempt to alleviate the 'problem'. Some young woman devastated by what they perceive to be 'severe' acne may demand repeated courses of isotretinoin.

What should I do?

- Avoid doing anything that might produce changes such as redness, scars, or pigment that will cause even more dissatisfaction. Cosmetic surgery is unlikely to satisfy the patient.
- Encourage the patient to see a psychologist or psychiatrist for mental health assessment, especially if cosmetic surgery is being considered.
- Sadly these patients are rarely satisfied with any treatment, have little psychological insight, and are most unlikely to accept that nothing is wrong.

Delusions of parasitosis

Patients with this rare disorder have a fixed, but false, belief that they are infested with an insect or parasite. Occasionally a close family member (usually a spouse) may be become convinced that he/she too is infested.

You will be shown the bumps or 'tracks' that have been produced by 'insects' under the skin (all signs are caused by scratching and picking) and patients will describe how they have extracted 'insects' from the skin.

You are likely to be presented with a container (often a matchbox) containing carefully collected specimens of the 'parasites'. These are usually fragments of skin scale, crust, dressings, or hair.

What should I do?

- Exclude other causes of thought disorders or formication (crawling sensations) including abuse of alcohol or recreational drugs such as cocaine or amphetamine.
- Try to convince the patient to seek the help of a psychiatrist (this will be difficult).
- Atypical antipsychotic drugs such as olanzapine (5–10mg/day) or risperidone (1–4mg/day), which are better tolerated and safer than other antipsychotics, are probably the treatment of choice. Aripiprazole (5–15mg/day) has also been recommended. Pimozide <6mg/day was the traditional treatment, but this drug has more extrapyramidal adverse effects and in higher doses is associated with cardiotoxicity including prolongation of the QT interval and sudden death.

Box 28.3 Terminology

Definitions

- *Hypochondriasis:* an excessive and persistent fear of having a serious physical illness. Fears usually develop in response to minor physical abnormalities. The person is amenable to reassurance, but the impact of reassurance is only temporary.
- *Delusion:* a false personal belief that is not subject to reason or contradictory evidence and is not explained by a person's usual cultural and religious concepts. A delusion may be firmly maintained in the face of incontrovertible evidence that it is false.
- *Delusions of hypochondriasis:* a fixed belief that a problem is due to a serious physical disease, despite evidence to the contrary.

Further reading

Lee CS *Dermatol Therapy* 2008; **21**:2–7.

Eating disorders and skin

Cutaneous symptoms or signs may be the first presentation of anorexia nervosa (restrictive type) or bulimia nervosa (restrictive with inappropriate compensatory behaviour such as self-induced vomiting or laxative and diuretic abuse), conditions in which patients, usually young women, fear fatness and pursue thinness. The cutaneous features may be caused by starvation (skin changes are most frequent in patients with a body mass index of ≤16kg/m^2), adverse effects of drugs taken to induce weight loss, or complications related to self-induced vomiting. Hypothyroidism and vitamin deficiency contribute to the changes and the cutaneous manifestations may resemble those seen in HIV infection.

Patients may also have other skin conditions related to an underlying psychiatric disease such as a self-induced dermatosis—see 🕮 p.524.

What should I look for?

Cutaneous signs of starvation

- Loss of subcutaneous fat.
- Pitting oedema (pretibial or pedal).
- Dry skin with fine scaling or asteatotic eczema—see 🕮 p.204.
- Generalized pruritus sometime with prurigo—see 🕮 p.206.
- Cheilitis.
- Acne.
- Generalized hyperpigmentation or melasma (pigment localized to the face—see 🕮 Box 30.1, p.539).
- Cold intolerance with acrocyanosis and perniosis.
- Paronychia, brittle nails, and/or interdigital intertrigo.
- Dry brittle scalp hair, diffuse hair loss (telogen effluvium), and/or hypertrichosis with fine lanugo-like body hair.
- Acquired striae distensae.
- Orange palms (carote-inoderma).
- Pellagra (niacin deficiency), scurvy (vitamin C deficiency), acrodermatitis enteropathica (zinc deficiency)—see 🕮 p.474.
- Petechiae and purpura in association with hypoplastic bone marrow and thrombocytopenia.
- Poor wound healing.

Drug-related adverse effects

- Fixed drug eruption (e.g. phenolphthalein-containing laxatives).
- Photosensitivity with thiazide diuretics.
- Finger clubbing associated with laxative abuse.

Complications of self-induced vomiting

- Single or multiple calluses on knuckles (Russell's sign).
- Dental enamel erosion and gingivitis.
- Benign, usually bilateral, painless parotid gland enlargement.
- Transient facial purpura from increased intrathoracic pressure.
- Subcutaneous emphysema and/or spontaneous pneumomediastinum.

Chapter 29
Skin in the elderly

Contents

Relevant pages in other chapters

Ageing skin

The changes observed in old skin are caused by a combination of intrinsic and extrinsic ageing. Skin undergoes genetically programmed senescence (intrinsic ageing), but exposed skin is also modified by environmental factors (extrinsic ageing), the most important of which is UV light (photoageing)—see 🕮 p.43. Mechanical trauma and chemicals such as nicotine also alter the skin. Compare the appearance of sun-protected intrinsically aged skin on a covered site such as the buttock with exposed extrinsically aged, photodamaged skin (face, forearm, back of hand).

Intrinsic ageing

- Variable epidermal thickness with loss of rete ridges reduces epidermal adhesion and predisposes to blistering.
- Reduced dermal collagen with degenerate elastin leads to inelasticity and fine wrinkles.
- Abnormal epidermal barrier function and abnormal lipids lead to increased permeability and water loss with dryness and fissuring.
- Fewer active melanocytes impair photoprotection.
- 50% decrease in Langerhans cells impairs cell-mediated immunity.
- Reduced dermal microvasculature contributes to delayed healing.
- Benign neoplasms, including cherry angiomas and seborrhoeic warts.

Photoageing

UV radiation is responsible for many of the signs we associate with old age, including coarse wrinkles, purpura, and dyspigmentation—see 🕮 Box 3.1, p.43.

Common skin conditions in the elderly

Old skin, much like the skin of neonates, is easily irritated or traumatized and should be handled gently. Although no one dies of old skin, skin disease lowers quality of life. Examine all the skin of your patients—see Box 29.1. Management may be challenging because older people may have difficulties bathing or using treatments—see Box 29.2.

The commonest skin conditions in the elderly are:

- Dry itchy skin.
- Eczema: asteatotic, varicose, seborrhoeic, contact (irritant >allergic).
- Skin infections, particularly fungal in skin creases.
- Toenail dystrophy: poor vision or reduced mobility may mean that patients cannot cut their toenails (filing is safer than cutting or clipping). Fungal infection may complicate problems such as onychogryphosis (thick distorted nails).
- Scabies.
- Adverse drug reactions.
- Leg ulcers, pressure sores or traumatic erosions, blisters, or ulcers.
- Premalignant changes and skin cancers, as well as benign skin tumours.

Box 29.1 Assessing elderly patients: a dermatological checklist

- Sun damage and skin cancer are common in older people: inspect all the skin but pay particular attention to sun-exposed skin on the face, scalp, and ears.
- Inspect the skin under wigs or hair pieces.
- Do spectacles or hearing aids fit comfortably without traumatizing skin? Look behind the ears.
- When were false teeth last checked by a dentist? Angular cheilitis is common in individuals with ill-fitting dentures.
- Inspect the nails: can the patient cut (or file—much safer!) their fingernails and toenails? Should the patient see a podiatrist or chiropodist? It is easier to cut thick nails if they have been softened by soaking in warm water, e.g. after a bath.
- Inspect skin folds and perineum: intertrigo is common in the elderly. Causes include irritant contact dermatitis secondary to incontinence as well as infection (*Candida* or tinea).
- Look at areas subjected to pressure, particularly the sacrum, and check cushions or wheelchairs, as well as shoes.
- Remove bandages: do not accept the diagnosis of 'leg ulcer' without examining the ulcer. BCCs on the leg are frequently misdiagnosed as 'ulcers'.
- Are compression bandages or stockings applied correctly so that they run smoothly from the base of the toes to just below the knee (and stay in place)? Is there ridging or blistering of the skin beneath the bandage suggesting poor bandaging technique? See 📖 Box 15.10, p.287; Box 33.3, p.591; Fig. 33.1, p.591.
- Are legs oedematous because the patient is immobile and spending much of the day in a sitting position ('armchair legs')? Would periods of elevation or compression stockings be helpful?
- Ensure that skin is not being traumatized by appliances such as in-dwelling urinary catheters or by adhesive tape.

Box 29.2 Practicalities of treatment in the elderly

- Impaired mobility may make it difficult to reach parts of the skin or to apply topical treatments.
- Difficulties bathing or showering or washing scalp.
- Risk of falls if bath is slippery.
- Reactions to topical treatments: irritancy is more common than allergy.
- Incontinence contributing to an irritant contact dermatitis.
- Immobility and obesity may contribute to intertrigo (sweating and irritation of skin in flexures).
- Poor vision may make it difficult to apply treatments correctly.
- Poor memory and difficulty following guidance.
- Interactions between systemic medicaments.
- Sedating antihistamines may cause confusion or falls.

Dry itchy skin and asteatotic eczema

Most elderly individuals have dry itchy skin (xerosis) that is easily irritated. Symptoms often deteriorate after admission to hospital because skin is dried out by enthusiastic washing with soap, a low humidity, and central heating. Some patients with very dry skin develop asteatotic eczema. Itch may be distressing, interfering with sleep—see 🕮 Fig. 10.2, p.204.

What should I ask?

- Find out precisely what the patient or carer is using to wash the skin or is putting in the bath.
- Is the patient putting anything on the skin? Check precisely how any treatments have been used—see 🕮 p.30.
- Take a full history including a drug history—see 🕮 p.18 and p.20.
- Is anyone else itchy? Remember the old lady with 'a rash' who is in the same nursing home, the spouse with 'hand dermatitis', or the grandchild with 'eczema' may well have scabies.

What should I look for?

- Dry slightly scaly skin.
- Asteatotic eczema: skin is very dry and has a network of shallow erythematous fissures in the epidermis that produce an appearance that resembles 'crazy paving' (eczema craquelé). Asteatotic eczema usually starts on the shins, but may spread in a patchy fashion to the thighs and trunk. Intensity of itch varies—see 🕮 Fig. 10.2, p.204.
- Some very itchy patients may have secondary changes such as excoriations or nodules (prurigo nodularis) where the skin is being scratched (the centre of the back is usually spared)—see 🕮 p.206 and Fig. 10.6, p.207.
- Look for evidence of an infestation such as scabies (burrows or crusting between fingers). Elderly patients with scabies may have a widespread crusted scaly rash—Norwegian scabies—see 🕮 Box 8.1, p.165.
- Signs of another skin disease e.g. bullous pemphigoid, an autoimmune blistering disease that presents in the elderly. Itchy erythematous 'urticated' papules may appear months before the tense blisters—see 🕮 p.250.

What should I do?

- Investigate to exclude a systemic cause for itch—see Box 29.3.
- Soap substitutes and emollients should be sufficient to settle irritation in most patients with dry skin—see Box 29.4, and 🕮 p.584.
- Prescribe a mild or moderately potent topical corticosteroid ointment to use ×2/day on inflamed skin—see 🕮 p.586.
- If itch persists despite these measures, check the treatment is being used correctly (is the skin still dry?), look for scabies again, and revaluate for a systemic disease before considering the possibility of a psychogenic component to the itch—see 🕮 Box 28.1, p.525.

Box 29.3 Causes of itch in the elderly

- Dry skin with asteatotic eczema particularly on shins.
- Another primary skin disease or infestation (scabies).
- Systemic disease:
  - Iron deficiency.
  - Thyroid disease.
  - Cholestatic jaundice.
  - Chronic renal failure.
  - Polycythaemia.
  - Lymphoma.
- Drugs:
  - Statins (also cause dryness).
  - ACE inhibitors.
  - Opiates.
  - Barbiturates.
  - Antidepressants.

Box 29.4 Managing dry itchy skin

- Trim nails to prevent damage to skin from scratching.
- Avoid soap or excessive bathing (water should not be too hot).
- Prescribe a creamy emollient for day-time use and a greasier emollient for the evening. Show the patient or carer how to use the treatment—see 🕮 p.584.
- Recommend a soap substitute such as Hydromol® ointment but beware of making the bath or shower slippery. Avoid other bath additives—see 🕮 p.584.
- Aqueous cream with 1% menthol may relieve itch if emollients are not effective.
- Occlude very itchy skin with a paste bandage or Zipzoc® stocking. This is soothing and protects the skin from fingernails—see 🕮 p.590.
- Consider prescribing a sedating antihistamine, but this may cause confusion or falls in the elderly.

Chapter 30

Skin and pregnancy

Contents

Relevant pages in other chapters

Subacute cutaneous LE 📖 Box 19.7, p.373
Antiphospholipid syndrome 📖 Box 20.8, p.419

Skin in pregnancy

The changes in skin and hair that occur during pregnancy are linked to the physiological hormonal changes during gestation including:

- Synthesis of human chorionic gonadotrophin (peaks at week 12).
- Production of progesterone and oestrogen from the corpus luteum.
- Alterations in thyroid function and increased output of gonadotrophins and adrenocorticotrophic hormone (ACTH).

What skin signs should I look for?

- Hyperpigmentation: more marked in women with dark hair. Some pigment tends to persist postpartum in dark-skinned women.
  - Nipples, areolae, axillae, vulva, perianal, and scars.
  - Abdomen: a central line of pigmentation (linea nigra) that is usually most marked below the umbilicus but may extend higher.
  - Face: the 'mask of pregnancy' (melasma)—see Box 30.1.
  - Increased numbers of melanocytic naevi (moles) and darkening or enlargement of pre-existing melanocytic naevi and freckles. Apply the ABCDEF rule—any suspicious changing or new melanocytic naevus should be excised—see 🕮 p.330. Pregnancy has no effect on survival in women diagnosed with localized cutaneous melanoma.
  - Generalized hyperpigmentation (less common than focal).
- Vascular: increased vascular permeability and proliferation:
  - Palmar erythema.
  - Cutis marmorata, purpura, and petechiae affecting legs.
  - Spider naevi predominantly in area drained by the superior vena cava (face, neck, arms, and hands). Capillary haemangiomas usually on head and neck. Also pyogenic granulomas of oral mucosa.
  - Varicose veins: lower legs, vulva (also haemorrhoids).
- Connective tissue:
  - Striae gravidarum ('stretch marks') predominantly on abdomen, and breasts. Appear in the 3rd trimester. Initially pink or purple and fade leaving white depressed bands. Never disappear entirely.
  - Skin tags (molluscum fibrosum gravidarum) on neck and axillae. Involute partially after delivery.
- Hair:
  - Thickening of hair during pregnancy.
  - Diffuse loss (telogen effluvium) 2–4 months postpartum causing thinning of hair (not baldness). Shedding continues for 6–24 weeks and then hair regrows—see 🕮 p.24 and p.44.
- Excoriations:
  - 18% of pregnant women develop itching which may be localized or generalized—see 🕮 p.540.
  - A shift to T-helper 2 (Th2) cytokines in pregnancy may trigger atopic eczema even in patients with no previous history of atopy.

Box 30.1 More about melasma

Synonym: chloasma.

- Melasma is increased pigmentation that is most often centrofacial (forehead, cheeks, upper lip, chin) or malar (cheeks) but may involve the mandibular ramus or the forearms. Pigment is brown and distributed in blotchy smooth flat patches.
- Exposure to sunlight increases pigmentation.
- Melasma occurs most often in pregnancy or in women taking oral contraceptives, but may be seen in men (particularly Asian men) and women who are not taking any hormones.
- The melanin pigment may be mainly epidermal (contrast is accentuated by examination of the skin using Wood's light), dermal (no accentuation under Wood's light), or mixed—see 📖 p.568.
- The differential diagnosis includes postinflammatory hyperpigmentation including pigmentation secondary to contact dermatitis. Ask if a rash or itching preceded the colour change.
- Melasma tends to fade postpartum, particularly in fair-skinned women.
- Rigorous photoprotection (hats, sunblock creams) is crucial in management—see 📖 p.316.
- Avoid irritating the skin, particularly dark-coloured skin, as this may increase hyperpigmentation (postinflammatory hyperpigmentation).
- Persistent epidermal melasma may be treated for 6–12 months with 20% azelaic acid cream or 0.05% tretinoin cream (may irritate) or creams containing 2–4% hydroquinone in combination with tretinoin and a mild corticosteroid to prevent irritation, but the response may be disappointing. Sun protection must be continued during treatment and even when pigment has faded.
- Avoid prolonged treatment with creams containing >4% hydroquinone as these can cause exogenous onchronosis with permanent hyperpigmentation, particularly in dark-skinned patients.
- Cosmetic camouflage may be helpful.
- Dermal melasma is unresponsive to treatment.

Pregnancy-specific dermatoses

What should I ask?

- When did symptoms start: before or after onset of 3rd trimester?
- Is there a rash: where did it start, e.g. in striae? Any blisters?
- Any past or family history of skin problems or atopy?
- Any rash in previous pregnancies or when taking the contraceptive pill?

What should I look for?

Evidence of scratching without a primary rash

Excoriations or firm erythematous nodules (prurigo), but background skin is not inflamed or scaly. The centre of the back is usually spared.

- Search for other causes of itching such as scabies—see Box 30.2.
- Is the patient jaundiced? Intrahepatic cholestasis of pregnancy is associated with risk to fetus—see Box 30.3.

A primary rash

Erythematous scaly skin, wheals, or blisters. Consider:

- *Atopic eruption of pregnancy* (common). Starts earlier than other specific dermatoses (before 3rd trimester). The scaly erythematous eczematous rash is often flexural. Some patients also have prurigo or follicular papules. Commonly recurs in subsequent pregnancies.
- *Polymorphic eruption of pregnancy*. Starts late in pregnancy or immediately postpartum. Smooth erythematous 'urticated' papules and plaques (like wheals but do not come and go) appear in abdominal striae. ***Spares periumbilical skin***. May exhibit Köbner phenomenon (rash in scars). Occasional vesicles, usually associated with scratching. Rash spreads to distal sites. Most common in primigravidas and multiple gestation pregnancies. Settles within 2 weeks of delivery.
- *Pemphigoid (herpes) gestationis* (rare). Autoimmune blistering disease that usually starts in 2nd or 3rd trimester. Crops of urticated erythematous papules, vesicles, or tense bullae on the abdomen. ***Involves periumbilical skin***. Spreads to trunk and limbs. Usually settles 4 weeks postpartum but may persist for longer. May recur and be more severe in subsequent pregnancies. Associated with small-for-date babies. 10% of infants have a transient rash.

What should I do?

- Check LFTs and serum bile acid levels to exclude intrahepatic cholestasis—see Box 30.3.
- Take a skin biopsy for histology and direct immunofluorescence (IMF) to distinguish polymorphic eruption of pregnancy from pemphigoid gestationis. In pemphigoid gestationis, direct IMF shows linear deposition of C3 with or without IgG at the dermoepidermal junction. Direct IMF is negative in polymorphic eruption of pregnancy.
- Treat with emollients, potent topical corticosteroids (see 🕮 p.584 and p.586) and if needed, chlorphenamine. Prednisolone (0.5–1 mg/kg/day) may be required in pemphigoid gestations.

Box 30.2 Causes of itch in pregnancy

- Consider causes unrelated to pregnancy—see 📖 p.60 such as:
  - Infestations (scabies) or infections (viral, bacterial, or fungal).
  - Systemic disease (renal, hepatic, haematological, HIV).
  - Drugs.
  - Contact dermatitis.
  - Exacerbation of a pre-existing dermatosis.
- Intrahepatic cholestasis of pregnancy—see Box 30.3. Onset usually in 3rd trimester.
- A specific dermatosis of pregnancy (see 📖 p.540):
  - Atopic eruption of pregnancy (includes eczema in pregnancy, prurigo of pregnancy, and pruritic folliculitis of pregnancy). The most common dermatosis of pregnancy. Onset early in pregnancy.
  - Polymorphic eruption of pregnancy—common. Also known as pruritic urticarial papules and plaques of pregnancy = PUPP. Onset late in pregnancy or immediately postpartum.
  - Pemphigoid gestationis (rare). Onset 2nd or 3rd trimester.

Box 30.3 Intrahepatic cholestasis of pregnancy

- Intrahepatic cholestasis with raised serum bile acids causes itching. Itch may recur in subsequent pregnancies. Abnormal biliary transport is probably caused by a combination of genetic factors, the cholestatic effect of sex hormones (mainly oestrogens), and environmental factors (seasonal, dietary, geographic). May also be caused by the contraceptive pill.
- Itch usually commences around 25–32 weeks of gestation but clears promptly postpartum. Worse in twin pregnancies. Serum bile acids, alkaline phosphatase, and aminotransferases are raised. Jaundice occurs in 10–25% of patients.
- ⚠ Associated with placental insufficiency, premature labour, and sudden fetal death. Placental anoxia may be caused by decreased fetal elimination of toxic bile acids. Fetal monitoring is essential.
- Ursodeoxycholic acid alleviates itch, improves liver enzymes, and prolongs duration of pregnancy. Other options include emollients, 1% menthol in aqueous cream, and sedating systemic antihistamines (chlorphenamine).

Further reading

Arrese M *et al Expert Rev Mol Med* 2008; **10:**e9.

Geenes V and Williamson C. *World J Gastroenterol* 2009; **15:**2049–66.

Vaughan Jones SA *et al. Br J Dermatol* 1999; **141:**71–81.

Safety of treatments in pregnancy

Most drugs are not studied in pregnancy and we have very little data about the safety of commonly used medicaments in pregnancy. Congenital malformations may be produced during the 1st trimester—the greatest risk is from the 3rd to the 11th week of pregnancy. Drugs should only be prescribed if the benefits outweigh the risks, but remember that suboptimal treatment of the mother might also be harmful to the unborn child.

Topical medicaments

- Antifungals: safe when used topically.
- Corticosteroids: mild to potent topical corticosteroids are safe to use in pregnancy. Large amounts of very potent topical corticosteroids may be linked to low birthweight, but data are inconclusive.
- Calcipotriene (topical vitamin D): no data, probably safe when used topically.
- Coal tar: no data, probably safe when used topically.
- Retinoids: probably safe when used topically, but insufficient data.
- Tacrolimus: no data, probably safe when used topically.

Oral medicaments

- Antibiotics: penicillins, erythromycin, and clindamycin—appear safe.
- Antivirals: aciclovir, valaciclovir, famciclovir—appear safe.
- Antihistamines: chlorphenamine and loratidine—probably safe. Cetirizine appears safe in the 3rd trimester.
- Antifungals: avoid itraconazole. Risk of abortion. Terbinafine: no data.
- Azathioprine: risks not established but may be associated with low birth weight or spontaneous abortion. Avoid if possible.
- Ciclosporin: may be associated with prematurity, growth retardation, or impaired immune function. Avoid if possible.
- Dapsone: folic acid should be given throughout pregnancy. Risk of neonatal haemolysis and methaemoglobinaemia. May cause kernicterus—avoid in late pregnancy.
- Prednisolone: 88% of prednisolone is inactivated as it crosses the placenta. Short-term treatment is safe. Prolonged or repeated treatment may be associated with intra-uterine growth restriction.
- Methotrexate: teratogenic. Avoid in pregnancy. Males and females should use effective contraception during treatment and for at least 3 months after stopping the drug. May also reduce fertility.
- Retinoids: teratogenic. Females must use effective contraception during treatment. Acitretin: continue contraception for at least 2 years after withdrawing treatment. Isotretinoin: continue contraception for at least 1 month after withdrawing treatment.

Further reading

Chi CC *et al. Cochrane Database Syst Rev* 2009; **3:**CD007346 (reviews safety of topical corticosteroids in pregnancy).

Chapter 31

Skin in infancy and childhood

Contents

We do not attempt to address the whole of paediatric dermatology but have selected topics, generally with a medical overlap, that may concern doctors working in paediatrics or dermatology trainees.

Relevant pages in other chapters

Acne 📖 p.224
Acrodermatitis enteropathica 📖 p.475
Bacterial infections 📖 p.122
Bites 📖 p.170
Blistering disorders 📖 p.240
Capillary malformations 📖 p.520
Dermatitis artefacta 📖 p.524
Eczema herpeticum 📖 p.106
Epidermal naevi and epidermal naevus syndromes 📖 p.516
Incontinentia pigmenti, Goltz syndrome 📖 p.518
Melanocytic naevi 📖 p.322
Mosaicism 📖 p.514
Neonatal lupus erythematosus 📖 Box 19.7, p.373
Neurofibromatosis 📖 p.508
Photodermatoses including porphyria 📖 Box 16.7, p.307, p.312
Pigmentary mosaicism 📖 p.518 Scabies 📖 p.164
Skin biopsy in infants and children 📖 Box 32.4, p.577
Skin failure and emergency dermatology 📖 p.93
Tuberous sclerosis 📖 p.512
Viral exanthems including Kawasaki's disease 📖 p.142

Skin of the neonate: the first 28 days

The skin of a full term infant

- Fine desquamation at 24–48h of age. Increased desquamation in post-mature babies. WSP is a safe emollient.
- Increased heat loss with reduced vasoconstriction.
- Permeable, particularly if occluded or in high temperatures or humidity. Topical agents are easily absorbed and may be toxic. Wash with unperfumed, neutral pH cleanser. Rinse and dry completely. Aqueous chlorhexidine is a safe antimicrobial.
- Minimal eccrine sweating, more on forehead than trunk and limbs. Emotional sweating on palms and soles in response to pain or hunger.

The skin of a premature infant

- Thin, very fragile skin prone to mechanical injury. Injuries from tapes, electrodes, etc. may leave scars, only apparent after a few months. Protect injuries with occlusive dressings. Avoid adhesive tapes.
- Very permeable with large amounts of transepidermal water loss (20–50% body weight in 24h). Loss is increased by phototherapy and heat.
- Immature thermal homeostasis—loss of body heat. No sweating.

Some transient neonatal skin changes

- Vascular changes:
  - Cutis marmorata. A physiological net-like (reticulate) pattern of purplish red mottling that disappears on warming.
  - Capillary ectasia (salmon patch) on nape (stork bite), eyelids (angels' kisses), and/or glabella. Most resolve in months or years. May persist on nape of neck.
  - Petechiae on upper body caused by pressure during delivery.
  - Harlequin colour change (rare). Reddening of dependent side of body with sharp midline demarcation and blanching of upper side. Each episode last seconds to minutes. Seen most often in premature infants lying on one side. Episodes cease after 3 weeks.
- Sebaceous hyperplasia: creamy papules on nose. Last a few weeks.
- Milia: 1–2mm firm yellowish papules on face. Last a few months.
- Pigmented macules:
  - Mongolian spots (dermal melanosis). Blue grey macules on sacrum or low back. Most often in black or Asian neonates. May be multiple and can be confused with bruises. Disappear by age 4—see 🕮 Fig. 31.10, p.565.
- Blisters and pustules—see 🕮 p.546.
- Perianal dermatitis:
  - Erythematous macules, 2–3mm, that may be eroded or bleed. Occurs between days 4 and 7. More common in premature infants. Associated with feeds of formula milk.

⚠ More worrying signs

- Perinatal injury—see Box 31.1.
- Subcutaneous nodules or plaques—see Box 31.2.
- Purpuric macules or nodules—see Box 31.3.

Box 31.1 Cutaneous signs of perinatal injury

- Caput succedaneum: swelling over presenting part of scalp caused by pressure on the head during labour. Vacuum extraction—haematoma and oedema. Forceps—facial erythema or abrasions.
- Needle marks: hypopigmented speckles. Heel pricks may leave calcified nodules. Scalp electrodes may leave cuts, superficial ulcers, or, uncommonly, abscesses.
- Ring of alopecia 'halo scalp ring' caused by pressure during labour. Usually over vertex and associated with caput succedaneum. Sometimes necrosis. If severe, may leave permanent scarring alopecia.
- Amniocentesis scars: more apparent after a few weeks. 1–5mm cutaneous dimple-like scars. Most often on extremities.

Box 31.2 Subcutaneous nodules or plaques in neonates

Neonate appears well

Subcutaneous fat necrosis. 1 or more circumscribed firm mobile subcutaneous nodules in first few months of life. Sign of preceding fetal stress or difficult labour with ischaemic fat injury. Persist for up to 6 months. Prognosis good, but monitor for hypercalcaemia.

Sick neonate

⚠ Sclerema neonatorum. Generalized yellowish hardening of skin that occurs in very sick preterm neonates. Treat underlying condition and, if infant survives, hardening resolves.

Box 31.3 ⚠ Blueberry muffin baby

Bluish-purple, non-blanching (purpuric) macules, papules and/or nodules are produced by extramedullary erythropoiesis in the dermis. Usually involves head, neck, and trunk. Causes include:

- Congenital infections, e.g. Toxoplasmosis, Other, Rubella, Cytomegalovirus (commonest), Herpes simplex ('TORCH').
- Haematological disease, e.g. haemolytic disease of the newborn, hereditary spherocytosis, twin–twin transfusion syndrome.
- Malignancy/proliferative diseases, e.g. leukaemia, neuroblastoma, congenital rhabdomyosarcoma, Langerhans cell histiocytosis.

Investigate to determine the cause (including skin biopsy) (see 🕮 p.577) and manage the underlying condition.

Pustules and blisters

Blisters are discussed in detail in 📖 Chapter 13, p.240, but here we consider some problems specific to infants and children. Blisters may evolve into pustules. Consider infection, infestation, dermatitis, or trauma before much less common or very rare blistering diseases.

What should I ask?

- Is the child sick—any fever, lethargy, loss of appetite?
  - Could blisters or pustules be caused by a systemic disease or drug?
- When did problem start—neonatal or childhood?
- Is the problem localized or generalized?
- What triggers blisters or pustules?
  - Are sun-exposed sites affected more than covered sites?
  - Is skin fragile? Do blisters occur at sites of friction, e.g. feet? Or in any particular season? (Sweating may exacerbate EB.)
- Are mucosal surfaces affected?
- Any postinflammatory pigment, scarring, or milia?
- Is there a family history of skin problems? E.g. maternal autoimmune blistering disease—IgG autoantibodies cross the placenta and may cause transient blisters in the neonate.

Neonatal vesicles, pustules, or papulopustules See Box 31.4.

Vesicles, pustules, or papulopustules in childhood

- Infections and Infestations
  - Scabies: vesicopustules on palms and soles in infants usually at least 4 weeks of age. Is mother itchy? See 📖 p.164.
  - Virus: HSV, including eczema herpeticum (see 📖 p.133), VZV, cytomegalovirus, EBV, coxsackie virus (hand–foot–mouth disease).
  - Bacterial: *Staphylococcus aureus* (bullous impetigo, SSSS)—see 📖 p.128, streptococcus, *E. coli*, *H. influenzae*, *K. pneumoniae*.
- Contact dermatitis including phytophotodermatitis—see 📖 Box 16.6, p.305.
- Trauma: including burns—see 📖 p.104.
- EM—see 📖 p.104
- Drug-related:
  - Phototoxic or photoallergic—see 📖 p.304.
  - SJS or TEN—see 📖 p.110.
- Mastocytosis—see Box 31.5.
- Rare: EB (see 📖 Box 13.1, p.244), photosensitivity (see 📖 Box 16.7, p.307), acrodermatitis enteropathica (zinc deficiency—unusual before age 4 weeks)—see 📖 p.475, autoimmune—see 📖 p.250, p.252, and p.254.

What should I do?

- Identify the primary lesions: vesicle or pustule. Remember these may evolve into erosions or ulcers.
- Exclude infection: culture fluid or pus for bacteria, *Candida*, and herpesvirus.
- A Tzank smear may help you to make the diagnosis—see 📖 p.575.

Box 31.4 Vesicular and pustular eruptions in neonates

Swabs sterile

- Erythema toxicum neonatorum: onset age 1–3 days. Mainly trunk. 1–2mm yellowish papules or pustules with an erythematous halo (like flea bites). Fluctuates. Resolves in 2–3 days. Eosinophils in smear (common).
- Transient pustular melanosis: usually in black neonates. Present at birth. Flaccid 1–2mm pustules on chin, neck, and trunk evolve into pigmented macules. Persists a few months. Neutrophils in smear.
- Miliaria: clear vesicles, papules, or pustules caused by occlusion of sweat ducts. Induced by heat and high humidity.
- Sucking blisters or trauma, including burns.
- Aplasia cutis congenita may resemble a blister—see 📖 Box 31.6, p.549.
- Acropustulosis of infancy: crops of very itchy vesicles and pustules on hands and feet. Usually in black neonates (neutrophils in Tzank smear) (uncommon). Differentiate from scabies—see 📖 p.164. Lasts 1–2 years.
- Neonatal 'acne' (benign cephalic pustulosis): pustules face, scalp. No comedones. Onset age 2 weeks. Resolves in about 2 months. May be a reaction to *Pityrosporum* yeasts.
- Rare: maternal immunobullous disease (IgG autoantibodies cross placenta), EB, incontinentia pigmenti (eosinophils in Tzank smear; look for linear pattern; examine mother)—see 📖 p.518.

⚠ ***Infection: neonate may not appear unwell***

- Bacterial infection: e.g. staphylococcal/streptococcal impetigo (common), SSSS (see 📖 p.128), listeriosis (rare cause of pustules and petechiae).
- Cutaneous candidiasis (may be congenital).
- HSV or VZV: look for scars (multinucleated giant keratinocytes in Tzank smear—see 📖 p.575).

Box 31.5 What is mastocytosis?

Mastocytosis is an uncommon group of conditions in which mast cells proliferate and accumulate in skin and other organs. Systemic mast cell disease (raised serum tryptase) is extremely rare in children.

Presentations in childhood:

- Mastocytoma: localized reddish-yellow macule, plaque, or nodule. Develops in infancy. Swells and may blister when rubbed. Blistering is less frequent with age. Nodule tends to resolve slowly.
- Urticaria pigmentosa: brown freckle-like macules that urticate (become erythematous and raised) if rubbed. Improves by adolescence.
- Diffuse cutaneous mastocytosis: very rare. Mast cells disseminated widely in skin. Skin may be erythematous, leathery, or normal. Generalized blistering in infants age <3, may mimic SSSS. Systemic symptoms include itch, flushing, hypotension, syncope, diarrhoea, and dyspnoea. Tends to improve with age.

Congenital cutaneous lesions

⚠ Midline congenital lesions on the nose, scalp, or spine may be a marker for occult neural tube defects. Some communicate directly with intracranial tissue. Is there any family history of neural tube defects? Check for neurological symptoms or signs. Consider imaging if clinically suspicious.

Spinal cutaneous lesions: what should I look for?

Congenital malformations are mostly due to the defective closure of the caudal neuropore at the end of week 4. The defects may involve the tissue overlying the spinal cord (meninges, vertebral arch, dorsal muscles, and skin). Spina bifida is non-fusion of the vertebral arches.

- Lumbosacral signs: midline dimple above gluteal cleft, hypertrichosis (faun's tail), sacral lipoma, telangiectatic patch, infantile haemangioma, or vascular malformation near midline. An underlying spinal defect is more likely in the presence of 2 or more cutaneous signs.
- Palpable vertebral defects.
- Asymmetrical curved gluteal cleft.
- Urogenital or anorectal abnormalities.

Facial cutaneous lesions: what should I look for?

- Midline dermoid cyst (firm subcutaneous nodule): those on nose or scalp are most likely to have intracranial extension.
- Nasal glioma: firm blue nodule on side of nose. May be connected to deeper structures.
- Midline nasal mass or pit.

Scalp cutaneous lesions: what should I look for?

- Midline dermoid cyst (occipital scalp): punctum with long hairs increases chance of intracranial connection.
- Midline 1–4cm bluish subcutaneous nodule or circular area of alopecia, with a translucent membrane (may look bullous). Usually on occipital or parietal scalp. Indications of possible intracranial involvement:
  - Pulsation or changing in size with crying.
  - Transillumination.
  - Overlying port-wine stain (PWS).
  - Hair collar sign: a rim of dark coarse hair around the bald patch. This marker for ectopic neural tissue is also seen in membranous aplasia cutis congenita. See Fig. 31.1.
  - If hair collar is present, image to look for a skull defect and to exclude an encephalocoele or a meningocoele. If no connection, lesion may either be heterotopic brain tissue or membranous aplasia cutis congenita—see Box 31.6.
- Sebaceous naevus: yellowish plaque with loss of hair. Occur on face as well as scalp. Most often oval. If linear (follow Blaschko's lines) may be associated with neurological problems—see 📖 p.516 and Fig. 31.2.

Box 31.6 What is aplasia cutis congenita?

In this rare condition, localized areas of skin are absent at birth. The aetiology is uncertain, but may relate to incomplete closure of embryonic fusion lines.

- Aplasia cutis congenita has been classified into 9 groups. All but group 1 have associated abnormalities.
- Most cases are sporadic, rarely inherited in an autosomal dominant or autosomal recessive pattern.
- Usually presents as 1–2cm circular or oval bald patch near vertex of the scalp. Rarely affects face (focal facial dermal hypoplasia) and other areas.
- Appearance of skin varies—most often bald patch appears to be covered by a shiny translucent membrane (membranous aplasia cutis) but skin may be eroded, deeply ulcerated, or scarred.
- Membranous aplasia cutis is usually surrounded by a hair collar—see 📖 Fig. 31.1 and p.548.
- On scalp, may be associated with an underlying skull defect.
- May be >1 lesion.
- Rarely associated with other congenital abnormalities.
- Extensive aplasia cutis of the trunk is associated with fetus papyraceus (defects may be caused by placental infarcts after death of a twin fetus). Also malformations in other organs.
- Differential diagnosis: obstetric trauma: e.g. forceps injury, herpes simplex or VZV infection, EB (rare).

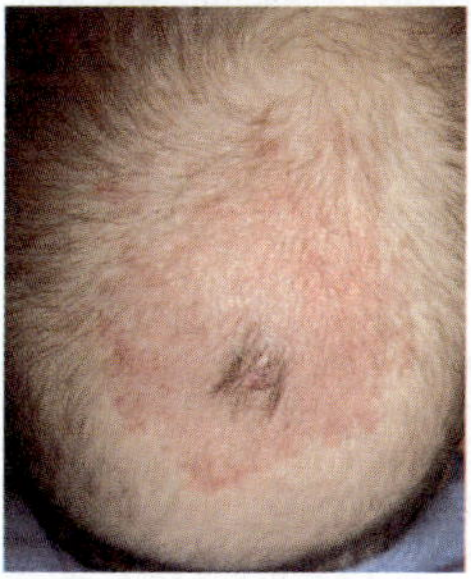

Fig. 31.1 Membranous aplasia cutis congenita with dark hair collar and surrounding capillary malformation.

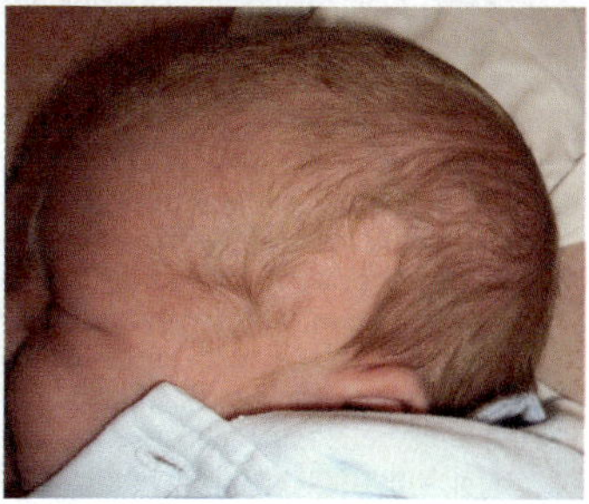

Fig. 31.2 Linear sebaceous naevus—yellowish smooth plaque and absence of overlying hair.

Further reading

Baselga E *et al. Pediatr Dermatol* 2005; **22:**13–17.

Drolet B *Pediatr Clin North Am.* 2000; **47:**813–23.

Drolet B *et al. Arch Dermatol* 1995; **131:**1427–31.

Frieden IJ. *J Am Acad Dermatol* 1986; **14:**646–60.

Guggisberg D *et al. Arch Dermatol.* 2004; **140:**1109–115.

Infantile haemangioma

Synonyms: strawberry haemangioma, capillary haemangioma.

Infantile haemangiomas are common benign proliferative tumours that present most often in girls and in preterm babies, when they may be multiple. The haemangiomas may be disfiguring and alarming. You should be able to differentiate haemangiomas from vascular malformations (see 📖 p.552); decide if further investigation is needed and discuss the likely outcome.

What should I look for?

- 50% occur on the head and neck. The tumours are not apparent at birth, but parents may notice a pale, telangiectatic or erythematous macule (may resemble a PWS).
- Bright red, dome-shaped nodules or plaques evolve in the first month of life. Some have a deeper bluish component (Fig. 31.3).
- Growth phase: rapid for 3–4 months; slow for 6–18 months. Deep components grow for longer.
- Involution. Colour slowly fades, nodules soften and shrink. 50–60% involute completely by age 5 years; 70–75% by age 7 years and 90% by age 9 years. Residual changes may include pallor and lax skin.
- Deeper components may persist.

⚠ When to worry (Boxes 31.7 and 31.8)

- Ulceration: often painful. Occurs in growth phase. Looks alarming but blood loss minimal unless there is a coagulopathy—see Box 31.7.
- Organ compromise—needs urgent treatment:
  - Periocular: may obstruct vision and lead to permanent amblyopia. Refer for urgent visual assessment. MRI if displacement of globe or thickening of lid.
  - Mandibular or neck area: internal haemangiomas may cause airway obstruction. If noisy breathing, stridor or difficulty breathing when feeding, refer for urgent ENT assessment.
  - Lips: may interfere with ability to suck.
- Plaque-like facial haemangioma may be associated with PHACE (**P**osterior fossa malformations, **H**aemangioma, **A**rterial abnormalities, **C**oarctation of the aorta and **E**ye abnormalities). Called PHACES if also **S**ternal clefting and/or **S**upraumbilical raphe.
- Plaque-like lumbosacral haemangioma: look for tags or dimples in genital and sacral area. May be associated with spinal dysraphism, tethered cord syndrome, and/or multiple congenital anomalies.
- 5 or more cutaneous haemangiomas: rarely associated with disseminated haemangiomatosis (liver, heart, and other internal organs). Most not life threatening. Age >6 months: unlikely to be problems.

Management (Boxes 31.7 and 31.9)

- Clinical photographs are useful to document evolution and resolution.
- Plaque-like haemangiomas covering a large area are more likely to be associated with systemic problems. Investigate with imaging, e.g. MRI.

Box 31.7 Ulcerated infantile haemangiomas: what to do

- Large haemangiomas growing rapidly may ulcerate. Haemangiomas affecting anogenital skin, flexures, or lip area are particularly prone to ulceration.
- Ulceration may be painful, particularly in anogenital region.
- Ulcers usually heal in 2–3 weeks, but deep ulcers cause scarring.
- Bleeding is usually minimal.
- Monitor for infection—spreading erythema, warmth, and pain—and swab for bacterial culture.
- Treatment options:
  - Wound care: soak off crusts, apply petrolatum to protect skin.
  - Antibiotic ointments. Occlusive dressings.
  - Topical lidocaine has been advocated for pain relief (pea-sized amount, no more than ×4/day).
  - Paracetamol for pain control.
  - Topical potent or very potent corticosteroid ointment may relieve pain and speed involution as well as re-epithelialization.
  - Pulsed dye laser surgery may relieve pain and speed re-epithelialization.
  - Propranolol has been recommended—see Box 31.9.
  - Oral prednisolone 2–3mg/kg/day gradually tailed off over months.

Box 31.8 Kasabach–Merritt phenomenon

- Definition: a rapidly enlarging vascular tumour associated with thrombocytopenia, microangiopathic haemolytic anaemia, and consumption coagulopathy.
- This rare phenomenon is virtually never seen in association with infantile haemangiomas, but may occur with other, much less common, enlarging vascular tumours presenting in infancy, e.g. tufted angioma or Kaposiform haemangioendothelioma.
- ⚠ Look for a purplish, tender, rapidly enlarging deep dermal nodule or plaque surrounded by petechiae or bruising as well as prolonged bleeding at other sites.
- Check FBC with film (low platelets, fragmented RBC) and fibrinogen level.

Box 31.9 Treatment for enlarging infantile haemangiomas

Most infantile haemangiomas do not need treatment. If an enlarging haemangioma is compromising organ function, options include:

- Propranolol appears to be a very promising treatment. The dose is gradually increased up to 2mg/kg/day. Treatment is continued for around 6 months.
- Intralesional corticosteroids; systemic corticosteroids (2–3mg/kg/day).
- Pulsed dye laser surgery.

Further reading

Haggstrom AN *et al. Pediatrics* 2006; **117**:698–703.

Lawley LP *et al. Paed Dermatol* 2009; **26**:610–14 (reviews the use of propranolol).

Vascular malformations

Malformations may be predominantly capillary, venous, lymphatic, arterial, and arteriovenous, or any combination of these. Distribution may be localized or diffuse. Malformations may be present at birth or only become apparent in childhood. Unlike infantile haemangiomas, most malformations do not involute but persist and may slowly worsen with age.

What should I look for?

- Port-wine stain (PWS): malformation with dilated capillaries that may be associated with complex vascular syndromes:
  - Limb PWS may be associated with Klippel–Trenaunay (varicose veins, capillary, or mixed capillary–lymphatic malformation) or Parkes–Weber (multiple arteriovenous shunts) syndromes. Look for varicosities, haemangiomas, lymphangiomas, and hypertrophy with gradual asymmetrical lengthening of affected limb.
  - ⚠ Facial PWS with distribution in V1 branch of trigeminal nerve (forhead, upper eyelid) is linked to Sturge–Weber syndrome—see Fig. 31.4, and 🕮 p.520. Epilepsy is a frequent complication and patients need regular ophthalmological review to detect glaucoma.
- Cutis marmorata telangiectatica congenita: very rare malformation with dilated capillaries and veins in dermis and subcutis.
  - A network of purplish-red bands with some telangiectasia. Persists when skin is warm.
  - Involved skin may be atrophic and may ulcerate.
  - Girth of involved limb may be reduced—less fat, muscles and/or bone.
  - Rarely associated with other congenital problems.
  - Fades partially over years.
- Venous—slow flow: elevated D-dimer levels.
  - Subtle bluish compressible vessels—no thrill or bruit.
  - May swell when dependent.
  - Can be associated with chronic localized or diffuse intravascular coagulopathy.
- Ateriovenous—fast flow: normal D-dimer levels.
  - Most often head and neck.
  - May be subtle initially, like a PWS.
  - Look for local warmth, subtle thickening. Rarely a thrill or bruit.
  - Potentially life-threatening haemorrhage.
- Lymphatic: normal D-dimer levels.
  - Cystic hygroma: mass, usually in neck or axilla, that presents in the neonate. Collections of dilated lymphatics in dermis with superficial vesicles that intermittently leak clear fluid.
  - Localized group of vesicles: lymphangioma circumscriptum. These appear during childhood. Most common on proximal limbs and limb girdle.

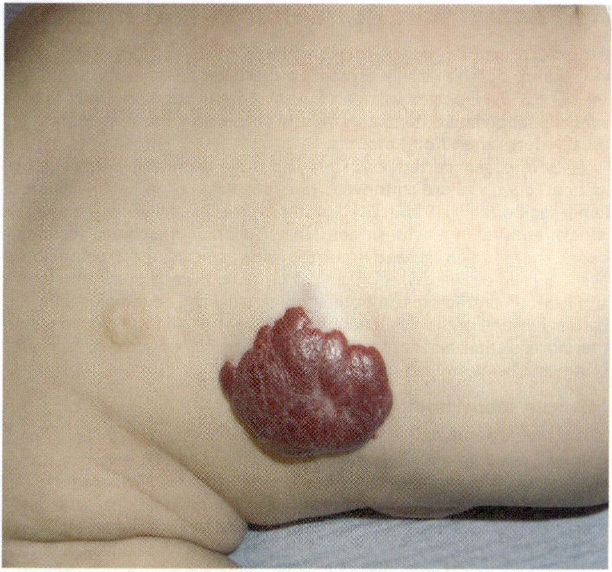

Fig. 31.3 Infantile haemangioma.

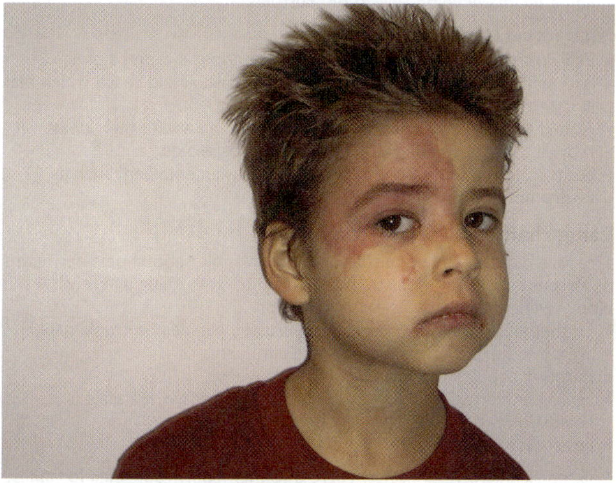

Fig. 31.4 Sturge–Weber syndrome: PWSs in the distribution of the V1 branch of trigeminal nerve may be associated with epilepsy and glaucoma.

Red scaly skin in neonates and infants

Atopic eczema (dermatitis), the commonest cause of redness and itching in children, doesn't usually present until around the age of 3 months—see 📖 p.558. Neonates with red scaly skin are much more likely to have infantile seborrhoeic dermatitis, which presents in the first month and usually clears after 3 or 4 months.

⚠ Severe generalized erythema and scale (neonatal erythroderma) associated with failure to thrive is rare, but suggests an underlying problem—see Boxes 31.10 and 31.11. In some forms of ichthyosis, the neonate is born encased in a tight, smooth, shiny collodion membrane (collodion baby). The tight skin causes dysmorphic features including ectropion (lower eyelid turned outwards), eclabium (lip turned outwards), malformed ears, and flexion contractures. In both erythroderma and collodion babies, the barrier function of the skin is abnormal leading to fluid loss, infection, poor thermoregulation, and absorption of topical agents. Care for the skin with bland emollients and control humidity.

Infantile seborrhoeic dermatitis

What should I look for?

- A well infant who is not particularly itchy (atopic eczema is very itchy).
- A greasy erythematous scaly orange-red papular rash involving the face, scalp ('cradle cap') and flexures. Look in skin folds, particularly around the neck and in the napkin area (usually spared in atopic eczema) (Fig. 31.6). Irritant napkin dermatitis involves convex surfaces and spares skin folds—see 📖 Box 31.12 and Fig. 31.5, p.557. Rash may be secondarily infected by *Candida*.
- Some infants develop tiny sterile pustules.

What should I do?

- Explain that the condition should clear by about 4 months of age.
- Bath with emollients to reduce scale and crust. Avoid soaps which may irritate the skin.
- A mild topical corticosteroid combined with an antifungal ×2/day will reduce redness. Avoid more potent corticosteroids.
- Scalp scale can be removed with olive oil or an emollient such as Hydromol® ointment.

Langerhans cell histiocytosis

This rare disease may be misdiagnosed as infantile seborrhoeic dermatitis. ⚠ Purpura and ulceration should alert you to 'something different'. A skin biopsy will confirm the diagnosis. Look for:

- Erythematous pink or brown, scaly, crusted papules on trunk, napkin area, and flexures that may become confluent.
- Purpuric papules that may ulcerate and weep.
- Scaling and crusting in the scalp. The scalp bleeds when scale is removed (a useful sign).
- Fever (sometimes).

Isolated skin involvement may regress spontaneously but refer for assessment and treatment.

Box 31.10 Red scaly skin—differential diagnosis

Common

- Atopic eczema—see 📖 p.558.
- Seborrhoeic dermatitis—see 📖 p.554.
- Scabies—see 📖 p.164.
- Keratosis pilaris: small scaly follicular papules on lateral aspects of arms and thighs and, sometimes, cheeks. Not itchy. Skin feels rough.
- Psoriasis (much less common than eczema in childhood)—see 📖 p.177. Usually a family history of psoriasis.
- Ichthyosis vulgaris: fine pale scale, increased skin markings on palms. Presents after age 3 months. Mutation in filaggrin gene.

Rare

- Langerhans cell histiocytosis—see 📖 p.554. Refer to a specialist for assessment and treatment.
- Netherton's syndrome: erythroderma (diffusely red and scaly), failure to thrive, hypernatraemic dehydration, and sparse hair. Mutations in *SPINK5* gene that encodes the lymphoepithelial Kazal-type 5 serine protease inhibitor (LEKTI), lead to uncontrolled proteolytic degradation of the corneodesmosomes and a thin, highly permeable stratum corneum. May find characteristic hair shaft abnormality—trichorrhexis invaginata (bamboo hair) in scalp or eyebrow and later a characteristic rash—ichthyosis linearis circumflexa. Also raised IgE, atopy, and food allergies. Skin very permeable—risk of infection and absorption of topical agents. Avoid topical corticosteroids or topical calcineurin inhibitors.
- Nutritional deficiency including:
  - Zinc deficiency (see 📖 p.475) well-demarcated perorifical and perineal glazed erythema, paronychia, dermatitis fingers and toes.
  - Cystic fibrosis: perorifical and perineal rash like zinc deficiency. (see 📖 Box 24.6, p.479)
  - Biotin deficiency: eczematous or psoriasiform rash around eyes, face, and perineum. Also vomiting, seizures, developmental delay, hypotonia, ataxia.
- Immunodeficiency—see 📖 p.562.

Box 31.11 ⚠ Features that should make you revaluate the diagnosis of atopic eczema or seborrhoeic dermatitis

- Congenital onset.
- Erythroderma, large scaling plaques, or indurated skin.
- Purpura or ulceration.
- Failure to thrive.
- Diarrhoea.
- Repeated infections.
- Poor response to treatment with emollients and mild or moderately potent topical corticosteroids.

Napkin rashes

Atopic eczema, the most common form of dermatitis in infancy, tends to spare the moist skin in the napkin area. Instead most napkin rashes are caused by urine and/or faeces irritating the skin (irritant dermatitis). The prevalence of irritant dermatitis has fallen because infants wear highly absorbent nappies that are designed to wick moisture away from the skin.

What should I look for?

- Irritant dermatitis occurs between the ages of 3 weeks and 2 years. The rash involves the convex surfaces (e.g. buttocks) in contact with the napkin and spares skin folds. The erythematous skin may have a rather glazed shiny appearance (Fig. 31.5). Severe chronic irritant dermatitis may be associated with well-demarcated erosions (Jacquet's dermatitis) or extensive papules.
- Candida napkin dermatitis, in infants aged 6–24 months, starts in skin folds but may extend to involve the entire perineum. Look for satellite papules (less often pustules) and oral candidiasis.
- Infantile seborrhoeic dermatitis is an asymptomatic rash that usually presents around age 4–6 weeks. Look for well-demarcated erythematous patches, without much scale, in skin folds. Inspect scalp, face, and axillae—see 🕮 p.554 and Fig. 31.6. May be difficult to differentiate from napkin psoriasis—see Box 31.12.
- Erosive perianal eruption is caused by diarrhoea, often in breastfed infants aged 6 weeks to 3 months. The rash is characterized by erythema with well-demarcated superficial erosions.
- Staphylococcal impetigo may present with flaccid bullae in the napkin area often in the first few weeks of life.
- Group A streptococcal dermatitis in older infants, >6 months, causes a painful perianal erythema that may involve inguinal folds—see 🕮 p.124.

What should I do?

- Culture skin swabs for *Candida* and bacteria.
- Minimize irritation of the skin:
  - Wash skin with plain water and a soap substitute.
  - Ensure that baby wipes are alcohol- and fragrance-free.
  - Change napkin as soon as it is soiled by faeces.
  - Avoid talcum powders which may irritate the skin.
- Paraffin-based ointments such as Hydromol® or 50% WSP in liquid paraffin hydrate the skin and act as a barrier to external irritants.
- Treat inflamed skin with twice daily applications of an ointment containing 1% hydrocortisone in combination with an antifungal agent such as miconazole or clotrimazole.
- Treat bacterial infection with oral antibiotics.
- Rashes unresponsive to treatment: think again—see Box 31.12.

Box 31.12 Napkin rash unresponsive to standard treatment

- Find out exactly how skin in napkin area is being washed, how often napkin is being changed, and what ointments are being applied.
- Take skin swabs and culture for *Candida* and bacteria … again.
- Psoriasis responds poorly to treatments used for napkin dermatitis. The well-demarcated, but asymptomatic, erythema has minimal scale. Napkin psoriasis tends to start on the convex surfaces of the buttocks, but may spread to flexures, trunk, face, and scalp. Most infants do not have evidence of psoriasis in nails. Any family history of psoriasis? The rash is difficult to differentiate from infantile seborrhoeic dermatitis, but seborrhoeic dermatitis is usually controlled after 2–4 weeks of treatment. Aim to keep the skin comfortable using emollients and mild topical corticosteroids, rather than clear psoriasis.
- Dermatophyte infection ('ringworm') presents with well-demarcated scaly erythematous papules and plaques, usually in toddlers rather than infants. Sometimes there are pustules. Often involves thighs and lower abdomen as well as napkin area. Has anyone in the family got tinea pedis? Take a skin scrape for mycology—see 📖 p.156.
- Any blisters or erosions? SSSS, caused by a circulating exfoliative exotoxin, presents with a tender peeling erythema sometimes limited to the napkin area—see 📖 p.106. Allergic contact dermatitis is uncommon but may present as a vesicular eruption in infants age >6 months. Rare autoimmune blistering diseases may present in the napkin area in infancy.
- ⚠ Any purpura or ulceration? Langerhans cell histiocytosis involves the flexures and the napkin area but may also affect scalp, skin behind the ears, and the trunk—see 📖 p.554.
- ⚠ Zinc deficiency presents with psoriasiform dermatitis around mouth as well as in napkin area. Look for paronychia, sparse hair, and failure to thrive as well as recurrent candida infections—see 📖 p.475.

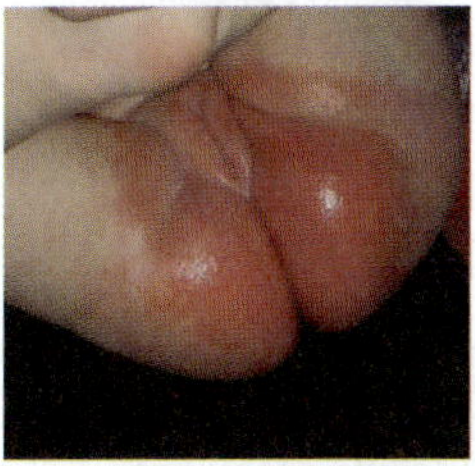

Fig. 31.5 Painful irritant dermatitis with a shiny glazed erythema that spares skin folds.

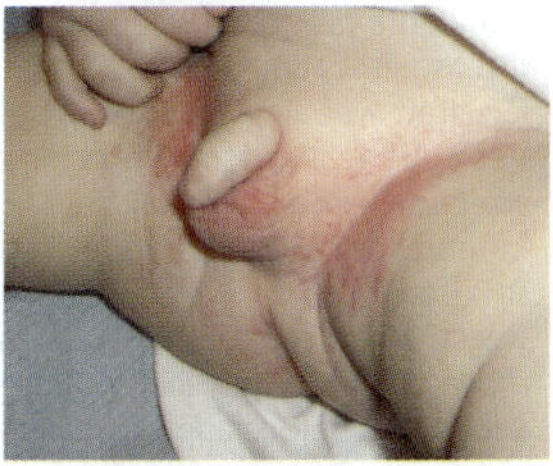

Fig. 31.6 Seborrhoeic dermatitis favours skin folds.

Atopic eczema (atopic dermatitis)

Atopic eczema is a chronic itchy skin condition that affects 20–25% of children in Western Europe. Prevalence is increasing. Eczema usually starts around age 3 months. Eczema clears in about 50% of children by puberty, but in others the disease is chronic and recurrent. Pathogenesis is complex—see Box 31.13. The prevalences of bronchial asthma and allergic rhinitis are increased in patients with atopic eczema. Skin prick tests to many common environmental allergens are positive in atopic patients.

What should I ask?

Explore these areas:

- Age of onset, pattern, and severity of the eczema.
- Response to previous and current treatments.
- The impact of eczema on children and their parents or carers.
- Growth and development.
- Dietary history including any dietary manipulation.
- Immediate reactions (urticaria, wheeze, angio-oedema) to foods.
- Contact with potential trigger factors including irritants such as soaps, shampoos, bubble baths, and shower gels. Contact allergic dermatitis is unusual in children, but irritant reactions to creams are common.
- Personal and family history of atopy (e.g. asthma, allergic rhinitis).

What should I do?

- Confirm diagnosis; for diagnostic criteria see Box 31.14 and Figs. 31.7, 31.8, 31.9, p.561.
- Make a global assessment:—mild, moderate, or severe—based on symptoms (such as itching and sleep disturbance); the quantities or strengths of treatment, clinical signs, and the area affected by eczema.
- Record impact on quality of life of the child and family.
- Using 'POEM', (a simple 'patient-orientated eczema measure') get the patient's view (see www.nottingham.ac.uk/dermatology/POEM.htm).
- You may wish to try using SCORAD ('SCORing Atopic Dermatitis'), a detailed index comprising an assessment of clinical features, extent of disease, itch, and sleep loss.
- Crusted weeping eczema or pustules: take swabs for bacterial culture.
- Vesicular rash or small erosions: take swabs to exclude herpes simplex infection—see p.106.
- Immediate reactions to foods: refer for further investigation—see Box 31.15.
- Reactions to topical preparations: irritation of inflamed skin is much more common than allergy. Suggest trying out creams on normal skin for a few days before applying to eczematous skin. If the normal skin does not react, allergy is unlikely. Refer for patch testing if you suspect allergy.
- The approach to management is discussed on p.560.

Further reading

Werfel T. *J Invest Dermatol* 2009; **129:**1878–91.

Cork MJ *et al. J Invest Dermatol* 2009; **129:**1892–908.

Box 31.13 Pathogenesis of atopic eczema

- Genetic and environmental factors interact.
- Atopic diseases are common in the family of affected individuals. Risk is more closely related to inheritance of maternal than paternal genes.
- No single atopic gene has been identified but potential loci have been mapped to chromosomes 1q, 3q, 3p, 17q, and 20p amongst others.
- Defective barrier function and innate immunity seem likely to play a role in pathogenesis. Loss of function variants in the gene encoding the epidermal barrier protein, fillagrin, predispose to atopic eczema. A defective stratum corneum may allow pathogens/allergens to penetrate the skin and trigger a hyperactive immune response with activation of T-lymphocytes, dendritic cells, macrophages, keratinocytes, mast cells, and eosinophils. Pro-inflammatory cytokines and chemokines may perpetuate disease.
- *Staphylococcus aureus* enterotoxins with superantigenic activity may play some part by activating T-cells and macrophages.

Box 31.14 UK criteria for diagnosis of atopic eczema

A child with an itchy skin condition in last 12 months plus 3 or more of the following:

- Visible flexural dermatitis involving the skin creases, such as the bends of the elbows or behind the knees (or visible dermatitis on the cheeks and/or extensor areas in children aged <4 years).
- History of flexural dermatitis.
- History of dry skin.
- Personal history of asthma or allergic rhinitis (or history of atopic disease in a first-degree relative if child aged <4 years).
- Onset before age of 2 years (not used in children <4 years of age).

Reference: www.nottingham.ac.uk/dermatology/eczema/index.html (includes excellent pictures).

Box 31.15 Food allergy

Most children with mild eczema do not need investigation for food allergies.

Consider food allergy in children with atopic eczema who have reacted previously to a food with immediate symptoms (e.g. urticaria, wheeze, angio-oedema), or in infants and young children with moderate or severe atopic eczema that has not been controlled by optimum management, particularly if associated with gut dysmotility (colic, vomiting, altered bowel habit) or failure to thrive. Refer to a paediatric allergist.

Most children will grow out of food allergies except allergy to nuts. Food allergy is very unlikely to play any part in the pathogenesis of atopic eczema in adults.

Atopic eczema: management

Step 1: the explanation (this will be time well spent)

- Discuss the cause, particularly the abnormal skin barrier.
- Provide written information about eczema and support groups.
- Explain that treatment can control but not cure eczema.
- Reassure parents that most children improve as they grow older.
- Explain that eczema will fluctuate and can be frustrating to treat.
- Discuss how to recognize flares of eczema and skin infections.
- Answer questions about food allergy—investigation is not indicated in most children with mild to moderate atopic eczema—see 🕮 Box 31.15, p.559.
- Involve a dermatology nurse to provide education and support.

Step 2: emollients and soap substitutes

- Emollients are the cornerstone of management and should be used all over the body, even when eczema has cleared. Give the patient a range of unperfumed emollients to try. The best emollient is the one the patient likes. Creamy emollients, rather than ointments, may be preferred for daytime use. Prescribe emollients in large quantities (>500g/week) to be used liberally and frequently—see 🕮 p.570.
- Eliminate irritants such as soap; use an emollient as a soap substitute.
- Reduce bacterial colonization with antibacterial emollients e.g. products containing benzalkonium chloride and/or chlorhexidine.

Step 3: topical corticosteroids and other treatments

- Discuss the use of topical corticosteroids and reassure that these are safe if used as prescribed. Explain how to step up and step down the strength of treatment. Steroid phobia and under-use are common.
- Show how to measure the application in fingertip units—see 🕮 Box 33.2, p.587.
- Explain that topical corticosteroids, unlike emollients, should only be applied to eczematous skin. Apply 20–30min after emollient.
- Most infantile atopic eczema can be controlled with mild to moderate corticosteroid ointments used once or twice daily. Ointments are preferable to creams as they are less likely to irritate the skin. Mild corticosteroid ointments can be used safely on the face.
- Potent corticosteroids may be needed for 7–14 days in children or for longer in adults. Very potent corticosteroid ointments should not be prescribed without the guidance of a specialist.
- Wraps or paste bandages can help children with very itchy skin—see 🕮 Box 33.4, p.593 and p.590.
- A topical calcineurin inhibitor (pimecrolimus, tacrolimus) may be indicated if eczema is not controlled with topical corticosteroids.
- Treat secondary bacterial infection with antibiotics.
- Treatments such as UVB, PUVA, azathioprine, or ciclosporin may be indicated in severe chronic atopic eczema.
- Prednisolone should be avoided except for acute severe flares.

Step 4: general measures for itch

- Minimize itching by using cool cotton clothing and keeping the bedroom cool.
- A sedating antihistamine may be helpful at night.

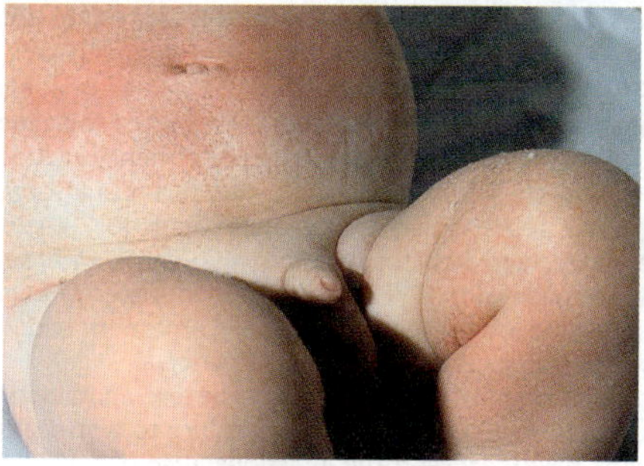

Fig. 31.7 Atopic eczema typically spares the napkin area.

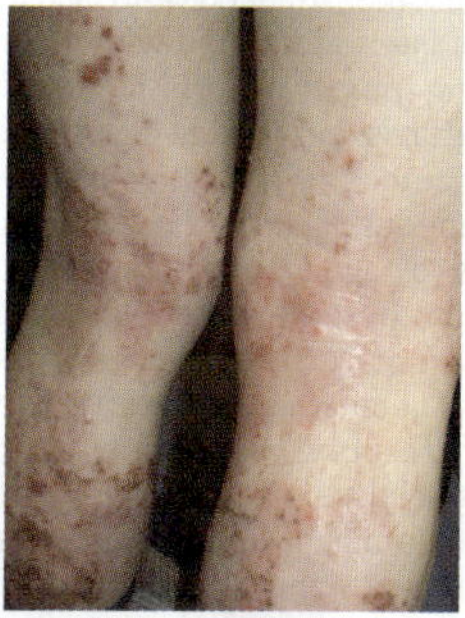

Fig. 31.8 Atopic eczema with secondary bacterial infection causing crusting and weeping.

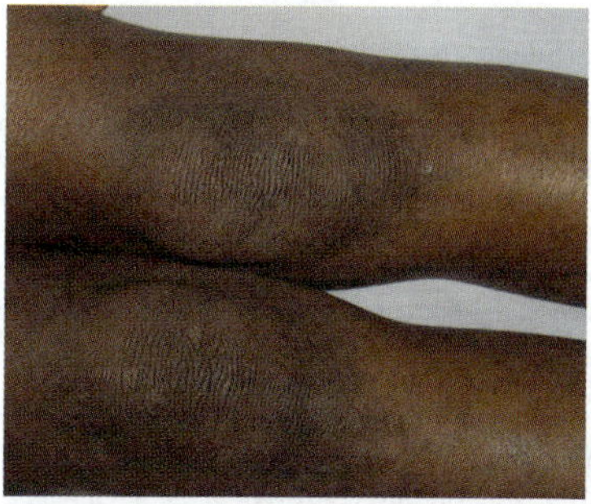

Fig. 31.9 Lichenification with increased skin markings secondary to chronic rubbing.

Further reading

Management of atopic eczema in children. NICE clinical guideline, December 2007. Available at: http://www.nice.org.uk/CG57

Cutaneous signs in rare syndromes

Immunodeficiency syndromes

⚠ Cutaneous signs may provide a valuable early clue to the diagnosis of these rare syndromes. Problems suggesting immunodeficiency include recurrent, prolonged, or severe infections, infections with unusual organisms, and infections poorly responsive to antibiotics. Look for failure to thrive, chronic diarrhoea, and hepatosplenomegaly. Infants with severe T-cell immunodeficiency develop GVHD secondary to maternal engraftment at or around the time of delivery and may become erythrodermic. These patients also have an increased risk of malignancy.

- Omenn's syndrome: autosomal recessive. Severe combined immunodeficiency. Generalized eczema, failure to thrive, alopecia, eosinophilia, diarrhoea, repeated infections. Also hepatosplenomegaly and lymphadenopathy.
- Wiskott–Aldrich syndrome: X-linked disorder. Severe atopic eczema in first few months of life is associated with recurrent pyogenic infections and bleeding (petechiae, bruising) due to thrombocytopenia. May present with epistaxis and bloody diarrhoea.
- Ataxia telangiectasia: autosomal recessive disorder. Ataxia noticed in infancy. Oculocutaneous signs develop from age 3, conjunctival bulbar telangiectasias (by age 6), and cutaneous telangiectasias (ears, eyelids, malar, anterior chest, flexures). Also premature ageing of skin (loss of fat), café-au-lait macules, hypertrichosis, chronic seborrhoeic dermatitis, and painful cutaneous granulomas (non-infectious). May have sinopulmonary infections, growth retardation, mental retardation, and endocrine abnormalities.
- Hyper IgE: autosomal dominant disorder. Includes Job's syndrome. Recurrent severe cutaneous and sinopulmonary infections in association with papulopustular dermatitis in first few months of life. 'Cold' abscesses with limited erythema. Also repeated fractures and retained primary teeth. Elevated IgE levels (>2000IU/L) and eosinophilia.
- Chronic mucocutaneous candidiasis. Most do not have positive family history. Progressive *Candida* infections of skin, nails, and mucous membranes. May be associated with polyglandular autoimmune syndrome type 1 (autoimmune polyendocrinopathy–candidiasis–ectodermal dystrophy=APECED)—see p.450.
- Chronic granulomatous disease: X-linked or autosomal recessive. Chronic staphylococcal infections of skin, suppurative lymphadenitis, bronchopneumonia, hepatosplenomegaly, chronic diarrhoea, and malabsorption.
- Chediak–Higashi syndrome: autosomal recessive. Silvery sheen to hair, partial albinism (strabismus and nystagmus), photophobia, hyperpigmented exposed skin, severe recurrent infections, and progressive neurological deterioration.

Multiple lentigines

What is a lentigo? (plural: lentigines or lentigos)

Lentigines are small (1–3mm diameter), well circumscribed, flat, brown to black 'freckles' that may appear on any body site. Lentigines do not fade when skin is no longer exposed to sun and are not necessarily triggered by sun exposure.

Some normal individuals have numerous lentigines but in a child with numerous 'freckles' you should consider:

- Xeroderma pigmentosum: premature sun damage with many lentigines mainly on sun-exposed skin. High risk of early onset skin cancers, including malignant melanoma—see 🕮 p.314.
- Peutz–Jegher's syndrome: freckling on vermillion borders of lips, oral mucosa, perioral, perianal, and periorbital skin, over joints, and on palms and soles—see 🕮 p.501.
- LEOPARD syndrome: **L**entigines (hundreds of freckle-like spots all over skin), **E**lectrocardiographic cardiac conduction defects, **O**cular telorism, **P**ulmonary stenosis, **A**bnormalities of genitalia, **R**etardation of growth, **D**eafness.
- Carney complex (includes NAME and LAMB syndromes): mucocutaneous pigmentation (lentigines on lips, conjunctiva, inner or outer canthi, vaginal and penile mucosa, blue naevi. May have small café au lait spots that tend to fade with age), myxomas (cardiac, cutaneous—eyelid, external ear, nipple), breast myxomatosis or ductal adenoma, endocrine tumours (primary pigmented nodular adrenocortical disease, pituitary adenoma, testicular neoplasms, thyroid adenoma or carcinoma, ovarian cysts), psammomatous melanotic schwannoma, osteochondromyxoma.
- Neurofibromatosis 1: freckling in skin folds—see 🕮 p.508.
- Segmental neurofibromatosis 1: unilateral lentigines in axilla or groin—see 🕮 p.510.

This list is not exhaustive and other rare syndromes are associated with multiple lentigines, either in a generalized or localized distribution.

Physical and sexual abuse

Sadly some children are abused and it is important to recognize cutaneous signs that may indicate abuse—but it is equally important to realize that some dermatoses can be confused with abuse. Record all signs and refer urgently to a paediatrician with expertise in this area if you suspect abuse. The welfare of the child should be your primary concern.

What should I look for?

- Carer has delayed seeking medical help.
- Inconsistent history, incompatible with the injury or signs.
- Parental hostility or lack of interest.
- Sad, withdrawn, or frightened child.
- A child displaying frequent sexualized behaviour.
- Physical abuse—the upper head and body are frequently targeted in cases of deliberate physical injury. Look for:
  - Many bruises of different ages, often in clusters.
  - Pinch marks on the ear or petechiae on the pinna.
  - Linear slap marks, belt marks, finger impressions, or buckle marks.
  - Cigarette burns to face or hands or burns to lower limbs (child held forcibly in scalding water).
- Sexual abuse:
  - Pregnancy.
  - HIV infection or another sexually transmitted disease in absence of perinatal acquisition. Anogenital warts in children may be acquired by autoinnoculation, but the possibility of sexual abuse should be considered, particularly in children <2 years.
  - Signs of acute penetrating anogenital trauma including acute hymenal injury, laceration, bruising, or perianal lacerations.
  - Genital abrasions, lacerations, bites, suction marks, or burns.

Dermatological conditions that may simulate abuse

- Mongolian spots may simulate bruises—see 🕮 p.322 and Fig. 31.10, p.565.
- Bullous impetigo may simulate cigarette burns—see 🕮 Fig. 6.1, p.122.
- SSSS, as the name suggests, can simulate scalds—see 🕮 Fig. 6.2, p.123.
- Phytophotodermatitis with blistering in linear streaks may simulate burns or the residual pigmented streaks may simulate linear bruising—see 🕮 Fig. 31.11 and Box 16.5, p. 305.
- Angio-oedema with swelling of the face or lips may simulate an early bruise—see 🕮 p.98.
- Cutaneous vasculitis with purpura may simulate bruises—see 🕮 p.408.
- Group A streptococcal perineal infection with itch, pain, erythema, discharge, and localized bleeding may suggest sexual abuse—see 🕮 p.124.
- Lichen sclerosus with haemorrhage may suggest sexual abuse—see 🕮 p.268.
- EB (rare) with skin fragility and blistering may suggest physical injury—see 🕮 p.244.

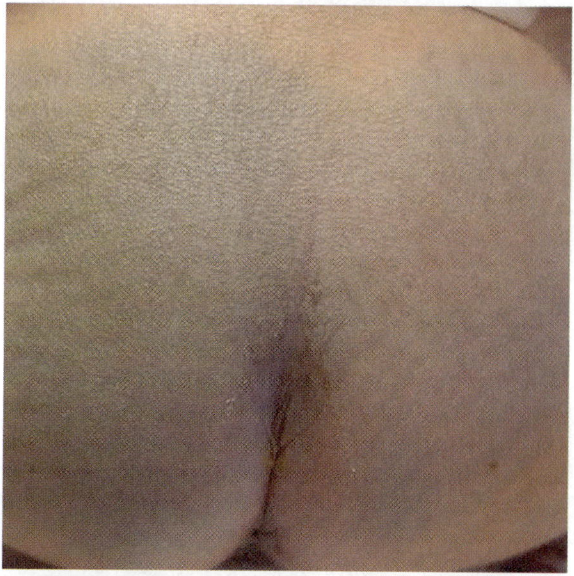

Fig. 31.10 Mongolian spot.

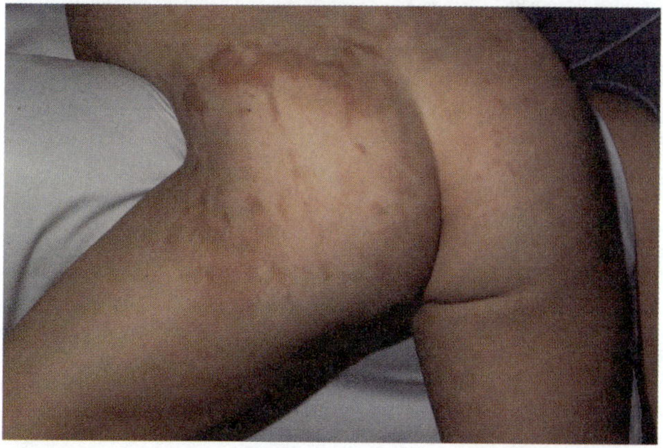

Fig. 31.11 Phytophotodermatitis. Linear pigmentation was preceded by streaky erythema and blisters where the sun-exposed skin had been in contact with the juice of a plant that contained psoralen.

Chapter 32

Special tools and investigations

Contents

Tools in the clinic

Dermoscopy

Synonyms: dermatoscopy, epiluminescence microscopy, skin surface microscopy.

- The dermoscope is a hand-held instrument with a bright halogen beam that illuminates and magnifies (10×) intra- and some subepidermal structures, including the superficial vascular plexus.
  A smear of alcohol, water, or mineral oil on the surface of the lesion eliminates surface reflection and makes the horny layer translucent.
- Dermoscopy was developed as a non-invasive aid for assessing melanocytic skin tumours *in vivo*. Certain features in the pigment network correlate with malignancy.
- The appearance under a dermoscope may also help in the diagnosis of some non-pigmented skin tumours such as haemangiomas or BCCs.
- Dermoscopy has an increasing role in medical dermatology. For example, the extra magnification has been advocated to visualize nail fold capillaries in patients with possible vasculitis or a connective tissue disorder (see 🕮 Box 19.19, p.385), find the mites in suspected scabies (see 🕮 Box 8.2, p.165), and assess the cause of alopecia (see 🕮 p.454).
- Dermoscopy may also be used to screen hair shafts for abnormalities in conditions such as Netherton's syndrome (see 🕮 Box 31.10, p.555).

See http://www.dermoscopy.co.uk for more information.

Wood's light (black light)

- The light emits UV radiation in the long-wave UVA region.
- Hypopigmentation is more obvious under Wood's light and examination may be particularly helpful in assessing a child with possible tuberous sclerosis for the presence of hypopigmented macules—see 🕮 Box 27.6, p.513.
- Depigmented skin, e.g. vitiligo, fluoresces a bright ivory-white unlike hypopigmented skin which just looks pale.
- Epidermal hyperpigmentation is accentuated by Wood's light, but pigment that is mainly in the dermis is not accentuated—see 🕮 Box 30.1, p.539.
- Some cutaneous infections fluoresce:
  - Tinea capitis caused by *Microsporum audouini* or *Microsporum canis*: light bright green fluorescence
  - Pityriasis versicolor: yellow fluorescence
  - Erythrasma: coral pink fluorescence
  - *Pseudomonas*: green fluorescence
- Urine containing porphyrins fluoresces pink—see 🕮 p.308.

Diascopy

A diascope is a flat glass plate (most often a microscope slide) through which one examines superficial skin lesions after applying gentle pressure to reduce or remove erythema.

- Diascopy distinguishes between inflammatory and haemorrhagic lesions. A glass slide pressed down on the skin will blanch the erythema of an inflammatory lesion or the redness of a vascular tumour. Bleeding into the skin (petechiae or purpura) does not blanch.
- Diascopy is recommended for assessing the reddish-brown granulomatous lesions in sarcoid (see 🕮 p.486) or cutaneous TB (see 🕮 p.136). Gentle pressure enhances the yellow-brown 'apple jelly' colour of the dermal nodules by removing the background erythema.
- Diascopy will also differentiate a naevus anaemicus (where vasoconstriction gives the skin a pale colour—see 🕮 p.520) from a patch of hypopigmented or depigmented skin, e.g. vitiligo. A naevus anaemicus is no longer detectable when a glass slide is pressed down gently onto the skin. The naevus anaemicus merges into the normal surrounding skin which is blanched by gentle pressure. Hypopigmented or depigmented skin is still detectable.

Testing for allergy

What is patch testing?

- Dermatitis may be caused by delayed (type IV) hypersensitivity and this type of allergy is detected by patch testing.
- Hypersensitivity is confirmed by development of allergic contact dermatitis under a patch containing the allergen to which the individual is sensitized. The reaction develops gradually over several days.
- The screening battery of patch tests contains standardized dilutions of allergens such as rubber allergens, neomycin and other medicaments, fragrance allergens, lanolin, and nickel (a very common allergen).
- Patch tests are generally put onto the skin of the back (day 0) and are usually read on day 2 and again on day 4.
- Photopatch testing may be required in suspected photoallergic dermatitis. 2 identical batteries of allergens are applied to the skin, but 1 side is irradiated with UVA after 24–48h.
- It takes expertise to select the correct allergens for testing and to read the tests, but especially to determine the significance of the results.

Who should I refer for patch testing?

- Patients with persistent eczematous eruptions, particularly long-standing facial dermatitis, hand dermatitis, or perianal pruritus.
- Patients with chronic leg ulcers who may become sensitized to the constituents of dressings, bandages, or topical medicaments.

What is skin prick testing?

- Skin prick testing detects immediate (type I) hypersensitivity.
- Patients should stop taking anti-histamines 48h before the test.
- Drops of allergens in standardized dilutions are placed on marked areas on the forearm and gentle intradermal punctures are made through each drop with separate sterile fine needles. Positive and negative controls are performed with histamine and saline respectively.
- Type I hypersensitivity is manifested by an urticarial wheal of 4mm or more that is usually apparent after 10–15min.
- The risk of anaphylaxis is a small, but tests should only be carried out by an experienced individual with facilities for resuscitation.
- Specific IgE quantification is an alternative investigation—see Box 32.1.

Who should I refer for skin prick testing?

- Prick testing is used in the investigation of some patients with acute urticarial reactions, but the relevance of positive results may be difficult to interpret—see 🕮 p.217.
- Prick testing is not indicated in most patients with dermatitis, apart from those with hand dermatitis, who may have a type I hypersensitivity to natural rubber latex in addition to delayed (type 4) hypersensitivity to natural rubber latex or rubber additives.

Box 32.1 What is specific IgE quantification?

- The test is used to measure total and specific IgE levels to inhaled and ingested antigens.
- The test is performed on a blood specimen, so, unlike skin prick tests, does not present a risk of anaphylaxis.
- Specific IgE quantification may be indicated in patients with suspected food allergies, e.g. immediate reactions such as urticaria, lip swelling, or wheeze.
- Like skin prick tests, the significance of positive results may be difficult to interpret, particularly in atopic individuals who tend to have multiple type 1 reactions.

Specimens for bacterial or viral culture

Surface swabs will identify harmless resident surface microbial species, e.g. coagulase-negative staphylococci such as *Staphylococcus epidermidis*, micrococcus species, and some subsurface organisms, as well as pathogenic organisms, e.g. *Staphylococcus aureus* or group A beta-haemolytic streptococci. Inevitably you only sample a small area of skin.

How to take a skin swab for bacterial culture

- Whenever possible take your sample from pus, exudates, eroded skin or tissue (see Box 32.2) rather than from the surface of intact skin.
- In individuals with recurrent skin infections, you may also wish to sample uninvolved skin, nose, axillae, and groins.
- To maximize pick up from dry areas, first moisten the head of the swab with sterile saline or sterile water.
- Apply reasonably firm pressure to the skin with the swab.
- Put the swab into transport medium designed for bacterial culture.
- Label your sample and complete the labelled request form. Provide clinical details and, if necessary, ask for the culture of specific organisms, e.g. anaerobes.

Surface swabs in chronic leg ulcers

Any chronic cutaneous ulcer will be colonized by large numbers of organisms. In most cases 'routine swabs for culture' are unhelpful. The role of bacteria in delaying healing or causing pain is controversial, but surface culture may be indicated in specific situations:

- Heavy malodorous exudate.
- Painful ulcer.
- Non-healing ulcer.
- Cellulitis (even in this situation, surface swabs may not be very informative).

How to take a skin swab for viral culture

In general you will be trying to prove if the patient has cutaneous infection with HSV or VZV.

- Please check that you have the right culture medium before you start (usually a small bottle of pink fluid that should be kept in a fridge in the ward or outpatient department). The commonest mistake is to put the swab into transport medium designed for bacteria.
- Put on sterile gloves.
- Look for a fresh vesicle and gently de-roof with a scalpel. Try to retain some of the roof on the scalpel blade and wipe this onto your swab.
- Collect a sample of the fluid on the swab and rub the swab firmly across the base of the vesicle.
- Place the swab in the viral culture medium.
- Alternatively you can aspirate some fluid using a needle and syringe. Put the fluid directly into the viral culture medium.
- Label your sample, complete the request form and provide clinical details. PCR can usually provide a rapid result.

Box 32.2 Culture of a skin biopsy

Culture of tissue is more informative than surface swabs when dealing with deep cutaneous infections. Consider the need to exclude infection and obtain suitable culture media (or sterile saline) before you start the biopsy, particularly if dealing with immunosuppressed patients. It may be helpful to obtain advice about suitable media from a microbiologist.

Send a sample for histological examination as well as sending tissue for culture in these situations:

- ⚠ Any persistent undiagnosed skin lesion (nodule, plaque, blister, ulcer) in an immunosuppressed patient.
- Pyoderma gangrenosum.
- Granulomatous inflammation to exclude deep fungal infection or mycobacterial infection (TB, atypical mycobacteria).
- Chronic non-healing ulcers, particularly in immunosuppressed patients. Virology (herpes simplex) is as important as bacteriology in this situation.

Skin scrapes and smears

Superficial fungal infections

Skin scrapes or brushings in scaly rashes

- Use a glass slide or a No. 15 scalpel blade and gently scrape the active scaly edge rather than the centre of the lesion. You are just trying to scrape off scale, not to draw blood.
- Scrape onto dark paper so you can see the sample and also scrape some scale onto a glass slide so you can inspect this for hyphae yourself—see later in this section.
- Fold up and seal the paper containing your sample—no transport medium is required. Label the specimen and complete the request form providing clinical details.
- In suspected tinea capitis, pluck hair and brush scale off scalp with a disposable (unpasted!) toothbrush. The toothbrush in its container can be sent directly to the laboratory.
- Microscopy (see later in this section) will provide a rapid result but it will probably take 4–6 weeks for results of culture.

Sampling dystrophic toenails

- Nails infected by fungus are discoloured, thickened, and fragile.
- Clip off samples of the crumbling nail using nail clippers and also scoop out some of the soft debris beneath the nail.
- Transport the samples in paper just as you do for skin scrapes.
- In superficial white onychomycosis, scrape a sample from the discoloured surface of the nail.

Microscopy in clinic

Scrapes or nail clippings may be examined for hyphae using light microscopy after dissolving scales, hairs, or nails in potassium hydroxide.

- Place the scrapings, hair, or nail clippings onto a glass slide and cover with a coverslip.
- Drop a few drops of a solution of 20% KOH with 40% DMSO in distilled water on to the slide and allow it to spread under the coverslip. (No heat is needed if DMSO is included.)
- Leave the sample in suspension for a few minutes (nails are thicker than skin or hair and should be left for a couple of hours).
- Examine for branching fungal hyphae running across the sheets of keratinocytes using a low power (×25) objective lens with the iris diaphragm closed down and the condenser lowered to increase contrast.

Deep fungal infection

- You will need to take a skin biopsy and culture tissue—see 📖 Box 32.2, p.573.

Tzank preparation (smear for cytology)

Cytology may be helpful in blistering rashes, particularly if you suspect infection with HSV or VZV. If you are experienced, you can get a preliminary result in the outpatient room. Tzank preparations (cytological smears) are used infrequently in the UK.

How to make a Tzank preparation

- You will need a glass slide and a No. 10 or 15 scalpel blade.
- Put on sterile gloves.
- De-roof a fresh blister and gently scrape the base (you only need tissue fluid and keratinocytes—try not to contaminate the smear with blood). Smear the contents of your blade onto a glass slide.
- Air dry, fix with methanol, and stain with Giemsa, toluidine blue, or Wright's stain.
- Examine under a light microscope ×40.
- HSV or VZV infection: multinucleated giant keratinocytes confirm the diagnosis, but laboratory tests such as PCR are a more accurate diagnostic tool and have supplanted Tzank preparations.
- Tzank preparations may be a help to differentiate subepidermal from intraepidermal blistering in autoimmune blistering diseases such as bullous pemphigoid (subepidermal, no keratinocytes in Tzank preparation) or pemphigus vulgaris (intraepidermal, acantholytic rounded-up keratinocytes in Tzank preparation). The gold standard is histology with immunofluorescence studies—see 📖 Box 13.3, p.247.
- Tzank preparations have been advocated to differentiate SSSS from TEN. The presence of keratinocytes in the smear suggests SSSS (the blister is in the granular layer and some intact epidermis is retained in the floor of the blister). In TEN, the blister is subepidermal so there are no keratinocytes on the floor of the blister and a Tzank preparation from the base of the blister will not have any keratinocytes. The preparation must be made from freshly denuded dermis, because once the epidermis starts to regenerate, keratinocytes will be found in the smear. In practice, it is not usually difficult to differentiate the diseases particularly if the patient has mucosal involvement (a feature of TEN not SSSS)—see 📖 p.106, p.110.

Skin biopsy in inflammatory conditions

Taking a skin biopsy is not technically difficult, but it may be more challenging to provide the pathologist with a differential diagnosis, to know what sort of biopsy to take, and to chose the right site for the biopsy.

What sort of biopsy

- Pathologists prefer elliptical biopsies—see Box 32.3—because they provide more tissue than a punch biopsy—see Box 32.4—but a deep (uncrushed) 4mm punch biopsy is adequate in some situations.
- Take an elliptical biopsy in panniculitis, when you need to examine fat lobules. The fat often shears off in punch biopsies.
- Punch biopsies are particularly suitable for investigating alopecia (ensure you insert the punch deeply along the length of the hair follicle) and in the investigation of blistering diseases—see 📖 Box 13.3, p.247.

Where to take the biopsy

- Generally choose a well-developed primary lesion, avoiding secondary changes such as excoriations. If the rash has a variety of morphologies, you may wish to take several biopsies.
- Try to avoid taking biopsies from the leg (poor healing) or the cape area, i.e. shoulders, upper back, and central chest (risk of keloid).
- If taking a biopsy from the face, use wrinkles to disguise the scar. Scars are particularly easy to hide in sun-damaged wrinkled skin. Ask the patient to screw up his/her face to help you to decide on the direction of the incisional biopsy or position of the punch biopsy.
- In blistering diseases, take the biopsy from a small early intact blister. If you select a large blister, the roof of the specimen may be lost during processing. In old blisters, re-epithelialization at the base of subepidermal blisters can mimic intraepidermal blisters.
- If you suspect a condition such as cutaneous T-cell lymphoma it is worth taking >1 biopsy. Be prepared to repeat the biopsies on several occasions over a number of years before your clinical suspicions are confirmed.

Working with the pathologist

- You are not setting a mind-reading exercise for your pathology colleague! You had the advantage of seeing the patient, so describe the rash on the request form and tell the pathologist what diagnoses you are considering, what sort of lesion you have biopsied (fresh, well developed, blister, papule, etc.), and from where the biopsy was taken.
- Become familiar with the terms commonly used to describe pathological changes in the skin—see 📖 p.578.
- Histopathology, like all of medicine, is an art as well as a science. If you think that the diagnosis provided by the pathologist does not fit the clinical findings, you both need to think again. Ideally you should sit down with the pathologist to review the skin biopsies alongside the clinical photographs. You will learn a lot by discussing the case.

Box 32.3 Elliptical biopsy: how to do it

- The biopsy should either remove an entire lesion or extend from normal skin into the centre of the lesion. The longitudinal axis of the incision should run parallel to wrinkle lines (face) or Langer's lines (trunk, limbs—see 📖 p.8) and measure at least 1cm in length.
- Mark out an elongated diamond shape with a sterile skin marker prior to infiltration of local anaesthetic.
- Clean skin and infiltrate local anaesthetic (see Box 32.4).
- Incise vertically down into subcutaneous tissue using a No. 15 scalpel blade. Lift up the specimen at a corner and peel back cutting the base with the scalpel. Do not crush the specimen.
- Close with interrupted or intradermal sutures.

Box 32.4 Punch biopsy: how to do it

- Mark the biopsy site.
- In children, 2.5% lidocaine plus 2.5% prilocaine cream (EMLA®) applied under occlusion for 40–60min reduces the pain of infiltration.
  - Infants <3 months: maximum dose = 1g.
  - Infants >3 months: maximum dose = 2g.
- Consider restraining infants by wrapping firmly in a sheet.
- 1% lidocaine with adrenaline 1 in 200 000 is suitable for most sites (avoid in digits). Warm local anaesthetic to body temperature prior to infiltration and infiltrate slowly to minimize discomfort.
- Local anaesthetic in infants:
  - 1% lidocaine without adrenaline: up to 3mg/kg (maximum for a 5kg infant = 1.5mL).
  - 1% lidocaine with adrenaline 1 in 200 000: up to 5mg/kg (maximum for a 5kg infant = 2.5mL).
- Allow 20–30min for the anaesthetic and adrenaline to act before taking the biopsy. Go away and do something else.
- Do not attempt to check if the skin is numb by jabbing with a needle. Instead ask an adult patient to tell you if the procedure is uncomfortable.
- Stabilize the skin. Insert the punch slowly down into fat, watching the patient's face. (The expression will soon tell you if it is painful.)
- Minimal pressure is needed, particularly in children or elderly people with thin skin. Disposable punches are very sharp.
- Depress the skin firmly on each side of the wound so the specimen pops up and lift it out on the tip of your scissors—you may need to cut the base with a sharp pair of scissors. Do not damage the specimen by crushing it with forceps or spearing it with a needle!
- Usually sutures are not required if you have used adrenaline. Haemostasis can be obtained using topical 20% aluminium chloride or a piece of calcium alginate dressing in the wound and pressure.

What does the pathologist mean?

Epidermis

- ***Acanthosis:*** thickening of the epidermis.
- ***Papillomatosis:*** projections of the dermal papillae and the overlying epidermis above the surface of the surrounding skin.
- ***Hyperkeratosis:*** increased thickness of the stratum corneum.
- ***Dyskeratosis:*** abnormal keratinization of keratinocytes.
- ***Parakeratosis:*** flattened nuclei retained within the stratum corneum. Linked to hyperproliferation and altered differentiation, e.g. psoriasis.
- ***Scale crust:*** a mix of serum, variable numbers of inflammatory cells, and parakeratotic cells in the stratum corneum.
- ***Spongiosis:*** intercellular oedema causes widening of spaces between keratinocytes. The adhesion junctions between keratinocytes rupture and vesicles form in the epidermis. Common in eczema.
- ***Acantholysis:*** loss of cohesion between keratinocytes. The individual keratinocytes round up and separate from each other. For example in the autoimmune blistering disease, pemphigus.
- ***Ballooning degeneration:*** swelling and vacuolization of keratinocytes is followed by acantholysis (see earlier). Common in cutaneous herpes simplex and VZV infections.
- ***Necrosis:*** cell death resulting from acute cellular injury, e.g. ischaemia.
- ***Apoptosis:*** programmed cell death. Excess apoptosis causes atrophy; insufficient apoptosis is linked to uncontrolled cell proliferation.
- ***Colloid or Civatte body:*** an eosinophilic round body in the basal layer of the epidermis or in the upper papillary dermis. The end result of apoptosis of a keratinocyte. Seen in lichenoid reactions—see below.
- ***Epidermotropism:*** lymphocytes in the lower layers of the epidermis.
- ***Vesicle:*** fluid-filled cavity either within or just below the epidermis.

Dermis

- ***Lichenoid reaction or interface dermatitis:*** a band-like infiltrate of inflammatory cells in the papillary dermis which is often associated with basal keratinocyte apoptosis—see earlier in this section—and pigment incontinence—see next in this section.
- ***Pigment incontinence:*** melanin released from basal keratinocytes is deposited in the upper dermis. The pigment may be found within macrophages (melanophages) or free in the dermis. Pigment incontinence is a sign of damage to the basal layer of the epidermis.
- ***Fibrinoid necrosis:*** extravasation of fibrin into the wall of a blood vessel or its immediate surroundings. A feature of cutaneous vasculitis.
- ***Leucocytoclasis:*** disintegration of white blood cells, usually neutrophils, with small dark staining nuclear fragments in the dermis (nuclear dust). Associated with activation of neutrophils in conditions such as such as small-vessel cutaneous vasculitis (leucocytoclastic vasculitis), neutrophilic dermatoses, or dermatitis herpetiformis.
- ***Granulomatous inflammation:*** see Box 32.5.
- ***Necrobiosis:*** indistinct appearance of collagen fibres associated with accumulation of mucopolysaccharides. (The term necrobiosis is also used to mean death of cells.)

Box 32.5 Granulomatous inflammation

Chronic dermal inflammation in which collections of histiocytes are organized into relatively discrete granulomas, sometimes in the presence of multinucleate giant cells. The pattern of inflammation and the presence of features such as necrobiosis or suppuration will provide clues to the underlying diagnosis. The pathologist will use polarized light to detect birefringent foreign material and will perform special stains for organisms. You should consider sending material for culture.

Types of granuloma include:

- ***Sarcoidal granuloma*** (few lymphocytes, 'naked' granuloma). Consider sarcoidosis and some types of foreign body reaction (silica, tattoo pigments, zirconium, and beryllium).
- ***Tuberculoid granuloma*** (granulomas surrounded by a cuff of lymphocytes): think of TB, leprosy, leishmaniasis, or cutaneous Crohn's disease.
- ***Necrobiotic granuloma*** (altered collagen surrounded by histiocytes and sometimes multinucleated giant cells). Consider rheumatoid nodule, granuloma annulare, or necrobiosis lipoidica.
- ***Suppurative granuloma*** (neutrophils in the centre of the granuloma). Think of *Mycobacterium marinum* and deep fungal infections.
- ***Foreign body granuloma*** (a granuloma forms around the foreign body material). Localized granulomatous inflammation may be triggered by exogenous foreign bodies or endogenous material such as a ruptured hair follicle or cyst.

Chapter 33

Medical management

Contents

We cannot provide more than a brief introduction to the principles of treatment. Patient information leaflets about most of the topical and systemic treatments mentioned here can be downloaded from the website of the British Association of Dermatologists (http://www.bad.org.uk). This information may also help carers, including ward nurses unfamiliar with managing skin problems.

Relevant pages in other chapters

Management of leg ulcers p.286
Photoprotection p.316
Management of atopic eczema in children p.560

General principles of topical treatment

Undertreatment is more common than overuse of topical medicaments. Patients (and ward nurses) are most likely to adhere to simple treatment plans that have been negotiated and explained. Provide a written treatment plan if you can, in addition to the prescription.

What to tell the patient and/or carer

- Explore anxieties and reassure (steroid phobia is common).
- Explain how often to apply the treatment and when to apply the treatment—particularly if using >1 medicament. Should both be applied at once or should applications be separated?
- Ensure that the patient understands what to use where (provide a written treatment plan).
- Explain how much to use and demonstrate how to use the treatment.
- Explain the adverse effects and how these may be minimized.
- Discuss the expected outcome of treatment—when might something happen and how much improvement is likely?
- Explain how long to continue treatment.
- Ensure the patient knows how and when to step up or step down the strength of treatment (if this is an option).

The prescription

- Specify the base (ointment, cream, gel, lotion, foam) and quantity—see 📖 Box 33.1.
- Prescribe tubs (500g) not tubes (25–30g) of emollient.
- Specify the site and frequency of application. You may need to provide >1 strength or type of treatment for different body sites.
- The potency of a topical corticosteroid preparation is dependent on the formulation as well as the corticosteroid, so it is acceptable to prescribe using proprietary names rather than the generic names of steroid molecules. This will also ensure that you know exactly what else is in the preparation including the vehicle and preservatives—important in patients with allergies.
- Inpatients: if the patient needs regular applications of an emollient or a topical corticosteroid, please do not write the prescription on the 'when necessary' (prn) part of the drug chart. Ensure that the nurses understand the importance of the topical treatment and that someone helps the patient to apply the treatment as prescribed (most often ×2/day but emollients may be required ×3 or 4/day).

Box 33.1 Quantities required in adults for a single daily application for 2 weeks

• Face and neck:	15–30g
• Both hands:	15–30g
• Scalp:	15–30g
• Both arms:	30–60g
• Both legs:	100g
• Trunk:	100g
• Groins and genitalia:	15–30g

Moisturizers and soap substitutes

Indications: dry flaky itchy skin, e.g. eczema, psoriasis.

Emollients (moisturizers)

- Emollients soothe dry itchy skin, but effects are short-lived so apply frequently and liberally to all the skin.
- Best applied after a shower or bath when the skin is moist.
- The best emollient is the one the patient likes! Offer a selection.
- Preparations
  - Light creams (e.g., Dermol® cream, Cetraben® cream, Diprobase® cream, Doublebase®) or lotions (Dermol 500®).
  - The Dermol® products contain benzalkonium chloride and may be useful if secondary infection is a problem, e.g. in atopic eczema.
  - Greasy preparations (e.g. Hydromol® ointment, Epaderm® ointment, emulsifying ointment, 50% WSP in liquid paraffin, Emollin® or Dermamist® spray).
- Adverse effects:
  - Ointments are less likely to irritate or sensitize skin than creams.
  - Ointments are messy to use and some patients find that greasy preparations make them hot and itchy.
  - Irritants in creams may cause transient burning or erythema.
  - Allergy to emollients is uncommon, but patients occasionally become allergic to excipients in creams such as cetostearyl alcohol, parabens, and sodium metabisulphite or to fragrances.
  - Folliculitis. Smear the emollient onto the skin in the direction of hair growth and allow it to soak into the skin. Advise patients not to rub the emollient into the skin, to minimize irritation or blockage of hair follicles.
  - Fire hazard: emulsifying ointment or 50% liquid paraffin in WSP can be ignited by a naked flame. The risk is greater when these preparations are applied to large areas of the body, and if clothing or dressings are soaked with ointment.

Soap substitutes

- Useful in dry itchy skin conditions.
- Aqueous cream is a better soap substitute than an emollient.
- Hydromol® ointment or Epaderm® ointment are greasy and effective soap substitutes.

Bath additives

- Patients (and carers) like to add oils to the bath. Most contain emollients that help to soothe dry itchy skin, e.g. Balneum® range, Dermol® range, Oilatum® range.
- It is easy to moisturize all the skin with a bath oil.
- Emollient ointments and creams applied directly to the skin are probably more effective than bath additives in patients with very dry skin.
- Bath oils may make the bath very slippery—a problem in the elderly and the very young.

Topical corticosteroids

Indications: inflammatory conditions such as insect bites, acute or chronic eczema, localized psoriasis including flexural and scalp psoriasis. Topical corticosteroids are of no value in the treatment of urticaria.

Potency

Prescribe a corticosteroid strong enough to control the problem and aim to gradually reduce the strength and frequency of application. Absorption is greatest where the skin is thin and in intertriginous areas, e.g. vulva, groins, and axilla. Use a milder corticosteroid in these areas. Avoid potent or very potent corticosteroids on the face except in special circumstances, e.g. acute contact dermatitis, chronic cutaneous LE.

Commonly used topical corticosteroids include:

- Mild:
  - Hydrocortisone 0.5%, 1%, or 2.5%.
  - Hydrocortisone with antibiotic.
  - Hydrocortisone with antifungal (used for inflamed flexural rashes when candidiasis may complicate treatment with a corticosteroid).
- Moderate:
  - Betamethasone valerate cream 0.025%, clobetasone butyrate 0.05%.
  - Moderate with antibacterials and antifungals (clobetasone butyrate 0.05%, oxytetracycline 3% [as calcium salt], nystatin 100 000 units).
- Potent:
  - Betamethasone valerate 0.1%, mometasone furoate 0.1%, hydrocortisone butyrate 0.1%.
  - Potent with antimicrobials.
  - Potent with salicylic acid, e.g. betamethasone 0.05% with salicylic acid 3%.
- Very potent:
  - Clobetasol propionate 0.05%, diflucortolone valerate 0.3%.

How to apply

- No more frequently than twice daily; once daily is often sufficient.
- Spread thinly on the affected skin. One fingertip unit (approximately 500mg) is sufficient to cover an area that is twice that of the flat adult palm—see Box 33.2.
- Apply about 20–30min after (or before) any emollient that has been supplied.
- Undertreatment because of steroid phobia is a common cause of treatment failure. Show the patient how to use the treatment.

See 📖 p.560 for more information about treatment of children.

See 📖 p.588 for adverse effects.

Box 33.2 Rough guide to the amount of topical corticosteroid

1 fingertip unit (FTU) is the amount of cream or ointment squeezed from a standard tube (5mm nozzle) along the palmar surface of the distal phalanx of an adult index finger from the very tip to the crease of the DIP joint.

1FTU weighs approximately 0.5g and will cover a surface area equivalent to the palmar surface of 2 adult hands (including the fingers).

In children the FTU of cream or ointment is measured on an adult index finger before being rubbed onto a child. 1FTU treats an area of skin on a child equivalent to twice the size of the palmar surface of an adult's hand with the fingers together. Estimate the amount of topical steroid to use by using your (adult) hand to determine the area of skin affected on the child.

Tubes usually contain 30g (60FTUs) or 100g (200FTUs). All measurements assume the tube has a standard 5mm nozzle.

3–6-month-old child

- Entire face and neck: 1FTU
- An entire arm and hand: 1FTU
- An entire leg and foot: 1.5FTUs
- The entire front of chest and abdomen: 1FTU
- The entire back including buttocks: 1.5FTUs.

1–2-year-old child

- Entire face and neck: 1.5FTUs
- An entire arm and hand: 1.5FTUs
- An entire leg and foot: 2FTUs
- The entire front of chest and abdomen: 2FTUs
- The entire back including buttocks: 3FTUs.

3–5-year-old child

- Entire face and neck: 1.5FTUs
- An entire arm and hand: 2FTUs
- An entire leg and foot: 3FTUs
- The entire front of chest and abdomen: 3FTUs
- The entire back including buttocks: 3.5FTUs.

Adult

- A hand and fingers (front and back): 1FTU
- A foot (all over): 2FTUs
- Front of chest and abdomen: 7FTUs
- Back and buttocks: 7FTUs
- Face and neck: 2.5FTUs
- An entire arm and hand: 4FTUs
- An entire leg and foot: 8FTUs.
- Entire body about 40FTUs.

Adverse effects of topical corticosteroids

- *Mild* and *moderately potent* topical corticosteroids are associated with few side effects and are safe to use in children and on the thin skin of the face and flexures.
- *Potent* and *very potent* topical steroids—local side effects include:
  - Spread and worsening of untreated skin infection including dermatophyte infections (tinea incognito)—see 🕮 p.156.
  - Thinning of the skin which may be restored over a period after stopping treatment, but the original structure may never return. More common on flexural skin where the skin is already thin. In general, avoid potent and very potent corticosteroids in the flexures.
  - Irreversible striae atrophica and telangiectasia—also more common in flexures.
  - Acne, worsening of acne or rosacea or perioral dermatitis—see 🕮 p.236. In general, avoid potent or very potent corticosteroids on the face.
  - Hypopigmentation which may be reversible. More often the loss of colour is secondary to the skin condition (postinflammatory hypopigmentation) than the treatment.
  - Rarely, prolonged topical treatment with large quantities of a very potent corticosteroid has been reported to cause adrenal suppression or Cushing's syndrome.
  - Absorption with the risk of adverse effects is increased by occlusion.

Occlusion

Occlusion cools and soothes itchy skin as well as protecting the skin by preventing the damage wrought by fingernails, particularly at night. Consider occlusion in chronically itchy conditions when endless rubbing has thickened the skin (lichenification—see Fig. 31.9, p.561) or resulted in nodules (prurigo—see 🕮 p.206). Occlusion softens scaly skin and enhances the penetration of topical corticosteroids applied under the dressing or bandage. Do not occlude infected skin.

Occlusive dressings

- For a localized area of chronic irritation, prescribe a self-adhesive hydrocolloid dressing such as Granuflex® or DuoDERM® in combination with a potent or very potent topical corticosteroid ointment.
- Apply the ointment thinly to the active area.
- Cut a piece of the sticky hydrocolloid to cover the affected area and 1cm of surrounding skin. Trim the corners so it is an oval shape.
- Apply the dressing and hold it in place firmly for several minutes until it warms up, becomes tacky and sticks firmly to the skin.
- Advise the patient to leave the dressing in place for about 6 days (the patient can bath or shower as normal) and then remove it to give the skin a 24-h 'breathing' period. Then the patient should apply more ointment and another dressing.
- Continue treatment until itch and inflammation settle. This may take a few weeks or several months.

Medicated stockings

- Zipzoc® are tubular rayon stockings impregnated with ointment containing 20% zinc oxide. Zipzoc® were developed for patients with chronic leg ulcers, but the stockings have proved extremely useful in patients, including children, with chronic eczema.
- The stockings are easy to use. Simply cut to length and pull on.
- Corticosteroid ointment may be applied beneath the stocking.
- An overlying cotton tubular bandage (e.g. Tubifast®) will prevent staining of clothing or bedding.
- It may be possible to remove and reuse a Zipzoc® on several consecutive nights.

Medicated paste bandages

- The bandage may be impregnated with coal tar, icthammol, calamine, or zinc paste. Paste bandages are particularly useful for managing gravitational eczema associated with chronic venous leg ulcers, when they can be used under compression bandages—see Fig. 33.1.
- An emollient or topical corticosteroid ointment may be applied to areas of eczema beneath the bandage.
- Paste bandages, unlike Zipzoc®, are tricky to apply properly—see Box 33.3.

Box 33.3 Applying a paste bandage

- Paste bandages are an old-fashioned but effective method of occluding a whole limb.
- Clean the skin and apply an emollient and/or a topical corticosteroid ointment if required.
- If the paste bandage is simply wrapped around the limb in a continuous spiral, as it dries, it may tighten and restrict the blood supply.
- Either cut up the bandage and wrap around the leg in single overlapping strips or use the pleating method of bandaging—see Fig. 33.1. Wrap the bandage around the limb once in one direction until the ends meet and then fold the bandage back upon itself and apply in the opposite direction slightly overlapping the previous turn of the bandage. Continue up the limb reversing the direction of each turn of the bandage to avoid a circumferential band.
- A cohesive elastic bandage, such as Coban®, applied over the paste bandage will hold everything in place.
- Leave for up to 1 week.
- The patient should use a clean polythene bin liner to protect the bandage in the shower or bath.

Further information

http://www.bdng.org.uk/news/patients/How_to_Apply_Paste_Bandages BDNG.pdf

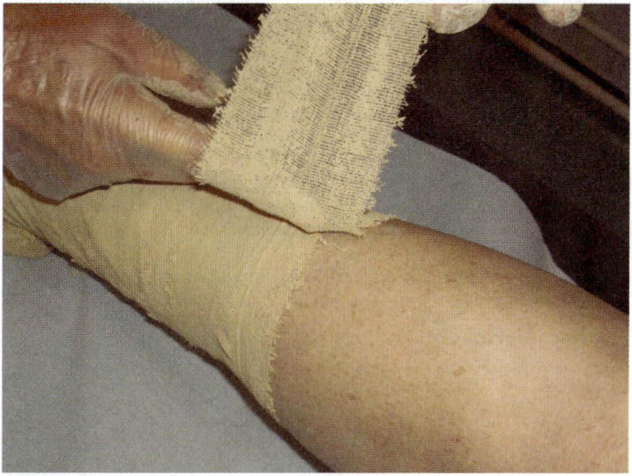

Fig. 33.1 Bandaging technique.

Soaks, wet dressings, and 'wet wraps'

Astringent lotions are used to clean, dry, and soothe weeping eczema or blistering eruptions. Solutions are antiseptic and are also used to reduce bacterial contamination in chronic ulcers. The limb is soaked for 10–20min once or twice a day. You do not need anything more complicated than a plastic bucket and a bin liner, but you will have to explain to patient and/or carer exactly what to do.

Wet dressings are a cooling and antiseptic alternative to soaks that may be used on an area that is difficult to soak in a bucket. Dip clean gauze in the solution and apply as a compress to the affected skin several times a day.

Solutions also may be added to a bath, but some will stain the bath.

'Wet wraps' may be used to relieve itching in conditions such as acute atopic eczema—see Box 33.4.

Preparations for weeping eczematous skin or blistering

- Potassium permanganate (available in the UK as Permitabs®). Line a bucket with a clean bin liner and half fill with tap water. Put on gloves, add 1 Permitab® to the water and agitate to ensure the potassium permanganate dissolves completely. Undissolved crystals at the bottom of the container could burn the skin. Dilute with more water, continuing to stir, until you have a uniform pale pink solution, the colour of rosé wine (1 Permitab dissolved in 4L of water = 0.01% solution). The solution will stain fabric, skin, and nails brown. Coat nails with petroleum jelly prior to soaking to avoid staining. Remove brown stains on the skin with lemon juice. Potassium permanganate solution may be added to a bath—but the bath will be stained permanently!
- Silver nitrate 0.5% solution.
- Aluminium acetate solution 0.13–0.5% (Burrow's solution). This is available in the USA as tablets or powder for dissolving in water.

Preparations for chronic leg ulcers (also see 📖 p.286)

- Potassium permanganate solution—discussed earlier in this section.
- Acetic acid—2 tablespoonfuls of vinegar to 1 pint of tap water—is useful for chronic leg ulcers colonized with *Pseudomonas* (indicated by malodorous bright green dressings).
- Wet gauze dressings soaked in the antiseptic solution may be applied to the ulcer and kept wet for 20min.

Further information

Patient information leaflets on the website of the British Association of Dermatologists: http://www.bad.org.uk

Box 33.4 Wet wrap dressings

Infants and children

'Wet wraps' may be used for short periods to treat infants with acute flares of atopic eczema that have not responded to standard treatment. The wraps reduce itch by cooling the skin but also enhance the effect of topical treatments, including moisturizers, and protect itchy skin from finger nails.

Do not use wet wraps if there are any signs of cutaneous infection.

How do you apply a wet wrap?

- Make a suit out of lengths of cotton tubular bandage, e.g.Tubifast®. Washable cotton garments (long-sleeved vests and tights in different sizes) are also available for use as wraps.
- Affected skin—apply a mild topical corticosteroid ointment, e.g. 0.5% hydrocortisone in infants <1 year or 0.0025% fluocinolone acetonide (1 in 10 Synalar®) in older children.
- Apply 50% WSP in liquid paraffin (or another emollient) liberally to unaffected skin.
- Then apply a suit of wet cotton tubular bandages. Cover this with a dry layer of tubular bandages.
- The wraps can be left in place overnight or longer if tolerated by the child. Keep the wet layer damp with a sponge or spray.

Adults

Wet dressings have been advocated as an inpatient treatment to relieve severe itching, recalcitrant to standard therapy, caused by inflammatory dermatoses such as eczema. Generally symptoms are relieved within 24h.

Do not use wet wraps if there are any signs of cutaneous infection.

- The patient bathes in the morning.
- Topical treatment is applied e.g. a moderately potent corticosteroid ointment to inflamed skin and emollients elsewhere.
- Gauze dampened with tap water is applied to all the body and covered with a dry cotton cloth.
- Warm cotton blankets are placed over the patient.
- Dressings are removed every 3h for 30–45min so that the patient may use the bathroom or walk around and then dressings are reapplied.
- Dressings are applied ×5–6 every 24h.
- Oral hydroxyzine 10–25mg is taken every 4–6h as needed.

Further reading

Bingham LG *et al. J Am Acad Dermatol* 2009; **60:**792–800.

Systemic drugs in dermatology

We provide no more than pointers to using these drugs—please read detailed prescribing guidelines and local protocols. Involve the patient in any decision about his/her treatment. Discuss how long the drug will take to act and what the outcome might be, but offer written as well as verbal information. Explain the importance of monitoring. Provide a hand-held record for recording results of tests. The patient should bring this to clinic visits. Generally you will share monitoring with the GP according to a local protocol—read this so you know what is expected of you. In many departments, specialist nurses monitor patients on systemic treatment, but the prescriber is responsible for minimizing the likelihood of problems.

Oral antihistamines

- Non-sedating: chronic urticaria, e.g. fexofenadine, cetirizine.
- Sedating: for itching, e.g. hydroxyzine, chlorphenamine, but treat any underlying skin problem or systemic disease causing the itch.

Azathioprine

Azathioprine is an anti-inflammatory and immunosuppressant drug that is converted to 6-mercaptopurine (6-MP). Some 6-MP is catabolized to inactive metabolites by enzymes such as thiopurine methyltransferase (TPMT). Other pathways produce 6-MP metabolites that interfere with cell division and function of T- and B-cells. Dose: 2–2.5mg/kg/day.

What should I do?

- Measure TPMT activity or check genotype before starting treatment. A mutation in the TPMT gene lowers enzyme activity and increases risk of myelosuppression. Approximately 1 in 10 of the population is heterozygous (intermediate activity) and 1 in 100 homozygous (low activity) for the mutation. Prescribe low dose if TPMT activity reduced.
- Warn about nausea and diarrhoea. Limit alcohol intake.
- Warn about increased risk of malignancy, including skin cancer, with long-term treatment. Advise patient to use sun protection—see 🕮 p.316.
- Monitor for hepatotoxicity and myelosuppression, initially with weekly FBC and LFT. Increased risk of pancytopenia with allopurinol.
- Avoid live vaccines, e.g. oral polio, BCG, rubella. Influenza and pneumococcal vaccines are safe and are recommended.

Ciclosporin

Ciclosporin is an immunosuppressant drug that blocks calcineurin, thus preventing the activation of T-cells. It is metabolized by the cytochrome P450 pathway and is susceptible to interaction with other drugs inhibiting or inducing these enzymes. Duration of treatment should be <2 years whenever possible. Dose: 2.5–5mg/kg/day.

What should I do?

- Exclude contraindications: hypertension, renal impairment, active infection, or malignancy except cured non-melanoma skin cancer.
- Urinalysis, FBC, renal function, LFTs, and fasting lipids.
- Measure blood pressure and creatinine twice before starting treatment.

- Warn about hypertension and nephrotoxicity, as well as nausea, diarrhoea, gum hypertrophy, hirsutism, tremor, and burning sensation in hands and feet.
- Warn about increased risk of malignancy, including skin cancer, with long-term treatment (particularly if previous PUVA). Advise patient to use sun protection—see 📖 p.316. Advise cervical smear if appropriate.
- Warn about drugs or foods which may increase (e.g. cimetidine, erythromycin, grapefruit juice) or decrease (e.g. carbamazepine, phenytoin, St John's wort) ciclosporin levels. Avoid nephrotoxic drugs, e.g. NSAIDs and ACE inhibitors or potassium-sparing diuretics (increase risk of hyperkalemia). Ciclosporin increases the risk of statin-induced myositis.
- Avoid live vaccines e.g. oral polio, BCG, rubella. Influenza and pneumococcal vaccines are safe and are recommended.
- Prescribe 1 brand as different preparations differ in bioavailability.
- Monitor BP and renal function 2-weekly initially. Once stable, monitor monthly. Reduce dose if creatinine rises 30% above baseline. Treat hypertension with a calcium antagonist, e.g. nifedipine or amlodopine.

Colchicine

Colchicine is extracted from the autumn crocus, *Colchicum autumnale*. Colchicine has anti-inflammatory effects and decreases neutrophil degranulation. Dose: 0.5–2mg/day.

What should I do?

Warn patients about diarrhoea, the most common adverse effect. Gastrointestinal adverse effects are related to higher doses. Other adverse effects include bone marrow suppression, peripheral neuropathy, myopathy, and hair loss.

Corticosteroids

Corticosteroids are potent anti-inflammatory drugs that exert their effects by binding to intracellular glucocorticoid receptors and regulating anything from 10–100 genes involved in inflammation. Short-term courses of prednisolone 20–30mg/day, tapered over 2–3 weeks, may control acute inflammation. Some conditions require long-term treatment, high doses (up to 60mg/day), or pulses of IV methylprednisolone. Do not stop topical treatments, including emollients and topical corticosteroids, if you prescribe oral corticosteroids for a skin problem.

What should I do?

- Patients will be worried about adverse effects—discuss these and help the patient to weigh up risks and benefits. Adverse effects are related to dose and duration of treatment. The most common are weight gain, osteoporosis, dyspepsia, easy bruising, thinning of skin, myopathy, mood changes, cataracts, menstrual irregularity, diabetes, hypertension, susceptibility to infections, and, in children, growth suppression.
- Advise patients on long-term treatment not to stop medication suddenly and to carry a steroid treatment card.
- Monitor weight, blood pressure, and blood glucose while on treatment.

- Live vaccinations are not recommended if taking high doses of oral corticosteroids (40mg prednisolone daily for >1 week), but encourage influenza and pneumococcal vaccination.
- Consider bone protection with a bisphosphonate and calcium/vitamin D. Check Royal College of Physicians guidelines for patients who are starting a course of at least 3 months of corticosteroids (http://www.rcplondon.ac.uk). Bone protection (oral bisphosphonate with calcium and vitamin D supplements) should be given to high-risk patients (e.g. aged ≥65, or a previous fragility fracture), without bone densitometry. In other patients, measure bone density and start a bisphosphonate if T score is −1.5 or lower. Consider calcium and vitamin D supplementation in all patients, but particularly if photosensitive and using sun blocks, e.g. patients with SLE.

Dapsone

Dapsone is a sulphone drug with antineutrophilic properties (inhibits neutrophil myeloperoxidase). Dose: 50–150mg/day.

What should I do?

- Ask about allergy to sulphonamides (dapsone contraindicated).
- Check for glucose-6-phosphate dehydrogenase (G6PD) deficiency in people of Mediterranean, African, and Asian ancestry.
- Warn about nausea, headache, or blue discoloration of fingertips and lips (methaemoglobinaemia). More serious but rare problems include agranulocytosis, peripheral motor neuropathy (weak hands and feet) and hypersensitivity ('DRESS'—fever, rash, lymphadenopathy 1–2 months after starting treatment—see p.114).
- Contraindications include liver disease, anaemia, allergy to sulphonamides, porphyria, G6PD deficiency.
- Start with a low dose (50mg/day) and increase slowly if tolerated.
- Monitor FBC, and liver and renal function. Initially the haemoglobin will fall. Dapsone always causes some haemolysis.
- Monitor for motor neuropathy by asking patient to walk on tip-toes and then on heels.

Hydroxychloroquine

Hydroxychloroquine is an antimalarial with anti-inflammatory properties. Dose: 200–400mg/day. Maximum dose = 6.5mg/kg/day.

What should I do?

- Advise to take with food to reduce nausea.
- Retinal toxicity is a rare adverse effect that is avoided by using a dose no more than 6.5mg/kg daily. Patients should see an optician annually. Refer to an ophthalmologist if patient develops visual problems.
- Check FBC, and renal and liver function before starting. Reduce dose in renal and hepatic impairment.

Mepacrine

Mepacrine is another antimalarial. Dose: 50–100mg/day.

What should I do?

- Warn about transient orange discoloration of the skin and urine (disappears on stopping the drug), dizziness, nausea, diarrhoea, and headache. Liver and bone marrow toxicity are rare. No retinal toxicity.
- Contraindications include porphyria and liver disease.
- Check FBC and LFTs twice a year.

Methotrexate

Methotrexate is a folic acid analogue with anti-inflammatory properties. It inhibits the enzyme dihydrofolate reductase, which reduces dihydrofolate to tetrahydrofolate. Tetrahydrofolate is required for the synthesis of DNA precursors. Methotrexate is thought to inhibit the proliferation of lymphocytes involved in inflammation. Dose: 5–25mg ***once a week***.

What should I do?

- Contraindications include excessive alcohol intake, significant renal or hepatic impairment, active acute infection, immunodeficiency, blood dyscrasias, breastfeeding, pregnancy, and lactation.
- Prior to starting therapy check FBC, liver function, and renal function. Enquire about alcohol use—recommend limiting or, ideally, avoiding entirely.
- Check CXR if any risk of prior lung disease.
- UK dermatologists recommend screening for liver fibrosis by measuring the PIIINP. Many patients with arthritis have a raised PIIINP despite a normal liver biopsy, so PIIINP is not helpful in this population.
- Methotrexate is teratogenic—men and women should use contraception and stop the drug for at least 3 months before conception.
- Warn about common adverse affects, e.g. nausea, diarrhoea, hair loss, and less common serious adverse effects: mouth ulcers, bone marrow or liver or lung toxicity (lung toxicity is very uncommon in psoriasis).
- Ensure the patient has 2.5mg tablets not 10mg tablets, which look the same. Prescribe a test dose (5mg) and check FBC after 1 week. If normal, prescribe the full weekly dose (usually 12.5–15mg/week). Reduce the dose in renal impairment or the elderly.
- Prescribe folic acid (≥5mg/week) to reduce mucosal and GI toxicity.
- Monitor FBC and LFTs, ideally weekly, while dose is adjusted. Once dose is stable, check FBC and liver function 1–3-monthly.
- Check renal function and PIIINP 6-monthly.
- Consider liver biopsy if LFTs are persistently elevated.
- Nausea may limit the dose. Take with food, try splitting the dose over 12h, take at night or try ondansetron (antiemetic) prior to methotrexate. Subcutaneous methotrexate may be tolerated better than oral.
- Patients with mouth ulcers, sore throat, fever, epistaxis, unexpected bleeding, or bruising should have urgent FBC and LFTs. Investigate breathlessness with CXR to exclude pneumonitis.
- Avoid co-trimoxazole and trimethoprim (antifolate effects).
- Avoid live vaccines, e.g. oral polio, BCG, rubella. Influenza and pneumococcal vaccines are safe and are recommended.

Mycophenolate mofetil

Mycophenolate mofetil is an immunosuppressant that is converted to the active agent mycophenolic acid, which inhibits lymphocyte proliferation and antibody production. Dose: 1–3g/day.

What should I do?

- Check FBC, and renal and liver function before starting and monitor during treatment (weekly initially and then every 1–3 months).
- Warn patients about adverse effects of nausea, diarrhoea, and anaemia.
- Advise patients to use sun protection (risk of skin cancers).
- Avoid pregnancy during treatment and for 6 weeks after stopping.

Retinoids

The retinoids are analogues of vitamin A that regulate gene transcription via intracellular nuclear receptors. They have diverse effects on cell differentiation and proliferation, immune function, and embryonic development. Acitretin (a metabolite of etretinate) is used in disorders of keratinization, e.g. severe psoriasis, and oral isotretinoin is used in severe acne. Dose: 0.25–1mg/kg/day.

What should I do?

- Oral retinoids are teratogenic and must be avoided in pregnancy. You will be expected to follow a protocol for prescribing, dispensing, and monitoring these drugs. Women of childbearing age must sign a consent form, agree to use secure contraception (2 types are recommended), and agree to have monthly pregnancy tests. Contraception should be continued for at least 1 month after stopping isotretinoin and 2 years after stopping acitretin. In practice, acitretin is rarely used in women of childbearing age.
- Common adverse effects include dryness of mucous membranes and skin, muscle aches and pains, photosensitivity, raised serum triglycerides or cholesterol, and raised liver enzymes.
- Check plasma lipids (fasting) and liver function prior to starting treatment and then monitor 1–3 monthly depending on the retinoid prescribed.

Thalidomide

Thalidomide was used in the 1950s as a sedative and antiemetic, but phocomelia was a tragic adverse effect and by 1961 the drug had been withdrawn worldwide. Thalidomide has anti-inflammatory and immunomodulatory actions that may be mediated by inhibition of TNFα.

What should I do?

- The risk of birth defects is 100% if the drug is taken in the first 21–36 days of gestation. Prescribers, pharmacists, and patients must register with the Pharmion Risk Management Programme (🔗 http://www.prmp.com).
- Follow the protocol for prescribing, dispensing, and monitoring thalidomide.
- Patients must give written consent. Women of childbearing age must use 2 forms of contraception and have monthly pregnancy tests.

- Another serious adverse effect is a peripheral sensory neuropathy that may be irreversible. Patients have painful paraesthesiae of the hands and feet. Refer for pre-treatment nerve conduction studies and monitor 6-monthly during treatment.

Further reading

British National Formulary: http://www.bnf.org/bnf/bnf/current/index.htm

Patient information leaflets on the website of the British Association of Dermatologists: http://www.bad.org.uk

Wakelin SH. *Handbook of Systemic Drug* Treatment *in Dermatology*, 2002. London: Manson Publishing.

Chapter 34

Resources

Contents

Resources

The British Association of Dermatologists

http://www.bad.org.uk

The British Association of Dermatologists (BAD) is the professional organization for dermatologists in the UK and Irish Republic. The website has excellent resources for doctors as well as for patients—check it out!

Clinical standards

Guidelines of the BAD (published in the *British Journal of Dermatology*), can be accessed here as PDF documents. You will also find a list of unlicensed dermatological preparations, 'Specials'.

Public information

The public information section has patient information leaflets that not only explain many skin conditions, but also include information about drugs and topical treatments. The leaflets are easy to download. Nurses without specialist training in dermatology may also find some of this information helpful. The 'how to' section discusses how to use treatments such as the EpiPen®, paste bandages, and potassium permanganate soaks, as well as introducing what happens during surgical procedures such as skin biopsy. A large section is devoted to skin cancer and sun safety. Information addresses topics such as sunbeds, sunscreens, and vitamin D as well as specific skin cancers. Links to the published BAD guidelines for management of skin cancers are provided here. The site also provides an extensive list of local, national, and international patient support groups.

Education

Look here for information on academic dermatology, training, and careers in dermatology in the UK. The resources for teaching and assessment include the 'BAD Recommendations for Dermatology in the UK Undergraduate Medical Curriculum'. You can also access a dermatology handbook written by a junior doctor for medical students. The content of the handbook is mapped to the BAD recommendations for the undergraduate curriculum.

Specialist groups

Find out more about subspecialty interests such as paediatric dermatology and dermatological surgery. There are also links to websites of societies such as the Scottish Dermatological Society, the Primary Care Dermatology Society, and the British Dermatological Nursing Group.

British Society for Medical Dermatology (BSMD)

http://www.medderm.org.uk

American Academy of Dermatology

http://www.aad.org/

Explore the Academy's website for more educational resources including clinical guidelines and fact sheets about skin conditions.

Box 34.1 Online atlases

- Primary Care Dermatology Society: http://www.pcds.org.uk/image-atlas
- NZ Derm Net: http://www.dermnetnz.org/
- DermIS: http://www.dermis.net/dermisroot/en/home/index.htm
- Dermatoweb.net: Spanish text. http://dermatoweb2.udl.es/
- Dermatology Image Atlas: Johns Hopkins University http://dermatlas.med.jhmi.edu/derm/
- Loyola University Dermatology Medical Education Website: http://www.meddean.luc.edu/lumen/MedEd/medicine/dermatology/melton/atlas.htm
- eMedicine http://emedicine.medscape.com/dermatology
- Online Dermatology Quiz: http://dermatlas.med.jhmi.edu/derm/quiz.cfm
- Text and self-assessment quiz: www.health.auckland.ac.nz/courses/dermatology/

Box 34.2 Miscellaneous information

- NHS Evidence—skin disorders is an excellent resource with information on all aspects of skin disorders. http://www.library.nhs.uk/skin/
- British Skin Foundation (BSF): a charity committed to raising funds for research into skin disease. Includes real life stories—what it is like to live with a skin disease. http://www.britishskinfoundation.org.uk/
- Skin cancer: http://www.cancerhelp.org.uk/
- Clinical guidelines published by the National Institute for Health and Clinical Excellence (NICE): http://www.nice.org.uk/guidance/index.jsp?action=byType&type=2&status=3
- The Cochrane Collaboration—an international independent organization dedicated to providing accurate information about effective healthcare. The Cochrane Library includes reviews of the management of some common skin problems. http://cochrane.co.uk/en/collaboration.html
- Dermoscopy: images and training: www.dermoscopy.co.uk
- The Electronic Textbook of Dermatology http://www.telemedicine.org/stamford.htm
- Centre of Evidence Based Dermatology http://www.nottingham.ac.uk/SCS/divisions/evidencebaseddermatology/index.aspx
  Includes links to Cochrane Skin group, UK dermatology clinical trials network, UK diagnostic criteria for atopic eczema manual and NHS Evidence—skin disorders. Also provides access to Dermatology Health Care Needs Assessment Report (2009)
- www.medscape.com for review articles in Medscape CME and eMedicine. Registration is free.
- www.nature.com. Sign up to selected journal alerts published by the Nature group. The contents and abstracts come straight to your email address.

Dermatology textbooks

Reference textbooks

Braverman I. *Skin Signs of Systemic Disease*, 3rd edn, 1998. Philadelphia: WB Saunders (*well worth dipping into if you can find it*).

Bolognia J, Jorizzo J, and Rapini R. (eds.) *Dermatology*, 2nd edn, 2008. London: Mosby Elsevier Ltd.

Burns T, Breathnach S, and Cox N *et al.* (eds.) *Rook's Textbook of Dermatology* 8th edn, 2010. Oxford: Wiley-Blackwell.

Ogg G. Diseases of the skin (Chapter 23). In Warrell D, Cox T, Firth J, *et al.* (eds) *Oxford Textbook of Medicine*, 5th edn, 2010. Oxford: Oxford University Press.

du Vivier A and McKee PH. *Atlas of Clinical Dermatology*, 3rd edn, 2002. London: Mosby Elsevier Ltd.

Specialist dermatology

Archer CB. *Ethnic Dermatology*, 2nd edn, 2008. Inform Healthcare.

Baran R, Dawber RPR, de Berker DAR, *et al. Baran and Dawber's Diseases of the Nails and their Management*, 3rd edn, 2001. Blackwell Science Ltd.

Ferguson J and Dover J. *Photodermatology*, 2006. Oxford: Wiley-Blackwell.

Irvine A, Höger P, Yan A. *Textbook of Pediatric Dermatology*, 3rd edn, 2010. Oxford: Wiley-Blackwell.

Lewis-Jones S. *Paediatric Dermatology* (Oxford Specialist Handbooks) 2010. Oxford: Oxford University Press.

Neill S and Lewis F. *Ridley's The Vulva*, 3rd edn, 2009. Oxford: Wiley-Blackwell.

Olsen EA (ed.). *Disorders of Hair Growth: Diagnosis and Treatment*, 2nd edn, 2003. New York: McGraw-Hill.

Rietschel R, Fowler J, and Fisher A. *Fisher's Contact Dermatitis*, 6th edn, 2008. New York: McGraw-Hill Medical.

Management

Lebwohl MG, Heymann WR, Berth-Jones J, *et al. Treatment of Skin Disease*, 3rd edn, 2010. London: Saunders Elsevier Ltd.

Wakelin S. *A Handbook of Systemic Drug Treatment in Dermatology*, 2002. Oxford: Wiley-Blackwell.

Williams H, Bigby M, Diepgen T, *et al. Evidence-based Dermatology*, 2nd edn, 2008. Oxford: Blackwell Publishing.

Introductory textbooks

Gawkrodger D. *Dermatology: An Illustrated Colour Text*, 3rd edn, 2002. London: Elsevier Science Ltd.

Graham-Brown R and Burns T. *Lecture Notes: Dermatology*, 9th edn, 2006. Oxford: Wiley-Blackwell.

Weller R, Hunter JAA, Savin J, *et al. Clinical Dermatology*, 4th edn, 2008. Oxford: Wiley-Blackwell.

Index

D

E

F

N

O

P

Q

R